Community Nursing

PROMOTING CANADIANS' HEALTH

SECOND EDITION

EDITED BY

MIRIAM J. STEWART

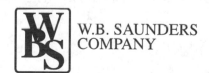

W.B. SAUNDERS COMPANY

A Harcourt Canada Health Sciences Company

Toronto Montreal Fort Worth New York Orlando
Philadelphia San Diego London Sydney Tokyo

Canadian Cataloguing in Publication Data

Main entry under title:
Community nursing : promoting Canadians' health

2nd ed.
Includes bibliographical references and index.
ISBN 0-920513-38-7

1. Community health nursing—Canada. I. Stewart, Miriam.

RT98.C66 1999   610.73'43'0971   C99-930786-X

New Editions Editor: Liz Radojkovic
Developmental Editor: Liz Radojkovic
Production Editor: Stephanie Fysh
Production Coordinator: Cheryl Tiongson
Copy Editor: Francine Geraci
Permissions Editor: Cindy Howard
Cover Design: Sonya V. Thursby, Opus House Incorporated
Interior Design: CJ Design & Desktop Publishing/Steve Eby Production & Design
Typesetting and Assembly: Steve Eby Production & Design
Printing and Binding: Transcontinental Printing Inc.
Cover Art: *The Boardwalk at Toronto Beaches* by William Kurelek, 1974. Mixed media on masonite. 54.6 x 43.2 cm. Courtesy Duncan E. Meyer. Copyright courtesy The Estate of William Kurelek and The Isaacs Gallery, Toronto. Photographer: Simon Glass.

Harcourt Canada
55 Horner Avenue, Toronto, ON, Canada M8Z 4X6
Customer Services
Toll-Free Tel.: 1-800-387-7278
Toll-Free Fax: 1-800-665-7307

This book was printed in Canada.

1 2 3 4 5   03 02 01 00 99

Contents

Foreword

Consumers, the health sector, and the nursing profession should encourage and appreciate up-to-date, comprehensive contributions to community nursing literature. Since 1978 and the declaration of Alma Ata, the World Health Organization has acknowledged the goal of Health for All by the Year 2000 and Primary Health Care as the strategy toward its achievement. Nursing—because of its history, perspective, and potential—has an important role to play in a community- and family-centred system emphasizing health promotion and disease prevention, public participation, accessibility, appropriate personnel and technology, and multidisciplinary and multisectoral cooperation.

Since Alma Ata, the nursing profession has reinforced the view that Primary Health Care become the key function and focus of a country's health system and has recommended that it be accorded a correspondingly central place in nursing curricula. A 1989 joint World Health Organization and International Council of Nurses report on *Nursing in Primary Health Care: Ten Years After Alma Ata and Perspectives for the Future* described Primary Health Care roles as requiring "new attitudes and orientations, . . . patterns of practice incorporating epidemiological, biostatistical, psychological, cultural, political, and socioeconomic elements, as well as a good knowledge of modern communication techniques and educational technology." We hope, therefore, that community nursing texts will embrace these essentials, as is the case with the second edition of *Community Nursing: Promoting Canadians' Health*.

Margretta Madden Styles
Past President, International Council of Nurses

Foreword

It is indeed a pleasure to write a Foreword for the second edition of *Community Nursing: Promoting Canadians' Health*. The text's emphasis on Primary Health Care and its health promotion orientation is timely and appropriate. Indeed, its content is relevant beyond Canadian borders, and instrumental for a purposeful debate on Primary Health Care and nursing in the 21st century.

Primary Health Care is a key element recommended by the World Health Organization in its Health for All strategy. The need to reorient health services, and to put more "health" on the health policy agenda, has been taken up strongly in the health strategy pursued within the framework of the 1986 *Ottawa Charter for Health Promotion*. Primary Health Care and strategies for health promotion represent main goals in the Ninth General Program of Work of the World Health Organization globally for 1996–2001. In this respect, Canada continues to play an important role in the shift toward community-based health promotion on the international scene.

It is significant, therefore, that this text focusses on promotion of the health of Canadians. It is appropriate, too, that Dr. Miriam Stewart, as former Director of the Atlantic Health Promotion Research Centre and current Director of the Centre for Health Promotion Studies, University of Alberta, is the editor of this book.

Community Nursing: Promoting Canadians' Health (2nd edition) should make a major contribution to Canadian health promotion literature and will have implications for international initiatives.

Erio Ziglio
Regional Adviser for Health Promotion and Investment
World Health Organization Regional Office for Europe

Preface

The World Health Organization and the International Council of Nurses recognize the urgency of orienting nurses to Primary Health Care as a key to attaining Health for All by the Year 2000. As in other countries, community health nurses in Canada are pivotal to the achievement of health for all Canadians in the 21st century. It has been 14 years since the publication of *Community Health Nursing in Canada*, whish was the only Canadian text to depict the unique nature of community health nursing since Florence Emory's book in 1953. Four years have passed since the first edition of *Community Nursing: Promoting Canadians' Health* in 1995. This updated text is timely as the nursing profession prepares to implement this Canadian goal of Health for All in the new millennium.

In Part 1 of this book, forces shaping the historical evolution of community health nursing in Canada are reviewed, and systemic and societal changes are analyzed for their impact on community-based nursing. In Part 2, core theoretical premises and principles underpinning community health nursing are delineated, and the five principles of Primary Health Care are highlighted as the framework for the book. These principles ground health system reform initiatives across the country and have implications for policy, as illustrated in Part 3. The focus in Part 4 shifts to contemporary perspectives for community health nursing practice, and current trends and accomplishments are explored. The richness of the geographical, cultural, linguistic, educational, and social diversity of target populations and practice settings is portrayed, and pertinent community health nursing knowledge, attitudes, roles, and skills are explicated. In Part 5, the links between practice and research, the status and contributions of community health nursing research in Canada, and appropriate methodologies are analyzed. Administrators can also guide community health nurses into the next era of Primary Health Care reform (Part 6). Finally, new challenges for community health nursing theory, practice, research, education, and policy are projected in Part 7, together with a vision of the future.

Acknowledgements

It is gratifying to acknowledge W.B. Saunders's invitation to write a second edition of *Community Nursing: Promoting Canadians' Health*. The first edition (1995) provided an update to the 1985 book *Community Health Nursing in Canada*. The current book would not have been possible without the superb contributions of the 44 authors, acknowledged experts in the themes of their chapters.

I am delighted that Dr. Margretta Styles, past president of the International Council of Nurses, contributed an insightful Foreword from a nursing perspective, and that Dr. Erio Ziglio, Regional Advisor for Health Promotion, World Health Organization (Regional Office for Europe), also lent his support for this book from a health promotion viewpoint in the second Foreword. Dr. Alice Baumgart, former Member-at-Large for the International Council of Nurses and past President of both the Canadian Nurses Association and the Canadian Association of University Schools of Nursing, contributed the thoughtful and timely Afterword.

Leona Laird's skill and perseverance in typing my communications with authors and my contributions to this publishing venture are greatly appreciated.

This book is dedicated to my daughters, Evelyn and Shauna, and to my parents, Dorothy and Ross Mortimer.

Part 1
Historical Evolution

Community health nurses have made significant strides over the past century. The authors of this section reveal that past accomplishments and challenges have paved the way to recent times.

Allemang's impressive review of the historical evolution of community health nursing, which introduced the 1985 book Community Health Nursing in Canada and the 1995 version of this textbook, once again sets the stage for an in-depth look at community health nursing in Canada. Her extensive examination of changing health care contexts and health concerns provides an excellent backdrop to the analysis of the expanding contributions of community health nurses that follow throughout this book. It is striking that many health problems are not new. The health challenges faced by the poor, cultural minorities, and isolated people, and the social causes of illness, persist today. These difficulties reflect barriers to accessibility, a key Primary Health Care principle.

In this context, the pioneer nursing sisters provided accessible care to all clients. Early in the 19th century, Canadian nursing leaders urged government-sponsored health care plans and free, accessible public health services, and public health workers increasingly included in their work prevention of disease and promotion of health—another Primary Health Care principle. Visiting nurses changed with the advent of nursing schools. Later, community nurses joined agencies interested in health promotion and disease prevention, and the family and community became the key focus of community nursing. This raised the question of appropriate education for community health nurses. Since the 1970s, the baccalaureate degree has been espoused.

The historical introduction to this book continues in Chapter 2, with emphasis on the reawakened interest in the early principles of community health care. Rodger and Gallagher review the key leadership role that nurses and nursing associations played in the shift to Primary Health Care over the past 15 years. The significant 1980 submission, Putting Health into Health Care by the Canadian Nurses Association (CNA), influenced amendments to the Canada Health Act in 1984. Health reform committees and commissions issued recommendations that implicitly promoted Primary

Health Care principles. The CNA (1988) document, Health for All Canadians: A Call for Health Care Reform, *was followed by numerous position statements and projects.*

Most provincial nursing associations developed Primary Health Care position statements and documents on nurses' relevant roles. Health promotion and disease prevention were emphasized by nurses after 1984. The nursing profession also advocated accessibility and the role that nurses can play us an entry point to the health care system. However, two other principles, related to appropriate technology and intersectoral collaboration, received the least attention by nurses. Rodger and Gallagher surveyed university nursing programs about integration of Primary Health Care concepts and the varied associations for community health nurses in Canada about integration in the diverse roles and settings for practitioners.

These two chapters, which trace the development of community health nursing, provide a sound foundation for the sections to follow.

CHAPTER 1

Development of community health nursing in Canada

Margaret M. Allemang

An examination of the past may provide the gifts of historical study: greater clarity in understanding contemporary ideologies and more precision in projecting trends. This chapter traces the development of community health nursing in Canada and identifies some of the influences that shaped this field of health care.

LEARNING OBJECTIVES

In this chapter, you will learn:

- how Canada's changing culture influenced the development of community nursing and health care from the 17th century to the present
- how definitions of health and health services changed during the 19th and 20th centuries in response to secular trends, scientific advances, and new legislation
- how nursing was conceptualized and practised, and how hospital nursing schools gave way to a university-based nursing curriculum
- the major problems and issues (philosophical and financial) that currently challenge Canada's comprehensive federal–provincial health plan

Introduction

Paradoxically, a historical account takes its frame of reference from contemporary thought patterns, in themselves the outcome of historical change. Thus, what is perceived as relevant to the study of community health nursing is determined in part by contemporary concepts that structure and give meaning to its domain. The historian's task is to discover the circumstances, thought patterns, and supporting activities leading to the identification and professional acceptance of what is now known as community health nursing.

Hazards in this undertaking include too limited a perspective; seeing in the past only what the historian wants to see or is conditioned to see; and a tendency to judge by present-day values rather than by those of the years under examination. A further limitation is the scope of the subject: it is difficult to meet the demands for critical examination and synthesis of credible evidence considering the many themes affecting community health nursing in Canadian society, one marked by multiculturalism and regionalism and influenced by natural geographical divisions and unique historical events.

During the past century, goals of health workers have developed to include prevention of disease, promotion of health, and rehabilitation of the sick and disabled. Recently, their specific aims encompass reduction in risk factors, strengthening of self-care abilities, and maintenance or improvement in the quality of life. Since the early 1980s, community health nursing in Canada has moved increasingly toward the goals of Primary Health Care.

This account provides an overview of Canadian history and highlights the integral nature of community health nursing in societal continuity and change. Briefly identified are the main historical events, threats to health, developing resources, and the responsive nursing values and activities in the early French and British regimes, through the years immediately before and after Confederation (1867), to the close of the 20th century. Although community health nursing enters the picture in prodromal forms in this history, over time its meaning has become increasingly more complex and more precisely defined.

Community nursing: French and British regimes

Historical perspectives on community health nursing in Canada would be incomplete if attention were not focussed on New France. The period dramatically illustrates a comprehensive type of community service in a precarious environment, conducted by women motivated by strong beliefs in Christian charity. This early model of community nursing developed at a time when two alien cultures met, medical science and technology were unknown, and trained nurses did not exist. Intuitive concepts of community nursing may be recognized in the relationship between the persons giving and receiving care, in the attention given to people without community supports, and in the stark political and financial problems that had to be confronted.

The beginning of organized community-style nursing in New France may be attributed to the Duchesse d'Aiguillon (1604–1675), who organized and financed a small group of Augustinian Hospitallers of Dieppe to bring health care to the settlement of Québec in 1639. The first three sisters almost immediately established a hospital and also carried out work within the community, sending their members to surrounding villages and, whenever possible, supervising care in the homes. Jeanne Mance (1606–1673), co-founder with Paul de Chomedey de Maisonneuve of Ville Marie (Montréal) in 1642, had been a member of the Dames de Charité in Langes, France, her birthplace, before deciding to found a hospital in New France. As a leading figure in the colony, politically astute and personally concerned over its survival and the quality of life of the settlers and the Native people, Jeanne Mance returned to France three times seeking financial assistance and resolution of political issues undermining the colony and its hospital (Gibbon & Mathewson, 1947). As administrator of the Hôtel-Dieu of Ville Marie until her death, she assumed many roles, including those of nurse, pharmacist, physician, and surgeon. She changed the course of events for the small colony and left a legacy of committed community service, broad in scope and appropriate to the age in which she lived.

In the Hôtel-Dieu, the type of hospital that became established in New France, care was extended not only to the sick but also to those in need of shelter and attention. Families just arriving in the new country were housed at the Hôtel-Dieu, fed, comforted, and instructed about life in New France while awaiting construction of their houses. Survival in the small settlements was precarious. The Indian Wars, fought over the issue of the fur trade, regularly brought an influx of casualties to the hospitals. Smallpox routinely took its toll among colonists, Indians, and nursing staff. Epidemics of typhoid fever resulted from sick crews and infested ships coming to port. And victims of yellow fever entered the colony as a result of trade with the West Indies. At the Hôtel-Dieu, unconditional care was given to all who arrived for help: settlers, seamen, Natives—friend or foe—and to the British, to whom the French surrendered in 1760 and formalized their agreements in the Treaty of Paris in 1763.

Canada's first community nursing order—the Grey Nuns—was established in New France. Started in 1738 by Marguerite d'Youville (1701–1771), a widow and philanthropist of Montréal, the sisterhood was uncloistered, accepted women regardless of social distinction, and required a three-year novitiate (Gibbon & Mathewson, 1947). The innovative work of the Grey Nuns, in the name of Christian love, spread far and wide as explorers extended frontiers north and westward. Their distinctive contribution was in the visiting of the sick in their own homes to provide care, treatment, and instruction. They also organized houses of refuge for the elderly and the infirm and hospitals for the acutely ill. Like the cloistered orders, their care was unconditional and beyond distinctions based on race, creed, culture, or nationality.

Roots of regionalism

From 1763, when New France was ceded to Britain, to 1867, when the *British North America Act* established the Dominion of Canada, the regionalism that was to become so distinctive in Canada's emerging identity took form.

The trend affected not only events but also the health of all people and the possibilities for health services. Human life was threatened by wars, hazards of immigration, dangers of pioneer life, epidemics of infectious diseases, and scarcity of health care and services. Health, illness, and death were in large measure beyond human control. Yet, in these years health- and life-threatening circumstances lessened to some extent, at least regionally, as political, economic, and social forces influenced the structure of society and changed the pattern of people's lives.

In 1763, the British Empire in North America extended from Hudson Bay to the Gulf of Mexico. Within the boundaries now known as Canada existed only four British possessions: the Province of Québec, Nova Scotia, Rupert's Land, and Newfoundland (Careless, 1970). In the next century, differences in these four regions were heightened dramatically by events primarily influencing the Province of Québec and the colony of Nova Scotia. During the American Revolutionary War (1775–1783), Montréal and Québec were attacked, but Nova Scotia, despite its population of New Englanders, remained neutral. The most profound regional changes as a result of the war came with the influx of Loyalists. Most of the 30 000 who went to Nova Scotia settled along the St. John River and the Bay of Fundy. The enlarged population and new cultural elements led to partition to form New Brunswick. Similarly, migration of 10 000 Loyalists and of settlers moving westward for land brought settlement to the area of the Lower St. Lawrence and Great Lakes. In 1791, the Province of Québec became the Province of Canada with two divisions—Upper Canada (later Ontario) and Lower Canada (later Québec).

The War of 1812–1814, fought over unresolved fishing and fur trading issues and underlined by the Americans' desired liberation from possible British influences, brought new hardships to Canada. Americans attempted to attack Montréal, and the Niagara Peninsula became a battleground. The most significant consequences for the future of Canada were stronger British bonds and a sense of difference between the people of British North America and the United States (Careless, 1970).

After 1820, British immigration brought new elements into the changing society of the Maritimes and the Province of Canada. This movement scarcely affected Newfoundland and Rupert's Land. In the waves of immigration, lasting into the 1850s, 800 000 people entered British North America. The majority were from the poor and displaced segments of society, although some members of the middle and upper classes arrived to seek whatever fortunes the new country might offer. By 1850, Upper Canada's population was almost a million, approximately one-third of the population of British North America at that time.

In these years, the Maritimes entered their most prosperous period as lumbering, ship building, and trade flourished. Upper Canada also prospered as land was cleared; farming was successful; roads, canals and later railways were built; and towns and cities came into existence with their banks, libraries, newspapers, schools, and other facilities supported by growing wealth. Lower Canada gained much of its prosperity from rising commercial interests centred in Montréal, which controlled sea traffic and trade. As these regions emerged from the pioneer age, political conflicts forced movement toward responsible government. Partisan interests became expressed in reform elements arising from frustrated assemblies blocked by oligarchies, composed of British government officials, wealthy bankers and merchants, and other persons of privilege according to the society of the time.

By 1860, Newfoundland had shown development. Here, too, an oligarchy had risen in St. John's, where wealthy commercial houses controlled the marketing of goods to the outports as well as the handling of the yearly catch of cod for export. Sealing had become a source of livelihood, but farming remained restricted. Although a stable government had become possible, the political scene remained turbulent as most of the island's population remained poor and continued debts plagued the government and blocked development.

Remarkable developments of a different nature took place in Rupert's Land and in the vast uncharted area extending to the Arctic and Pacific Oceans. Just around 1800, explorers discovered the great rivers to these oceans and opened surrounding country to the fur trade. A planned settlement of Scottish Highlanders on the Red River in 1811 suffered tragedy, yet survived (Careless, 1970). By 1850, the settlement's heterogeneous population of 5000 included a majority of French Métis supplemented by Scottish Indian Métis, English and Scottish settlers, some Americans moving westward for land, and some Upper Canadians who desired annexation of the settlement (McInnis, 1969). On the West Coast, settlement was only gradually appearing to threaten the fur trade. In 1849, Vancouver Island became a Crown colony in an attempt to further stabilize British control through settlement. After the gold rushes of the 1850s along the Fraser River, the British Columbia mainland became part of the colony as fears of annexation by Californian prospectors arose (McInnis, 1969). Further rushes to the Cariboo gold fields brought the building of roads and the nucleus of settlement, and in 1866 Vancouver Island and the mainland became the Province of British Columbia despite a future clouded by a dwindling population and huge debts (McInnis, 1969).

Thus, by the 1860s, these regions, eventually to become the Canada of the future, showed disparate environmental conditions and stages of societal development, all demanding untold motivation, energy, and wealth if barriers to a more mature society were to be overcome. It would seem that development of health services could only have low priority in these circumstances. Nevertheless, health and welfare of the population was of concern to some people in all regions. Throughout the 1800s, concern grew as trends and events gave support to those motivated to deal with the mounting issues of health, sickness, and death.

Threats to health in the 1800s

In a land dominated by the fur trade, Aboriginals and newcomers alike suffered from trauma, nutritional disorders, mental illness, tumours, and epidemics of smallpox, influenza, measles, scarlet fever, and other fevers of unknown origin (Ray, 1981). Introduced by the immigrants, infectious diseases, particularly smallpox, brought high mortality to Aboriginal tribes. As family life became more firmly established, childbearing complications and diseases of children were further causes of suffering and death.

The events that moved the Maritimes and the Province of Québec into and beyond the pioneer period of development also endangered people's lives. Wars brought not only military casualties and sickness among officers and ranks but also disruption of families. Widows, orphans, and abandoned children required care and welfare services. Poverty-stricken, malnourished immigrants, who had been crowded into the holds of wooden ships used for carrying timber or furs on the return trips, frequently arrived in the new country without worldly possessions (Carroll, 1979). Many were ill on arrival or dying from typhus fever, cholera, and other infectious diseases. The cholera epidemics of 1832 and 1834 created states of panic and emergency as the disease spread and victims died within hours or days of becoming ill. In 1832, the disease killed 3851 in Québec and 4000 in Montréal and its surrounding villages (Heagerty, i, 1928). The hardy settlers also had their crises as clearing the land, logging, working in the timber industry, and building roads, bridges, canals, and railways took their toll in injuries and death among the male population. For women, complicated childbirth remained hazardous.

As towns and cities appeared, so did dichotomous scenes of wealth and power. The back streets and the waterfronts had slums with shanties, barns, privies, and manure-strewn dirt roads. Cities had high death rates, thought to be caused by unsanitary conditions among the poor, inadequate nutrition, and contaminated food and water. The cities received the homeless, disorganized, sick, and poverty-stricken immigrants and harboured the unemployed and the abandoned women and children.

Resources and preventive medicine before Confederation

In the sparsely settled areas of Canada before Confederation, health care was left mainly to the individual with little involvement from governments. Missionaries entered the relatively underdeveloped regions to provide caring activities in times of sickness and distress as well as religious services. Trained physicians and medical attendants were included in many explorations of discovery and were also part of the military and naval establishments. Often in developing settlements and outposts, they acted as government officials, law givers, and agents of social reform.

The growth of hospitals as curative as well as custodial institutions and as a means of protecting people from contagious diseases was associated with the increasing complexity of society in the pioneer period. Some of the new hospitals were started by religious sisterhoods, others by United Empire Loyalists, benevolent societies, church groups, physicians, and local government authorities. Some started as houses of refuge for the sick poor or as tent hospitals to care for cholera patients. Asylums were built to permit transfer of the mentally ill from cells outside hospital walls or from the city jail. At the time, sick people of means did not readily enter hospitals, since mortality was generally high and care often less than humane.

A resource that would become highly significant in future health care and preventive medicine was the opening of medical schools in Upper and Lower Canada and in the Maritimes. The first to be founded was in Montréal in 1824. Before that, qualified physicians and surgeons received their education and training in the schools of the British Isles or in the United States. Many practising medical doctors had been trained only as apprentices to local physicians.

The science of medicine was still in an early phase of development. Although surgery had advanced, medical treatment was not based on well-grounded theories and scientific facts. For example, a popular theory of disease was that miasmas (noxious materials in the form of vapours and odours from decaying matter, body excreta, polluted water, or filth) were causative factors. Observation and shrewd hunches had also led to the belief that disease could be spread by person-to-person contact and indirectly by clothing and other materials used by infected persons. Although in England the sanitary movement was advancing consistently with these beliefs, treatment of the sick still included bleeding, purging, medications, and use of leeches and blistering.

The women of religious sisterhoods and untrained lay nurses continued as essential resources in underdeveloped regions and in hospitals in the larger cities and towns. Authorities concerned about the health and spiritual needs of their people often requested the specialized services of the Order of the Grey Nuns or other religious orders, such as the Sisters of Saint Ann and the Sisters of Providence. Travelling by whatever means possible (foot, horseback, ox cart, canoe, or barge), these sisters pioneered health care development along Canada's frontiers.

As pioneers in health services to the Red River Settlement in 1844, the Grey Nuns made 6000 visits during the next 10 years to sick people. In 1847, they opened a hospital in St. Boniface (in what is now Manitoba). A call to Bytown (later Ottawa) in 1845 resulted in the founding of a community hospital and visits to the poor; here, two years later, among the Irish immigrants, the Grey Nuns gave emergency nursing services to 578 typhus fever victims. By 1860 their work had extended to a Native settlement 400 miles north of Saskatoon and by 1867 to Fort Providence on Great Slave Lake. Their activities brought education, nursing services, and a hospital to the area (Gibbon & Mathewson, 1947).

Women designated as nurses in the pioneer rural communities were also available to provide care in the home in times of sickness or distress. Generally, they were respected for their skill and remedies derived from experience and for their devotion and courage in travelling day and night over treacherous roads. Competent unmarried or widowed women with nursing and managerial interests frequently became matrons in the new secular hospitals. The scarce numbers of women to provide direct nursing care in these institutions meant that caregivers were often of lower social standing and of questionable interests and abilities.

Early formal attempts to control disease and protect the health of communities resulted from the cholera epidemic of 1832. When Britain's Colonial Office in 1831 alerted Québec officials to the possible arrival of immigrants with cholera, a Sanitary Commission and a Board of Health were immediately appointed and issued directives for the protection of people. The Act of 1831 giving legal status to these directives was revised in 1849 to apply to both Canada West and Canada East. Framed to prevent malignant, contagious, and infectious diseases, the act detailed regulations for personal and environmental cleanliness; quarantine of infected persons; attention to contaminated clothing by boiling, baking, or burning; and private and immediate burial of the dead (Bryce, 1910). The regulations were logical in view of generally accepted theories of disease and were in agreement with the sanitary movement in England.

Confederation: New attitudes, new health services

Attitudes shifted during the last decades of the 1800s from fatalism concerning survival to belief in the possibility of control and prevention of communicable diseases, and then to hope for a healthy life. The changed attitude was not widespread; rather, it was possessed mainly by those aware of discoveries in the biological and medical sciences and by social reformers anxious to ameliorate the health and social problems of the poor in cities and of people in remote and isolated areas.

Political factors played their part. The *British North America Act* of 1867 established Canada as a nation but left legislative power related to health and social welfare to the provincial governments for administration. Under this

Act, now known as the *Constitution Act, 1867*, the federal government retained powers of taxation as well as responsibilities for census and statistics, quarantine, and marine hospitals. The Act addressed only briefly social and health matters, a fact criticized by those deeply concerned about public health in the country (Bryce, 1910). The provinces therefore assumed responsibilities for hospitals, asylums, and charities and other matters related to health care.

Canada becomes a nation

Confederation did not come from a vision of nationhood; in fact, many people were ambivalent toward the idea. But politically, Confederation was a reasonable solution for regional problems: the failing economy and political instability of the Atlantic provinces; the unworkable political structure of Canada West and Canada East (formerly Upper and Lower Canada); the need of the Western plains for settlement and agricultural development; and British Columbia's burgeoning debt and desire for trade and commerce from a transcontinental railway. Adding weight to regional decisions for Confederation was the matter of defence, brought home to many people by internal and external pressures for annexation by the United States. Britain had changed its attitude and wanted its North American possessions to take greater responsibility for conduct of their own affairs, particularly defence.

The new Dominion of Canada only gradually enlarged its domain. Nova Scotia, New Brunswick, Québec, and Ontario were charter members in 1867. In 1870, the vast holdings of the Hudson's Bay Company were transferred from British to Canadian jurisdiction to become Canada's Northwest Territories (later divided into the Prairie provinces and the northern territories). In the same year, the Canadian government secured the Red River Settlement, giving the tiny area provincial status and rights as the province of Manitoba (later enlarged). With British Columbia entering Confederation in 1871 and Prince Edward Island in 1873, the land previously known as British North America became a Dominion stretching from sea to sea.

A worldwide depression beginning in 1873, abating from 1879 to 1883 only to return and continue into the 1890s, threatened the economic benefits projected at the time of Confederation. Ontario and Québec fared best in these circumstances, since they sold minerals, farm machinery, and asbestos to world markets and their manufactured goods and farm produce were required by people in the proliferating towns and small cities and in the rapidly growing commercial centres of Montréal and Toronto. In 1891, Montréal had a population of 250 000 and Toronto 181 000. Urban population in the older provinces that year showed a 50-percent increase since 1881; rural populations remained stationary or declined slightly (McInnis, 1969). The federal government's commitment to protective tariffs and the building of railways favoured these provinces' industrial growth and marketing of their goods across Canada.

The Maritimes were not as fortunate economically as was Central Canada. Their population patterns also showed a shift from rural to urban living, but growth was minimal. New Brunswick barely maintained its numbers. Protective tariffs were not to the advantage of the east coast provinces; their own industries failed to develop. Goods from Ontario and Québec were sold in their stores. With the coming of steamships, their shipbuilding industry had declined. Since goods for world markets could be shipped more reasonably from Montréal to American seaports than by railway to the ports of Halifax and St. John, their carrying trade was reduced, and the Maritime railways failed to bring projected profits.

Although Manitoba had a difficult time during the early years after Confederation, public enthusiasm for the wealth to be derived from railways, homesteading, and wheat farming made Winnipeg a boom city. Its population grew from 250 in 1871 to 20 000 in 1886 (Batten, 1977; Leacock, 1941). Hardship came to homesteaders as a world depression closed in, but Winnipeg survived and even increased its wealth and culture as the Gateway to the West. Meanwhile, unresolved issues existed between the province and the federal government over the monopoly of railway traffic, high transportation rates, and the federal government's power to override provincial decisions, culminating in the dispute over the *Manitoba Act* of 1890 calling for a single government-supported, non-sectarian school system. Deeper issues were the rights of minorities, especially those of French Canadians, to their language and religion.

British Columbia was fairly content within Confederation after completion of the Canadian Pacific Railway in 1885, although the federal government's failure to meet time commitments for its building had angered provincial authorities and brought threats of secession. Chinese immigration was another contentious issue, since the federal government opposed British Columbia's desire for its curtailment. After 1885, the future looked brighter; Vancouver became the western terminus for transcontinental trade, commerce, and travel, and American capital and initiative opened the interior to exploration of its mineral and timber resources (Saywell, 1967).

The most profound social changes probably occurred in the territory from Manitoba to the Rockies, in the fertile land marked for railways, settlement, and agricultural development. Sparsely populated in 1871 with Indian tribes, Métis, Hudson's Bay Company employees, a few white settlers, and missionaries from Ontario, by 1891 the territory had a population of 50 000 (McInnis, 1969, p. 396). Anticipating the magnitude of the required social changes and the need for law and order to entice settlers, the national government organized the North-West Mounted Police in 1873 and dispatched the force to the western plains in the following year. Several physicians accompanied the force to work in its hospitals and with the people in the surrounding territory.

The North-West Mounted's most critical role came with the North-West Rebellion of 1885. Fearful of encroachment by government-sponsored settlement on their riverside farms, the Métis brought back Louis Riel, who had fled to the United States after an earlier rebellion, to be their leader. A clash with the Mounted Police resulted in the federal government's sending 5000 militia from Ontario and Québec to end the rebellion. Canada's first military field hospitals were used in this brief war effort.

Threats to health in the late 1800s

In the difficult decades following Confederation, life in Canada continued to be hazardous for people of all ages. Contagious diseases still brought sickness and death, except that cholera had been brought under control as a result of preventive measures, declining immigration, replacement of wooden sailing ships with the more sanitary and faster steamships, and worldwide attention to reported cases. Mortality from smallpox epidemics was high, particularly among the Western tribes and in Montréal, statistically the unhealthiest city in North America. Montréal's smallpox epidemic of 1885 claimed more than 3000 lives, with 90 percent of the deaths in children under 10 years of age. Poverty-stricken French Canadians seemed most vulnerable. The anti-vaccination protests, contributing to the bleak statistics, ceased only as the demonstrated high cost in lives among the unvaccinated overruled people's fear of possible harmful effects from vaccination (Bliss, 1991). Typhoid fever became prevalent in these years as the excreta of the sick and the carriers spread the causative organism in the poor sewage disposal and impure water supply systems. Diphtheria caused a particularly high death rate among children until antitoxin was introduced in 1894 (Heagerty, i, 1928). High mortality also accompanied scarlet fever, measles, and influenza.

Tuberculosis, generally known as "consumption," "the white plague," or "phthisis," was common. It was believed to be hereditary until 1865, when it was classified as infectious. Hopeless attitudes lessened somewhat after the causative organism was identified in 1885 and a sanatorium regime of fresh air, rest, diet, and graded exercise was found to be a relatively successful treatment.

The plight of the mentally ill, now an enlarged and more visible element in society, worsened in these decades as asylums increased in number, remained overcrowded, and provided few attendants for custodial care (Francis, 1981). Asylums did not appear in British Columbia until 1870 or in the Prairies until the late 1880s.

High maternal death rates continued, although birth rates declined in all provinces (McLaren, 1981). Both in urban and in rural areas, most confinements were at home, with the assistance of midwives, neighbours, or physicians; the medical profession generally found no fault in this practice if conditions were favourable. In cities during the early years of this period, most single, poverty-stricken women without proper accommodation had their babies in small lying-in or maternity cottages where professors of midwifery gave lectures, attended deliveries, and had their students follow the mother's labour (Cosbie, 1975). By the 1880s and 1890s, obstetrical units had become attached to general hospitals and were used for the education and training of medical students. In the 1890s, the maternal and infant deaths among the immigrant groups in remote settlements and among the industrial poor in the growing towns and cities of the west were of much concern to the National Council of Women (Buckley, 1979).

Advances in knowledge and new legislation

Scientific knowledge advanced in the decades following Confederation, bringing new theories of health and disease. Although many of the require ments of the people for health care in the developing regions of the country remained unaffected, this knowledge influenced legislation and resources for health care.

In the 1870s, Pasteur's confirmation of the germ theory of disease, Lister's application of the theory in antiseptic surgery, and Koch's development of precise methods of studying micro-organisms provided a scientific foundation for prevention of infection in hospitals and prevention of contagious diseases through use of sera and vaccines. Most, but not all, proponents of the sanitary movement changed their rationale for sanitary procedures from elimination of miasmas to destruction and control of causative organisms. Consequently, authorities became more precise in their recommendations for cleaner towns and cities, sewage disposal, purification of water and milk, preparation and marketing of meat and other foods, and standards of cleanliness in the workplace and in the home.

Physicians and scientists at British and European medical centres and laboratories continued to link pathology and clinical symptoms and to identify disease entities. Investigations of insanity by post-mortem brain examination had resulted in general acceptance that pathology of the brain and nerves, hereditary in origin, was the cause of disturbed behaviour. Hysteria in women, however, was postulated to result from reflex disturbances between the reproductive system and the brain. Neurologists thought that neuroses were caused by brain exhaustion resulting from strain, worry, and hereditary traits (Brown, 1981). Despite these uncertain conclusions, the science of pathology, disease, and diagnosis advanced; the science of therapeutics remained negligible. As faith was lost in bleeding, purging, and blistering, practitioners turned to naturalistic methods of healing by rest, diet, fresh air, and encouragement, but they also embraced many unproven new technologies based on hydrotherapy and electrotherapy.

Of interest is the recognition of promotion of health as a value in itself. The new and developing sciences of physiology, psychology, and pathology led some reformers to believe in a science of hygiene as the greatest conquest of medicine, permitting not only prevention of disease and ill health but also advance of physiological, intellectual, and moral development. Broadly conceived as the art of preserving health and the achievement of perfect mind–body interaction, the science and art of hygiene recommended healthful work and community relationships and self-control of thoughts, feelings, desires, and habits ("Remarks on the Antiquity," 1875).

In this era, medical schools increased in number, standards of education were raised, and apprenticeship was ruled out as a means of entry into the medical profession. Growing interest in sanitary science permitted its inclusion in the curriculum. Specialization now extended to ophthalmology and otology. By the 1890s, well-trained surgeons had the knowledge and skill to perform a broad range of surgical procedures successfully. These developments, however, did not preclude the existence of unlicensed practitioners, many of whom were in the underdeveloped territories of the West (Neatby, 1981).

Of much significance to community health care was the opening of training schools for nurses in Canada based on an adaptation of the Nightingale model. Florence Nightingale's fame was widespread in the 1860s as the heroine of the Crimean War, a foremost sanitarian and social reformer, and an authority on the management of hospitals and the training of nurses. Her *Notes on Nursing*, published in 1859, was a bestseller at home and abroad. The text made explicit a philosophy of nursing based on the belief that the nurse could help or hinder the healing processes of nature. For Nightingale, the art of nursing lay in creating a clean, well-ventilated environment and providing proper diet, rest, diversion, conversation, and companionship (Nightingale, 1859). She also believed that nurses should "intelligently," "competently," and "faithfully" execute the physician's orders (Dock, 1901).

In view of the advances in surgery, medical education, and specialization and the close association of Canadian physicians and their British mentors, it is understandable that physicians initiated the beginning of Nightingale nursing schools in this country. After the successful founding of the first training school at the General and Marine Hospital in St. Catharines, Ontario, in 1874, nursing schools became an essential part of the organization of all large and small hospitals. Although the early schools began before the germ theory was accepted and antiseptic surgery practised, the first nurses prepared the way for the scientific practice of medicine and surgery as their activities brought cleanliness to hospitals, humane care, and disciplined commitment in their endeavours (Allemang, 1974). Graduates of the new training schools for nurses became superintendents of these schools and of hospitals, private nurses in the homes of the sick, and military nurses in the North-West Rebellion of 1885.

Visiting nursing entered a new phase with the development of nursing schools. Graduate nurses became part of the missionary movement, taking their skills to the still sparsely settled areas of the country. Of lasting importance was the work of Lady Aberdeen, wife of the Governor General of Canada from 1894 to 1898, who travelled extensively across the Dominion. As President of the National Council of Women, she learned of the lack of health services for women in the isolated settlements, particularly during childbirth, and saw the need for health care for the people in the shack towns by the railways and near the mining areas of British Columbia. She suggested that an Order, similar to the "Queen's Nurses" in the United Kingdom, was needed to supply visiting nurses and cottage hospitals to small communities.

The project suggested by Lady Aberdeen was staunchly supported by local branches of the Council of Women but blocked by medical men fearing lowered standards of care from unqualified workers. She arranged for support from Dr. Alfred Worcester, professor of hygiene at Harvard University and founder, in 1886, of the Waltham Training Home for District Nurses in Massachusetts, who visited Canada to interpret the plans to opposing Ontario physicians. Consequently, in 1897, general approval for the proposed plan was forthcoming and Charlotte Macleod, a Canadian from New Brunswick, trained at Waltham and then superintendent of the Waltham school, became the first superintendent of the Victorian Order of Nurses (VON) for Canada (Gibbon, 1947; Gibbon & Mathewson, 1947; Pringle & Roe, 1992). Nurses working with the VON were required to be graduate nurses and have six months' additional training in district nursing at a VON centre (later reduced to four months). This private, non-profit, voluntary nursing organization, which has modified its role many times, helped illustrate the benefits of community nursing and primary care offered in the community (Pringle & Roe, 1992).

Of significance for future health care was legislation passed in 1882 in Ontario for the first permanent provincial Board of Health. The board had responsibilities for public education and advisory functions to municipal councils. Recognition of the lack of legislation requiring municipal boards of health was quickly followed by the *Public Health Act* of 1884, which overcame this omission (Bryce, 1911). Similar legislation was soon enacted in most other provinces (Heagerty, i, 1928).

Thus, by the turn of the century the public health movement was under way. Pioneering tasks in health education would lead to new demands on the trained nurse.

The 20th century: Every nurse a public health nurse

In the years between the turn of the century and the close of the third decade a world emerged based on new values, a new social structure, new sources of wealth, and changed political relationships. Equally remarkable was the new perspective of some nurses that every nurse should be a public health nurse. The ideal was consistent with the new program of health education espoused by public health authorities in addition to those of sanitary reform and prevention of disease defined before the turn of the century (Burton & Smith, 1970).

By the close of the first decade of the 20th century a spirit of optimism pervaded the country as economic prosperity returned and continued to flourish. Railway systems expanded and criss-crossed the Western plains. A dynamic program of immigration, reaching a peak of 400 000 immigrants during 1913, brought settlement to the West (Craig, 1977). Development of the wheat industry made Canada the world's leading country in the export of this grain. Industrialism advanced, particularly in Central Canada, which now produced three-quarters of the country's manufactured goods. The lumber industries of British Columbia, Ontario, and Québec fared well as Western settlers built their houses with B.C. lumber and the countries of the world bought Canada's pulpwood. Increasing wealth also came with discovery of mineral deposits in the Canadian Shield, a development advanced by generation of electricity from water power.

Many outward features of society indicated this growing national prosperity. In the large cities, grand hotels, well-designed city halls, libraries, churches, university buildings, imposing hospitals, large department stores, ornate theatres, and stately houses reflected opulence. The Prairie provinces also showed their increasing wealth in large grain elevators, roads and railway lines linking small towns and creating new ones, and mechanized equipment in use on successful farms (Phillips, 1977). Canada's enlarging population was partly responsible for these developments. Between 1896 and 1914 approximately 2.5 million people emigrated to Canada. Almost all the nationalities of the world appeared in the Western provinces. By 1905, population growth permitted provincial status for Alberta and Saskatchewan. When World War I began in 1914, settlement had extended to the Peace River area, and by 1920 Canada no longer possessed an agrarian frontier.

Of interest are the population shifts and the distribution of the population that emerged across Canada. Despite the influx of settlers on farmlands and an increasing rural population, by 1911, 45 percent of the Canadian population was urban (McInnis, 1969). Industrial development showed itself not only in working-class neighbourhoods in cities and towns and in employment for those able to work but also in the entry of women into the labour force. Although 90 percent of those employed were male, young women from the farms and those entering Canada as immigrants found ready work in domestic service, and as secretaries and clerks in developing business, industrial, and cultural enterprises. In 1930, Canada's population had risen to slightly more than 10 million. Ontario and Québec, with 6.2 million, had twice the combined population of the Prairie provinces and British Columbia. The Maritimes had just over a million people and Newfoundland approximately 275 000.

Economic prosperity and accompanying optimism were reflected in the social philosophy of the period, a belief in the power of the individual to master circumstances. Of interest in view of this belief is the beginning organization of labour unions desiring a shorter work week, fewer hours of work, better pay, and improved working conditions.

Many of these trends continued during the years of World War I (1914–1918). The Allies, now deprived of many former trading countries, increased their demands for wheat, other food supplies, and pulpwood as well as for armaments. Mining and lumbering industries expanded to provide metals for shells and other armaments and wood for ships and aircraft. Toward the close of the war, Canada had a large industrial force, with women contributing substantially to its operation and efficiency when men were recruited into military service. New trends emerged, however, to accompany this economic growth: national debts, inflation showing a 60-percent rise in the cost of living, and the first Dominion income tax in 1917.

All these events and trends had their effect on what was required and on what was possible in health services.

New threats to health

These decades of prosperity had a dark side. Personal and environmental situations threatened health and brought accidents, sickness, and death. The West also had unsuccessful newcomers with large families, living in poverty, unaccustomed to the rigorous climate and without sufficient money to buy land or knowledge to make the land produce. Transients employed in railway construction went to the cities in the winter months and worked in slaughter houses, in sweatshops, or in construction work required to provide paved streets, sewage disposal, and safe water supplies. All the large cities had people living in boarding-house slums and in overcrowded tenement houses, and had those who went to brothels and used the services of back-street abortionists.

In 1901, tuberculosis was a leading cause of death in the cities and among the poor and had a death rate of 180 per 100 000. The disease continued as a major killer in succeeding decades. A high incidence of communicable diseases was still evident. Native people living on reserves were victims of epidemics of typhoid fever, measles, smallpox, and tuberculosis. Although prevention of smallpox and diphtheria was possible by vaccination and inoculation, strong prejudices persisted and parents often evaded professional attempts to control disease by quarantine and care in isolation hospitals. The social effects of venereal disease were known to be widespread, but reticence to openly discuss on the subject prevented concerted action. A worldwide epidemic of Spanish influenza in 1918, attacking one-sixth of the Canadian population and killing approximately 30 000 people, caused untold suffering and anxiety and dramatically revealed Canada's uncoordinated and scarce health services (McGinnis, 1981). Public attitudes toward mental deviations and illness, now recognized as rooted in psychological and social as well as physical and hereditary causes, were seen as detrimental to prevention and treatment. Maternal death rates and the high incidence of abortions as a cause of death were likewise of growing concern.

As in other centuries, war resulted in bereaved and broken families and disabled veterans suffering from physical and emotional illness of immediate and long-term consequence. Of the 400 000 recruits who went overseas in World War I, 50 000 became casualties. A new insight came to those examining Canadian youth for military service. Too large a number failed to meet acceptable standards for army duty because of physical defects and emotional disabilities. Authorities concluded that more had to be done to raise the general level of health of Canadian society.

Developing resources

Advancing medical science in these decades and the need for its application justified health education as an aim of the public health movement. Smallpox and diphtheria were now preventable, and increasing knowledge of tuberculosis permitted more control of its incidence and mortality. Hope for the prevention of syphilis and its long-term neurological complications was realistic after the Wasserman test was perfected in 1906 and salvarsan and bismuth were discovered in 1909 and 1921 as specific therapeutic agents. The scientific study of nutrition and identification of vitamins permitted control of some deficiency diseases, including rickets in children. Promotion of mental health and the prevention of "psychopathic behaviour" became credible goals with advancing knowledge of normal and abnormal personality development and descriptive studies on the effect of infant and childhood experiences on later social and personal adjustment. The new skill of intelligence testing became useful in the diagnosis of the "feeble-minded" and their need for special services and facilities.

Belief in the ordinary citizen and concern for health were shown in the Dominion and provincial governments' new legislation for improved health and social welfare and their shared funding of special programs. After years of unsuccessful effort, an Act was passed in 1919 creating a national department of health. This centralized the fragmented public health responsibilities previously assigned to various departments. The Act also created a Dominion Council of Health, composed of provincial officers of health and lay representatives, to act in an advisory and liaison capacity to the national department. As part of the postwar readjustment plans, the Dominion and provincial governments cooperated to provide unemployment relief and employment services. Pensions were given to disabled veterans and bereaved families, and rehabilitation and retraining programs became available. Military hospitals provided long-term care for physically and mentally disabled veterans (Nicholson, 1975).

The organization of significant voluntary agencies, national in scope, also demonstrated Canada's growing nationalism and a unified perspective on health and welfare. New associations focussed their attention on the creation of public enlightenment and on the need for increased responsibility by private citizens and official agencies for vulnerable groups showing high morbidity and mortality. Of special importance to the development of public health nursing in Canada was the extension of the work of the Canadian Red Cross Society at the close of the 1914–1918 war; the Society incorporated aims, based on an article of the League of Nations' Covenant, for promotion of health, prevention of disease, and relief of suffering in time of peace as well as war. The extended aims required provincial divisions to work with official provincial agencies for health promotion (Heagerty, ii, 1928).

In the early decades of the 1900s, the growth of large and small hospitals continued in response to Canada's growing population and the services these institutions could now offer as a result of medical specialization and new beliefs about the hospital's social responsibility. Specialty hospitals increased in number to include sanatoria for tuberculosis patients, isolation hospitals, children's hospitals, and those for the mentally ill. University teaching hospitals enlarged their outpatient departments and developed liaison services to homes in the belief that effective sick care required social and health care for patients and families (Allemang, 1974; Reid, 1913).

In rural and isolated areas, many small hospitals managed by such voluntary organizations as the Victorian Order of Nurses, Canadian Red Cross Society, religious sisterhoods, and mission boards extended services into the homes of people many miles distant, as well as giving in-hospital care. Many new facilities likewise became available for the promotion of health, prevention of disease, and early detection of defects. Large industries, insurance companies, and department stores developed health services to keep employees well, assist in preventing accidents, render first aid, and give nursing care and health teaching. To benefit employees and their families, some companies maintained home nursing and maternity services. Toward the close of the first decade, school systems expanded medical supervision of children to include nursing supervision and health teaching of the children and their families (Gibbon & Mathewson, 1947; Sutherland, 1981).

All these developing resources had their effect, both direct and indirect, on what was conceived and demonstrated as nursing.

The nurse becomes a
community health worker

By the turn of the century the nurse had firmly established her role in Canadian society as an essential person in the care of the sick in hospitals and at home. Nurses assumed positions of responsibility as superintendents of nursing departments in large and small hospitals and as teachers in each hospital's nursing school. Nurses in training still provided most of an institution's patient care and in isolated areas might be sent to give nursing care in the home in dire circumstances. Most trained nurses worked in private practice, attending those who were financially able to procure their services either at home or in private patient pavilions. Such care was not readily available to people of moderate means or to those in isolated areas or in the class of the sick poor.

But this pattern of a community's nursing services began to change gradually as nurses became part of all the new agencies and institutions interested in health promotion and prevention of disease. Of major importance in the transition were the enlarging views and attitudes toward the social causes of disease and suffering, particularly among a city's poor and working classes. If the new bacteriological discoveries and new knowledge on the prevention of various diseases could be applied, it was believed a better and healthier society would emerge. At the same time, the enlarging possibilities of sick care for assisting patients and their families in recovery also brought new forms of nursing service and expanding concepts of visiting nursing. The possibility of control of tuberculosis brought the social service or health nurse into outpatient departments for case finding and follow-up home visiting (Allemang, 1974; Emory, 1945). In the isolated areas, the small community hospital often had visiting nurses as part of its staff, a contemporary and modified version of the services offered in past centuries by the Grey Nuns.

Also advancing the work of the nurse in community health, and gathering momentum thereafter, was the trend toward amalgamation of nursing services dealing with health and social matters. Divisions of Public Health Nursing were formed within the structure of provincial and municipal health departments. Further moves toward generalized services came with the transfer of school health services from boards of education to health departments (Sillars, 1983). The timing of the moves varied from province to province, as did the complexity of the services offered under the aegis of public health nursing.

In these circumstances, public health work became generalized as the family, the home, and the community, rather than just the individual, became the primary focus of attention. For example, Manitoba employed and paid nurses from public funds for a demonstration of generalized health services as early as 1916 (Gibbon & Mathewson, 1947). Soon after observing

Manitoba's scheme of providing public health nursing services to its rural communities, Alberta developed its plan for an official district nursing service; in 1919, the provincial health ministry gave official sanction to its district nurses in remote areas to act as midwives (Cashman, 1966). In the same year, British Columbia developed a health centre for a district composed of several adjoining communities, using a staff of public health nurses. The advance of official public health nursing services in the rural communities of Nova Scotia and New Brunswick came as a result of demonstration projects by the Canadian Red Cross Society. In both provinces in 1921, the Society appointed and financed public health nurses on an experimental basis for one year. The success of the projects led to public and private funds and government subsidies to continue these services. In the 1920s, Saskatchewan also initiated and developed generalized nursing services in cities and rural areas.

Efforts toward development of public health nursing services in Newfoundland were blocked by lack of finances and the isolated living conditions of half the population in distant outposts without municipal structures to support health services. Child care and maternity services were primary concerns of voluntary groups seeking to provide essential services. The work of the international Grenfell Association, organized in 1912, and the Newfoundland Outpost Nursing and Industrial Association, organized in 1926, brought maternity and nursing services to many isolated communities. However, a Royal Commission's report in 1933 still showed many settlements without resources for health care apart from the help the people themselves gave to each other. On the recommendation of the Commission, a reorganization of health service was initiated and a chain of government-supported health services spread across the island (Nevitt, 1978).

Education for public health nursing

The new role of the public health nurse, with emphasis on health teaching, case finding, and preventive care in a variety of community settings, brought to the foreground many professional issues, some clearly identified, others only vaguely defined. One issue was the education of nurses for public health nursing; a deeper issue was whether public health nursing was a specialty or an integral part of all nursing.

As nurses assumed extended responsibilities in public health, employing agencies provided short preparatory courses for their nurses, and some organized a form of continuing instruction and supervision. In 1914, nurses with Toronto's Health Department were required to take the newly organized course in Medical Social Work at the University of Toronto during their first year of employment (Risk, 1973). At the same time, discontent grew over the inadequate training of nurses in the hospital nursing schools for their new roles and responsibilities in public health.

In 1913, Mary Ard MacKenzie, national superintendent of the Victorian Order of Nurses and president of the Canadian National Association of Trained Nurses, suggested that a committee study the training of nurses and recommend improvements. The committee, which included two university presidents and nurses from across Canada, drew attention to the limited focus in the curriculum to requirements of hospital nursing and the schools' failure to develop and educate nurses for the broad scope of professional work and for their personal growth. The committee recommended nursing schools or colleges in connection with the educational system; the schools would offer a general course and an honours course with specialization options. One specialty was to be district and public health nursing.

After the postwar readjustment period, the issue again emerged of who was a public health nurse and what should be expected from a hospital school of nursing. Nurses in leadership positions in nursing education and in public health nursing seem to have been the prime movers in raising crucial questions that surfaced over the statement that "every nurse should be a public health nurse," an idea forcefully expressed in new educational trends in the United States. Annie W. Goodrich, dean of the School of Nursing at Yale University, claimed that the whole field of nursing received its fullest expression in public health nursing. The curriculum of Yale's nursing school, started in 1923, integrated the concept of health throughout the program in the belief that public health nursing was not a specialty but an integral part of all nursing. The Committee on Education of the National League of Nursing Education in the United States stated in its curriculum guide, published in 1927, that the nurse was essentially an "agent and teacher of health" and that nursing programs should emphasize the social, preventive, and teaching aspects of nursing (National League of Nursing Education, 1927).

In Canada, Margaret Moag, a district supervisor with the Victorian Order of Nurses, wrote on this theme and pointed out that opportunities existed for health promotion in every patient contact and in every occupational field that a nurse might enter. At the same time, she criticized hospital nursing schools for the nursing curriculum's limited scientific content, particularly in regard to psychology and sociology, and for acceptance of a narrow and technically based clinical program that frustrated the likelihood of any interest in nursing as a family service dealing with childbearing, child care, and other health matters over extended periods of time (Moag, 1924). In 1926, the Canadian Nurses Association appointed Jean I. Gunn, director of nurses at the Toronto General Hospital, as convenor of a committee to consider possible modification of the nursing curriculum to meet the needs of public health nursing (Gunn, 1926; Riegler, 1992).

E. Kathleen Russell, director of the department of public health nursing at the University of Toronto, was distressed over the inadequacy of the scientific knowledge that graduate nurses brought to the study of this subject in the new university certificate program in public health nursing, which opened in 1920. She did not, however, believe that hospital schools of nursing should prepare public health nurses. This type of school, she thought, should only prepare nurses for the fine "art" of bedside nursing, although the goal for the sick patient in hospital should be health, not just relief of symptoms. She pointed out that what was taught about health and public health nursing should be related directly to the patient's particular requirements at that time (Russell, 1920, 1926).

Baccalaureate nursing education in Canada was stimulated partly as a result of the Canadian Red Cross Society's funding of public health nursing certificate courses at six Canadian universities (Toronto, Western Ontario, McGill, Dalhousie, Alberta, and British Columbia) in 1920–1921. University-based degree programs for nurses had started in the United States in 1909. In 1919, the University of British Columbia opened Canada's first degree program in nursing, a five-year course that offered two years of liberal and scientific education, two years in hospital, and a final year on campus (Zilm & Warbinek, 1994). The final year offered preparation for nursing in a field of the student's choice, either in public health nursing (an expansion of the 1919 certificate course) or in teaching and supervision.

The pattern of the degree program for nursing at the University of British Columbia and at most other Canadian universities throughout the 1920s and 1930s was eventually criticized. The transfer of educational control of the student body from the university to the hospital for the clinical practice portion allowed students to fall heir to most of the shortcomings of the traditional training schools for nurses. Furthermore, the university was granting a degree when a large proportion of the students' time was spent in experiences outside the university's jurisdiction.

Some justification may exist for the arrangement during this period of nursing education. The theory and practice of bedside nursing probably could not be conceived as an appropriate university subject without losing much of the richness of hospital experiences through direct patient care. Likewise, the question of academic standards for teaching bedside nursing probably was troublesome to the university. Although these anxieties could not readily be resolved, the less than desirable arrangement brought positive outcomes. The leadership component, taught at the universities, advanced the numbers of qualified nurses for nursing administration, nursing education, and community health nursing. Furthermore, educational authorities in related fields became increasingly aware of nursing's contribution to the health of society and the expanding body of knowledge required for nursing services.

Demographic nursing statistics of the 1920s had also supported the need for change in nursing education. Data collected by Professor George M. Weir, head of the Department of Education at the University of British Columbia and director of the study of nursing education in Canada, showed that as of January 1, 1930, there was one active public health nurse for every 6500 persons in the population and, of the 10 530 registered nurses in Canada in active practice, only 1521 were classified as public health nurses. The findings recommended that the number of public health nurses be doubled in the next five to 10 years. Dr. Weir attributed the confused, chaotic picture of nursing education emerging from the survey to the uncontrolled growth of hospital training schools for nurses with little attention paid to the health needs of communities (Weir, 1932).

Despite the survey's negative findings, the 1920s had brought hope for the future. Initiation of the survey was, in itself, an indication of professional growth and recognition of nursing as a social force. Of significance for the future of community health nursing was the support of the Rockefeller Foundation, an American philanthropic organization chartered in 1913 to improve health care and promote well-being of people throughout the world. The previous success of visiting nursing in the United States permitted nurses to marshal convincing evidence of nurses' skills and abilities toward these goals through effective home visiting and health education. The debatable question concerned the proper education and training for all branches of essential nursing services. The Rockefeller Foundation's support of a study of nursing education in the United States and its subsequent financial assistance to university nursing schools for the education of public health nurses and as "pathfinders of professional education for nurses" furthered nursing's transition from apprenticeship training to professional education (Allemang, 1974).

In Canada, the support of the Rockefeller Foundation permitted implementation of Russell's plans, conceived during the 1920s, for an experimental school of nursing founded on sound educational principles. Her desire was for a unified three-year program that would interrelate curative and preventive aspects of nursing throughout a curriculum of closely aligned theoretical instruction and clinical practice. Although health was to be the focus of the program and the science of health its theoretical foundation, development of the "art" of bedside nursing was regarded as essential. Students would therefore have clinical practice in a wide variety of relevant services in appropriate hospitals, in community environments, and with families in their own homes (Russell, 1929, 1936).

In the development of Russell's thought, a legitimate claim was that the new school would offer a generalized preparation for nursing in the community, the hospital, and the home, a claim she could not support for the traditional school where, in actuality, specialized training solely for hospital work took place (Russell, 1932, 1933). Since the new school would be administered within the organizational structure of the university and possess financial resources not dependent on the services given by students, as heretofore required in hospital schools, freedom to experiment with and test a new design for nursing would be possible (Russell, 1938). The school came into being in 1933. Its general program qualified graduates for nurse registration examinations, public health nursing, and hospital nursing.

In 1942, the program was succeeded by a four-year undergraduate course leading to a bachelor of science in nursing degree. Russell's maturing conviction was that the future of professional nursing required advanced general education for a deeper understanding of human beings (Carpenter, 1982). The principles on which this degree course was established eventually became the model in Canada for what is known as generic baccalaureate nursing education. The baccalaureate nursing degree as the basis for entry to practice is a goal espoused since the 1970s by the national and most provincial nurses' associations (Bajnok, 1992). The belief that health is the aim and focus of professional nursing, wherever it is practised, continues as an underlying philosophy in keeping with the principles of Primary Health Care.

Diverging philosophies

Although university nursing education programs were incorporating public health principles and emphasized the health of individuals and communities, other events lessened the impact of these trends. The severe worldwide economic depression of the 1930s limited funds for health care advances. Hospitals continued to proliferate as medical science made advances, especially in the fields of surgery and anesthesiology. Hospitals needed workers, supplied mainly through the unpaid apprentice labour of student nurses, so hospital schools remained the norm. Major public health advances of clean water, better sewage systems, immunization programs, education, and improved communications systems led to vastly improved health in the general population and to longer lifespans and decreased infant mortality.

The Great Depression of the 1930s ended only with the outbreak of World War II (1939–1945). During the war and postwar years of the 1940s and 1950s, medical science made tremendous advances based mainly on development of antibiotics and other "wonder drugs." The belief became rampant that there would be a cure, probably through some magic drug, for every illness. The emphasis shifted from prevention and care to cure.

In the booming postwar years, governments turned their attention to development of social programs, including the establishment of hospital insurance plans (Storch & Meilicke, 1994). The first comprehensive, compulsory hospital insurance plan in North America was introduced in 1947 by the Saskatchewan government, followed closely by provincial governments in Alberta, British Columbia, and Newfoundland. Arrangements through federal–provincial negotiations led to the introduction of a federal Hospital

Insurance and Diagnostic Services plan in 1958, with all provinces joining the plan by 1961.

Saskatchewan again took the lead in the next major social policy development in health care; in 1962, despite fierce opposition from the medical profession, that province brought in a medical insurance plan. Other "have" provinces that could afford the cost soon followed suit. A 1964 Royal Commission on Health Services recommended that the federal government enter into cost-sharing agreements with the provinces so that a nation-wide, comprehensive, universal, portable, provincially administered medical insurance plan could be implemented; this was in place in 1968 (Storch & Meilicke, 1994).

During the boom years, the federal government also introduced several other health care social policies, including establishment of the National Health Grants in 1948. Although public health research was purportedly a main target of this grants-in-aid program, a large portion of attention was directed toward hospital construction and to development of medical technologies and pharmacological research. In 1967, the federal government separated the Medical Research Council from the National Research Council and earmarked health care research as a priority. However, this structure further affected the direction of health care, as research funding continued to be controlled by physicians and directed to medical priorities; few dollars went to public health or nursing research (see also Chapters 26 and 28). In the 1970s, the National Health Research and Development Program (NHRDP) assumed responsibility for the funding of health care research. Although this program has become the major source of funding for nursing research in Canada, a majority of its funds continued to go to medical and pharmacological research.

The resulting emphasis on hospitals, physician resources, and pharmacological cures seems, with hindsight, predictable; but in the boom years of the 1960s and early 1970s, the increasing costs for these services could be absorbed. By the mid-1970s, federal health ministers were looking at ways to have individuals once again assume more responsibility for health (Lalonde, 1974). By the 1980s, costs for health care were taking up to one-third of provincial budgets (see Chapter 8) and cost containment became a serious consideration. Health care policy makers once again began to look at principles espoused decades earlier by public health officials and nursing leaders. (This is explored further in Chapter 2.)

In perspective

When did community health nursing begin in this land now known as Canada? What forces shaped its course? If the past is to throw light on the present and point directions for the future, such questions require critical thinking.

In historical perspective, New France appears to have had its own form of community health nursing as religiously inspired agents of change answered their particular calls to assist and care for people experiencing vicissitudes of life in hazardous environments. Interrelated physical, social, and spiritual services, based on the values of the religious sisterhoods and their followers, laid the foundation of health care as a comprehensive service for all people, regardless of circumstances.

Under British rule, these religious organizations and their caring activities persisted. At the same time, secular authorities built hospitals, primarily for custodial reasons, and lay medical men attempted restorative care in outposts, towns, and cities. A significant contribution of the period was legislation for the control of contagious diseases, motivated primarily by the devastating and demoralizing effects of epidemics.

In the decades after Confederation and the turn of the century, a new frame of reference for health care captured the minds and imaginations of some people. The sanitary and humanitarian reforms of 19th-century England and new scientific knowledge resulting from laboratory and experimental study gave rise to the belief that controlled environmental conditions and personal health habits could alleviate suffering and promote health and that control of causative organisms could prevent disease. This justified the transfer of knowledge of health and disease into educative activities, a theme supported by trained and educated nurses.

Political, social, and economic forces since the early 1900s have led to national and provincial policies that markedly affected the direction that community health care in Canada has taken in recent decades (Storch & Meilicke, 1994). Among these forces are wars, depressions, regional political pressures, prosperous times with expanding economies, further recessions, a greater concern for the status of women, new waves of immigration, and improved worldwide communication and transportation systems. Further discussion of the effects and implications of these more recent events is provided in other chapters throughout this book.

Thus, an exploration of history helps to reveal how the past lies within every contemporary situation and how projected possibilities become part of present circumstances, eventually to take their place in the record of what has been thought, known, and experienced. The historical situation shapes not only what people conceive as worthy and possible but also determines the timing of change. Nevertheless, over time, the milieu will change, modified by many forces, including those arising from the ideas, values, motivations, and actions of persons who become agents of change (Collingwood, 1956; Tholfsen, 1967).

Acknowledgement
The author extends special thanks to Glennis Zilm, a fellow member of the Canadian Association for the History of Nursing, for editing this chapter,

which was originally written for the 1985 edition of *Community Health Nursing in Canada,* and for her analytical contribution, "Diverging Philosophies," presented in the later years of this continuing story.

QUESTIONS

1. What were some of the contemporary issues that helped introduce community health nursing in early Canada?
2. What are some of the epidemics that have plagued Canadians throughout the centuries, and what community health measures have been used to combat these epidemics?
3. How has federal government policy with respect to funding of research affected community health nursing in Canada?

REFERENCES

Allemang, M.M. (1974). Nursing education in the United States and Canada, 1873–1950: Leading figures, forces, views on education (Doctoral dissertation, University of Washington, Seattle, 1974). *Dissertation Abstracts International, 75,* 28308.

Bajnok, I. (1992). Entry-level educational preparation for nursing. In A.J. Baumgart & J. Larsen (Eds.), *Canadian nursing faces the future* (2nd ed.) (pp. 401–420). St. Louis: Mosby Year Book.

Batten, J. (1977). *Canada moves westward.* Toronto: McClelland & Stewart.

Bliss, M. (1991). *Plague: A story of smallpox in Montreal.* Toronto: HarperCollins.

Brown, T.E. (1981). Dr. Ernest Jones: Psychoanalysis and the Canadian medical profession, 1908–1913. In S.E.D. Shortt (Ed.), *Medicine in Canadian society: Historical perspectives* (pp. 315–360). Montréal: McGill-Queen's University Press.

Bryce, P. (1910). History of public health in Canada. *Canadian Therapeutist and Sanitary Engineer, 1,* 287–291.

Bryce, P. (1911). Evolution of local public health: County officers. *Public Health Journal, 2,* 103–105.

Buckley, S. (1979). Ladies or midwives? Efforts to reduce infant and maternal mortality. In L. Kealey (Ed.), *A not unreasonable claim: Women and reform in Canada 1880s–1920s* (pp. 131–149). Toronto: Women's Educational Press.

Burton, L.E., & Smith, H.H. (1970). *Public health and community medicine.* Baltimore: Williams & Wilkins.

Careless, J.M.S. (1970). *Canada: A story of challenge.* Toronto: Macmillan of Canada.

Carpenter, H.M. (1982). *A divine discontent: Edith Kathleen Russell—reforming educator.* Toronto: University of Toronto Faculty of Nursing.

Carroll, J. (1979). *Pioneer days 1840–1860.* Toronto: McClelland & Stewart.

Cashman, T. (1966). *Heritage of service: The history of nursing in Alberta.* Edmonton: Alberta Association of Registered Nurses.

Collingwood, R.G. (1956). *The idea of history.* Oxford: Oxford University Press.

Cosbie, W.G. (1975). *The Toronto General Hospital 1819–1965: A chronicle.* Toronto: Macmillan of Canada.

Craig, J. (1977). *The years of agony 1910–1920.* Toronto: McClelland & Stewart.

Dock, L.L. (1901, November). History of the reform in nursing in Bellevue Hospital. *American Journal of Nursing, 2,* 89–95.

Emory, F.H. (1945). *Public health nursing in Canada.* Toronto: Macmillan of Canada.

Francis, D. (1981). The development of the lunatic asylum in the Maritime provinces. In S.E.D. Shortt (Ed.), *Medicine in Canadian society: Historical perspectives* (pp. 93–114). Montréal: McGill-Queen's University Press.

Gibbon, J.M. (1947). *The Victorian Order of Nurses: 50th anniversary, 1897–1947.* Montréal: Southam Press.

Gibbon, J.M., & Mathewson, M.S. (1947). *Three centuries of Canadian nursing.* Toronto: Macmillan of Canada.

Gunn, J.I. (1926). To consider the possible modification of the curriculum and hospital service to meet the needs of public health nursing. *Canadian Nurse, 22,* 575–576.

Heagerty, J.J. (1928). *Four centuries of medical history in Canada* (Vols. i–ii). Toronto: Macmillan of Canada.

Lalonde, M. (1974). *A new perspective on the health of Canadians: A working paper.* Ottawa: Government of Canada.

Leacock, S. (1941). *Canada: The foundations of its future.* Montréal: Author.

McGinnis, J.D. (1981). The impact of epidemic influenza: Canada 1918–1919. In S.E.D. Shortt (Ed.), *Medicine in Canadian society: Historical perspectives* (pp. 447–477). Montréal: McGill-Queen's University Press.

McInnes, E. (1969). *Canada: A political and social history.* Toronto: Holt, Rinehart & Winston of Canada.

McLaren, A. (1981). Birth control and abortion in Canada, 1870–1920. In S.E.D. Shortt (Ed.), *Medicine in Canadian society: Historical perspectives* (pp. 285–313). Montréal: McGill-Queen's University Press.

Moag, M. (1924). Every nurse a public health nurse. *Canadian Nurse, 20,* 749–751.

National League of Nursing Education, Committee on Education. (1927). *Curriculum for schools of nursing.* New York: Author.

Neatby, H. (1981). The medical profession in the North-West Territories. In S.E.D. Shortt (Ed.), *Medicine in Canadian society: Historical perspectives* (pp. 165–168). Montréal: McGill-Queen's University Press.

Nevitt, J. (1978). *White caps and black bands: Nursing in Newfoundland to 1934.* St. John's: Jeperson Printing.

Nicholson, G.W.L. (1975). *Canada's nursing sisters.* Toronto: A.M. Hakkart.

Nightingale, F. (1859/1946). *Notes on nursing.* London: Harrison & Sons/Philadelphia: Lippincott.

Phillips, A. (1977). *Into the 20th century 1900–1910.* Toronto: McClelland & Stewart.

Pringle, D.M., & Roe, D.I. (1992). Voluntary community agencies: VON Canada as example. In A.J. Baumgart & J. Larsen (Eds.), *Canadian nursing faces the future* (2nd ed.) (pp. 611–626). St. Louis: Mosby Year Book.

Ray, A. (1981). Diffusion of diseases in the western interior of Canada, 1830–1850. In S.E.D. Shortt (Ed.), *Medicine in Canadian society: Historical perspectives* (pp. 45–73). Montréal: McGill-Queen's University Press.

Reid, H.R.G. (1913). Social service and hospital efficiency. *Canadian Nurse, 9*, 542–547.

Remarks on the antiquity of hygiene and its scope. (1875, July). *Public Health Magazine and Literary Review, 1*, 21–27.

Riegler, N.N. (1992). *The work and networks of Jean I. Gunn, superintendent of nurses, Toronto General Hospital 1913–1941: A presentation of some issues in nursing during her lifetime 1882–1941*. Unpublished doctoral thesis, University of Toronto.

Risk, M.M. (1973). *Origins and development of public health nursing in Toronto from 1890 to 1920*. Unpublished master's thesis, University of Toronto.

Russell, E.K. (1920). Public health field work for the undergraduate nurse. *Canadian Nurse, 16*, 462–464.

Russell, E.K. (1926). Public health nursing and the undergraduate nurse. *Canadian Nurse, 22*, 563–568.

Russell, E.K. (1929). The training of a public health nurse. *Canadian Nurse, 25*, 78–82.

Russell, E.K. (1932). The approved school for nurses. *Canadian Nurse, 28*, 528–532.

Russell, E.K. (1933). A new school of nursing. *Canadian Nurse, 29*, 285–290.

Russell, E.K. (1936). The new school carries on. *Canadian Nurse, 32*, 107–109.

Russell, E.K. (1938). The proposed curriculum in action: The story of a very young school. *Canadian Nurse, 34*, 498–505.

Saywell, J.T. (1967). The 1890s. In J.M.S. Careless & R.C. Brown (Eds.), *The Canadians 1867–1967* (pp. 108–136). Toronto: Macmillan of Canada.

Sillars, D.J. (1983). *The development of community mental health nursing in Toronto from 1917 to 1947*. Unpublished master's thesis, University of Toronto.

Storch, J.L., & Meilicke, C.A. (1994). Political, social, and economic forces shaping the health care system. In J.M. Hibberd & M.E. Kyle, *Nursing management in Canada*. Toronto: W.B. Saunders Canada.

Sutherland, N. (1981). To create a strong and healthy race: School children in the public health movement, 1880–1914. In S.E.D. Shortt (Ed.), *Medicine in Canadian society: Historical perspectives* (pp. 361–393). Montréal: McGill-Queen's University Press.

Tholfsen, T. (1967). *Historical thinking*. New York: Harper & Row.

Weir, G.M. (1932). *Survey of nursing education in Canada*. Toronto: University of Toronto Press.

Zilm, G., & Warbinek, E. (1994). *Legacy: History of nursing education at the University of British Columbia 1919–1994*. Vancouver: University of British Columbia School of Nursing.

The move toward Primary Health Care in Canada: Community health nursing from 1985 to 2000

Ginette Lemire Rodger and Sheila M. Gallagher

Despite the historical contributions of community health nurses to the development of the health system, in recent years the new demands to implement Primary Health Care (PHC) worldwide have been particularly challenging. This chapter examines the move toward Primary Health Care in Canadian nursing, and in particular in Canadian community health nursing, since the mid-1980s. This review allows reflection on the activities of this decade-and-a-half of movement toward a new paradigm in Canadian nursing and health services.

In this chapter, the sociopolitical context has been presented, and the movement toward a PHC paradigm from 1985 to 1998 is reviewed. As well, the authors present an overview of the international, national, and provincial evidence of political will and self-reported activities from the national, provincial, and territorial nursing associations, community health nursing associations, and university nursing programs. PHC projects planned for the period of 1998 to 2000 are identified. The final section analyzes the findings and offers an agenda for the future.

LEARNING OBJECTIVES

In this chapter, you will learn:

- the concept of Primary Health Care, and major international and national events that fostered its development
- five principles of Primary Health Care and the contribution made by nursing professional organizations, educators, and researchers toward the implementation of these principles in the Canadian health care system
- the contribution of community health nurses to the development and integration of Primary Health Care principles in their local communities
- strategies used by nursing groups to plan, implement, and forecast the route ahead for further implementation of Primary Health Care principles

Introduction

In 1985, the Director General of the World Health Organization (WHO) issued a challenge to nurses around the world:

If the millions of nurses in a thousand different places articulate the same ideas and convictions about primary health care, and come together as one force, then they could act as a powerhouse for change. I believe that such a change is coming, and that nurses around the globe, whose work touches each of us intimately, will greatly help to bring it about. (Mahler, 1985)

Canadian nurses took up this challenge. The profession as a whole took definite strides toward implementation of Primary Health Care (PHC) in the period from 1985 to 2000. During this period, which followed the passing of the *Canada Health Act* in 1984, the nursing profession turned its focus to the community and to community health nursing as the major player in the implementation of PHC.

This move to community nursing occurred without a corresponding shift of human resources. Between 1985 and 1996 there was an approximate two-percent increase in community health nurses (Statistics Canada, 1985, 1996). In 1992, Statistics Canada coding was revised to reflect the diversity of nursing roles in community health (CNA, 1994). The only area demonstrating an increase in human resources is home care, which expanded from 6901 nurses in 1992 to 9064 nurses in 1996 (Statistics Canada, 1992, 1996).

Definitions

The move toward PHC in Canada, particularly the move in community health nursing, is examined in this chapter using Lewin's (1951) Change Theory. Lewin suggests that change goes through three stages: the "unfreezing" stage, during which the individual or community is exposed to the idea of the need for change; the "moving" stage, which is a cognitive redefinition in which the change is planned and initiated; and the "refreezing" stage, in which change is integrated and stabilized. The years 1985 to 2000 qualify as Lewin's moving stage; Canadian nursing underwent a major shift from a medical model to a Primary Health Care model.

In this chapter, the definition of PHC is the one approved at the 1978 WHO Conference. Primary Health Care is:

essential health care based on practical, scientifically sound and socially acceptable methods and technology made universally accessible to individuals and families in the community through their full participation and at a cost that the community and country can afford to maintain at every stage of their development in the spirit of self-reliance and self-determination. It forms an integral part both of the country's health system, of which it is the central function and main focus, and of the overall social and economic development of the community. It is the first level of contact of individuals, the family and community with the national health system bringing health care as close as possible to where the people live and work, and constitutes the first element of a continuing health care process. (WHO, 1978, p. 21)

Based on this definition of PHC, the five principles that are discussed in this chapter are: health promotion; public participation; intersectoral and interdisciplinary collaboration; accessibility; and appropriate technology.

The term "community health nursing" in this chapter is defined broadly to mean nurses practising in a setting outside an illness care institution.

Search strategies

In the preparation of this chapter, several resources were used, including results of two surveys of all national, provincial, and territorial nursing associations and community health nursing associations identified through their respective professional nursing associations. In the first survey, in 1993, all 11 national/provincial nursing associations and one of the two territorial nursing associations responded. Of the 16 community health nursing groups contacted, nine replied. For the 1998 update, 10 of 11 national/provincial nursing associations, both territorial nursing associations, and six of the 13 community health nursing groups contacted replied. The first survey provided a review of self-reported PHC activities carried out between 1985 and 1995, and the second covered the years 1996 to 2000. An open-ended questionnaire was used for both surveys. The thematic content analysis of the responses is reported in this chapter.

Canadian university nursing programs were also surveyed. In the first survey, 30 university nursing programs were contacted and 25 replied. In the second survey, 23 of 34 universities responded. A computer online review of the literature from 1983 to 1998 was carried out using CINHAL, Star Health, Sociofile, and Medline. The following topics were reviewed: PHC and community health nursing (CHN); CHN and health promotion and illness prevention; CHN and public participation; CHN and intersectoral and interdisciplinary collaboration; CHN and accessibility; and CHN, appropriate technology, and determinants of health. Additionally, other published and non-published documents from universities were reviewed.

The division of this chapter is inspired by this book's framework as presented in Chapter 3. The first section presents a review of national and international events that occurred prior to 1985 and sets the stage for the decade to follow. These events positioned Canadian nurses for action in the movement toward PHC. The second section reviews events occurring between 1985 and 1998. An account of the activities of the associations of professional and community health nurses and university nursing programs is presented under the heading of the five principles of PHC. The next section highlights the projected plans of the nursing organizations surveyed for the years 1998 to 2000. The chapter concludes with an analysis of the movement toward PHC in Canadian nursing.

Positioned for action (pre-1985)

Many significant international and national events related to PHC occurred prior to 1985. The most important initiative was the 1978 WHO conference at Alma Ata, in the USSR, which identified PHC as the favoured strategy to achieve Health for All by the Year 2000 (WHO, 1978). Canada and all other member states of WHO agreed to work toward the principles of Health for All.

A Canadian precursor to Alma Ata was the 1974 report from the federal Ministry of Health (Lalonde, 1974), which emphasized health promotion and called for a redirection of health care. These two key events, along with the federal government's review of the national–provincial health program (Hall, 1980), provided the impetus for the Canadian nursing profession to articulate and begin to disseminate its vision of a future health care system. *Putting Health into Health Care*, the Canadian Nurses Association's submission to the federal government's commission (CNA, 1980), served as the basis for major lobbying efforts by nurses.

These efforts certainly affected the amendments made to the *Canada Health Act* in 1984. This new enabling legislation allowed nurses and health professionals other than physicians to be fully used in a reformed health care system inspired by PHC. A year later, in 1985, the World Health Organization recognized officially the importance of the leadership role that nurses could play in the implementation of PHC in the statement "Nurses Lead the Way" (Mahler, 1985). By 1985, the nursing profession in Canada was well positioned for action to follow.

Moving toward a paradigm shift (1985–1998)

Many of the international, national, and provincial events that occurred between 1985 and 1998 created a favourable sociopolitical context for nurses to assume a leadership position. A major WHO conference in Tokyo on "Leadership in Nursing for Health for All" marked the beginning of international recognition of the leadership role nurses could play and set the stage for more prominent support for the nursing agenda (WHO, 1986).

Political will

Internationally, WHO's activities helped shape the political will to implement Primary Health Care. The 1988 WHO assembly reviewed "progress and problems experienced in pursuing the goal of health for all and consider[ed] the reassessments that might be necessary in order to proceed more effectively toward the goal of health for all by the year 2000, and beyond" (WHO, 1988, p. 3). In 1989, a WHO progress report on the role of nursing and midwifery personnel in the strategy for Health for All (WHO, 1989) was tabled at the 42nd WHO Assembly. This report "reaffirmed that nursing and midwifery personnel were essential to the planning, implementation and evaluation of primary health care" (p. 3). WHO's member states were urged to work closely with the nursing profession toward achievement of the Health for All goal. Since 1990, eight United Nations world conferences focussed on problems related to health (WHO, n.d.), and three international conferences on health promotion (WHO, 1997a) were held to develop strategies for Health for All in the 21st century. These strategies are evident in the recent activities of Canadian nurses.

In 1986, two events in Canada manifested the political will for health care reform. These were the release of the federal health agenda in Health Minister Jake Epp's *Achieving Health for All* and the release of the WHO *Ottawa Charter for Health Promotion*. Canadian provinces responded by making preparations for major health care reform. All provinces struck advisory committees, task forces, and/or commissions to determine appropriate models of health care for their respective constituencies. All these committees and commissions produced recommendations that promoted the principles of PHC (even if the term was rarely used) and reflected the message of the nursing profession's submissions to these committees and commissions.

Mhatre and Deber (1992) reviewed and critically analyzed the policy options included in several of these provincial reports. Some recurring themes were: broadening the definition of health and intersectoral planning; emphasizing health promotion and disease prevention with a partial rejection of the medical model; shifting from institutional to community-based care; increasing public participation, particularly in planning; and developing regional authorities.

In 1997, the National Forum on Health released its report and made recommendations that clearly support four of the five PHC principles (to the exclusion of appropriate technology). The nursing profession contributed to this forum through the participation of Madeleine Doyon Stout, Margaret Rose McDonald, and Dr. Judith Ritchie.

Despite the evident political will, the barriers created by the dominant paradigm of the hospital/medical model in most Western industrialized countries, which is antithetical to the principles of a PHC model, remain a significant challenge for the Canadian nursing profession.

The nursing profession on the move

The leadership role of the Canadian Nurses Association (CNA) in the move toward PHC from 1985 to 1998 is impressive. CNA clarified its position on PHC in Canada and recommended strategies to attain this goal in *Health for All Canadians: A Call for Health Care Reform* (CNA, 1988). As a follow-up, CNA also produced documents including a five-year plan to guide the implementation of Canadian nursing PHC strategies. Implementation is also evident in adoption of PHC strategies for specific target populations, such as the elderly (CNA, 1989a) and urban Aboriginal people (CNA, 1995a), and issues such as mental health (CNA, 1991, 1992) and comprehensive school health (CNA, 1994). CNA's commitment to PHC was reaffirmed by the 1992 resolution of the CNA Board of Directors to coordinate and support provincial nursing PHC activities (CNA, 1992). In 1995, two policy statements, *A Framework for Health Care Delivery* (CNA, 1995b) and *The Role of the Nurse in PHC* (CNA, 1995c), incorporated the principles of PHC and the CNA vision for health care systems.

The implementation of these strategies is evident in the publications mentioned above, in regular reports of the CNA Board, and in briefs such as the submissions to the Standing Committee of the House of Commons on Health and Welfare, Social Affairs, Seniors, and the Status of Women (CNA, 1989b); to the Royal Commission on New Reproductive Technologies (CNA, 1990); and *Back to Basics* (CNA, 1997a), a CNA document on child health. It is also evident in the development of different instruments to facilitate political action for change, such as the compilation of research results on cost effectiveness (CNA, 1993a) and a political action handbook (CNA, 1993b, 1997b).

In addition, all provincial/territorial nursing associations have been involved in PHC-supporting activities, such as the development of public policies on health, political action for health system reform, and PHC projects. By 1993, every nursing association had representation on the provincial/territorial governments' task forces related to health system reform (see Table 2.1).

Although survey data compiled for this chapter revealed that few professional nursing activities were organized in the post–*Canada Health Act* period from 1984 to 1987, there are notable exceptions. For example, in the Northwest Territories and the Yukon, a PHC approach was used for several years in the delivery of nursing and health services, and nurses were recognized as leaders in the implementation of PHC in Canada. Another notable exception was the inception of the Newfoundland–Denmark Primary Health Care Nursing Model Project (1985). This project was the first PHC project in Canada during the 1985 to 1995 period. Since its inception it has served as an inspiration for other PHC projects. Documentation developed for the Newfoundland–Denmark project has been shared with more than 50 agencies and groups nationally and internationally. Other exceptions for this period were the Alberta Wellness Proposal (1984), the revision of the PHC

Table 2.1
Summary of information from provincial/territorial nursing associations related to Primary Health Care

Nursing Association	Year of Position Statement on PHC[1]	Has Position Statement on Role of Nurses in PHC[1] Document	Mentions PHC[1] in Scope of Nursing Practice	Has Nursing Representation on Gov't Task Force Related to HCR[2]
British Columbia	1994	x	x	x
Alberta	1991			x
Saskatchewan	1997	x	x	x
Manitoba	1993	x[3]	x	x
Ontario	1995		x[4]	x
Québec	1983	x		x
New Brunswick	1996	x	x	x
Nova Scotia	1990	x		x
Prince Edward Island	1993			x
Newfoundland	1994	x		x
Northwest Territories	developing			
Yukon				x

[1] PHC: Primary Health Care

[2] HCR: Health Care Reform

[3] For nurses employed by Aboriginal Health Authorities in Manitoba

[4] Primary Health Care Nurse Practitioner

Adapted from Canadian Nurses Association (1993), *Member Association Activities in Primary Health Care*. Ottawa: Author and Canadian Nurses Association (1993), *The Scope of Nursing Practice: A Review of Issues and Trends* (Appendix B). Ottawa: Author.

statement in Saskatchewan, and workshops on the development of competencies (including PHC) for nurses in Québec.

Between 1987 and 1993, a major professional mobilization occurred. Strategic activities during this mobilization ranged from multiple information sessions and workshops involving nurses, the public, government, other health professionals, and the media to the implementation of several PHC projects. Provincial nursing associations submitted briefs that promoted PHC to their respective governments. The Registered Nurses Association of Ontario (RNAO) and the Association of Registered Nurses of Newfoundland (ARNN) were exceptions. For the Northwest Territories Registered Nurses Association (NWTRNA), the submission to the NWT government took the form of written documents on how the principles of PHC may be used to enhance the well-being of people in the territory. ARNN already had the approval of its government for a PHC project, as the submission predated 1987.

Between 1993 and 1998, mobilization continued with a particular emphasis on collaboration, partnership, and proliferation of projects in the form of community health centres, outreach programs, nurse-managed clinics, and joint practice projects. The relationship with governments during this period moved from representation on health care committees to working with governments on a multitude of issues related to PHC including nurse practitioner legislation (RNAO, ARNN); nurse clinicians in PHC (RNANS, YRNA); extended health services (AARN); interdisciplinary delivery models (NANB, NWTRNA, RNAO); multi-organization promotion of Community Health Centres (RNABC); rural health, health reform, and health services (SRNA, RNABC); midwifery and occupational health (OIIQ); transfer of health services to First Nations and child health (YRNA); and devolution of health and social services to communities (NWTRNA). Regular meetings, representation on committees, and lobbying efforts with government continue to be reported, once again, as an ongoing part of PHC strategies.

Most provincial nursing associations developed, reviewed, revised, or updated their position statements on PHC, and seven associations developed or revised their documents on the nurse's roles in light of PHC (see Table 2.1). Newfoundland also developed a position statement on the *Advanced Practice Nurse Practitioner—Primary Health Care* (ARNN, 1997). It is interesting to note that the influence of PHC is also visible in the provincial revisions of statements on the scope of nursing practice. The scope of nursing practice refers to "the activities its practitioners are educated and authorized to perform" (CNA, 1993d, p. 3).

Primary Health Care principles: Canadian nursing contributions

When the multitude of provincial nursing activities is examined from the perspective of the five principles of PHC (CNA, 1988), the key contributions and gaps in the nursing profession's efforts are revealed.

Health promotion
By far, health promotion and disease/injury prevention have been the major thrust of nursing's PHC activities. This theme is evident in all PHC publications

and briefs to governments and highlighted in PHC projects, lobbying efforts, public information sessions, and public service announcements. For example, in the first survey, six provincial/territorial nursing associations had reported projects exemplifying the health promotion principle. Since 1993, a proliferation of these projects is evident. Eight professional organizations reported projects such as Brigus South to Cappahadden Community Health Centre Pilot Project (ARNN); Cheticamp Primary Health Care Project (RNANS); Community Health Centre Pilot Project and the Family Practice Collaboration Project (ANPEI); McAdam Community Health Centre Pilot Project and a project comprising three ambulatory care service delivery models (NANB); Beechy Collaborative Practice Pilot Project (SRNA); Bassano Community Health Centre (AARN); Comox Valley Nursing Centre (RNABC); and a network of 14 community health nursing centres, including services of the Outreach Community Health Nursing Program for at-risk populations in Whitehorse, which range from providing warm shelter and wool socks to lifestyles and addiction counselling (YRNA).

Public forums sponsored by nurses in Saskatchewan (11 communities) and British Columbia (15 communities), public displays and advertisements (YRNA), a position paper on health promotion in British Columbia, and lobbying efforts to increase public health services in New Brunswick and Manitoba are other initiatives in support of the principle of health promotion. The Nurses Association of New Brunswick (NANB) lobbied to increase the number of public health nurses, and the Manitoba Association of Registered Nurses (MARN) lobbied for immunizations to be considered part of wellness care. In 1993, the Registered Nurses Association of British Columbia (RNABC) studied the role of hospital nursing and health professionals in health promotion to demonstrate nursing's special contribution to promotion of the health. Between 1993 and 1998 there was a significant increase in nursing participation in projects addressing specific health promotion issues, such as bicycle helmet use and asthma (OIIQ); tobacco and bovine growth hormone (RNAO); tobacco, breast cancer, and AIDS (OIIQ, NWTRNA, CNA); school health (OIIQ, YRNA, NWTRNA, CNA); vulnerable populations (AARN, RNAO); children's and mental health (CNA); and community-based nutrition programs for healthy pregnancy (NWTRNA).

Public participation

The Canadian nursing profession supports the principle of public participation, both in words and in action. Nine provincial/territorial nursing associations carried out activities related to public participation. These diverse activities range in intensity from promotion of the concept of participation to actual partnership. These activities include communication of the concept of participation in a television series and videos (RNABC) and briefs (CNA, AARN, ANPEI, NWTRNA); public mobilization for quality health services

(RNAO); public consultation or membership on advisory boards for input in policies, strategies, and project development (AARN, NANB, ARNN, RNABC, OIIQ, NWTRNA); focus groups and discussions on community health needs (SRNA, NWTRNA); community needs assessment and community involvement processes culminating in public control of PHC demonstration projects (RNANS, ARNN); and direct public involvement in the provision of health promotion and prevention activities (OIIQ, ARNN). Yukon nurses are participating in the Health Partnership Development Committee, a community-driven forum for Yukon First Nations, government, and other parties to work together with respect to health and health care programs (YRNA).

Two examples highlight public involvement. The Registered Nurses Association of Nova Scotia (RNANS) describes the extent of public participation in the Cheticamp Primary Health Care Project as follows:

Data for the needs assessment were collected using multiple strategies to promote the maximum participation of the community. These methods included the use of [a] survey, focus groups, [a] community forum and kitchen table discussions. To date 23 per cent of the catchment area has participated in the needs assessment. Currently the findings of the needs assessment are being validated with members of the community through community forums. The community advisory board, which has played a major role in the needs assessment and oversees the development and implementation of strategies, is another forum for public participation. The advisory board is designed to reflect the profile of the community with emphasis on groups who are at risk of being underserved by the traditional system including the fishing industry, the elderly, the unemployed, single parents and adolescents etc. It is hoped that at the end of this three year project, the community will take ownership and sustain this initiative. (Personal communication, L.M. Lauzon, nursing practice consultant, RNANS, December 20, 1993)

In the project "Santé au coeur," members of a Québec community are directly involved in the delivery of preventive services. The key to this project, headed by a nurse from the local community health centre, Les Aboiteaux, is the training of community members to help fellow citizens gain increased control over their health. This project helps ordinary citizens to become more aware and responsible for their own health. The experience has been positive, and other communities want to join in the project. The project is described by the Ordre des infirmières et infirmiers du Québec (OIIQ) in the following way:

Ordinary people/citizens go from house to house to take blood pressure readings of their neighbours and also evaluate the level of cholesterol with the help of portable equipment. In other words, they help identify and prevent cardiovascular problems in their community. (Personal communication, P. Lange-Sondack, counsellor and associate secretary, OIIQ, March 16, 1994)

Intersectoral and interdisciplinary collaboration

CNA has underscored the importance of the principle of intersectoral and interdisciplinary collaboration and identified a series of strategies for implementation (CNA, 1988). Most of these strategies address interdisciplinary collaboration. The results of the initial survey done for this chapter indicated that nursing associations have been active in interdisciplinary initiatives over and above traditional collaboration with physicians and other health providers. Efforts to achieve broad interdisciplinary collaboration have extended from the provision of services and advice to lobbying efforts for health system reform, such as the Health Action Lobby (HEAL) ("HEAL on the move," 1991) and the National Forum on Health (1997). The results of the second survey (1993–1998) indicated that many nurse–physician collaborative practice projects have been initiated (RNANS, ANPEI, SRNA, NWTRNA, RNAO) as well as interdisciplinary teams/shared practice projects (NANB). Interdisciplinary collaboration was also evident through participation in working groups and committees with physicians, pharmacists, social workers, midwives, and others.

The nursing profession is more tentative in the area of intersectoral collaboration. Only four professional associations reported activities that promote collaboration outside the traditional health professions and outside the health system. For example, RNABC has participated in bicycle helmet and safe drinking water projects. In Newfoundland, nurses are involved with several local groups, such as school personnel, the Royal Canadian Mounted Police, and a community substance abuse program. In Québec, nurses contribute to multiple-community projects that use intersectoral models (Guérin & Martin, 1990) and maintain an ongoing exchange with the Chamber of Commerce, seniors' associations, and the Commission on the Status of Women, among others. RNAO also reported their work with the Older Women's Network and the Senior Citizens Coalition.

Accessibility

The principle of accessibility was strongly supported by nurses during the *Canada Health Act* debate (CNA, 1984a, 1984b). Nurses confirmed their readiness to provide additional points of entry to the health care system and condemned any barriers that would reduce accessibility to the system, such as extra billing or user fees. Between 1985 and 1998, professional nursing associations lobbied against these barriers. The nursing profession used public statements and publications to advocate for increased accessibility and more efficient use of nurses as a point of entry.

All projects reported in the surveys conducted for this chapter promoted increased accessibility to health care services and reduced some geographic and financial barriers faced by at-risk populations. Two projects with particular emphasis on accessibility are the Northwest Territories' Ranklin Inlet

Birthing Project, which facilitated local birthing rather than transport to southern health care centres, and the AARN's 1991 Increased Direct Access to Nursing Services project, which promoted nurses as one of the points of entry to the health care system in all communities in the province. A recent project in Québec titled The Virtual Nurse is increasing accessibility to nursing services through the Internet (Salette, 1998).

Appropriate technology

Five nursing associations indicated that they were concerned with the PHC principle related to appropriate technology. RNABC and OIIQ have promoted this principle through their publications, identifying examples of appropriate technology and requesting evaluations of new technology. The Saskatchewan Registered Nurses Association (SRNA) has had a representative on the Saskatchewan Health Ministry's Technology Advisory Committee since 1990. This committee reviews a wide range of new technologies and advises the Minister of Health regarding dissemination of technology. RNAO also participated in discussions with the Ministry of Health on issues of appropriate technology for health care reform. The Alberta Association of Registered Nurses (AARN) developed an internal background paper on the issue and recommends strong links between technological assessment and health policy through the coordinated input of a broad range of professions and significant public representation. The Nurses Association of New Brunswick (NANB) also used examples of appropriate technology in its lobbying effort for health care reform in provincial and federal elections. In the second survey, CNA reported the development of a policy statement on the use of health care technology.

Movements of community
health nursing associations

Nurses who work in community health practice in Canada have formed varied associations, including the Community Health Nursing Association, Occupational Health Nursing Association, Home Care Nursing Association, Nurse Practitioner Association, Independent Practice Association, and other regroupments.

G. Cradduck, past president of the Community Health Nurses Association of Canada (CHNAC), believed that the members of these diverse CHN associations were actively involved in the movement toward PHC between 1985 and 1993, through numerous initiatives (personal communication, January 3, 1994). Most of the community health nursing associations lack the infrastructure (such as human, material, financial, and organizational resources) required to support intense activities focussed on PHC. This may explain, in part, their 45-percent response rate to both surveys and the limited nature of their organizational activities, with one exception. The Community Health Nursing Interest Group of Ontario (CHNIG) reported activities in relation to the five principles of PHC that parallel an active organized professional regroupment. Some of these CHNIG activities include direct lobbying to the Minister of Health for PHC initiatives; representation on an advisory committee to the Ministry of Health for the development of community health frameworks; input to Ministry of Health guidelines for healthy growth and development programs; active contribution to RNAO documents and policy statements (e.g., Healthy Babies, Healthy Children Program; Shortened Length of Obstetrical Stay); funding and representation to the Public Health Nurse Effectiveness research project at McMaster University; a public information campaign; and newsletters to members.

During the period studied, CHNAC was involved with the Canadian Public Health Association (CPHA) Task Force in developing a document, *Community Health Public Health Nursing in Canada: Preparation and Practice*, based on a PHC framework (CPHA, 1990). Provincially, the NWT chapter of CPHA, B.C. Community Health Nurses Group (BCCHNG), B.C. Home Care Nurses Professional Practice Group, Alberta Community Health Nurses Society (ACHNS), Alberta Occupational Nurses Health Association (AONHA), and Nurse Practitioner Association of Ontario were active in presenting briefs to their respective health care reform commissions or committees. CHNAC, BCCHNG, the New Brunswick Public Health Nurses Interest Group (NBPHNIG), and CHNIG supported the PHC position statement of their respective professional nursing associations (CNA, RNABC, NANB, RNAO).

The information received from most community health nursing associations focussed on the work of community health nurses instead of the activities of the association. When these data are examined from the perspective of the five PHC principles, it is difficult to identify discrete activities that relate to only one principle. CHNAC indicated that the five PHC principles are now incorporated in the practice and professional activities of most community health nurses. To illustrate, the Family Resource Centre in Dartmouth, Nova Scotia, focusses on health promotion, public participation, accessibility, and interdisciplinary collaboration. Public health nurses are actively involved in the program. Another example, the Early Childhood Initiative Program in New Brunswick, incorporates health promotion, intersectoral and interdisciplinary collaboration (e.g., nutritionists, public health nurses, home teachers, home economists, speech therapists), and accessibility for children aged 0–5 years, who are most at risk for physical and developmental problems.

There is no doubt that health promotion and disease/injury prevention have been the cornerstone for community health nursing to date, particularly in the area of public health. Immunizations, tobacco education, sexuality education, prenatal nutrition programs, wellness clinics, heart health, and disability management are just a few examples (ACHNS, AOHNA, NBPHNIG, CHNANS). "Nurses work with individuals, groups, communities, and to a lesser extent coalitions. They use a variety of approaches, such as education, community development, social marketing and advocacy to improve and maintain the health status of their clients. However, the shift to work beyond the level of individuals and incorporate approaches beyond more traditional ones such as education has been recent" (Personal communication, Denise Tardif, NBPHNIG, March 25, 1998). The initiative of a public health nurse going door-to-door in a rural community to offer parenting classes is one innovative example. This initiative resulted in a play group and periodic meetings with community leaders and health providers (NBPHNIG). Occupational health nurses in Alberta have noticed a reduction of health promotion efforts in favour of management of disabilities. This shift is driven by financial cutbacks to health care and pressures for early return to work (Personal communication, AONHA, March 10, 1998).

In 1994, G. Cradduck suggested that public participation may be the least utilized principle, owing to the difficulty experienced by nurses in moving away from their expert role. In the period from 1993 to 1998, many projects that include public participation in health services have been reported that are similar to the examples cited above. For some associations, the integration of public participation has been longstanding. The NWT chapter of the CPHA reported that each community has a local representative on the regional health board, which is responsible for planning, delivery, and management of health care services. Further, many communities have health committees that serve as a vehicle for local people to bring forward health concerns. Increased public participation and innovative modes of delivery of health services by community health nurses have contributed greatly to increase accessibility to new forms of health services.

As determinants of health become more widely accepted, the importance of interdisciplinary and intersectoral collaboration is increasingly visible. All projects included interdisciplinary and/or intersectoral activities. The only report received on the principle of appropriate technology related to better utilization of nursing personnel as human resources.

PHC in nursing education

Nursing academia also was active in promoting the principles of PHC during this "movement stage" between 1985 and 1998. Our survey of university nursing programs revealed that, of the 25 that responded to the first survey and of the 23 that responded to the second survey, half had integrated the concepts of PHC into several courses—in particular, in community health courses. The PHC principle mentioned most often was health promotion. This finding was echoed in Tenns's study (1995) of integration of PHC in the curricula of Canadian university schools of nursing. "The study reveals that schools are moving toward integrating PHC and that approximately 60% of them can be said to have a reasonable degree of integration" (p. 350).

During this period, all programs increased their PHC content. Some nursing programs added new courses (University [U.] of Calgary, Dalhousie U., Memorial U. of Newfoundland, St. Francis Xavier U., U. de Moncton, U. Laval, U. of Toronto, Ryerson Polytechnic U., McMaster U., Lakehead U., U. of Manitoba, U. de Montréal, U. of Ottawa), while others modified their clinical placements to be more congruent with PHC (McGill U., Memorial U. of Newfoundland, U. of Calgary, U. of New Brunswick, U. of Western Ontario, St. Francis Xavier U., Dalhousie U., Lakehead U., U. de Montréal). Some clinical placement included non-traditional and international experiences such as Interval House, James Bay, Moose Factory, and Barbados (Queens U.); a street youth storefront and a coffeehouse for the mentally ill (U. of Western Ontario); Primary Health Care centres in Finland (U. of Prince Edward Island); health promotion for children in India (U. de Moncton); Swift Street Clinic, William Head Jail, Intercultural Society, Homestead, and others (U. of Victoria and the 10 institutions that comprise the Collaborative Nursing Program); and internships in Haiti, Peru, and Cameroon (U. de Montréal).

Graduate programs where nurses major in PHC, or in CHN with a strong PHC content, were developed at Dalhousie U., U. of Calgary, U. of Manitoba, U. of Ottawa, and U. of Alberta. Several undergraduate programs and collaborative programs revised their curriculum to introduce a PHC component in their revised or new curriculum (McMaster U., U. of British Columbia, U. of Victoria and Collaborative Nursing Program, U. de Montréal, U. of New Brunswick, Dalhousie U., Queens U., McGill U., and U. de Sherbrooke). The University of PEI had a curriculum built around the principles of PHC. Recently, they developed a conceptual model for nursing based on the principles of PHC as the foundation of their baccalaureate program.

A number of universities indicated that they offered courses with majors or options in PHC or CHN with a strong PHC component. For example, U. de Montréal and U. Laval offer a certificate in CHN or community health (multidisciplinary). Graduate programs at the master's level with a major or advanced practicum in PHC, CHN, and public health nursing (PHN) are offered at Dalhousie U. (PHC), U. of Manitoba and Memorial U. of Newfoundland (CHN), U. of Ottawa (CHN—French and English), U. of Calgary (PHN), and U. of Alberta (CH–PHN). U. de Sherbrooke offers an advanced practicum in community health in its graduate diploma program.

Additional PHC activities were reported in the second survey. These activities included delivery of services by faculty and students in projects such as breast cancer screening (St. Francis Xavier U.); asthma clinic (McGill U.); asthma clinic and health fair (U. of PEI); student projects involving high-risk groups, ethnic minorities, and public health promotion campaigns (McGill U.); and development of such tools as a PHC clinical guide for preceptors (U. of New Brunswick) and a resource manual for mothers of children with disabilities (St. Francis Xavier U.). Finally, St. Francis Xavier U. and McGill U. reported increased faculty involvement in community-based organizations and boards.

PHC in unpublished research

In order to appreciate the current scholarly work by nurses in PHC in Canadian universities, the authors submitted a request to nursing education programs for information on unpublished research or studies conducted by either faculty members or graduate students. Nineteen of the 23 universities responding provided information. The number of citations per university varied from one to 201 items and covered work-in-progress by their faculty members or graduate students. Of the 410 research items submitted, 136 were considered (by both authors) relevant to one or more of the five PHC principles: health promotion (87); public participation (22); accessibility (20); interdisciplinary collaboration (8); intersectoral collaboration (4); and appropriate technology (2). Nine research items focussed on the development of tools to measure the elements of PHC. The most frequently reported topic areas were smoking (13); seniors (13); AIDS/HIV (10); communities (9); breast cancer (7); health professionals' roles, responsibilities, and education (5); and adolescents (5). Other topics reported less frequently included poverty, homelessness, family, empowerment, violence, heart health, drugs, sex, and asthma.

Nurses plan ahead (1998–2000)

In the first survey, all professional nursing associations and some of the CHN associations identified activities for implementation between 1993 and 1996. This was part of their continued pursuit to make PHC a reality in Canada. These plans included initiation of PHC projects; active participation in health care reform and in lobby and discussion groups to promote PHC; revision of position statements on PHC; continuing education; incorporation of PHC in standards, criteria, and scope-of-practice documents; support and assistance to members working in PHC and nursing clinics in public places. In the second survey, nursing associations reported that all these forecasted activities have been accomplished.

The activities predicted between 1998 and 2000 are similar to the previous forecast, with greater emphasis on collaboration with other organizations. NBPHNIG expects that the same activities in each of their seven health regions will continue for the period 1998 to 2000. By far the most frequently cited activities still involve PHC projects. The provincial/territorial nursing associations in New Brunswick, Prince Edward Island, Ontario, Yukon, and Northwest Territories indicated plans to implement, evaluate, or contribute to PHC projects.

The second largest effort of the nurses' associations involves plans to lobby for PHC—either lobbying the government (CNA, RNAO, RNABC, CHNIG) or the universities for graduate studies (ARNN). Further, the lobby effort is identified as an interdisciplinary and intersectoral collaborative venture (CNA, RNABC, YRNA, NWTRNA).

The continued need for policy statements and educational activities represented the third largest area of projected activities by the nurses' associations. Examples include revision of the policy statement on PHC (CNA); development of a position statement on PHC for developed countries (CHNAC); development of guides for community health practice and for nurses practising in "Info-Santé" (OIIQ); and revision of a document on scope of practice for the expanded role of the nurse (YRNA). RNABC plans include educational workshops to promote community health centres and a national think tank about PHC for nurses. AARN plans an interdisciplinary workshop to discuss their systematic review of research on clinical topics. Both CNA and AARN have identified target populations as potential foci of future PHC initiatives, specifically, children and vulnerable populations.

Finally, two associations identified outcomes in their forecast: (a) by 2000, there will be more registered nurses in advanced practice in PHC settings (SRNA); and (b) disability management will be the priority in occupational health (AOHNA).

In the first survey, 18 university programs forecasted either development of new programs or integration of PHC into their programs through increased focus, courses, changes of curricula, framework, or clinical practice experience. All these forecasted activities have been accomplished, with the possible exception of U. of Manitoba, which developed three community health courses at the graduate level instead of a full program.

In the second survey, 14 university programs foresee further integration of PHC. Additionally, three universities plan to develop relevant graduate programs: a master's degree in community and PHC as advanced practice (Memorial U.); an advanced practice stream (U. of Manitoba); and a proposed interdisciplinary PhD program (U. of Ottawa). Further, some projects and tools have been projected: U. of Western Ontario plans a nurse-managed family health centre and a medicine–nursing collaboration project on the care of young families; and U. of PEI will be testing a PHC model in a demonstration practice setting. Researchers at U. of Manitoba will use their newly developed PHC questionnaire to implement a comparative evaluation with similar programs in the United Kingdom. St. Francis Xavier U. will integrate a new theoretical framework that includes self-care, empowerment, and social action into all scholarly work.

Critical analysis of the movement toward PHC

Although the information presented previously represents only a glimpse of the increased activities by community health nurses to promote and implement Primary Health Care in Canada, it is evident that Canadian nurses are on the move. In the second survey, the concept of primary care, meaning the first contact with a health professional, was mentioned several times. Federal and provincial governments have been promoting the concept of primary care, which creates confusion with the global concept of Primary Health Care. Our surveys' data also indicated a significant increase in the implementation of the PHC principles of health promotion and illness/injury prevention, accessibility, and interdisciplinary collaboration. Public participation also is more visible than ever in the planning of health care and direct involvement in specific projects and programs. However, the principles related to appropriate technology and intersectoral collaboration have received the least attention to date.

MacIntosh and McCormack (1994) recommended that "primary health care requires that all five principles be implemented simultaneously. The absence of any one of these principles will change the intended shape of the health care delivery system" (p. 10). Based on this premise, the review of progress to date, and an analysis of recent literature, an agenda for the future can be created.

The increased focus on health promotion and illness/injury prevention has been integrated throughout all the reported nursing activities. Nevertheless, many of these projects are time limited; the next step for the nursing profession is to ensure integration of these activities into the health system. To facilitate integration, the Alberta Nurses' Association has developed *Guidelines to Anchor a Nursing Clinic Project* (AARN, 1994). Chambers (1989) reiterates the need for more integration when he cautions about intraorganizational barriers to health promotion and calls for changes conducive to population-based health promotion.

Public participation in planning of health or nursing services, particularly in the needs-assessment phase, has been reported by seven provinces— ANPEI, RNANS, NANB, OIIQ, SRNA, AARN, and RNABC. This is congruent with the WHO report on Primary Health Care in industrialized countries

(WHO Regional Office for Europe, 1985). However, some authors believe that simple consultation is not sufficient for the goal of full public participation. Charles and DeMaio's (1992) model of citizen participation incorporates three levels: consultation, partnership, and dominant decision making. Respondents have confirmed that consultation and, more recently (since 1993), partnership are prevalent. The integration of this principle into community health nursing can only be underscored as one of the next areas for emphasis.

There is no doubt that the activities since 1985 increased accessibility by making nurses available as a point of entry into the health care system. The principle of accessibility challenges the profession to take a hard look at the remaining barriers to accessibility to the health system. There is a need to intensify consideration of all barriers to accessibility, including geographic, financial, cultural, functional (WHO, 1978), and policy and legislative barriers. In Canada, even though the principle of accessibility is recognized in the publicly funded health care system, the principle does not apply to community-based services. As the gap between the haves and the have-nots increases, the nursing profession must pay more attention to vulnerable populations in the community (Sebastian, 1992) and should work diligently with other partners to ensure that the five principles of the *Canada Health Act* apply equally to community-based services as they do to hospital-based services.

Technology can be broadly defined as the people, tools, and techniques used during interactions to achieve human goals (Bush, 1983). In our view, although people cannot be considered technology, the application of their arts and skills can. The implementation of the principle of appropriate technology does not apply only to high technology. This broad interpretation is more congruent with the use of technology by the nursing profession, ranging from low-technology applications (in which interpersonal skills are the primary tools) to high-technology use (in which machines are the main tools). The profession must participate in discussions of the nature and appropriateness of technology (Sandelowski, 1993).

Clearly, interdisciplinary collaboration has increased over the decade and a half from 1985 to 1998. The reform of the health care system, driven by major funding reductions, has created hardships for many professionals. At the same time, reform has created opportunities for community health nurses to become more skilful in building effective partnerships. These skills must continue to be refined. Intersectoral collaboration requires the greatest effort by CHN and nursing at large. Despite nursing's belief that the determinants of health are broader than health care, the present focus on an illness care industry and on bureaucratic compartmentalization of society has mitigated against significant movement in intersectoral initiatives. WHO (1997b) confirmed that intersectoral action for health was the least successful principle of PHC. This must be the focus of the next concerted effort.

Conclusion

There is no doubt that Canadian nurses, and community health nurses in particular, have accepted Mahler's challenge to assume a leadership role and have made definite strides toward implementation of PHC in Canada. There is a fit between CHN and PHC (Goeppinger, 1984). If the nursing profession continues to devote as much attention to PHC in the next 10 years as has been demonstrated in the past decade, there is no doubt that the goal of PHC will be realized.

Endnote

The information in this chapter is not exhaustive. The limitations include the low response rate by the CHN groups to the questionnaire, the uneven representation of provincial community health nursing groups, and the difficulty in accessing data on a rapidly evolving subject. The review of unpublished research was limited by an incomplete listing of studies. Some faculties refused to share the information and some respondents provided partial lists. Further limitation includes inconsistency in the information shared (e.g., titles, topics, brief descriptions). Even with these limitations, however, the information must be considered abundant.

QUESTIONS

1. Obtain a copy of the nursing association's position statement on Primary Health Care (PHC) developed for your province/territory (or, if your province does not have one, from another province). How are the five principles of PHC defined, and how are they currently being applied locally?
2. Identify all community health nursing associations active in your province. What are their views on the five PHC principles?
3. What are the barriers to accessibility to health care in your local community? How could local community health nurses form partnerships to overcome these barriers?

REFERENCES

Alberta Association of Registered Nurses. (1994). *Guidelines to anchor a nursing clinic project*. Edmonton: Author.

Association of Registered Nurses of Newfoundland. (1997). *Advanced practice nurse practitioner—Primary Health Care*. St. John's: Author.

Bush, C.G. (1983). Women and assessment of technology: To think, to be, to unthink, to free. In J. Rothschild (Ed.), *Machina ex dea: Feminist perspectives on technology* (pp. 151–170). New York: Pergamon Press.

Canada Health Act, 1984—Bill C-3. (1984). Ottawa: Government of Canada.

Canadian Nurses Association. (1980). *Putting health into health care: Submission to the Health Services Review.* Ottawa: Author.

Canadian Nurses Association. (1984a). *Brief to the House of Commons Standing Committee on Health, Welfare and Social Affairs in response to the proposed* Canada Health Act. Ottawa: Author.

Canadian Nurses Association. (1984b). *Brief to the Senate Committee on Social Affairs, Science and Technology in response to the amended Bill C-3.* Ottawa: Author.

Canadian Nurses Association. (1988). *Health for all Canadians: A call for health care reform.* Ottawa: Author.

Canadian Nurses Association. (1989a). *Health care reform for seniors.* Ottawa: Author.

Canadian Nurses Association. (1989b). *Submission to the Standing Committee of the House of Commons on Health and Welfare, Social Affairs, Seniors and the Status of Women: Select issues in health care delivery.* Ottawa: Author.

Canadian Nurses Association. (1990). *New reproductive technologies: Accessible, appropriate, participative.* Brief to the Royal Commission on New Reproductive Technologies. Ottawa: Author.

Canadian Nurses Association. (1991). *Mental health care reform.* Ottawa: Author.

Canadian Nurses Association. (1992). Annual meeting minutes. Ottawa: Author.

Canadian Nurses Association. (1993a). *Nurses make the difference: A brief on cost-effective nursing alternatives.* Ottawa: Author.

Canadian Nurses Association. (1993b). *Nurses know nurses can—An election handbook.* Ottawa: Author.

Canadian Nurses Association. (1993c). *Member association activities in Primary Health Care.* Ottawa: Author.

Canadian Nurses Association. (1993d). *The scope of nursing practice: A review of issues and trends.* Ottawa: Author.

Canadian Nurses Association. (1994). *Comprehensive school health.* Ottawa: Author.

Canadian Nurses Association. (1995a). *Health in Canada: Perspectives of urban Aboriginal people.* Ottawa: Author.

Canadian Nurses Association. (1995b). *A framework for health care delivery.* Ottawa: Author.

Canadian Nurses Association. (1995c). *The role of the nurse in Primary Health Care.* Ottawa: Author.

Canadian Nurses Association. (1997a). *Back to basics.* Ottawa: Author.

Canadian Nurses Association. (1997b). *Getting started. A political action guide for registered nurses.* Ottawa: Author.

Canadian Nurses Association Research Department. (1994). *Guidelines to assist with the collapsing of the 1992 data in order to compare with previous years.* Ottawa: Author.

Canadian Public Health Association. (1990). *Community health—Public health nursing in Canada: Preparation and practice.* Ottawa: Author.

Chambers, L. (1989). Individual client care and public policy: The dual challenges for public health nurses. *Canadian Journal of Public Health, 80*(5), 315–316.

Charles, C., & DeMaio, S. (1992). Lay participation in health care decision making: A conceptual framework. *Journal of Health, Policy, Politics and Law, 18,* 881–904.

Epp, J. (1986). *Achieving health for all: A framework for health promotion.* Ottawa: Health & Welfare Canada.

Goeppinger, J. (1984). Primary Health Care: An answer to the dilemmas of community nursing? *Public Health Nursing, 1*(3), 129–140.

Guérin, D., & Martin, C. (1990). *La promotion de la santé: Les acteurs en promotion de la santé. Concertation et action inter-sectorielle.* Santé société (Cahier 3). Québec: Ministère de la santé et des services sociaux, Gouvernement du Québec.

Hall, E.M. (1980). *A commitment for renewal: Canada's national–provincial health program for the 1980's.* Ottawa: Health & Welfare Canada.

HEAL on the move. (1991). *CNA Today, 1*(3), 1–2.

Lalonde, M. (1974). *A new perspective on the health of Canadians: A working paper.* Ottawa: Government of Canada.

Lewin, K. (1951). *The nature of field theory.* New York: Macmillan.

MacIntosh, J., & McCormack, D. (1994). Primary Health Care: Interpreting the concepts. *Info Nursing, 25*(1), 10–11.

Mahler, H. (1985). Nurses lead the way. *WHO Features* (No. 97). Geneva: World Health Organization.

Mhatre, S.L., & Deber, R. (1992). From equal access to health care to equitable access to health: Review of Canadian provincial commissions and reports. *International Journal of Health Services, 22*(4), 645–668.

National Forum on Health. (1997). *Canada health action: Building on the legacy* (Vol. 1). Ottawa: Author.

Ordre des Infirmières et Infirmiers du Québec. (1988). *Professional inspection.* Montréal: Author.

Registered Nurses Association of British Columbia. (1993). *The role of the hospital nurse in health promotion.* Vancouver: Author.

Salette, H. (1998). L'infirmière virtuelle. *L'infirmière du Québec, 5*(3), 49.

Sandelowski, M. (1993). Toward a theory of technology dependency. *Nursing Outlook, 41*(1), 36–42.

Sebastian, J.G. (1992). Vulnerable populations in the community. In M. Stanhope & J. Lancaster (Eds.), *Community health nursing: Process and practice for promoting health* (pp. 374–379). St. Louis: Mosby Year Book.

Statistics Canada. (1985). *Revised registered nurses data series* (Table 5). Ottawa: Author.

Statistics Canada. (1992). *Registered nurses management data 1992* (Table 5). Ottawa: Author.

Statistics Canada. (1996). *Registered nurses management data 1996* (Table 5). Ottawa: Author.

Tenns, L. (1995). Primary health care nursing education in Canadian university schools of nursing. *Journal of Nursing Education, 34*(8), 350–357.

World Health Organization (WHO). (n.d.). *Health for All in the 21st century—Draft.* Geneva: Author.

World Health Organization (WHO). (1978). *Primary Health Care: Report on the International Conference on Primary Health Care, Alma Ata, USSR, 6–12 September 1978.* Geneva: Author.

World Health Organization (WHO). (1986). *Why leadership for Health for All? Leadership in nursing for Health for All conference, Tokyo, April 7.* Geneva: Author.

World Health Organization (WHO). (1988). *From Alma Ata to the year 2000: Reflections at the midpoint.* Geneva: Author.

World Health Organization (WHO). (1989). *The role of nursing and midwifery personnel in the strategy for Health for All*. Geneva: Author.

World Health Organization (WHO). (1997a). *Health promotion: Milestones on the road to a global alliance* [WHO Homepage: http://www.who.int/]. Geneva: Author.

World Health Organization (WHO). (1997b). *Intersectoral action for health: Addressing health and environment concerns in sustainable development*. Geneva: Author.

World Health Organization Regional Office for Europe. (1985). *Primary health care in industrialized countries*. Copenhagen: WHO Regional Office of Europe.

World Health Organization (WHO), Health and Welfare Canada (HWC), & Canadian Public Health Association (CPHA). (1986). *Ottawa charter for health promotion*. Ottawa: Canadian Public Health Association.

Part 2
Theoretical Premises and Core Principles

The theoretical foundations of community health nursing must be defined. The embryonic evolution of community health nursing theory could be guided by the principles of Primary Health Care. Therefore, the authors in this section examine these principles for their relevance to community health nursing and analyze concepts congruent with the principles of public participation and health promotion. Community health nurses will need to collaborate with consumers and focus on promotion of Canadians' health.

The five Primary Health Care principles—accessibility, public participation, intersectoral collaboration, appropriate technology, and health promotion and illness prevention—form the theoretical framework for this book (delineated in Chapter 3). Accessibility to health services and health determinants is problematic for poor, rural, and stigmatized persons. Self-care, lay support, mutual aid, and empowerment are public participation mechanisms. Intersectoral collaboration recognizes that health is influenced by diverse determinants and necessitates interdisciplinary and intersectoral teamwork. Appropriate technology is adaptable to local needs and resources and should be used for illness prevention and health promotion. Public participation and accessibility are key components of the Canadian health promotion framework. Indeed, the five Primary Health Care principles are interrelated and create foundations for community health nursing roles.

Chapter 4 elucidates concepts pertinent to the principles of public participation—social support, coping, and self-care. Social support is a significant concept because it influences health status, health behaviour, and health services use. Support can moderate the impact of stress on health, and integration in a social network can maintain health and facilitate physical recovery. Moreover, social network members may influence clients' health behaviour, use of health services, and coping strategies, while the ways in which clients cope affect the support they receive. Emotional, instrumental, informational, and/or affirmational support can be provided by lay and professional sources such as nurses. Community health nurses should assess types of support required for different stressors; sources of support; associated costs and benefits; underuse and overuse of resources; timing and duration of support; behaviours perceived as supportive or non-supportive; reciprocity within relationships and client satisfaction.

In Chapter 5, Laffrey and Craig illuminate the principle of health promotion and emphasize aggregates and communities as clients. To shift from the predominant individual-oriented care to aggregate- and community-oriented care, community health nurses require a broader framework that incorporates interdisciplinary theories. They could view the community as the setting, the unit, or the target of their practice; the community-as-target is particularly pertinent. The community includes individuals and families, and aggregates include individuals; aggregate care should be differentiated from individual care. Laffrey's health promotion model conceptualizes nursing care as illness care, prevention of illness or injury, and health promotion; health promotion is central.

Health promotion concepts and Primary Health Care principles could bridge gaps in community health nursing theory, as noted later in Chapter 31.

CHAPTER 3

Framework based on Primary Health Care principles

Miriam J. Stewart

Primary Health Care is the key to attaining health for all Canadians and the core of community health nursing in Canada. Primary Health Care is based on five principles—accessibility, public participation, intersectoral and interdisciplinary collaboration, appropriate technology, and increased health promotion and illness prevention. These interlocking principles form a framework for community health nursing and for this book.

LEARNING OBJECTIVES

In this chapter, you will learn:

* the relevance of Primary Health Care principles to community health nursing
* key barriers to accessibility to health and health care in Canada
* mechanisms for promoting public participation
* the value of collaboration with other disciplines and sectors outside the health system
* the role of community health nurses in health promotion and in illness and injury prevention.

Introduction

In Chapter 2, Rodger and Gallagher traced the evolution of Primary Health Care nationally and provincially. Nurses and nursing associations have played a key leadership role in the shift toward a system based on Primary Health Care principles. The International Conference on Primary Health Care declared that "primary health care is the key to attaining this target—health for all" (WHO, 1978).

Primary Health Care (PHC) is a philosophy of health care (Beddome, Clarke, & Whyte, 1993) that emphasizes community-based health promotion and maintenance rather than curative care of individuals. Cost effectiveness and capacity to benefit people in greatest need make Primary Health Care compelling politically and economically (Primary Health Care Round Table, 1990). Primary Health Care involves decentralization, social participation, adjustment of financing, and development of new models (Collado, 1992). Regrettably, Primary Health Care is sometimes confused with primary nursing and primary medical care (Baines, 1995; Buxton, 1996; Dykeman & Ervin, 1993; Shoultz & Hatcher, 1997).

Lack of conceptual clarity and inadequate theory development in community health nursing have been criticized (Beddome et al., 1993). Clarke, Beddome, and Whyte (1993) point to the relevance of PHC principles to community health nurses' roles and changing context.

The effort to develop a theory for community health nurses will be guided by the five principles embodied in the definition of Primary Health Care: (a) equitable accessibility of health services to all populations, (b) maximum individual and community involvement in the planning and operation of health services, (c) increased emphasis on services that are preventive and promotive rather than curative only, (d) the use of appropriate technology, and (e) the integration of health with sectors involved in social and economic development (CNA, 1988, 1993). This book is founded on a framework encompassing these five PHC principles.

Accessibility of health and health care

Accessibility implies health care that is geographically, financially, and culturally within easy reach of the whole community. The care has to be appropriate and acceptable to people (CNA, 1988). A key issue in Primary Health Care is to make the best use of resources. There may be conflict, however, between cost effectiveness and equity, as the people most in need are often the most costly to reach (Smith & Bryant, 1988). The indicators for acceptable and accessible health services are sociocultural, economic, political, technological, and geographic (Hickman, 1990). Yet, barriers to accessibility persist in Canada.

Poverty
Access to health services and health status is particularly problematic for the poor (Stewart, 1990a). The poor and non-poor differ widely in their perception of susceptibility to health conditions, severity of conditions, coping, and effectiveness of health services (Singh & Pandey, 1990). Billings, Anderson, and Newman (1996) examined disparities in health outcomes for low-income populations in the United States and Canada, and concluded that Canadian

universal health coverage may help to reduce barriers to care. Nevertheless, equality of opportunity provided by national health insurance does not yield equality of access, and a review from the perspectives of the poor is needed (Badgley, 1991). A study of homeless adults in Toronto revealed that although almost 40 percent had health insurance, seven percent had been refused care and 25 percent received instructions inappropriate to their living circumstances (Crowe, 1993). Access to health care for those with poverty-related ill health has been referred to as the "health divide" (Hoskins & Lakey, 1997). Chapter 9 provides a comprehensive analysis of the barriers faced by the poor to health, health behaviour, and health services use.

Community health nurses should provide services that are responsive to the needs of poor families to help them cope with and avoid the worst effects of poverty. The working poor (Primas & Mileham, 1995), poor urban women (Chalich & White, 1997), and teen mothers (SmithBattle, 1995) are particularly vulnerable. Nurses should monitor the level and distribution of poverty-related problems, evaluate the effectiveness of services, and work for social change (Blackburn, 1991). There are a few reports of community interventions designed to enhance accessibility for the poor. One program, in a poor rural county, involved community outreach and education through diverse mechanisms (e.g., transportation system, Healthy Baby Week, computerized infant tracking system, home visits, minority self-help group, donation of equipment). After two years of the program, prenatal visits increased dramatically, and low birth-weight babies and teen births decreased (Boettcher, 1993). In another project that focussed on low-income housing for the elderly, seniors identified problems of undernutrition, crime, and safety, and then engaged in leadership training and community organization to overcome these problems. For example, they organized a cooperative weekly breakfast program (Minkler, 1992). A recent study revealed that public health nurses with skills in networking, fund raising, and public relations could provide comprehensive care in a community-based program for poor urban women (Chalich & White, 1997). Ervin and Young (1996) noted that a nursing centre in a medically underserved community could increase access when practice was tailored to the specific community. In Arizona, a nursing system of health care was proposed as one way to break the cycle of disadvantage (Primas, Mileham, Toronto, & McCoy, 1994). Poor communities should define their own needs, and services should integrate indigenous knowledge and be culturally relevant (Stone, 1992).

Cultural minorities

Cultural biases can pose a barrier to accessibility and have an impact on a community's health status and program development (Anderson & Yuhos, 1993). Access to health care for some cultural minority groups such as Aboriginal people is problematic (Ferris, 1994; Morewood-Northrop, 1994).

The health insurance system needs to be examined from the perspective of Indian and Inuit people living in isolated northern communities (Badgley, 1991). Immigrants such as Asians (Wallace, Awan, & Talbot, 1996), Hispanics (Juarbe, 1995), and Vietnamese (Lam & Green, 1994) could also benefit from PHC initiatives. Hoff's (1992) review revealed health professionals' ignorance of recognition of the traditional healers' role in cultural accessibility and the need for cooperation and mutual referral. Blending professional practices with the cultural beliefs and practices of laypersons is germane to the implementation of Primary Health Care (CNA, 1988). Community health nurses should not negate "culturally relevant folk treatment and implement a totally unfamiliar regimen" (Bushy, 1992a) in their provision of Primary Health Care. The community health nurse needs to understand community norms, values, knowledge, beliefs, resources, and power structure (Hickman, 1990). Chapter 10 (on culturally diverse communities) and Chapter 28 (on participatory research) emphasize cultural considerations for programs and research.

Rural communities

The health problems faced by rural communities are associated with limited resources and inaccessible and inappropriate services (Anderson & Yuhos, 1993; Boettcher, 1993). For example, Atlantic Canada has high rates of poverty and unemployment, as well as smoking, cardiovascular disease, cervical cancer, lung cancer, obesity, high blood pressure, and low rates of physical activity compared with other regions of the country. Atlantic Canada also differs considerably from the remainder of the country in terms of the rural nature of all four provinces—ranging from 46 percent to 60 percent compared with a Canadian average of 23 percent (Statistics Canada, 1993). The rural nature of the region contributes to social isolation and difficulty in accessing services (Stewart, Reed, et al., 1996). Thus, in Atlantic Canada and in the North, geographic barriers to access necessitate unique community health programs and community health nurses' roles such as outreach. Rural PHC initiatives include a health delivery model for rural Saskatchewan (Shanks, 1996), rural nurse practitioners (Hickey, 1996), and advanced nursing practice programs in rural areas (Schmidt, Brandt, & Norris, 1995). Leipert and Reutter (1998) reviewed community health nursing in geographically isolated settings from a Canadian perspective.

Stigmatized populations

Like cultural bias, bias toward some populations with health problems that evoke stigma is yet another barrier to access. For example, a review of U.S. home health care programs for AIDS patients found fragmentation of community services, discriminating responses, refusal to provide care (Combs, 1996), and inadequate professional knowledge. In our Canadian study, persons with hemophilia and AIDS and their family caregivers reported insensitivity, prejudice, and avoidance from nurses, physicians, and other health professionals (Stewart, Hart, & Mann, 1995). Community health nurses in Canada working in AIDS care face fears and anxieties related to drug consumption by the increased numbers living with addictions (Tomblin-Murphy, Ritchie, Stewart, & Johnson, in press). Persons with HIV/AIDS need community nursing services (Brocklehurst & Butterworth, 1996) and home nursing care (Brennan, Ripich, & Moore, 1994). Gay and lesbian clients (Harrison & Silenzio, 1996), especially teens (Nelson, 1997), also need PHC initiatives. Other stigmatized groups include people with learning difficulties (Rodger, 1994) and the mentally ill (Danielson, 1995; Van Hook, 1996).

Access to health care is also discussed in relation to correctional (prison) nursing (Sullivan, 1995), palliative and cancer care (Lake, 1995), care of the homeless (Lewis, 1996; Plumb, 1997), and services for older people (Summer, 1997). McGuire, Gerber, and Clemen-Stone (1996) advocated appropriate and timely referrals of clients from an institution, such as a hospital, to community services.

Community health nurses need to enhance accessibility to health determinants and to health care for the poor, cultural minorities, isolated people, and stigmatized populations.

Public participation

Clearly, the evolving health needs and accompanying service delivery constraints in Canada cannot be addressed by professional resources alone. Accordingly, Primary Health Care, which reflects a philosophy of citizen involvement, is espoused increasingly by professionals. Consumer control, support by volunteers, mutual aid, self-care, partnership with lay helpers, professional–client interactions, consumer perceptions, client participation, and empowerment are all compatible with the public participation principle of Primary Health Care.

Consumer control and volunteers

There has been an increase in consumer-control movements and in tensions in professional–layperson relationships. There is likely to be tension between professional knowledge and experiential knowledge (Borkman, 1990) and between professional and lay control (Stewart, 1990b). Health professionals need to acknowledge that impediments to public participation include consumer vulnerability in bureaucratic organizations, stigmatization of some illnesses, and tokenism in some health boards.

Participation of clients at individual and collective levels can be promoted by volunteers, self-help mutual aid groups, and self-care, as professional roles are not rigidly defined (Mezzina, Mazzuia, Vidoni, & Impagnatiello,

1992). Gottlieb and Peters (1991) reported that 27 percent of Canadians volunteered through a group or organization, but that volunteers are more advantaged in socioeconomic terms than non-volunteers.

Self-care and mutual aid

Mutual aid and self-care are key mechanisms for promoting health (Epp, 1986; Romeder, 1990). Furthermore, self-help mutual aid groups, which exist for every conceivable health condition, are significant sources of support (Katz, 1993) and provide a cost-effective complement to professional services. Groups led by professionals and those led by peers are equally supportive and effective in improving coping, self-efficacy, and psychological functioning (Toseland, Rossiter, Peak, & Hill, 1990) and in identifying priority needs (Meissen, Gleason, & Embree, 1991). In Chapter 4, health professionals are reported to perceive that referral, educator, and facilitator roles were conducive to partnerships with self-help mutual aid groups, and to believe that partnership is desirable (Stewart, Banks, Crossman, & Poel, 1996). Professionals should play roles conducive to partnership, such as referral, education, consultation, liaison, and facilitation (Chesler, 1991; Katz, 1993; Stewart, 1990b). This has implications for community health nursing roles.

Self-help mutual aid group membership may foster individual and collective efficacy, empowerment (Stewart, 1990b), and self-care. Self-care by clients involves setting goals for health and developing strategies to implement those goals (Holzemer, 1992). (Self-care is discussed further in Chapter 4 in relationship to social support.) One study indicated that "mutual goal setting and decision making between the client and the nurse are dependent upon shared perception of the clients' self-care agency" (Ward-Griffin & Bramwell, 1990). "Mutual participation relationships" between providers and clients can facilitate self-care through negotiation of mutual goals, plans to meet goals, and joint evaluation (Pesznecker, Zerwekh, & Horn, 1989).

Provider–client partnerships

Nurse practitioners' interactions with women clients involved a negotiable agenda and exchange of information (Johnson, 1993). In the PHC project in Newfoundland (see Chapter 2), social, mental, and physical health outcomes were mutually identified by the community health nurse and client (Hall, Ross, Edge, & Pynn, 1991). Kristanson and Chalmers's (1990) observations of nurse–client interactions in community-based practice revealed that interactions were either nurse controlled or joint controlled (Kristanson & Chalmers, 1990). (This study is described in Chapter 26.) Successful collaboration in client–community health nurse relationships requires active and committed involvement and joint effort (Paavilainen & Astedt-Kurki, 1997). One nursing centre model involved the community in determining the priority of health care needs; participation, support, and cost-effective outcomes were greater if residents were involved (Ruka, Brown, & Procope, 1997). More study of community health nurses' interactions with clients may be needed to promote public participation and elicit public perceptions (e.g., Powell-Cope, 1994).

Client perceptions and participation

There are few studies of consumer perceptions of community health nursing services. In one study, elderly clients perceived benefits from community health nurses' encouragement, support, education, and advice, such as increased health knowledge, health awareness, self-confidence, and self-care (Laffrey, Renwanz-Boyle, Slagle, Guthmiller, & Carter, 1990). In another study, elderly people who consulted a nurse for health assessments, blood pressure checks, flu injections, and similar reasons were very positive about their relationships with the nurse (Jones, Edwards, & Lester, 1997). Cancer patients reported that home visits by community nurses helped them deal with physical, psychological, and social problems; met their needs for information; and provided emotional support (van Harteveld, Mistiaen, & Dukkers van Emden, 1997). Poulton (1996) found that people rated their satisfaction with professional care from community nurses more highly than that from general practitioners. Larrabee (1997) revealed that community clients were highly satisfied with nurse practitioner care.

Women's perceptions of health care are unique. Welch (1996) found that most women were satisfied with nurse midwives as PHC providers and preferred a female practitioner for intimate health care needs. Gender as well as the personal approach of the health care provider are important to women (Brooks & Phillips, 1996). A Breast Health Centre in Ottawa responded to women's requests for changes in care (Gray, 1997).

Clients can participate directly in community health program evaluation and research. Clarke et al. (1993) report the use of client interviewers in participatory research. Chapter 28 (on participatory research) delineates the challenges and contributions of client participation and empowerment in research. When client participation in community mental health services through advisory committees was encouraged, families appreciated the accessibility, accountability, availability, flexibility, and coordination of services and perceived that empowerment was particularly important (Marchenko, Herman, & Hazel, 1992).

Empowerment

Client empowerment is promoted through consumer control movements, self-help mutual aid groups, self-care, partnership relationships and reciprocal interactions with clients, elicitation of client perceptions, and client participation. Empowerment implies that clients have the authority to influence decisions and interventions (Wallerstein, 1992) and have control and collective efficacy (Stewart, 1993). Empowerment involves participation, choice, support, negotiation (Connelly, Kleinbeck, Schneider, & Cobb, 1993), and advocacy. Community health nurses promote personal advocacy of individual clients and facilitate small groups, which can evolve into larger community organizations for change (Labonte, 1989). Social advocacy enables people to increase control over and improve their health. In political advocacy, the community health nurse interprets government priorities to the community and community priorities to the government (McMurray, 1991). Zerwekh (1992) studied the practice of empowerment by public health nurses in high-risk maternal–child care who sought to foster client responsibility and self-care. The nurses listened, expanded the family's vision of their options, and provided feedback (Zerwekh, 1992). Chapter 24 illustrates other empowering communication strategies. A client-held care record can also help clients achieve greater autonomy and empowerment (Stafford & Hannigan, 1997).

Community empowerment is another important component of community health nurse practice and of Primary Health Care (Eng, Salmon, & Mullan, 1992). The community can be empowered through advocacy, social planning, social action, and consciousness raising. In the PHC project in Newfoundland (see Chapter 2), community health nurses conducted community needs assessment and public forums (Remkes, 1992). Courtney (1995) described a community partnership model involving community development and community empowerment activities. (Chapter 21 delineates other community development strategies.) Primary care to the underserved involved community empowerment strategies (Bushnell & Cook, 1995). Although public involvement in the creation of Centres locaux de services communautaires (CLSCs) in Québec was strong, the power of citizens dwindled significantly once the CLSCs were formalized, illustrating that community participation and community empowerment differ (O'Neill, 1992). Furthermore, when the community is invited to be a participant, only some sectors may participate (O'Neill, 1992; Rousseau, 1993). Fundamental constraints lie in institutional processes designed to control power. A shift from hierarchical processes of control to horizontal processes of partnership in health services is needed to enable empowerment (Townsend, 1994). Community health nurses need to work with community organizers, community leaders, self-help groups, and professionals in other disciplines and sectors to empower communities and community members.

Intersectoral and interdisciplinary collaboration

Intersectoral collaboration is a key mechanism in the implementation of Primary Health Care. A broader approach to the determinants of health necessitates attention to areas outside traditional health services (National Forum on Health, 1997). Health cannot be examined in isolation from the education and economic condition of a community. Thus, there is a need to involve sectors outside the health sector (Ritchie, 1994). Furthermore, the health infrastructure interacts with the social and economic infrastructure in initiatives ranging from policy analysis, legislation and regulation, and social marketing to collaborative development of educational programs or coordinated community development at the local level (Holzemer, 1992). Intersectoral linkages are central to resolving many community health problems.

Interdisciplinary PHC teams face changing patterns of health needs, shifting populations, new developments in health care, and changing expectations of consumers. PHC teams require common objectives, clear understanding of members' roles, mutual respect for others' roles and skills, a flexible approach (Poulton & West, 1993), and shared leadership (Pearson, 1992). The skills of advocacy, mediation, and negotiation are also essential in intersectoral and interdisciplinary collaboration (Ritchie, 1994). However, multidisciplinary team-building interventions in the health arena have been rare. Facilitators are needed "to achieve a position of trust with the members of the primary health care team and to encourage synergy between dissimilar professionals" (Hooker, 1994). Interdisciplinary teams could be developed through workshops, models of team effectiveness, and undergraduate professional education (Poulton & West, 1993). Multidisciplinary meetings also promote collaboration because they foster greater awareness among various disciplines of the range of services (Bennett-Emslie & McIntosh, 1995). However, multidisciplinary teams in Primary Health Care face issues of hierarchy in leadership, interpersonal conflicts (Long, 1996), and organizational, professional, and interpersonal challenges (Barr, 1997; Cook, 1996). Measures of effectiveness for PHC teams include consumer outcomes, quality of care, team viability, and organization (Poulton & West, 1994).

Sheer (1996) suggested that nurses will collaborate in an egalitarian manner on multidisciplinary teams when they become empowered. Alliances between nursing and medicine should ensure broader services and quality care (Mundinger, 1996). To illustrate, collaboration of advanced practice psychiatric nurses with psychiatrists has improved client outcomes and job satisfaction and contained health care costs (Bailey, 1996). A model of geriatric primary collaborative care between nurses and physicians was successfully implemented in a large group practice setting (Schraeder, Britt, Dworlak, & Shelton, 1997). One U.S. study focussed on professional identities, roles, and relationships of nurses, social workers, educators, and other community-based providers (Netting & Williams, 1997). A new interdisciplinary model, the Canadian Integrated Delivery System, could foster alliances with community agencies and other health care services (Leatt, Pink, & Naylor, 1996).

There are a few reports of interdisciplinary educational initiatives that could prepare future community health nurses for intersectoral and interdisciplinary collaboration. In one community centre, nursing, medical, dental, and other health professional students worked as a team to involve the community, to identify health problems, and to design and evaluate interventions (Klevens, 1992). In another interdisciplinary educational initiative for community-based Primary Health Care, medical students and nursing students learned about the priorities, skills, and knowledge of the other discipline (Zungolo, 1994).

The important contributions by nurses and nursing associations to interdisciplinary collaboration were reviewed in Chapter 2. Indeed, nurses provide comprehensive care and assist people to use other professionals appropriately (Berland, 1991). However, community health nurses will need to pay greater attention to collaboration with other sectors essential to Primary Health Care.

Appropriate technology

Technology should be adapted to the community's social, economic, and cultural development, directed toward priority needs of high-risk groups, and maintained by resources that the community can afford (WHO, 1978). Appropriate technology is scientifically sound, adaptable to local needs, acceptable (CNA, 1993), compatible with constraints, and results in desirable outcomes (Parette & Parette, 1992). In community health, any technology can be considered appropriate depending on the nature of the problem, the state of knowledge, and the availability of resources (McKinlay, 1993).

The PHC principle of appropriate technology refers broadly to the appropriate use of all health care resources such as funds, facilities, equipment (CNA, 1990), tools, and techniques (Sandelowski, 1993). In this context, appropriate technology includes counselling, information services, educational technology, therapies, immunization, essential drugs, prevention and treatment of endemic diseases, and research tools (CNA, 1990; Cohen, 1989). Therefore, a broad interpretation of appropriate technology encompasses the interpersonal relationship skills discussed in Chapter 24 and the epidemiological research examined in Chapter 29.

Requisite research

The need for health-services research and health-focussed research is indisputable. Required research includes evaluation studies of PHC activities, controlled studies to test new interventions, identification of benefits and hazards of participation and collaboration, studies of health providers' behaviour, investigations of community health needs, and outcome measures for Primary Health Care and health promotion strategies (CNA, 1988). Research should focus on the non-medical determinants of health and test non-medical interventions (National Forum on Health, 1997). Research is needed to analyze human factors that affect appropriate use of technology, as well as the appropriateness of specific technological techniques.

Validated information is needed on the usefulness and limitations of health technology and its appropriateness for particular people. Information systems can foster rational allocation of resources and ensure more effective, equitable health systems. Information systems can also be used to link information needs to interventions and to translate human and material resources into interventions (Cohen, 1989). The relationships among health outcomes, utilization of health care services, and the determinants of health (e.g., socioeconomic status, employment status, work environment, social and physical environment) can be analyzed by matching health data to socioeconomic data (e.g., census or labour force survey) and to environmental data bases. For example, the Nova Scotia Health Survey (1995) collected data on socioeconomic variables, labour force activity, and psychosocial variables associated with health status. Modern information technology can improve communication between hospitals and community practitioners (Copland, 1994) and promote cost containment of home care services (Russon, 1997).

Technological innovation

Innovations in communications and computer technology can promote efficiency and relevance of health services. In New Brunswick, a telephone information line has eased demand at emergency departments (Robb, 1996). Nurses are using computer software that provides protocols for client complaints and helps them direct clients to the most appropriate community care. Clients using computers for prevention purposes were satisfied with this system of providing health information (Williams, Boles, & Johnson, 1995).

There is a need to document expenditures associated with technology and to assess quality of care (Sandiford, Annett, & Cibulskis, 1992). Values that centre on quality of life require re-evaluation of the costs and benefits of technology (Holzemer, 1992). Indeed, the role of technological innovation should be "subordinate to the goal of improving people's health" (Sandiford et al., 1992).

Nevertheless, there is a continuing professional, public, and government fascination with high technology. This is depicted in the media's reporting of new transplants, diagnostic equipment, advanced laboratory tests, and complicated surgical techniques. Governments often favour high-technological secondary and tertiary care and lack faith in lower-cost community-based alternatives (Beddome et al., 1993). Monies have been directed primarily toward building and renovating hospitals, nursing homes, and other institutions. In contrast, Canadian multiservice centres, community health centres, and CLSCs include within their objectives an implicit PHC philosophy of appropriate technology.

Clearly, there is a need for informed public opinion of realistic health technology in the context of the community's social and economic constraints and resources (Cohen, 1989). Therefore, the CNA (1990) recommended access to information about technology, public participation in decision making regarding development and use of technology, and creation of a data base on the social and clinical implications of technology. Technology should be used for prevention and promotion as well as treatment (CNA, 1990). Furthermore, the CNA (1988) "recognizes the need to develop alternatives to expensive, highly technical health care services." For example, nursing research that focussed on technologically dependent clients living in the community (Sandelowski, 1993; Parette & Parette, 1992) indicates that "frequently the most appropriate choice is a low technology solution that requires little training and minimal assistance" (Parette & Parette, 1992). Recently, the CNA developed a policy statement on appropriate use of health care technology.

The authors of Chapter 2 reported that only five provincial nursing associations have acknowledged appropriate technology in their publications, committee work, or lobbying, and community health nursing associations rarely address technology. Furthermore, the community health nursing literature appears to have neglected this PHC principle. Community health nurses need to understand the community's technology (Hickman, 1990) and to foster appropriate use of technology.

Health promotion and illness prevention

Some sectors of the Canadian health care system continue to be preoccupied with cure and treatment rather than illness prevention and health promotion. In contrast, the Canadian government's commitment to health promotion research was reflected in the 1992 creation of six nationally funded health promotion research centres in Atlantic Canada, Québec, Ontario, Saskatchewan, Alberta, and British Columbia (Stewart, 1997).

Canadian health promotion research and programs reflect other PHC principles. Community participation and multidisciplinary collaboration were key themes in the first national conference on health promotion research in Toronto (Eakin & MacLean, 1992). These themes persisted in subsequent conferences in Vancouver (1993), Calgary (1994), Montréal (1996), and Halifax (1997). Edwards, Ciliska, Habert, & Pond (1992) reported on a health promotion program for immigrants that fostered accessibility through cultural interpretation and community advocacy. A health promotion program in Saskatchewan also emphasized barriers to accessibility (e.g., poverty, unemployment, inadequate formal education) and the need for culturally acceptable strategies of community participation (Feather et al., 1993). Self-efficacy, social support (i.e., public participation), and accessibility were associated with participation in a workplace health promotion program (Alexy, 1991). Thus, accessibility, multisectoral collaboration, and public participation are key themes in health promotion initiatives in Canada.

Despite the importance of public participation, some health promotion priorities continue to be professionally defined by community participation rather than community control (Farrant, 1991; Grace, 1991). There may also be excess emphasis, in some health promotion programs, on individuals' lifestyles and health behaviours with inadequate consideration of social systems, organizational priorities, professional behaviours, and other environmental factors. Thus, health promotion efforts need to move from the individual to the social system (McKinlay, 1993). The book *Health Promotion in Canada* (Pederson, O'Neill, & Rootman, 1994) reflected the shift from a focus on the individual's lifestyle to the social, physical, and economic environments.

Environmental hazards and industrial products and by-products continue to cause concern to health promotion practitioners. Ecological illness and immunological disorders emerged as diseases of the 1980s and 1990s. Airtight buildings have been associated with increased infections and recirculation of smoke and fumes (CNA, 1988). These environmental problems signal the need for prevention.

Prevention

In developed countries, prevention efforts focus on ill health that results from pollution of the environment and unhealthy lifestyles (CNA, 1993). Indeed, six of the eight essential elements of Primary Health Care (WHO, 1978) are preventive: health education, nutrition, sanitation, maternal and child health care, immunization, and prevention and control of endemic diseases.

Health promotion and illness prevention initiatives occur with diverse populations in varied settings. "Preconception" health promotion includes assessment, intervention, and education (Perry, 1996). For children, health promotion and prevention initiatives have focussed on violence (Beauchesne, Kelley, Lawrence, & Farquharson, 1997) and chronic childhood illnesses (Broughton & Lutner, 1995). For adolescents, health promotion and prevention activities included prevention of alcohol use (Werch, Carlson, Pappas, & DiClemente, 1996) and promotion of physical activity (DuRant & Hergenroeder, 1994) and cardiovascular health knowledge (MacDonald, 1995). Other foci for health promotion efforts include the working poor (Primas & Mileham, 1995), poor urban women (Chalich & White, 1997), and sexual health of women (MacLaren, 1995; Ruston, 1996).

Role of community health nurses

Community health nurses assess and prioritize preventive and health promotion needs of clients and identify and implement strategies to address these needs (Collado, 1992; Edwards et al., 1992). Community health nursing diagnoses can focus on health maintenance (i.e., protecting against illness and preserving health) or health seeking (i.e., increasing health, wellness, and quality of life). These two diagnoses distinguish illness prevention and health promotion activities of community health nurses (Tripp & Stachowiak, 1992). (See Chapter 19.) A survey of community-based nurse practitioners in the United States revealed that they met most of the Healthy People 2000 national objectives for illness prevention (Lemley, O'Grady, Rauckhorst, Russell, & Small, 1994). Community health nursing programs for adolescents focussed on prevention of pregnancy, parenting problems, and at-risk lifestyle behaviours (Bushy, 1992b). Leipert (1996) described health promotion and prevention roles and activities of community health nurses in Vancouver, British Columbia. In the United States, health promotion is a role of advanced practice nurses who work with homeless women and children (Norton & Ridenour, 1995), in rural family practice (Goodyear, 1995), and in partnerships with healthy cities and communities (Flynn, 1997). Community health nurses have an increased understanding of health promotion and of their mandate to implement population-based health promotion strategies (Halbert, Underwood, Chambers, Ploeg, Johnson, & Isaacs, 1993). Nursing students preparing for a health promotion role in the community were catalysts for change, evaluators, researchers, advocates, referral agents, and consultants (Smillie, 1992).

The authors of Chapter 2 reported that most PHC activities by Canadian nurses have focussed on health promotion and illness prevention. This trend is illustrated in Chapter 5 (on a health promotion model for aggregates and communities), Chapter 12 (on adolescent health promotion), and Chapter 16 (on health promotion). Chapter 13 (on prevention of adolescent pregnancies), Chapter 15 (on prevention of seniors' falls), and Chapter 17 (on prevention of injuries) are also congruent with this PHC principle.

Primary Health Care framework for this book

Clearly, public participation and interdisciplinary/intersectoral collaboration are integral to health promotion, illness and injury prevention, and accessibility. Mutual aid, coping, self-care, other forms of public participation, and accessibility are key components of the Canadian health promotion framework (Epp, 1986). The appropriate use of resources and technology is consistent with the premise of accessibility, as bureaucratic structures and technological complexity pose barriers to accessibility. Thus, the five principles of Primary Health Care are interrelated (see Figure 3.1). Furthermore, all principles of Primary Health Care are foundations for community health nurses' roles and functions (CPHA, 1990). Nevertheless, as shown in Chapter 2, nursing has placed greater emphasis on health promotion, public participation, and accessibility than on intersectoral collaboration and appropriate technology. This emphasis is reflected in the content of the chapters of this book.

Challenges for community health nurses

The impact of health system reform on community health nursing and the practice of Primary Health Care requires study. More Canadian research is needed on how community health nurses engage in the principles of Primary Health Care, in diverse settings, and with various clients and populations. Intervention studies based on PHC principles are timely.

The continuing challenge for community health nurses is to attend to the links between PHC theory and practice; to promote community health nursing programs as cost-effective and accessible alternatives (Beddome et al., 1993); to deal with clients as equal participants; and to interact with other disciplines and non-health sectors (Berland, 1991). Community health nurses must also implement interventions that promote health and prevent illness of individuals, families, aggregates, and communities (Pender, Barkauskas, Hayman, Rice, & Anderson, 1992) in practice. Finally, community health nurses need to contribute to PHC research (Collado, 1992) and to commit to all five principles of Primary Health Care.

One survey revealed that nurses did not emphasize interdisciplinary and intersectoral collaboration and were not familiar with environmental or social issues (Dykeman & Ervin, 1993). Community health nurses should address the needs of the wider community (Caraher & McNab, 1996). PHC roles neglected by nurses include advocacy, coordination of care, and negotiation in social action (Neufeld & Harrison, 1990). Community health nurses need to play a more extensive role in social change and health policy development (Murphy, 1993). The policy development role of community health nurses is discussed in Chapter 8. This emerging political role means that community nurses in Canada need to develop skills relevant to community development, coalition building, teamwork, networking, advocacy, group facilitation, empowerment, and public education and relations (English & Hicks, 1992; Leipert, 1996; Stone, 1993). These challenges point to the need for education.

Figure 3.1
Primary Health Care framework for community health nurses

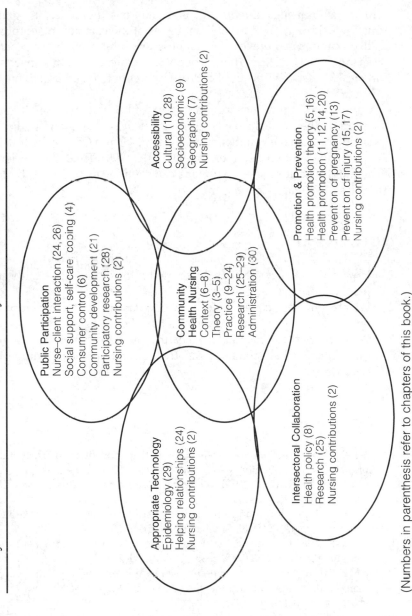

Public Participation
Nurse–client interaction (24, 26)
Social support, self-care coping (4)
Consumer control (6)
Community development (21)
Participatory research (28)
Nursing contributions (2)

Accessibility
Cultural (10, 28)
Socioeconomic (9)
Geographic (7)
Nursing contributions (2)

**Community
Health Nursing**
Context (6–8)
Theory (3–5)
Practice (9–24)
Research (25–29)
Administration (30)

Promotion & Prevention
Health promotion theory (5, 16)
Health promotion (11,12,14, 20)
Prevent on of pregnancy (13)
Prevent on of injury (15,17)
Nursing contributions (2)

Appropriate Technology
Epidemiology (29)
Helping relationships (24)
Nursing contributions (2)

Intersectoral Collaboration
Health policy (8)
Research (25)
Nursing contributions (2)

(Numbers in parenthesis refer to chapters of this book.)

To prepare nursing students for community-based practice, integration of Primary Health Care within different levels of the curriculum, emphasis on health promotion and prevention of illness, and interdisciplinary experiences (Oermann, 1994) are important. Continuing education is also needed. For example, workshops for public health practitioners focussed on policy change (Badovinac, 1997).

As nurses constitute the largest category of health personnel, it is important to orient them to Primary Health Care as the key to attaining health for all Canadians in the new millennium. Primary Health Care is the foundation of community health nursing practice (CPHA, 1990). Thus, the reorientation of community health nurses in Canada can continue to be guided by the five principles of Primary Health Care.

QUESTIONS

1. How can PHC principles be integrated into community health nursing practice, research, and theory?
2. Which PHC principles have been emphasized by community health nurses in Canada? Which principles have been neglected?
3. What barriers to health and health care are experienced by some Canadians? What strategies can the community health nurse use to enhance accessibility?

REFERENCES

Alexy, B.B. (1991). Factors associated with participation or nonparticipation in a Workplace Wellness Center. *Research in Nursing and Health, 14,* 33–40.

Anderson, J., & Yuhos, R. (1993). Health promotion in rural settings. *Nursing Clinics of North America, 28*(1), 145–155.

Badgley, R.F. (1991). Social and economic disparities under Canadian health care. *International Journal of Health Services, 21*(4), 659–671.

Badovinac, K. (1997). Policy advocacy for public health practioners: Workshops on policy change. *Public Health of Nursing, 14*(5), 280–285.

Bailey, M.K. (1996). Preparing for prescriptive practice: Advanced practice psychiatric nursing and psychopharmacotherapy. *Journal of Psychosocial Nursing and Mental Health Services, 34*(1), 16–20.

Baines, L. (1995). Community care: Let the clients choose their care. *Nursing Standard, 9*(38), 14–20.

Barr, O. (1997). Interdisciplinary teamwork: Consideration of the challenges. *British Journal of Nursing, 6*(17), 1005–1010.

Beauchesne, M.A., Kelley, B.R., Lawrence, P.R., & Farquharson, P.E. (1997). Violence prevention: A community approach. *Journal of Pediatric Health Care, 11*(4), 155–164.

Beddome, G., Clarke, H.F., & Whyte, N.B. (1993). Vision for the future of public health nursing: A case for PHC. *Public Health Nursing, 10*(1), 13–18.

Bennett-Emslie, G., & McIntosh, J. (1995). Promoting collaboration in the primary care team—the role of the practice meeting. *Journal of Interprofessional Care, 9*(3), 251–256.

Berland, A. (1991). Primary health care: What does it mean for nurses? *Canadian Nurse, 87*(9), 25–26.

Billings, J., Anderson, G.M., & Newman, L.S. (1996). Recent findings on preventable hospitalizations. *Health Affairs, 15*(3), 239–249.

Blackburn, C. (1991). Family poverty: What can health visitors do? *Health Visitor, 64*(11), 2–4.

Boettcher, J.H. (1993). Promoting maternal infant health in rural communities: The rural health outreach program. *Nursing Clinics of North America, 28*(1), 199–209.

Borkman, T. (1990). Self-help groups at the turning point: Emerging egalitarian alliances with the formal health care system? *American Journal of Community Psychology, 18*, 321–332.

Brennan, P.F., Ripich, S., & Moore, S.M. (1991). The use of home-based computers to support persons living with AIDS/ARC. *Journal of Community Health Nursing, 8*(1), 3–14.

Brocklehurst, N., & Butterworth, T. (1996). Establishing good practices in continuing care: A descriptive study of community nursing services for people with HIV infection. *Journal of Advanced Nursing, 24*(3), 488–497.

Brooks, F., & Phillips, D. (1996). Do women want health workers? Women's views of the primary health care service. *Journal of Advanced Nursing, 23*(6), 1207–1211.

Broughton, B.K., & Lutner, N. (1995). Chronic childhood illness: A nursing health–promotion model for rehabilitation in the community. *Rehabilitation Nursing, 20*(6), 318–322.

Bushnell, F.K.L., & Cook, T. (1995). Primary care to the underserved through community empowerment. *Nurse Practitioner: American Journal of Primary Health Care, 20*(8), 21–23.

Bushy, A. (1992a). Cultural considerations for primary health care: Where do self-care and folk medicine fit? *Holistic Nursing Practice, 6*(3), 10–18.

Bushy, A. (1992b). Preconception health promotion: Another approach to improve pregnancy outcomes. *Public Health Nursing, 9*(1), 10–14.

Buxton, V. (1996). Visions for the future . . . the future of primary care. *Nursing Times, 92*(25), 26–27.

Canadian Nurses Association (CNA). (1988). *Health for all Canadians: A call for health care reform.* Ottawa: Author.

Canadian Nurses Association (CNA). (1990). *New reproductive technologies: Accessible, appropriate, participative.* Brief to the Royal Commission on New Reproductive Technologies. Ottawa: Author.

Canadian Nurses Association (CNA). (1993). Five guiding principles for primary health care. *Journal of Nursing Administration, 23*(5), 4, 10.

Canadian Public Health Association (CPHA). (1990). *Community health–public health nursing in Canada: Preparation and practice.* Ottawa: Author.

Caraher, M., & McNab, H. (1996). The public health nursing role: An overview of future trends. *Nursing Standards, 10*(51), 44–48.

Chalich, T., & White, J.P. (1997). Providing primary care to poor urban women. *Nursing Forum, 32*(2), 23–28.

Chesler, M.A. (1991). Participatory action research with self-help groups: An alternative paradigm for inquiry and action. *American Journal of Community Psychology, 19*(5), 757–768.

Clarke, H.F., Beddome, G., & Whyte, N.B. (1993). Public health nurses' vision of their future reflects changing paradigms. *International Nursing, 25*(4), 305–310.

Cohen, J. (1989). Appropriate technology in primary health care: Evolution and meaning of WHO's concept. *International Journal of Technology Assessment in Health Care, 5*, 103–109.

Collado, C.B. (1992). Primary health care: A continuing challenge. *Nursing and Health Care, 13*(8), 408–413.

Connelly, L.M., Kleinbeck, S.V.M., Schneider, J.K., & Cobb, A.K. (1993). A place to be yourself: Empowerment from the client's perspective. *Image: Journal of Nursing Scholarship, 25*(4), 297–303.

Cook, R. (1996). Paths to effective teamwork in primary care settings. *Nursing Times, 92*(14), 44–45.

Combs, E.W. (1996). Home health, AIDS, and refusal to care [Review]. *Home Healthcare Nurse, 14*(3), 188–194.

Copland, G. (1994). How can modern information technology be used to improve communication between hospitals and community practitioners? *Informatics in Healthcare Australia, 3*(4), 165–168.

Courtney, R. (1995). Community partnership primary care: A new paradigm for primary care. *Public Health Nursing, 12*(6), 366–373.

Crowe, C. (1993). Nursing research and political change: The Street Health Report. *Canadian Nurse, 89*, 21–24.

Danielson, E. (1995). An integrated cooperation model for long-term mentally ill in the community. *Journal of Psychosocial Nursing and Mental Health Services, 33*(8), 29–35.

DuRant, R.H., & Hergenroeder, A.C. (1994). Promotion of physical activity among adolescents by primary health care providers. *Pediatric Exercise Science, 6*(4), 448–463.

Dykeman, M., & Ervin, N.E. (1993). Nurses' attitudes toward primary health care: Development of an instrument. *Journal of Advanced Nursing, 18*, 1567–1572.

Eakin, J.M., & MacLean, H.M. (1992). A critical perspective on research and knowledge development in health promotion. *Canadian Journal of Public Health, 83*(1), S72–S76.

Edwards, N., Ciliska, D., Halbert, T., & Pond, M. (1992). Health promotion and health advocacy for and by immigrants enrolled in English as a Second Language classes. *Canadian Journal of Public Health, 83*(2), 159–162.

Eng, E., Salmon, M.E., & Mullan, F. (1992). Community empowerment: The critical base for primary health care. *Family Community Health, 15*(1), 1–12.

English, J.C.B., & Hicks, B.C. (1992). A systems-in-transition paradigm for Healthy Communities. *Canadian Journal of Public Health, 83*(1), 61–64.

Epp, J. (1986). *Achieving health for all: A framework for health promotion.* Ottawa: Health & Welfare Canada.

Ervin, N.E., & Young, W.B. (1996). Model for a nursing center: Spanning boundaries. *Journal of Nursing Care Quality, 11*(2), 16–24.

Farrant, W. (1991). Addressing the contradictions: Health promotion and community health action in the United Kingdom. *International Journal of Health Services, 21*(3), 423–439.

Feather, J., Irvine, J., Belanger, B., Dumais, W., Gladue, R., Isbister, W., & Leach, P. (1993). Promoting social health in northern Saskatchewan. *Canadian Journal of Public Health, 84*(4), 250–253.

Ferris, L.E. (1994). Detection and treatment of wife abuse in aboriginal communities by primary care physicians: Preliminary findings. *Journal of Women's Health, 3*(4), 265–271.

Flynn, B.C. (1997). Partnerships in healthy cities and communities: A social commitment for advanced practice nurses. *Advanced Practice Nursing Quarterly, 2*(4), 1–6.

Goodyear, R. (1995). Concern, continuity, and choice: A health promotion formula for advanced practice nurses. *Advanced Practice Nursing Quarterly, 1*(3), 41–49.

Gottlieb, B.H., & Peters, L. (1991). A national demographic portrait of mutual aid group participants in Canada. *American Journal of Community Psychology, 19*(5), 651–666.

Grace, V.M. (1991). The marketing of empowerment and the construction of the health consumer: A critique of health promotion. *International Journal of Health Sciences, 21*(2), 329–343.

Gray, C. (1997). One-stop care at breast centre another sign of patients' increasing influence. *Canadian Medical Association Journal, 157*(10), 1419–1420.

Halbert, T.L., Underwood, J.E., Chambers, L.W., Ploeg, J., Johnson, N.A., & Isaacs, S.M. (1993). Population-based health promotion: A new agenda for public health nurses. *Canadian Journal of Public Health, 84*(4), 243–245.

Hall, D.C., Ross, A.S., Edge, D., & Pynn, G.A. (1991). Primary health care—a nursing model: A Danish–Newfoundland (Canada) project. In P.G. Norton, M. Stewart, F. Tudiver, M.J. Bass, & E.V. Dunn (Eds.), *Primary care research, traditional and innovative approaches: Research methods for primary care* (Vol. 1) (pp. 195–208). London: Sage.

Harrison, A.E., & Silenzio, V.M. (1996). Comprehensive care of lesbian and gay patients and families. *Primary Care: Clinics in Office Practice, 23*(1), 31–46.

Hickey, J.V. (1996). Reformation of health care and implications for advanced practice nursing. In J.V. Hickey, R.M. Ouimette, & S.L. Venegoni (Eds.), *Advanced practice nursing: Changing roles and clinical applications* (pp. 3–21). Philadelphia: Lippincott-Raven.

Hickman, P. (1990). Community health and development: Applying sociological concepts to practice. *Sociological Practice, 8*, 125–132.

Hoff, W. (1992). Traditional healers and community health. *World Health Forum, 13*, 182–187.

Holzemer, W.L. (1992). Linking primary health care and self-care through case management. *International Nursing Review, 39*(3), 83–89.

Hooker, J.C. (1994). Guest editorial. *Journal of Advanced Nursing, 19*, 1–3.

Hoskins, R., & Lakey, T. (1997). Till death us do part . . . Measures to deal with poverty-related ill health in England. *Nursing Times, 93*(32), 24–26.

Johnson, R. (1993). Nurse practitioner–patient discourse: Uncovering the voice of nursing in primary care practice. *Scholarly Inquiry for Nursing Practice: An International Journal, 7*(3), 143–157.

Jones, D., Edwards, J., & Lester, C. (1997). The changing role of the practice nurse. *Health and Social Care in the Community, 5*(2), 77–83.

Juarbe, T.C. (1995). Access to health care for Hispanic women: A primary health care perspective. *Nursing Outlook*, 43(1), 23–28.

Katz, A.H. (1993). *Self-help in America: A social movement perspective* [Irwin T. Sanders, Ed.]. New York: Twayne Publishers.

Klevens, R.M. (1992). Special contribution: Transforming a neighborhood health center into a community-oriented primary care practice. *American Journal of Preventive Medicine*, 8(1) 62–65.

Kristanson, L., & Chalmers, K. (1990). Nurse–client interactions in community-based practice: Creating common ground. *Public Health Nursing*, 7(4), 215–223.

Labonte, R. (1989). Community and professional empowerment. *Canadian Nurse*, 85(3), 24–26.

Laffrey, S.C., Renwanz-Boyle, A., Slagle, R., Guthmiller, A., & Carter, B. (1990). Elderly clients' perception of public health nursing care. *Public Health Nursing*, 7(2), 111–117.

Lake, L. (1995). Tonsillitis on the tall ships. *Nursing Standard*, 9(44), 18–20.

Lam, T., & Green, J. (1994). Primary health care and the Vietnamese community: A survey in Greenwich. *Health and Social Care in the Community*, 2(5), 293–299.

Larrabee, J.H., Ferri, J.A., & Hartig, M.T. (1997). Patient satisfaction with nurse practitioner care in primary care. *Journal of Nursing Care Quality*, 11(5), 9–14.

Leatt, P., Pink, G.H., & Naylor, C.D. (1996). Integrated delivery systems: Has their time come in Canada? *Canadian Medical Association Journal*, 154(6), 803–809.

Leipert, B.D. (1996). The value of community health nursing: A phenomenological study of the perceptions of community health nurses. *Public Health Nursing*, 13(1): 50–57.

Leipert, B., & Reutter, L. (1998). Women's health and community health nursing practice in geographically isolated settings: A Canadian perspective. *Healthcare for Women International*, 19(6), 575–588.

Lemley, K., O'Grady, E., Rauckhorst, L., Russell, D., & Small, N. (1994). Nurse practitioner. *American Journal of Primary Health Care*, 19(5), 57–63.

Lewis, J. (1996). Primary health care for homeless people in A&E. *Professional Nurse*, 12(1), 13–14.

Long, S. (1996). Primary health care team workshop: Team members' perspectives. *Journal of Advanced Nursing*, 23(5), 935–941.

MacDonald, S.A. (1995). An assessment of the Cardiovascular Health Education Program in primary health care. *Applied Nursing Research*, 8(3), 114–117.

MacLaren, A. (1995). Primary care for women: Comprehensive sexual health assessment. *Journal of Nurse-Midwifery*, 40(2), 104–119, 159–164.

Marchenko, M.O., Herman, S.E., & Hazel, K.L. (1992). A comparison of how families and their service providers rate family generated quality of service factors. *Community Mental Health Journal*, 28(5), 441–449.

McGuire, S.L., Gerber, D.E., & Clemen-Stone, S. (1996). Meeting the diverse needs of clients in the community: Effective use of the referral process. *Nursing Outlook*, 44(5), 218–222.

McKinlay, J.B. (1993). The promotion of health through planned sociopolitical change: Challenges for research and policy. *Social Science and Medicine*, 36(2), 109–117.

McMurray, A. (1991). Advocacy for community self-empowerment. *International Nursing Review*, 38(1), 19–21.

Meissen, G.J., Gleason, D., & Embree, M. (1991). An assessment of the needs of mutual help groups. *American Journal of Community Psychology*, 19, 427–442.

Mezzina, R., Mazzuia, P., Vidoni, D., & Impagnatiello, M. (1992). Networking consumer's participation in a community mental health service: Mutual support groups, "citizenship" and coping strategies. *International Journal of Social Psychiatry, 38*(1), 68–73.

Minkler, M. (1992). Community organizing among the elderly poor in the United States: A case study. *International Journal of Health Services, 22*(2), 303–316.

Morewood-Northrop, M. (1994). Overview: Nursing in the Northwest Territories. *Canadian Nurse, 90*(3), 26–31.

Mundinger, M.O. (1996). New alliances: Nursing's bright future. *Nursing Administration Quarterly, 20*(3), 50–53.

Murphy, N.J. (1993). An upstream approach to health care: The education of nurses for policy change. *Journal of Nursing Education, 32*(6), 285–287.

National Forum on Health. (1996). *Canada health action: Building on the legacy. Final report of the National Forum on Health* (Vol. 1.) Ottawa: Minister of Public Works and Government Services.

Nelson, J.A. (1997). Gay, lesbian, and bisexual adolescents: Providing esteem-enhancing care to a battered population. *Nurse Practitioner, 22*(2), 94–103.

Netting, F.E., & Williams, F.G. (1997). Case manager–physician collaboration: Implications for professional identity, roles, and relationships. *Health and Social Work, 21*(3), 216–224.

Neufeld, A., & Harrison, M.J. (1990). The development of nursing diagnoses for aggregates and groups. *Public Health Nursing, 7*(4), 251–255.

Norton, D., & Ridenour, H. (1995). Homeless women and children: The challenge of health promotion. *Nurse Practitioner Forum, 6*(1), 29–33.

Nova Scotia Health Survey. (1995). *Community health and epidemiology, Dalhousie.* Halifax: Public Health Section, Department of Health, Government of Nova Scotia.

Oermann, M. (1994). Reforming nursing education for future practice. *Journal of Nursing Education, 33*(5), 215–219.

O'Neill, M. (1992). Community participation in Quebec's health system: A strategy to curtail community empowerment? *International Journal of Health Services, 22*(2), 287–301.

Paavilainen, E., & Astedt-Kurki, P. (1997). The client–nurse relationship as experienced by public health nurses: Toward better collaboration. *Public Health Nursing, 14*(3), 137–142.

Parette, H.P., Jr., & Parette, P.C. (1992). Young children with disabilities and assistant technology: The nurse's role on multidisciplinary technology teams. *Journal of Pediatric Nursing, 7*(4), 237–245.

Pearson, P. (1992). Defining the primary care team. *Health Visitor, 65*(10), 358–361.

Pederson, A., O'Neill, M., & Rootman, I. (1994). *Health promotion in Canada: Provincial, national and international perspectives.* Toronto: W.B. Saunders Canada.

Pender, N.J., Barkauskas, V.H., Hayman, L., Rice, V.H., & Anderson, E.T. (1992). Health promotion and disease prevention: Toward excellence in nursing practice and education. *Nursing Outlook, 40*(3), 106–120.

Perry, L.E. (1996). Preconception care: A health promotion opportunity. *Nurse Practitioner: American Journal of Primary Health Care, 21*(11), 24, 26, 32.

Pesznecker, B.L., Zerwekh, J.V., & Horn, B.J. (1989). The mutual-participation relationship: Key to facilitating self-care practices in clients and families. *Public Health Nursing, 6*(4), 197–203.

Plumb, J.D. (1997). Homelessness: Care, prevention, and public policy. *Annals of Internal Medicine, 126*(12), 973–975.

Poulton, B.C. (1996). Use of the consultation satisfaction questionnaire to examine patients' satisfaction with general practitioners and community nurses: Reliability, replicability and discriminant validity. *British Journal of General Practice, 46*(402), 26–31.

Poulton, B.C., & West, M.A. (1993). Effective multidisciplinary teamwork in primary health care. *Journal of Advanced Nursing, 18*, 918–925.

Poulton, B.C., & West, M.A. (1994). Primary health care team effectiveness: Developing a constituency approach. *Health and Social Care in the Community, 2*(2), 77–84.

Powell-Cope, G.M. (1994). Family caregivers of people with AIDS: Negotiating partnerships with professional health care providers. *Nursing Research, 43*(6), 324–332.

Primary Health Care Round Table (1990). What still needs to be done? *World Health Forum, 11*, 359–366.

Primas, P.J., & Mileham, T.L. (1995). Reaching out to the working poor: A collaborative effort. In B. Murphy (Ed.), Nursing centers: The time is now. *National League for Nursing Publications, 41*(2629), 181–201.

Primas, P.J., Mileham, T., Toronto, C., & McCoy, B.J. (1994). Breaking the cycle of disadvantage: A nursing system of health care. *Nursing and Health Care, 15*(1), 10–17.

Remkes, T. (1992). Primary health care in Newfoundland. *Canadian Nurse, 88*(5), 14–15, 47.

Ritchie, J.E. (1994). Education for primary health care: Accommodating the new realities. *World Health Forum, 15*(2), 147–149.

Robb, N. (1996). Telecare acting as an "electronic grandmother" for New Brunswickers. *Canadian Medical Association Journal, 154*(6), 903–904.

Rodger, J. (1994). Primary health care provision for people with learning difficulties. *Health and Social Care in the Community, 2*(1), 11–17.

Romeder, J.M. (1990). *The self-help way: Mutual aid and health.* Ottawa: Canadian Council on Social Development.

Rousseau, C. (1993). Community empowerment: The alternative resources movement in Quebec. *Community Mental Health Journal, 29*(6), 535–546.

Ruka, S.M., Brown, J.A., & Procope, B. (1997). Clinical exemplar. A blending of health strategies in a community-based nursing center. *Clinical Nurse Specialist, 11*(4), 179–187.

Russon, N. (1997). Linking the healthcare continuum with technology. *International Journal of Health Care Quality Assurance Incorporating Leadership in Health Services, 10*(1), S-vii–S-ix.

Ruston, A. (1996). Women and "safer sex" promotion: Perceptions of risk and provision of effective interventions in different health care settings. *Health Education Journal, 55*(4), 404–412.

Sandelowski, M. (1993). Toward a theory of technology dependency. *Nursing Outlook, 41*(1), 36–42.

Sandiford, P., Annett, H., & Cibulskis, R. (1992). What can information systems do for primary health care: An international perspective. *Social Science and Medicine, 34*(10), 1077–1087.

Schmidt, L., Brandt, J., & Norris, K. (1995). The advanced registered nurse practitioner in rural practice. *Kansas Nurse, 70*(9), 1–2.

Schraeder, C., Britt, T., Dworak, D., & Shelton, P. (1997). Management of nursing within a collaborative physician group practice. *Seminars for Nurse Managers, 5*(3), 133–138.

Shanks, J. (1996). A health delivery model for rural Saskatchewan. *Concern, 25*(2), 11–12.

Sheer, B. (1996). Reaching collaboration through empowerment: A developmental process. *Journal of Obstetric, Gynecologic, and Neonatal Nursing, 25*(6), 513–517.

Shoultz, J., & Hatcher, P.A. (1997). Looking beyond primary care to primary health care: An approach to community-based action. *Nursing Outlook, 45*(1), 23–26.

Singh, A., & Pandey, J. (1990). Social support as a moderator of the relationship between poverty and coping behaviors. *Journal of Social Psychology, 130*(4), 533–541.

Smillie, C. (1992). Preparing health professionals for a collaborative health promotion role. *Canadian Journal of Public Health, 83*(4), 279–282.

Smith, D.L., & Bryant, J.H. (1988). Building the infrastructure for primary health care: An overview of vertical and integrated approaches. *Social Science and Medicine, 26*(9), 909–917.

SmithBattle, L. (1995). Teenage mothers' narratives of self: An examination of risking the future. *Advances in Nursing Science, 17*(4), 22–36.

Stafford, A., & Hannigan, B. (1997). Client-held records in community mental health. *Nursing Times, 93*(7), 50–51.

Statistics Canada. (1993). *Profile of urban and rural areas—Part A: Canada, provinces and territories.* Ottawa: Minister of Industry, Science & Technology. (Cat. No. 930339)

Stewart, M.J. (1990a). Access to health care for economically disadvantaged Canadians: A model. *Canadian Journal of Public Health, 81*(6), 450–455.

Stewart, M.J. (1990b). Professional interface with mutual-aid self-help groups: A review. *Social Science and Medicine, 31*(1), 1143–1158.

Stewart, M.J. (1993). *Integrating social support in nursing.* Newbury Park, CA: Sage.

Stewart, M. (1997). Health promotion research centres in Canada. *Canadian Journal of Nursing Research, 29*(1), 133–154.

Stewart, M., Banks, S., Crossman, D., & Poel, D. (1996). Partnerships between health professionals and self-help groups: Meaning and mechanisms. *Prevention in Human Services, 11*(2), 199–240.

Stewart, M., Gillis, A., Brosky, G., Johnston, B., Kirkland, S., Leigh, G., Pesaud, V., Rootman, I., Jackson, S., & Pawliw-Fry, B.A. (1996). Smoking among disadvantaged women: Causes and cessation. *Canadian Journal of Nursing Research, 28*(1), 41–60.

Stewart, M., Hart, G., & Mann, K. (1994). Living with hemophilia and HIV/AIDS: Support and coping. *Journal of Advanced Nursing, 22,* 1101–1111.

Stewart, M., Reed, G., Jackson, S., Buckles, L., Edgar, W., Mangham, C., & Tilley, N. (1996). Community resilience: Strengths and challenges *Health and Canadian Society, 4*(1), 53–81.

Stone, L. (1992). Cultural influences in community participation in health. *Social Science and Medicine, 35*(4), 409–417.

Sullivan, N.M. (1995). Primary health care and correctional nursing—the link. *Info Nursing, 26*(1), 8–9.

Sumner, P. (1997). Elderly care counts. Primary concerns . . . Links between primary health care services and older people . . . in the community and in residential homes. *Nursing Times, 93*(8), 54–55.

Tomblin-Murphy, G., Ritchie, J.A., Stewart, M.J., & Johnson, A. (in press). *Social support, work satisfaction, and coping among Canadian nurses in HIV/AIDS care.* Funded by NHRDP and the Dalhousie Research and Development Fund.

Toseland, R.W., Rossiter, C.M., Peak, T., & Hill, P. (1990). Therapeutic processes in peer-led and professionally led support groups for caregivers. *International Journal of Community Psychology, 40,* 279–303.

Townsend, E. (1994). *Enabling empowerment or managing medical cases? Occupational therapy's mental health work.* Doctoral thesis, Dalhousie University, Halifax, Nova Scotia.

Tripp, S.L., & Stachowiak, B. (1992). Health maintenance, health promotion: Is there a difference? *Public Health Nursing, 9*(3), 155–161.

van Harteveld, J.T., Mistiaen, P.J., & Dukkers van Emden, D.M. (1997). Home visits by community nurses for cancer patients after discharge from hospital: An evaluation study of the continuity visit. *Cancer Nursing, 20*(2), 105–114.

Van Hook, M.P. (1996). Challenges to identifying and treating women with depression in rural primary care. *Social Work in Health Care, 23*(3), 73–92.

Wallace, P., Awan, A., & Talbot, J. (1996). Health advice for Asian women with diabetes. *Professional Nurse, 11*(12), 794–796.

Wallerstein, N. (1992). Powerlessness, empowerment, and health: Implications for health promotion programs. *American Journal of Health Promotion, 6*(3), 197–205.

Ward-Griffin, C., & Bramwell, L. (1990). The congruence of elderly client and nurse perceptions of the clients' self-care agency. *Journal of Advanced Nursing, 15,* 1070–1077.

Welch, H. (1996). Nurse midwives as primary care providers for women. *Clinical Nurse Specialist, 10*(3), 121–124.

Werch, C.E., Carlson, J.M., Pappas, D.M., & DiClemente, C.C. (1996). Brief nurse consultations for preventing alcohol use among urban school youth. *Journal of School Health, 66*(9), 335–338.

Williams, R.B., Boles, M., & Johnson, R.E. (1995). Patient use of a computer for prevention in primary care practice. *Patient Education and Counseling, 25*(3), 283–292.

World Health Organization (WHO). (1978). *Report of the international conference on Primary Health Care in Alma Ata, USSR.* Geneva, Switzerland: Author.

Zerwekh, J.V. (1992). The practice of empowerment and coercion by expert public health nurses. *Image: Journal of Nursing Scholarship, 24*(2), 101–105.

Zungolo, E. (1994). Interdisciplinary education in primary care: The challenge. *Nursing and Health Care, 15*(6), 288–292.

C H A P T E R   4

Social support, coping, and self-care as public participation mechanisms

Miriam J. Stewart

As public participation is a key principle of Primary Health Care, and as social support, coping, and self-care are important mechanisms of public participation, community health nurses need to mobilize social support, foster coping, and promote self-care. This chapter focusses on social support, its relationship to coping and self-care, and its impact on health, health behaviour, and health services use. These associations are illustrated by examples from assessment and intervention projects in the Social Support Research Program at Dalhousie University School of Nursing. The implications for community health nursing practice are highlighted.

LEARNING OBJECTIVES

In this chapter, you will learn:

* why social support, coping, and self-care are forms of public participation
* the impact of social support on health outcomes
* factors that influence support interventions by community health nurses
* community nursing interventions that could foster coping and self-care

Introduction

As shown in Chapter 3, public participation is a key principle of Primary Health Care. Support, coping, and self-care are important mechanisms of public participation; thus, they are critical concepts for community health nurses to understand and apply in practice. The structure, function, and appraisal of social support; its conceptual relationship to coping with stress and to self-care; and its impact on health, health behaviour, and health services use are illustrated by examples from the assessment and intervention projects conducted in the Social Support Research Program (SSRP), Dalhousie University School of Nursing (see Table 4.1).

Table 4.1
Social Support Research Program, Dalhousie University
School of Nursing

Type of Support	Assessment	Intervention
Chronic illness & family caregivers	Mothers of children with chronic illness	Telephone support intervention for parents of children with chronic illness
	Children with chronic illness Children with stressful health care encounters	Mutual aid via computer for adolescents with chronic conditions
	Persons with heart failure/ stroke and family caregivers myocardial infarction	Support groups for couples coping with myocardial infarction
Support for professional caregivers	Support, stress, job satisfaction, and coping by nurses in HIV/AIDS care	Telephone support groups for community and hospital nurses in HIV/AIDS care
	Support, stress, and satisfaction experienced by community health nurses	
Peer & professional support	Partnership between self-help groups and health professionals	Education manual for health professionals

Social support

Social support is a significant concept for community health nurses because it influences health status, health behaviour, and health services use. Some argue that a global concept of social support should be replaced by precise concepts and models (Coyne & Bulger, 1990; Dunkel-Schetter & Bennett, 1990).

Social support is defined here as interactions with family members, friends, peers, and health care providers that communicate information, esteem, aid, and emotional help. These communications may improve coping, moderate the impact of stressors, and promote health and self-care (Stewart, 1993, p. 7). Social support occurs as a by-product of people's ongoing interactions. However, we cannot assume that it is always accessible or beneficial. Instead, it is important to understand how supportive interactions are elicited with different people, how social support can be expressed in different forms, and how it can be miscarried or dissipate over time (Stewart, 1993). The three dimensions of the construct of social support include *structure, function,* and *appraisal.*

Structure of support

The structure of social support comprises lay sources such as partners/ spouses, family members, friends, neighbours, co-workers, volunteers, and self-help groups, as well as professional sources such as health professionals. Professionals can provide temporary, specialized support, or can enable and mobilize lay support (Stewart, 1993).

Consistent with other research on support providers (e.g., Dakof & Taylor, 1990), the studies in the Dalhousie Social Support Research Program (SSRP) revealed that most support is provided by family and close relationships. Mothers of children with chronic illness revealed that most support came from family members, spouses or partners, and friends. Children with chronic conditions reported that their key supporters were their parents and family members. Partners were named as the primary source of support for individuals who had recently experienced a myocardial infarction. Thus, intimate relationships are important sources of support (Johnson, Hobfoll, & Zalcberg-Linetzy, 1993). Principal sources of support for persons on the waiting list for cardiac transplantation in four Canadian transplant centres were family, friends, and health professionals; peers were identified less frequently (Hirth & Stewart, 1994). Similarly, an investigation of the support experienced by men with end-stage renal disease revealed that their networks consisted primarily of family members, followed by friends, health professionals, and a few peers (Cormier-Daigle & Stewart, 1997).

The support provided by or desired from health professionals and peers emerged as a common theme in several studies in our research program. Although most mothers of chronically ill children referred to health professionals as key members of their support networks, they reported inadequate and deficient support from some health professionals. Health professionals were identified infrequently as sources of support by persons with ischemic heart disease and by seniors with chronic cardiac illness or stroke and their family caregivers. Moreover, men with hemophilia and HIV/AIDS, their family caregivers, and bereaved caregivers experienced insensitivity and prejudice from professionals.

Persons with AIDS and their caregivers desired support from identical peers—that is, persons with hemophilia and AIDS, *not* persons with AIDS only. The top-ranked support interventions in other assessment studies also involved disease-specific peers in dyadic or group relationships. For example, mothers of children with cystic fibrosis wanted support groups consisting of other mothers of children with cystic fibrosis, not of mothers of children with any chronic illness. Children with chronic conditions had much less peer support than their healthy counterparts and almost no contact with children who had the same condition. In a related study, during an acute stressful situation—venipuncture—young children sought and received support from nurses.

All these studies have implications for support interventions, in particular for those using professionals and peers. Although peers and peer groups can supplement the support from deficient or depleted natural networks and from professionals (Katz, 1993; Stewart, 1990), groups have been overlooked as providers of support (Felton & Berry, 1992). Respondents' preferences for meeting with similar peers who can provide affirmational support (i.e., interactions that involve feedback and appraisal) have implications for interventions by community health nurses. Community health nurses who create support groups or dyads should recognize that it is not sufficient to match participants on the basis of the shared problem or affliction only. These studies have taught us to look more closely at other dimensions, such as length of time since diagnosis, gender, age, marital status, and how the illness was contracted.

Functions of support

The four functions of support are emotional, instrumental (practical), informational, and affirmational (House & Kahn, 1985). Types of support functions should be specific to stressors encountered (Cutrona, 1990). Furthermore, specific types of support are most helpful when they are provided by particular sources (Dakof & Taylor, 1990). People waiting for cardiac transplantation indicated that families provided the most emotional and practical support, and that health professionals usually provided information about the procedure and their health status. Some professionals also offered affirmational support (feedback) and emotional support (encouragement and reassurance) (Hirth & Stewart, 1994). Mothers of children with chronic illness usually received informational support from health professionals; however, they wanted, but did not typically receive, feedback and reassurance from them.

Health professionals provided informational support for hemophiliacs with AIDS and their caregivers; relatives provided practical aid; and spouses and close family members were primary sources of emotional support. Our investigation of self-help groups revealed that health professionals were identified as educators and referral resources (i.e., informational support providers), while peers were valued for both emotional support and for their knowledge based on first-hand experience (affirmational support). This study and the study of hemophiliacs with AIDS indicated that joint leadership of self-help groups and support groups by peers and professionals was desired. Therefore, the telephone support groups for hemophiliacs with AIDS and their caregivers and for parents of children with chronic conditions, and the face-to-face support groups for couples coping with myocardial infarction, were co-facilitated by peers and professionals.

It is striking that a consistent pattern of specialization in support emerged across these studies: many participants perceived that family members specialized in practical support, health professionals in informational support, spouses/partners in emotional support, and peers in affirmational support. This suggests that support figures cannot readily be substituted for one another and that community health nurses should assess clients' and caregivers' unmet expectations for particular kinds of support from particular sources. This could help community health nurses plan strategies to augment or compensate for deficiencies in the support provided by the client or family caregiver's social network.

Appraisal of support

Social support may be perceived as potentially available from the social network, or may be actually delivered and received (Sarason, Sarason, & Pierce, 1990). It is important to distinguish the psychological sense of support from the actual expression and exchange of support (Dunkel-Schetter & Bennett, 1990). Support received from providers is appraised or evaluated with respect to its duration, direction, and drawbacks or benefits. Therefore, community health nurses should assess clients' receipt of support as well as their perceptions of support availability.

Duration. Support can endure or dissipate over time, depending on the stressor (Stewart, 1993). The changes that take place in an individual's social network over time (Bernard et al., 1990) in chronic stressful situations, such as illness or caregiving, should be examined. For example, there was a significant decrease in all types of support and in support from friends experienced by potential cardiac transplant recipients after 90 days on the waiting list (Hirth & Stewart, 1994). In the investigation of the role of social support in early readmissions of persons with cardiac disease, readmitted persons reported loss of more members from their social network than the non-readmitted group. For example, they reported less support from neighbours after more than one admission to hospital. The timing of support was a critical concern for mothers of children with chronic conditions who contended that support was needed at the time of diagnosis, but frequently was not available when required. Some mothers also described how support that was initially provided by others did not last.

These studies have implications for the timing of support interventions by community health nurses (as shown in Chapter 27, on intervention research). Accordingly, SSRP peer support intervention was directed at new family caregivers of seniors who had experienced a stroke for the first time and had recently been discharged from hospital to community. Similarly, the duration of support is important for determining intervention "dose." Thus, a peer (an experienced family caregiver) visited the home of the new family caregiver of a stroke survivor twice weekly over a period of 12 weeks, and the impact of the intervention was assessed, not only at the end of the 12 weeks, but also three and six months following the completion of the intervention. In the delayed post-test interviews, caregivers contended that they missed the peers when the visits terminated. Similarly, hemophiliacs with AIDS and their family caregivers indicated that they would have liked telephone support groups to continue longer.

Direction. Support can be unidirectional/non-reciprocal or bidirectional/reciprocal. Norms of equity and reciprocity (Tilden & Galyen, 1987) suggest that support should be bidirectional. As social exchange and equity theories indicate, support can involve benefits and costs for both recipients and providers. Yet, reciprocity has been neglected in many social support studies. In fact, most studies measure support provided by others, not support given to others (Winemiller, Mitchell, Sutcliff, & Cline, 1993). The ill experience non-reciprocal relationships with their social networks and with health professionals. For example, persons with chronic mental illness may have less reciprocity with network members than other people (Simmons, 1994).

In the SSRP, persons with severe heart disease and stroke were most concerned with their inability to reciprocate support to their spouse as their illness progressed. In contrast to previous research, which revealed that ill persons experience limited reciprocity, hemodialysis-dependent males with end-stage renal disease reported moderately high levels of reciprocity with network members. Unlike other research, which shows that many caregivers of the chronically ill experience lack of reciprocity (e.g., Gottlieb, 1989), family caregivers of persons with AIDS and mothers of chronically ill children did not express negative feelings of burden typically associated with inequitable relationships. This may be because, as spouses or as parents of children in long-term intimate relationships, they were committed and had less concern about immediate reciprocation. This seems to provide evidence of lifespan reciprocity (Antonucci & Jackson, 1990; La Gaipa, 1990).

In another project, a key characteristic of partnership and of a positive relationship between health professionals and self-help group members (peers) was reciprocity. As a social worker said, "I give and I get; it is very much a two-way street." Interventions that involve peers typically promote reciprocity. This assumption informed the design of the telephone support groups for persons with hemophilia and AIDS and their family caregivers and for parents of children with chronic illness.

Drawbacks and benefits. Finally, social interactions can have drawbacks and benefits. Indeed, most social relationships have supportive and stressful elements (Rook, 1990). Drawbacks of support affect both support providers and recipients. Overload, overexposure to chronic and acute stresses, overprotection, and overcommitment might be consequences of providing support. Difficulties for the support recipient include feared loss of support, advice that constrains options, learned helplessness, relational costs, diminished trust, and weak relationships (La Gaipa, 1990). Support provided may be perceived as unhelpful, particularly when it undermines the recipient's self-esteem.

Nevertheless, there has been insufficient research about the negative effects of social networks, and measures of support typically disregard the negative aspects of relationships. Reports of low support may reflect the absence of a supportive relationship, the presence of a negative, conflicted relationship (Coyne & Bulger, 1990), or lost support (Robinson, 1990). Conflict, inhibited communication, and negative interactions correlate more strongly than positive interactions with perceptions of low support (Coyne & Downey, 1991; Schuster, Kessler, & Aseltine, 1990). In one study in the SSRP, negative relationships between health professionals and self-help group members entailed conflicts, struggle for control, competitiveness, dominance, territoriality, and judgemental interactions. In another study, persons with hemophilia and AIDS experienced prejudice and insensitivity from health professionals and avoidance by friends. Conflict experienced by male hemodialysis patients with end-stage renal disease was associated with a large number of household members.

Even successful relationships involve lapses in support, miscarried support efforts (Sarason, Sarason, & Pierce, 1990), and failed support modes or functions (Eckenrode & Gore, 1990). Mothers of chronically ill children seemed more concerned about absent support and miscarried helping (i.e., support intended to be helpful but not) than about conflict. As all these drawbacks of support may have more powerful influences on health (Rook, 1990) and use of health services than the more general benefits of support, both the supportive and non-supportive features of clients' interactions and relationships should be assessed by community health nurses. Furthermore, community health nurses should test support interventions designed to alleviate negative interactions, through their research and practice.

Relationship between stress and social support

Stress and social support have bidirectional effects. In the previous section, it was noted that conflicted interactions, miscarried helping, and inadequate support can be stressful. Social exchange (reciprocity) and social comparison theories can inform interpretations regarding why support can have stressful effects and why stress can decrease the availability of support resources (Buunk & Hoorens, 1992). In our study of mothers of children with chronic illness, conflicts with spouses over the care of their child and absence of anticipated support were considered stressful. Hemophiliacs with AIDS and their family caregivers found insensitivity, prejudice, and avoidance by friends and by health professionals particularly stressful.

Conversely, support can mediate or moderate the impact of stress on health and functioning outcomes. Stressful situations, such as illness, can be chronic as well as acute. Virtually all intervention studies in the SSRP were based on the premise that support has a moderating effect on the stress of chronic illness and of caregiving. Stress-moderating processes determine a person's reaction to or appraisal of stress (Eckenrode & Gore, 1990). Instructive correlations between stress appraisal and social support were identified in a study of people with ischemic heart disease who were admitted to hospital. Persons admitted for the first time appraised the stress associated with the cardiac condition as less central and threatening, and received less emotional and affirmational support from health professionals, than persons with multiple admissions for cardiac illness. In the investigation of young children's coping with a stressful procedure (venipuncture), supportive nursing interventions were associated with reports of less pain. These two studies of stress appraisal in chronic and acute stressful situations reveal links to professional support that could have important implications for support intervention research as well as for community health nursing practice. In this context, it is noteworthy that increased support was related to decreased stress and burnout experienced by community health nurses (Stewart & Arklie, 1994) and by nurses in HIV/AIDS care working in community and hospital sites.

Social support and coping

Social support, as a coping resource or coping assistance (Thoits, 1995), modifies the impact of acute and chronic stressors on health outcomes. Support and coping have a reciprocal relationship. Supportive persons can alter appraisal of stressors, sustain coping efforts, and influence choice of coping strategies. Conversely, the ways in which an individual copes provide important clues to potential supporters about whether support is needed and, if it is, about the types of support required (Gottlieb, 1988).

Silver, Wortman, and Crofton (1990) demonstrate that coping strategies influence support received. People who use avoidance and distancing have fewer support resources, while support seeking has been linked to greater provision of support (Barbee, Gulley, & Cunningham, 1990; Dunkel-Schetter & Skokan, 1990). Dunkel-Schetter and Bennett (1990) suggest that the "nature and skill of a person's coping strategies, applied to particular stressful situations, may mediate the extent to which available support materializes." Although individuals who present themselves as coping effectively may generate positive responses from potential providers, they may not signal a need for support. In contrast, disclosure of distress, accompanied by evidence of coping efforts and indications that support is needed, can influence the appropriateness of support provided (Silver, Wortman, & Crofton, 1990).

Perceived availability of social support improves coping effectiveness (Bennett, 1993). Social support may augment coping resources available to deal with stressful encounters. Thus, social support influences coping abilities, and coping strategies influence support sought and received.

This research program recognizes the limitations of an individualistic perspective that ignores the social context of coping (Folkman et al., 1991). The links between coping and support were explored in several studies. The SSRP investigation of community and hospital-based Canadian nurses in HIV/AIDS care revealed that as social support and coping increased, work satisfaction also increased. In the case of persons waiting for cardiac transplants, support from transplant recipients (peers) and from health professionals was significantly related to coping effectiveness (Hirth & Stewart, 1994). The key coping strategy used by persons with hemophilia and AIDS and their family caregivers was "seeking support." Those who sought support from new friends wanted peer support in self-help groups. In contrast, hemophiliacs with AIDS who coped by withdrawing from others did so because of fear of negative reactions, concern about confidentiality, and associated reluctance to seek support. Escape–avoidance by men with end-stage renal disease was associated with a large number of household members. Similar to the study of men with hemophilia, seeking social support was the most common coping strategy used by males with end-stage renal disease and by individuals who had been admitted to hospital for cardiac illness. A higher than median score on "seeking social support" predicted readmission of persons with ischemic heart disease.

In contrast to the adults in these studies, coping behaviours used by young children experiencing a painful procedure less often included support seeking. Persons skilled at seeking support are more effective in obtaining social support; however, these coping skills may be learned later as adolescents and adults. It is noteworthy, however, that the coping behaviours of these young children were influenced by supportive interactions with nurses, again revealing links between coping and social support. According to post-intervention interviews, the SSRP support interventions for parents of children with chronic conditions, for hemophiliacs with AIDS and their family caregivers, for couples coping with myocardial infarction, and for family caregivers of stroke survivors enhanced participants' ability to cope with the demands of chronic health conditions and caregiving.

The Dalhousie researchers found that coping strategies, in addition to being emotion- or problem-focussed, may be relationship-focussed. In close support relationships, the coping of one partner influences the coping behaviours used by the other (Coyne & Downey, 1991; Gottlieb & Wagner, 1991). Mothers described their efforts to maintain their marriage and to cope with their spouses' lack of support for, and involvement in, the caregiving of their chronically ill child. They seemed to use "active engagement" (i.e., shared problem solving and open discussion) or "protective buffering" of stresses (Coyne & Downey, 1991) in interactions with their spouse to cope with these relationship stressors (Stewart, Ritchie, et al., 1997). Spouses of survivors coping with myocardial infarction used less protective buffering following a support group intervention.

Hemophiliacs with AIDS and their family caregivers used coping strategies aimed at keeping their personal relationships normal. Participants with end-stage cardiac disease and stroke, who were on average 69 years of age and married for 40 years, experienced stressors and support as a couple. They were satisfied with their relationship with their spouses, perhaps reflecting less need for relationship coping in long-term stable relationships.

Impact of social support on health, health behaviour, and health services use

Health

There is a bidirectional relationship between social support and health. Integration in a social network and support resources from the network can maintain health and facilitate physical recovery (Bloom, 1990). Kaplan and Toshima (1990) reviewed evidence that social support enhances health outcomes and reduces mortality, whereas stressful social relationships can prolong physical dysfunction. Epidemiological studies link social networks to morbidity and mortality. Socially integrated people are less likely to have tuberculosis, depression, hypertension, accidents, pregnancy complications, and schizophrenia (Ford & Procidano, 1990; House, Umberson, & Landis, 1988). However, these studies do not explain why social relationships enhance health. Current research focusses on three hypotheses: social support may prevent stress; social support buffers or cushions stress; and social support may have a direct positive effect on health unrelated to stress (Tilden & Weinert, 1987).

The *main-effect model* proposes that social support benefits well-being directly by fulfilling social needs and enhancing social integration (Cohen & Wills, 1985). The *buffering model* suggests that support protects individuals from harmful influences of stressful situations and enhances coping abilities. Quittner, Glueckauf, and Jackson (1990) indicate that the buffer model and the moderator model are similar. The *moderator model* predicts that perceived support interacts with stress to modify psychological adjustment; hence, social support is most beneficial under conditions of high stress. The *mediator model* predicts that social support acts as an intervening variable influencing indirectly the effects of stress on health. For example, parents reporting chronic caregiving burden might experience reduced or conflicted social interaction, which in turn would be associated with poorer mental health status (Quittner et al., 1990). Indeed, negative interactions are more predictive of depressed mood and poor emotional health than supportive interactions (Coyne & Downey, 1991; Rook, 1990; Schuster et al., 1990).

The SSRP intervention studies hypothesized that support would have a moderating impact on health outcomes in the context of chronic stressors. For example, it was anticipated that the support intervention for family caregivers of seniors with stroke would have a positive impact on the caregivers' psychological health, through decreased subjective burden; total burden as well as time, physical, and development burdens did decrease following the intervention. As predicted, face-to-face support groups for couples coping with myocardial infarction were associated with decreased negative affect. It was anticipated that telephone support groups for hemophiliacs with AIDS and for their caregivers would enhance psychological health by decreasing loneliness; social and emotional loneliness did diminish following the intervention. Finally, we predict that telephone support groups for parents of ill children will enhance their psychological health and perceived competence. These intervention studies can inform support interventions by community health nurses.

Support also influences health outcomes of community health nurses themselves. For example, total support and work-related support led to decreased burnout among community health nurses. Increased emotional support was associated with decreased emotional exhaustion (a component of burnout) experienced by nurses in AIDS care. Moreover, as affirmational and informational support increased, their burnout decreased.

Health behaviour
Support also has an impact on health behaviour. Social network members may influence health behaviour directly through motivation or provision of

information, and indirectly through encouragement to comply with regimes or to maintain health behaviours. Network members provide advice and role models and may constrain people from inappropriate behaviours (Bloom, 1990). Zimmerman and Connor (1989) found that the greatest influences on health behaviours were supportiveness, encouragement, and modelling by family members, friends, and co-workers. We anticipated, therefore, that a face-to-face support group intervention for couples coping with myocardial infarction would increase their perceived efficacy to make required lifestyle changes; spouses and survivors reported increased confidence during post-intervention interviews.

One form of health behaviour is *self-care*. Orem's (1991) individualistic theory of self-care can be adapted to community health nursing, as the community can foster self-care by protecting the "self-care agency" of individuals and by controlling environmental hazards (Taylor & McLaughlin, 1991). Braden's (1993) self-help model stresses the factors that enable people to engage in self-help behaviour. Self-help groups are important sources of support that enable self-care (Katz, 1993; Segal, Silverman, & Temkin, 1993; Stewart, 1993). Self-care practices can be taught or reinforced within self-help groups and other support networks. Moreover, self-care and self-help groups are manifestations of public participation. Community health nurses are faced with the challenge of developing meaningful partnerships with these informal helping networks.

In the assessment study of seniors with heart failure and stroke, there was considerable satisfaction with support and high self-care ability. The peer support intervention for family caregivers was predicted to have an indirect influence on stroke survivors' self-care because of the peers' experiential knowledge concerning strategies that foster it.

Interactions with network members may also yield negative outcomes, such as reinforcement of poor health behaviours or diminished self-care. For example, mothers expressed concern about the negative impact of peers on their adolescents' adherence to regimen and self-care.

Health services use

Finally, social network members can influence health services use by providing desired support, by acting as screening and referral agents, and by transmitting values about help seeking (Birkel & Repucci, 1983). Positive beliefs about help seeking are associated with support mobilization (Dunkel-Schetter & Bennett, 1990), and information on support seeking is related to social support skills (Hobfoll & Freedy, 1990).

It was anticipated that caregivers who had peer support would be less likely to seek expensive professional health services (e.g., take stroke survivors to hospitals). Visits to hospital emergency departments and outpatient departments did decline following the peer visitor intervention. In another study, mothers of children with chronic illness discussed their support needs associated with their child's health care, clinic appointments, and use of health services. Thus, support for family caregivers may influence health services use by ill persons. This indirect influence can be taken into account in planning community-based support interventions.

Health and illness affect availability and quality of social support. Illness can be a major stressor involving loss of social mobility, independence, capacity to work, status, and relationships. The continued need for social support in chronic stressful situations can deplete support and drain social network resources. Furthermore, chronic illness may produce alienation and estrangement from the network (Stewart, 1993). Thus, support can diminish over time in chronic stressful situations involving ill health.

Persons with hemophilia and AIDS and their family caregivers experienced isolation and avoidance by friends who were formerly supportive. Mothers of chronically ill children, particularly those with extensive physical caregiving demands, described absence of support that had been anticipated from network members. Persons with a history of admission to hospital for ischemic heart disease reported less support from neighbours than those admitted for the first time. As these studies target populations affected by chronic illness, these findings have implications for community health nursing practice. In chronic stressful situations, nurses need to assess duration of support, changes in types of support provided by specific sources, and alterations in appraisal of support to determine gaps in support experienced by their clients.

Implications for community health nursing interventions

Social support is an important protective factor in resilience (Egeland, Carlson, & Sroufe, 1993; Garmezy, 1993), and resilience is relevant to health promotion (Mangham, McGrath, Reid, & Stewart, 1994). Social support is discussed in relation to resilience of chronically ill children and adolescents (Brown, Doepke, & Kaslow, 1993), children living in poverty and other high-risk situations (Garmezy, 1993; Jessor, 1993), and families coping with illness (McCubbin & McCubbin, 1993). Social support is encompassed in interventions aimed at promoting resilience (e.g., Kumpfer & Hopkins, 1993).

Support programs
Social support, coping, and self-care have implications for community health nursing interventions. Many support programs have focussed on clients with chronic conditions and family caregivers. Ambulatory care centres provide opportunity for community health nurses to give emotional support

and information to cancer survivors and their families (Anderson, 1989). An education and support program for newly diagnosed cardiac clients and their families was implemented by community-based nurses in eastern Canada (Wiggins, 1989). Community health nurses also provide social support for clients with stroke (Richardson, Warburton, Wolfe, & Rudd, 1996), pulmonary disease (Dow & Mest, 1997), dialysis (Watson, 1996), injuries (Hemingway, 1996), myocardial infarction (Salisbury, 1996), and terminal illness (Hatcliffe, Smith, & Daw, 1996) and for older people with dementia and their family caregivers (Adams, 1996). Given that caregivers of mentally impaired elders who have low social support are at high risk for distress or depression, nurses should offer informational, practical, emotional, and spiritual support (Baillie, Norbeck, & Barnes, 1988; Doornbos, 1997). Community nurses provide information and practical help with vocational rehabilitation to psychiatric clients (Shepherd & Hill, 1996). Relapse rates of psychiatric clients were reduced when family-centred support included information, emotional support, and practical assistance (James, 1996). Families with chronically ill members (Sharkey, 1995; Zerwekh, 1995) and families with special needs (Cross & Marks, 1996) also need support from community health nurses.

Support interventions also focus on transitions across the lifespan. Community health nurses offered a unique breastfeeding support drop-in in Vancouver (Davidson, 1996). A joint program between the York Region Public Health Department and a social service agency provided support and education focussed on child sexual abuse (Breen, 1994). In a community development program for family caregivers in British Columbia, nurses offered education and support to families following a SIDS death (Baumer & McLinden, 1994). Community health nurses can include the friends of diabetic teenagers in teaching sessions and link their mothers with a mutual aid group (Dean, 1989). Community nurse visits to low-income teenage mothers emphasized education about parenting and health; recruitment of support from boyfriends, family members, and friends; and linkage to community agencies. Positive effects for the adolescent mother included improved health behaviour and interaction with children (Olds & Kitzman, 1990). Community health nursing support interventions focussing on seniors have involved senior companion/visiting nurse partnerships (Williams, 1995) and information for family caregivers of older adults (Mahoney & Shippee-Rice, 1994).

Social support for disadvantaged populations such as clients with HIV/AIDS or substance use problems (Willis, 1995), abused women (Dickson & Tutty, 1996), and people from minority cultures (DiMartile Bolla, DeJoseph, Norbeck, & Smith, 1996) or in rural settings (Hegney, 1996) is important. Community health nurses working in homes, schools, clinics, community centres, and occupational health settings can employ these support strategies with clients experiencing chronic conditions, caregiving, transitions, or stigma.

Community-based nurses in occupational health settings could use support to promote health behaviour change and ameliorate work-related stressors. For example, partner and group support in smoking-cessation and weight-loss programs (Cohen, 1988) and support training programs for the unemployed (Heller, Price, & Hogg, 1990) could be adapted as support interventions by nurses.

Coping interventions

Community health nurses foster coping of families experiencing bereavement (Kiberd, 1996; Webb, Roberts, & Grainger, 1995), homeless people (Killion, 1995), family caregivers (Grant, 1996), and people with chronic conditions (Martin, 1995). Burke et al. (1997) report that a community-based nursing intervention improved coping by families of children with chronic illness (this study is described in Chapter 11).

Self-help and self-care interventions

Other interventions by community health nurses focus on individual self-help and self-care. For example, one nursing intervention for women with systemic lupus erythematosus, which incorporated specific self-care activities (e.g., monitoring of symptoms, relaxation, exercise, pain management), increased their self-efficacy and self-worth and decreased depression (Braden, 1993). Community health nurses are in a key position to detect problems related to self-care practices such as over-the-counter medication use by the elderly (Conn, 1992). One self-care intervention for elderly clients with arthritis involved informational support about medications, exercise, depression, nutrition, sleep, relationships, and community resources, and encouraged active self-care (Albrecht et al., 1993; Goeppinger, Macnee, Anderson, Boutaugh, & Stewart, 1995). Other self-care programs involving community health nurses focussed on clients with diabetes (Mazzuca, Farris, Mendenhall, & Stoupa, 1997) or multiple sclerosis (Campion, 1996), client-controlled analgesia (Seaby & Roberts, 1996), smoking cessation (Utz, Shuster, Merwin, & Williams, 1994), and senior citizens (Wissman & Wilmoth, 1996).

Community health nurses enabled family self-help by praising the positive behaviours of the family, affirming the family's perspective, and helping the family anticipate a better future. These strategies developed the family's capacity for autonomy, responsibility, and self-care.

Implications for community health nurses

Social support can have implications for community health nurses themselves. Reutter and Ford (1996) found that public health nurses in Alberta believed their work is not well supported by others. In Nova Scotia, 90 percent of support for community health nurses came from spouses, family members, friends, and work associates; perceived lack of supervisor support was a major stressor. The primary types of support received by these nurses were emotional and affirmational (Stewart & Arklie, 1994). Nurses working in HIV care in the community and in hospital stressed the importance of emotional and affirmational support (Tomblin-Murphy, Stewart, Ritchie, & Johnson, in press). Clearly, community health nurses need support from colleagues (Billingham & Perkins, 1997). Support interventions for community nurses include burnout workshops (Schaufeli, 1995) and staff support groups (Thomas, 1995). Networking and support groups were important in the life of a public health nurse leader in Prince Edward Island (Baldwin, 1995). Another support intervention reduced stress experienced by community psychiatric nurses (Leary et al., 1995).

Self-care also has implications for nurses. One study found a positive relationship between community health nurses' "self-care agency" and their job satisfaction. Fostering nurses' self-care may promote job retention (Behm & Frank, 1992).

Conclusion

The impact of health system reform on Canadians' need for and ability to engage in social support, coping, and self-care should be examined. More research is needed on the support and coping of groups and communities, particularly those in rural and urban areas, from varied cultures, or with limited financial resources. The complex linkages among coping, social support, and self-care require further study. Furthermore, the impact of nursing interventions that mobilize social support, foster coping, and promote self-care should be tested. There is, however, evidence that community health nurses can promote public participation by integrating these concepts into their Primary Health Care practice.

Acknowledgements

The Dalhousie Social Support Research Program was made possible through a Scholar Award to the author from the Medical Research Council of Canada and the National Health Research Development Program. The contributions of the investigators and participants in all studies are gratefully acknowledged. The astute advice of Dr. Benjamin Gottlieb, the consultant, guided the development of this research program. An earlier version of the initial sections of this chapter appeared in Stewart, M., Ellerton, M., Hart, G., Hirk, N., Mann, K., Meghan-Stewart, D., & Tomblin-Murphy, G. (1997), "Insights from a Nursing Research Program on Social Support," *Canadian Journal of*

Nursing Research, 29(3), 93–110. This program of research is detailed in the book *Chronic Conditions and Caregiving in Canada: Sound Support Strategies?* (M. Stewart, Ed.), to be published by the University of Toronto Press in 2000.

QUESTIONS

1. Why are social support, coping, and self-care considered mechanisms of public participation?
2. How are social support, coping, and self-care related to health promotion?
3. What specific strategies could the community health nurse use to foster support, coping, and self-care of clients?

REFERENCES

Adams, T. (1996). Informal family caregiving to older people with dementia: Research priorities for community psychiatric nursing. *Journal of Advanced Nursing, 24*(4), 703–710.

Albrecht, M., Goeppinger, J., Anderson, M.K., Bautaugh, M., MacNee, C., & Stewart, K. (1993). The Albrecht nursing model for home health care: Predictors of satisfaction in a self-care intervention program. *Journal of Nursing Administration, 23*(1), 51–54.

Anderson, J.L. (1989). The nurse's role in cancer rehabilitation. *Cancer Nursing, 12*(2), 85–93.

Antonucci, T.C., & Jackson, J.S. (1990). The role of reciprocity in social support. In B.R. Sarason, I.G. Sarason, & G.R. Pierce (Eds.), *Social support: An interactional view* (pp. 173–198). New York: Wiley.

Baillie, V., Norbeck, J., & Barnes, L. (1988). Stress, social support and psychological distress of family caregivers of the elderly. *Nursing Research, 37,* 217–222.

Baldwin, D. (1995). Interconnecting the personal and public: The support networks of public health nurse Mona Wilson. *Canadian Journal of Nursing Research, 27*(3), 19–37.

Barbee, A.P., Gulley, M.R., & Cunningham, M.R. (1990). Support seeking in personal relationships. *Journal of Social and Personal Relationships, 7*(4), 531–540. [Special Issue: Predicting, activating and facilitating social support.]

Baumer, D., & McLinden, H. (1994). Support after cot death: The CONI Programme in action. *Professional Care of Mother and Child, 4*(5), 131–133.

Behm, L.K., & Frank, D.I. (1992). The relationship between self-care agency and job satisfaction in public health nurses. *Applied Nursing Research, 5*(1), 28–29.

Bennett, S.J. (1993). Relationships among selected antecedent variables and coping effectiveness in postmyocardial infarction patients. *Research in Nursing and Health, 16,* 131–139.

Bernard, H., Johnson, E., Killworth, P., McCarthy, C., Shelley, G., & Robinson, S. (1990). Comparing four different methods for measuring personal social networks. *Social Networks, 12,* 179–215.

Billingham, K., & Perkins, E. (1997). A public health approach to nursing in the community. *Nursing Standard, 11*(35), 43–46.

Birkel, R.C., & Repucci, N. (1983). Social networks, information seeking, and the utilization of services. *American Journal of Community Psychology, 11*(2), 185–205.

Bloom, J.R. (1990). The relationship of social support and health. *Social Science and Medicine, 39*, 635–637.

Braden, C.J. (1993). Research program on learned response to chronic illness experience: Self-help model. *Holistic Nursing Practice, 8*(1), 38–44.

Breen, H. (1994). Child sexual abuse: Parent group leads to community and social action. *Canadian Journal of Public Health, 85*(6), 381–384.

Brown, R.T., Doepke, K.J., & Kaslow, N.J. (1993). Risk–resistance–adaptation model for paediatric chronic illness: Sickle cell syndrome as an example. *Clinical Psychology Review, 13*, 119–132.

Burke, S.O., Handley-Derry, M.H., Costello, E.A., Kauffmann, E., & Dillon, M.C. (1997). Stress-point intervention for parents of repeatedly hospitalized children with chronic conditions. *Research in Nursing and Health, 20*(6), 475–485.

Buunk, B.P., & Hoorens, V. (1992). Social support and stress: The role of social comparison and social exchange processes. *British Journal of Clinical Psychology, 31*, 445–457.

Campion, K. (1996). Disease management: Living with multiple sclerosis. *Community Nurse, 2*(9), 27–29.

Cohen, R.Y. (1988). Mobilizing support through weight loss through work-site competitions. In B.H. Gottlieb (Ed.), *Marshalling social support: Formats, processes, and effects* (pp. 241–264). Newbury Park, CA: Sage.

Cohen, S., & Wills, T.A. (1985). Stress, social support and the buffering hypothesis. *Psychological Bulletin, 98*(2), 310–357.

Conn, V.S. (1992). Self-management of over-the-counter medications by older adults. *Public Health Nursing, 9*(1), 29–36.

Cormier-Daigle, M., & Stewart, M. (1997). Support and coping of male hemodialysis-dependent patients. *International Journal of Nursing Studies, 34*(6), 420–430.

Coyne, J.C., & Bulger, N. (1990). Doing without support as an explanatory concept. *Journal of Social and Clinical Psychology, 9*(1), 148–158.

Coyne, J.C., & Downey, G. (1991). Social factors and psychopathology: Stress, social support and coping processes. *Annual Review of Psychology, 42*, 401–425.

Cross, G., & Marks, B. (1996). Special families, special needs. *Nursing Times, 92*(13), 38–40.

Cutrona, C. (1990). Stress and social support—in search of optimal matching. *Journal of Social and Clinical Psychology, 9*(1), 3–14.

Dakof, G.A., & Taylor, S.E. (1990). Victims' perceptions of social support: What is helpful from whom? *Journal of Personality and Social Psychology, 58*, 80–89.

Davidson, M. (1996). A drop-in the right direction. *Nursing BC, 28*(4), 22–23.

Dean, P.G. (1989). Expanding our sights to include social networks. *Nursing and Health Care, 12*, 545–550.

Dickson, F., & Tutty, L.M. (1996). The role of the public health nurse in responding to abused women. *Public Health Nursing, 13*(4), 263–268.

DiMartile Bolla, C., DeJoseph, J., Norbeck, J., & Smith, R. (1996). Social support as road map and vehicle: An analysis of data from focus group interviews with a group of African American women. *Public Health Nursing, 13*(5), 331–336.

Doornbos, M. (1997). The problems and coping methods of young adults with mental illness. *Journal of Psychosocial Nursing and Mental Health Services, 35*(9), 22–26.

Dow, J.A., & Mest, C.G. (1997). Psychosocial interventions for patients with chronic obstructive pulmonary disease. *Home Healthcare Nurse, 15*(6), 414–420.

Dunkel-Schetter, C., & Bennett, T. (1990). Differentiating the cognitive and behavioral aspects of social support. In B.R. Sarason, I.B. Sarason, & G.R. Pierce (Eds.), *Social support: An interactional view* (pp. 208, 267–296). New York: Wiley.

Dunkel-Schetter, C., & Skokan, L. (1990). Determinants of social support provision in personal relationships. *Journal of Social and Personal Relationships, 7*(4), 437–450.

Eckenrode, J., & Gore, S. (1990). *Stress between work and family* (pp. 55–59). New York: Plenum.

Egeland, B., Carlson, E., & Sroufe, L.A. (1993). Resilience as a process. *Development and Psychopathology, 5*, 517–528.

Felton, B.J., & Berry, C. (1992). Groups as social network members: Overlooked sources of social support. *American Journal of Community Psychology, 20*(2), 253–261.

Folkman, S., Chesney, M., McKusick, L., Ironson, G., Johnson, D.S., & Coates, T.J. (1991). Translating coping theory into an intervention. In J. Eckenrode (Ed.), *The social context of coping* (pp. 240–260). New York: Plenum Press.

Ford, G., & Procidano, M. (1990). The relationship of self actualization to social support, life stress and adjustment. *Social Behavior and Personality, 18*(1), 41–51.

Garmezy, N. (1993). Children in poverty: Resilience despite risk. *Psychiatry, 56*, 127–136.

Goeppinger, J., Macnee, C., Anderson, M.K., Boutaugh, M., & Stewart, K. (1995). From research to practice: The effects of the jointly sponsored dissemination of an arthritis self-care nursing intervention. *Applied Nursing Research, 8*(3), 106–113.

Gottlieb, B.H. (1988). Support interventions. A typology and agenda for research. In S. Duek (Ed.), *Handbook of personal relationships* (pp. 519–541). Chichester, UK: Wiley.

Gottlieb, B.H. (1989). A contextual perspective on stress in family care of the elderly. *Canadian Psychology, 30*(3), 596–607.

Gottlieb, B.H., & Wagner, F. (1991). Stress and support processes in close relationships. In J. Eckenrode (Ed.), *The social context of coping,* (pp. 165–187). New York: Plenum.

Grant, J.S. (1996). Home care problems experienced by stroke survivors and their family caregivers. *Home Healthcare Nurse, 14*(11), 892–902.

Hatcliffe, S., Smith, P., & Daw, R. (1996). District nurses' perceptions of palliative care at home. *Nursing Times, 92*(41), 36–37.

Hegney, D. (1996). The status of rural nursing in Australia: A review. *Australian Journal of Rural Health, 4*(1), 1–10.

Heller, K., Price, R.H., & Hogg, J.R. (1990). The role of social support in community and clinical interventions. In B.R. Sarason, I.B. Sarason, & G.R. Pierce (Eds.), *Social support: An interactional view* (pp. 481–508). New York: Wiley.

Hemingway, S. (1996). Traumatic transitions . . . Counselling and support for people with disabilities. *Nursing Times, 92*(11), 42–44.

Hirth, A.M., & Stewart, M.J. (1994). Hope and social support as coping resources for adults waiting for cardiac transplantation. *Canadian Journal of Nursing Research, 26*(3), 31–48.

Hobfoll, S.E., & Freedy, J.R. (1990). The availability and effective use of social support. *Journal of Social and Clinical Psychology, 9*(1), 91–103.

House, J.S., & Kahn, R.L. (1985). Measures and concepts of social support. In S. Cohen & S.L. Syme (Eds.), *Social support and health* (pp. 83–108). Orlando, FL: Academic Press.

House, J.S., Umberson, D., & Landis, K. (1988). Structures and processes of social support. *Annual Review of Sociology, 14,* 293–318.

James, L. (1996). Family centred outreach for forensic psychiatry clients. *Australian and New Zealand Journal of Mental Health Nursing, 5*(2), 63–68.

Jessor, R. (1993). Successful adolescent development among youth in high-risk settings. *American Psychologist, 48*(2), 117–126.

Johnson, R., Hobfoll, S., & Zalcberg-Linetzy, A. (1993). Social support knowledge and behavior and rational intimacy: A dyadic study. *Journal of Family Psychology, 6,* 266–277.

Kaplan, R.M., & Toshima, T. (1990). The functional effects of social relationships on chronic illnesses and disability. In B.R. Sarason, I.B. Sarason, & G.R. Pierce (Eds.), *Social support: An interactional view* (pp. 427–453). New York: Wiley.

Katz, A.H. (1993). *Self-help in America: A social movement perspective.* New York: Twayne Publishers.

Kiberd, B. (1996). Helping parents to cope with SIDS. *World of Irish Nursing, 4*(6), 12–14.

Killion, C.M. (1995). Special health care needs of homeless pregnant women. *Advances in Nursing Science, 18*(2), 44–56.

Kumpfer, K.L., & Hopkins, R. (1993). Prevention: Current research and trends. *Recent Advances in Addictive Disorders, 16*(1), 11–20.

La Gaipa, J.J. (1990). The negative effects of informal support systems. In S. Duck (Ed.), *Personal relationships and social support* (pp. 122–139). London: Sage.

Leary, J., Gallagher, T., Carson, J., Fagin, L., Bartlett, H., & Brown, D. (1995). Stress and coping strategies in community psychiatric nurses: A Q-methodological study. *Journal of Advanced Nursing, 21*(2), 230–237.

Mahoney, D.F., & Shippee-Rice, R. (1994). Training family caregivers of older adults: A program model for community nurses. *Journal of Community Health Nursing, 11*(2), 71–78.

Mangham, C., McGrath, P., Reid, G., & Stewart, M. (1994). *Resiliency: Relevance to health promotion.* Unpublished discussion paper submitted to National Health Promotion Directorate.

Martin, S.D. (1995). Coping with chronic illness. *Home Healthcare Nurse, 13*(4), 50–54.

Mazzuca, K.B., Farris, N.A., Mendenhall, J., & Stoupa, R.A. (1997). Demonstrating the added value of community health nursing for clients with insulin-dependent diabetes. *Journal of Community Health Nursing, 14*(4), 211–224.

McCubbin, M.A., & McCubbin, H.I. (1993). Families coping with illness: The resiliency model of family stress, adjustment, and adaptation. In C.B. Danielson, B. Hamel-Bissell, & P. Winstead-Fry, *Families, health, & illness: Perspectives on coping and intervention* (pp. 21–61). St. Louis: Mosby.

Olds, D., & Kitzman, H. (1990). Can home visitation improve the health of women and children at environmental risk? *Pediatrics, 86*(1), 108–116.

Orem, D.E. (1991). *Nursing: Concepts of pratice* (4th ed.). St. Louis: Mosby.

Quittner, A.L., Glueckauf, R.L., & Jackson, D.N. (1990). Chronic parenting stress: Moderating versus mediating effects of social support. *Journal of Personality and Social Psychology, 56*(6), 1266–1278.

Reutter, L.I., & Ford, J.S. (1996). Perceptions of public health nursing: Views from the field. *Journal of Advanced Nursing, 24*(1), 7–15.

Richardson, E., Warburton, F., Wolfe, C.D., & Rudd, A.G. (1996). Family support services for stroke patients. *Professional Nurse, 12*(2), 92–96.

Robinson, K. (1990). The relationship between social skills, social support, self-esteem, and burden in adult caregivers. *Journal of Advanced Nursing, 15*, 788–795.

Rook, K. (1990). Parallels in the study of social support and social strain. *Journal of Social and Clinical Psychology, 9*(1), 118–132.

Salisbury, C. (1996). Rehabilitation after myocardial infarction: The role of the community nurse. *Nurse Standard, 10*(23), 49–51.

Sarason, R.B., Sarason, I.G., & Pierce, G.R. (1990). *Social support: An interactional view.* New York: Wiley.

Schaufeli, W.B. (1995). The evaluation of a burnout workshop for community nurses. *Journal of Health and Human Services Administration, 18*(1), 11–30.

Schuster, T., Kessler, R., & Aseltine, R. (1990). Supportive interactions, negative interactions and depressed mood. *American Journal of Community Psychology, 18*, 423–438.

Seaby, L., & Roberts, K. (1996). High dependency: Patient-controlled analgesia in the community. *Community Nurse, 2*(5), 16–17.

Segal, S.P., Silverman, C., & Temkin, T. (1993). Empowerment and self-help agency practice for people with mental disabilities. *Social Work, 38*(6), 705–712.

Sharkey, T. (1995). The effects of uncertainty in families with children who are chronically ill. *Home Healthcare Nurse, 13*(4), 37–42.

Shepherd, G., & Hill, R.G. (1996). Manic depression: Do people receive adequate support? *Nursing Times, 92*(26), 42–44.

Silver, R., Wortman, C., & Crofton, C. (1990). The role of coping in support provision: The self presentational dilemma of victims of life crises. In B.R. Sarason, I.B. Sarason, & G.R. Pierce. *Social support: An interactional view* (pp. 397–426). New York: Wiley.

Simmons, S. (1994). Social networks: Their relevance to mental health nursing. *Journal of Advanced Nursing, 19*, 281–289.

Stewart, M. (1990). Professional interface with mutual aid self-help groups: A review. *Social Science and Medicine, 31*, 1143–1158.

Stewart, M. (1993). *Integrating social support in nursing.* Newbury Park, CA: Sage.

Stewart, M., & Arklie, M. (1994). Work satisfaction, stressors and support experienced by community health nurses. *Canadian Journal of Public Health, 85*(3), 180–184.

Stewart, M., Ritchie, J.A., Ellerton, M.L., Salisbury, S., Sullivan, M., & Thompson, D. (1997). *Telephone support intervention for chronically ill children and their parents.* Proposal submitted to NHRDP, the American March of Dimes, and the Hospital for Sick Children Foundation.

Taylor, S.G., & McLaughlin, K. (1991). Orem's general theory of nursing and community nursing. *Nursing Science Quarterly, 4*(4), 153–160.

Thoits, P. (1995). Stress, coping, and social support processes; where are we? What next? *Journal of Health and Social Behaviour, (special number)*, 53–79.

Thomas, P. (1995). A study of effectiveness of staff support groups. *Nursing Times, 91*(48), 36–39.

Tilden, V., & Galyen, R. (1987). Cost and conflict: The darker side of social support. *Western Journal of Nursing Research, 9*(1), 9–18.

Tilden, V.P., & Weinert, C. (1987). Social support and the chronically ill individual. *Nursing Clinics, 22*(3), 613–620.

Tomblin-Murphy, G., Stewart, M., Ritchie, J., & Johnson, A. (in press). Support need of nurses: Telephone support for professional supporters. In M. Stewart (Ed.), *Chronic conditions and caregiving in Canada*. Toronto: University of Toronto Press.

Utz, S.W., Shuster, G.F., III, Merwin, E., & Williams, B. (1994). A community-based smoking-cessation program: Self-care behaviors and success. *Public Health Nursing, 11*(5), 291–299.

Watson, A.R. (1996). Home health and respite care. *Peritoneal Dialysis International, 16* (Suppl. 1), S551–S553.

Webb, J., Roberts, C., & Grainger, A. (1995). Helping families to cope. *Nursing Standard, 9*(27), 22–23.

Wiggins, N.C. (1989). Education and support for the newly diagnosed cardiac family: A vital link in rehabilitation. *Journal of Advanced Nursing, 14*, 63–67.

Williams, E. (1995). The senior companion/visiting nurse partnership: A marriage made in heaven. *Journal of Home Health Care Practice, 8*(1), 44–49.

Willis, J. (1995). A positive contribution . . . Mental health nurses are in a good position to give . . . Psychological support to groups of people who may be marginalised by society. *Nursing Times, 91*(48), 62–64.

Winemiller, D.R., Mitchell, M.E., Sutcliff, J., & Cline, D.J. (1993). Measurement strategies in social support: A descriptive review of the literature. *Journal of Clinical Psychology, 49*(5), 638–648.

Wissman, J.L., & Wilmoth, M.C. (1996). Meeting the learning needs of senior citizens and nursing students through a community-based pharmacology experience. *Journal of Community Health Nursing, 13*(3), 159–165.

Zerwekh, J.V. (1995). High-tech home care for nurses: Questioning technologies. *Home Healthcare Nurse, 13*(1), 9–14.

Zimmerman, R.S., & Connor, C. (1989). Health promotion in context: The effects of significant others on health behavior change. *Health Education Quarterly, 16*(1), 57–75.

CHAPTER 5

Health promotion for ~~mmunities and agg~~

Health Promot for communities
or Aggregates. Ch.5.

Shirl ig

In this chapter, the authors discuss the key concepts of aggregate and community, and their importance for community health nursing within a Primary Health Care framework. An integrated model is presented to guide community health nursing practice and research with four levels of client system (individual, family, aggregate, and community) and three types of care (illness care, illness prevention, and health promotion). Two clinical applications are presented to illustrate specific nursing activities for each client system and type of care. Community health nursing care is complex and continuous, and aims to promote the community's health. Community health nurses can identify and assess aggregates in the community with similar health characteristics and participate with consumers and other health providers to develop health programs that assist these aggregates and the community to attain optimal health.

LEARNING OBJECTIVES

In this chapter, you will learn:

- definitions of *community, aggregate,* and *community health nursing* relevant to Primary Health Care
- components of an integrated model of community health nursing
- community health nursing roles and activities appropriate for each level of client identified in the model
- community health nursing roles and activities appropriate for each focus of nursing care identified in the model

Introduction

The initial purpose of this chapter is to review community models and frameworks that reflect the responsibilities of community health nurses within Primary Health Care. The key concepts of *community, aggregate,* and

Primary Health Care are described and integrated within a model that depicts community health nursing practice at individual, family, aggregate, and community levels. The aggregate and community levels, which have received scant attention in practice and research, are emphasized throughout the chapter. Two applications of the integrated model are then presented.

As we move into the new millennium, nurses are increasingly challenged to expand their roles in community health and Primary Health Care. Traditionally, community health nurses have been a driving force in providing illness prevention and health promotion services to the community. However, the concept of community as client and the role of community health nurses in Primary Health Care require clarification.

The Canadian Public Health Association (CPHA, 1990) defined community health/public health as one of several specialties providing illness prevention and health promotion services in the community. Community health/public health nurses are described as diverse providers with multifaceted roles that encompass both nursing and public health. These roles include consultant, educator, community developer, facilitator, advocate, counsellor, communicator, coordinator, collaborator, researcher, evaluator, social marketer, and policy formulator (CPHA, 1990).

Most community health nurses accept that they have broad responsibilities for providing illness prevention and health promotion services to individuals, families, aggregates, and communities (Anderson & McFarlane, 1996; Williams, 1996). However, it is often difficult to determine how these responsibilities are carried out in day-to-day practice. Zerwekh (1992) argues that lack of role clarity has led to community/public health nurses' invisibility, isolation, and powerlessness. Community health nurses have been described as "translators or interpreters for clients, administrators, communities, and policymakers, and . . . the link between the data of epidemiology and the clinical understanding of health and illness as it is experienced in people's lives" (Wallinder, White, & Salveson, 1996, p. 1). Laffrey, Dickenson, and Diem's (1997) study of how community health nurses identify their professional roles included four groups: public health nurses working in health departments; nurses working in specialized programs such as schools, clinics, or prisons; home health care nurses; and nurses providing a combination of home health and generalized public health services. The nurses working in specialized programs tended to see their roles as more administrative, and rated their two most important roles as "planner/coordinator/organizer" and "resource person/referrer." The other three groups rated "educator" and "advocate" as their two most important roles. It is thus not surprising that the multiple roles of the community/public health nurse can lead many nurses to question whether every nurse is responsible for all roles.

Although community health nurses are expected to direct their efforts to health promotion and disease prevention at the community level, there is a constant tension between nurses' concern for human beings as individuals and their concern with the larger community and the aggregates of which it is composed. One study of community nursing competencies revealed that senior baccalaureate students, faculty, and administrators all ranked the students as more skilful in providing care to individuals than to groups or communities (Nickel et al., 1995). It is important to recognize that, although aggregates and communities include individuals and families, they also have an identity that extends beyond the sum of the individuals and families within them (Hanchett, 1988). Also, it is important to determine what nursing roles are most appropriate for each level of client system, i.e., individuals, families, aggregates, or communities.

Community as client

For an understanding of the complex definitions of community as client, let us turn to some earlier definitions of community.

Setting for practice. Community as the setting for practice takes the traditional view that community health nurses provide care outside the hospital (Sills & Goeppinger, 1985). Community settings include homes, schools, industry, neighbourhood clinics, and health centres. The community provides the context for nursing care and has an impact on the health of individuals and families. Despite the importance of the practice setting, distinguishing community health nurses solely by the setting in which they practise is inadequate, given today's complex community structures. Although many nurses have moved away from hospitals into community settings to provide care, this care often emphasizes persons who are either ill or at risk for illness, rather than health promotion, aggregates, or the community as a whole. The traditional strategies developed to guide nursing care of individuals and families in the community are inadequate to guide nursing care when the community is the focus of care (McKnight & Van Dover, 1994).

Unit of practice. Other community health nurses view the community as the unit of practice (Sills & Goeppinger, 1985). Within this view, the nurse would be concerned with the people, the place, and the functions of the defined community (Shuster & Goeppinger, 1996). The community unit would be a particular group of people and their characteristics, geographic location, living environment, and functions. Schools and workplaces could be defined as communities within this definition. If we define groups such as schools and workplaces as communities, we must also recognize that most individuals and families live in multiple communities at any given time.

Community as client. In Anderson and McFarlane's (1996) community-as-client model, interacting subsystems make up the community: physical environment; recreation; safety and transportation; communication; education; health and social services; economics; and politics and government. The focus of community health nursing practice is these interacting subsystems. Stewart (1985) also stressed the need to consider the community subsystems of health, communication, economy, education, law, politics, recreation, religion, and social life.

Energy field. Hanchett (1988) presents a more holistic definition of the community as an "energy field" that is integral with the environment and manifests dynamic patterns. Community health nurses would be concerned with overall community characteristics, such as movement of goods and people; changing patterns of culture; and daily rhythms of quiet, noise, and activity within the community (Hanchett, 1988). Recently, Hanchett (1998) enlarged on her community definition and urged nurses to think globally. Inherent in Hanchett's definition is a community of interacting individuals and groups. Their dynamic relationships, their adaptation and actions, and their effect on the whole environment become the focus of community care. For example, a nurse might be concerned with the effectiveness of community behaviours in response to an environmental occurrence such as a flood or a fire. This can assist community health nurses to understand the community as a whole.

Structural factors. Although earlier community definitions included geographic location, more recent definitions tend to focus on people in relationships. Understanding how the structural factors of the community influence the health of its members and understanding how the health of the people affects the structural factors in the environment are also important. Few studies have examined structural factors and have concentrated instead on how members influence each other and their communities. Preston and Bucher (1996) illustrate the necessity of understanding structural aspects of community in their study of educational levels and health within 18 communities undergoing rapid population changes. The communities with lower average education levels reported lower health levels than the communities with higher average education. Another study of environmental structural factors (Carruth, Gilbert, & Lewis, 1997) assessed the impact of an abandoned hazardous waste site on the health of residents. Extensive networking and door-to-door surveys were important in monitoring potential dangerous environmental conditions and reflect the definition of the community as a unit.

Target of practice. The perspective that the community is the target of practice (Sills & Goeppinger, 1985) is more complex because, regardless of where nursing care is provided or to whom (individual, family, aggregate, or

community), the goal of care is to achieve a healthier community. In this perspective, a health situation may be identified by an individual, a family, an
aggregate, or the total community. The health situation may be a problem, a
condition that could allow a problem to develop, a resource, or a strength.
The ultimate goal of the community health nurse is the greatest health for the
community.

For example, a prenatal client may confide in the nurse that she is living
with a partner who abuses her. The community health nurse assesses the
abuse and intervenes with the woman to change her situation. The nurse also
considers the impact of the abuse on all family members and assists the family unit to find appropriate care. Together with these individual and family
concerns, the community-as-target approach demands that the nurse also
consider other women in the community who are experiencing a similar
problem. By assessing the community, the community health nurse can
determine the extent of the problem, whether any community resources are
available to support abused women and their families, and whether there is
a need to encourage the community to initiate these resources. Viewing nursing care through the community-as-target perspective enables the nurse to
identify and assess populations at risk and to increase their involvement in
health promotion and disease prevention activities (Baldwin, Conger,
Abegglen, & Hill, 1998).

Thus, it is not only the setting and unit of practice, but also the perspective of practice that differentiates community health nurses. With the increasing complexity of communities and the consequent changes in nursing and
health care, the community-as-target definition provides an important
framework from which to view community health nursing practice.

Complexity of communities

Earlier in this century, communities and neighbourhoods were characterized
by individuals and families who knew each other, shared a common culture
and history, worked in proximity to one another, and were faced with the
same environmental stressors and resources. More recently, however, families, neighbourhoods, and communities have become much more varied and
complex. Frequently, a neighbourhood comprises people from diverse cultures, with a variety of lifestyles and living patterns, who may not even know
one another. As people travel farther to school and work, their life patterns
cut across several different kinds of communities. Support systems that had
been taken for granted are lacking in many communities, and families and
friends no longer live and work in proximity (see also Chapter 4).

Support often becomes an issue when illness prevents individuals from
developing needed support systems. As we move into the next century, there
is a trend to develop a greater sense of neighbourhood and community. This
may involve neighbourhoods and subsets of communities that include

geographic location, environmental conditions, people, and structures that influence health.

One community program that reflects a "community of caring" was developed by community health nurses in Scarborough, Ontario. The nurses identified an aggregate of caregivers in the community and developed a program to meet their support needs. The program consisted of eight weekly two-hour sessions, facilitated by a community health nurse. This nurse used information and resources appropriate to meet caregivers' learning needs and learning styles. The sessions were designed to encourage discussion and support among the group members. Because most caregivers were providing care to older adults, the weekly sessions provided information on the physical and emotional changes associated with aging. Caregivers learned about some aspects of the aging process through simulation exercises, such as experiencing what it is like to have joints that do not move easily or to be hearing-impaired or visually impaired. Group members shared successful strategies that they had used in their caregiving. Group discussions focussed on community resources, use and misuse of medications, alternative living accommodations, and communication techniques. Sharing experiences helped the members learn new ways to deal with the stress of caregiving.

After the eight sessions, some group members decided to continue meeting without the facilitator to guide them. Support and guidance were provided to one group as they made the transition from a professionally led to a peer-led group. The members felt very positive about assuming leadership roles in the group and requested the opportunity to call on the nurses for problem solving, if needed.

As this group continued to function, a network of community care evolved. Group members who lived in proximity assisted one another with caregiving tasks. For example, one man tended a woman's garden, and the woman cared for his wife when he needed to shop or have a short respite from caregiving. The group members were able to move from a formal, short-term educational and support program to develop their own community of caring.

Aggregate as client

The aggregate as client is another concern of community health nurses as they plan and deliver health care. An aggregate is a subgroup within the larger society whose members share characteristics related to their health needs. These characteristics can be a particular health problem, a health risk, or a nursing diagnosis (Hanchett, 1988; Schultz, 1987). Examples of aggregates are persons with hypertension, children who do not wear bicycle helmets and thus risk injury from bicycle accidents, and pregnant teenage girls.

Hanchett (1988) noted that the community is composed of aggregates, but that aggregates are composed of individuals. Similarly, Archer (1985) found that within an aggregate approach, it is individuals who are the "recipients of most community health nursing services, since all groups (families, aggregates, and communities) are composed of individuals" (p. 37).

These definitions are useful for community health nurses because they clarify that individuals are not separate from aggregates or communities. Aggregates have historically been considered an important concept for community health nursing. Care of aggregates is based, in part, on the community health nurse's concern with individual health risks, health needs, and health resources; yet, this concern transcends individual assessment and care by shifting the focus to the larger group of which the individual is a part. Aggregates, therefore, provide an important link between care directed to the individual or family and care directed to the total community.

Community health nurses identify high-risk aggregates in various community settings, such as schools, social gatherings, and street corners (Freeman & Heinrich, 1981). They play an important role in assessing communities for aggregates with health needs and developing programs to help them meet these needs. Assessing the community for high-risk aggregates requires a targeted approach that is designed to detect the presence of a particular health characteristic. Screening for a disease and measuring blood pressure of persons at health fairs or other community sites are examples of targeted assessments.

Community health nursing from an aggregate perspective is illustrated in the example of a nurse who develops educational and support services for persons in the community who have diabetes. Although the unit of service is the aggregate of diabetics, the actual recipients of the education and support are the individuals with diabetes. These individuals benefit from the education and support. However, at the aggregate level, outreach to the diabetic population within the community leads to developing programs and measuring improvements on a larger scale. These improvements can include fewer persons hospitalized with diabetic complications, fewer days lost from work or school, and fewer diabetes-related deaths within the community.

Another vulnerable aggregate is children who arrive at school hungry and are unable to benefit from class lessons. Within an individual approach, the community health nurse would provide food to each hungry child. In contrast, working from an aggregate approach could lead to the development of school breakfast and lunch programs. These interventions are usually developed in partnership with community leaders and residents and are based on an assessment of the needs of the aggregate of school children. By including the community residents, these programs are more likely to be congruent with their culture and resources.

The homeless population is an aggregate receiving increased attention in many communities. For example, the Toronto Coalition Against Homelessness

(1996) held an inquiry into homelessness and street deaths. Verbal and written information was received from homeless persons and front-line workers, including physicians and nurses. The health problems experienced by the homeless aggregate included infections, accidental injuries, injuries from assaults, sunburn, frostbite, and increased risk for HIV/AIDS and tuberculosis. These persons often lacked access to health care and were not well treated by health workers. Lack of a health card, due to loss or theft, frequently resulted in denial of health services. The coalition recommended that "everyone have access to an affordable home" (p. 13) and that homeless persons be included in developing strategies to meet their needs, to empower this aggregate.

As we can see from the above example, working with local residents to identify and determine solutions to the problems in their own communities can help to build stronger community support for those in need and increases the likelihood that resources will be relevant to the specific needs and culture of the community.

Health and illness paradigms

An integrated approach to nursing care is grounded in an understanding of two complementary paradigms (Kulbok, Laffrey, & Goeppinger, 1996; Laffrey, Loveland-Cherry, & Winkler, 1986). The *health paradigm* views humans and environment as continuously interacting with and affecting each other. Health care, within this view, is a dynamic process of promoting the harmony and growth of the interaction between humans and the environment. Recipients of care are involved in assessing and planning for their health care and are active partners. The health paradigm is reflected in the World Health Organization's (WHO, 1978) definition of health. This paradigm is most commonly seen in community development models, in which health professionals serve as consultants and facilitators, and community members assess their own health needs and develop health care resources (McKnight & Van Dover, 1994; Styles, 1994).

The second is the *illness paradigm*, based on the belief that health is the absence of illness and that illness results from the way in which humans react to factors in the environment. Health care is professionally directed and is aimed at preventing illness, disease, or disability. Health care measures include changing environmental stressors so they do not adversely affect the client or increasing the client's ability to react to the stimuli without illness or injury. Examples of care within the illness paradigm include diagnosis and treatment of an infection with appropriate medication (individual client) or epidemiological follow-up of an infectious disease to reduce its spread (family, aggregate, or community client). The illness paradigm is most commonly seen in the medical care system with individuals and in the public health system with aggregates and communities.

Community nursing in Primary Health Care

The concept of Primary Health Care (PHC) originated with the World Health Organization (WHO, 1978) conference, in which participants declared their intention to achieve Health for All by the Year 2000 (see also Chapter 2). Components of Primary Health Care have significance for community health nurses (see also Chapter 3). These components include essential health care services, acceptable and affordable care, universally accessible care, full participation of the community, and intersectoral collaboration (WHO, 1978).

- *Essential health care services* are relevant to meet identified health needs and are provided as a basic right to the entire population. The services might vary greatly from one community to another, based on specific health needs. Common essential health services include prenatal care, provision of clean water and air, health supervision of high-risk infants, and childhood immunizations.
- *Acceptable and affordable health services* are culturally acceptable and do not conflict with religious or ethnic beliefs of the population. They are provided at a cost the entire community can afford.
- *Universally accessible services* are provided for the entire community. Thus, no community members encounter barriers to obtaining essential services.
- *Public participation* means that health needs and services are assessed, planned, and developed by the population. This ensures that the services are relevant to their needs and congruent with their culture. Thus, a multidisciplinary and collaborative effort is required at each stage of health care, from the initial assessment of needs to the provision and evaluation of health care.
- *Intersectoral collaboration* among a variety of health care providers, with involvement of each sector of the population, ensures that essential services are accessible, acceptable, and affordable.

In the example of children arriving at school hungry, the inclusion of community residents from a variety of professional and citizen groups in the planning and development of the school lunch program illustrates community participation and intersectoral collaboration. The Toronto Coalition Against Homelessness (1996) is another good example of implementing these PHC concepts.

For community health nurses, these PHC components are not new. As early as 1860, Nightingale advocated using a community approach to achieve optimal health. Lillian Wald, in the early 1900s, emphasized community participation and community development as inherent to community health nursing (Buhler-Wilkerson, 1993). Characteristics of community health are remarkably similar to those of PHC nursing (Laffrey & Pagé, 1989). The components of essentiality—universality, acceptability, and affordability of health care—and total community participation are basic to community health nursing. Indeed, the Canadian Public Health Association (1990) noted that Primary Health Care addresses "the major health problems in the community, providing health promoting, preventive, curative, and rehabilitative services accordingly" (p. 3). The emphasis on "health promotion and maintenance, illness and injury prevention, community participation, and community development" (p. 4) provides the theoretical foundation for community health/ public health nursing.

Even though community health and Primary Health Care share many characteristics, several obstacles have stood in the way of community health nursing's contributions to the goal of Health for All by the Year 2000 (Laffrey & Pagé, 1989). One obstacle is the lack of a clear role identity, as mentioned at the beginning of this chapter. Consequently, the shift from individual and family care to aggregate and community care has been slow. Additionally, while nursing theories acknowledge environment and community, they provide little direction for nursing interventions aimed at changing the conditions within the environment that affect the health of the population (Bridges & Lynam, 1993). Social, political, and economic factors are as important as individuals' characteristics if positive changes in the population's health are to be achieved. To make the shift from individually oriented care to aggregate- and community-oriented care requires a broader framework that includes knowledge from fields such as social psychology, environmental health, and political science.

McKnight and Van Dover (1994) propose that baccalaureate programs emphasize "definitions of health and community, community assessment, community development, citizen participation and mobilization" (p. 14). The Canadian Public Health Association (CPHA, 1990) recommends an advocacy role for community health nurses so they may help "individuals, families, and groups who are disadvantaged by reason of socio-economic status, isolation, culture, lack of knowledge, etc., become aware of issues of significance to their health" (p. 9). Furthermore, the CPHA emphasizes the community developer role to identify and define community health issues, and work with consumers and other health providers to develop relevant health programs.

The provision of nursing care at the aggregate and community levels has increased during the past decade and will continue to increase (Bridges & Lynam, 1993). A major factor in this increase is a shift from expensive, institutionally based care to less expensive care in clients' homes and other community settings. Another important factor is the increasing recognition that health needs of individuals and families are a function of socioeconomic, cultural, and political factors in the community (Clemen-Stone, Eigsti, & McGuire, 1995). Moreover, community health care has been shown to empower the population to meet their health needs (Erickson, 1996).

Clearly identifying nursing care in relation to individuals, families, aggregates, and communities can assist community health nurses to define their unique roles within Primary Health Care. Community health nurses are concerned with all four levels of client. It is this unique perspective, providing the link between people's health and the broader community's health, that can move us toward the goal of achieving health for all.

Integrated model of community health nursing

A model of holistic community health nursing was proposed by Laffrey and Kulbok (1999) (see also Kulbok, Laffrey, & Goeppinger, 1996; Laffrey, 1994; Laffrey & Kulbok, 1994) to indicate the relationship and continuity among the various levels of clients and types of care with which community health nursing is concerned. This model (Figure 5.1) draws on concepts from both the health and illness paradigms. Community nursing care includes illness care; prevention of illness, disease, or injury; and health promotion. Illness care aims to reduce illness or disability and move the client toward a state of equilibrium. Prevention of illness, disease, or injury aims to identify and reduce known health risks. Health promotion aims to increase the physical, mental, emotional, spiritual, and functional well-being of the client. These three aspects of nursing care complement one another. However, although the actions may be similar, the aim of nursing care, the approach taken by the community health nurse, and the client's perception of the action would differ fundamentally.

For example, physical exercise could be performed by one who has had a myocardial infarction to strengthen the heart muscle following the attack (illness treatment) or by a person at risk for myocardial infarction (prevention). Others without any known illness or risk factors might perform physical exercise to increase their level of vitality and performance (health promotion). Although the action of physical exercise is the same, the goal of the exercise and the perceptions differ. Each of the three foci of care can be directed to any of the levels of client.

The individual is the most easily defined and concrete level of client, with family, aggregate, and community each becoming more abstract and complex. The spiral (Figure 5.1) indicates that care is continuous for the four client levels, and specific nursing activities are most appropriate for each level. Community health nurses are concerned with and have responsibilities for each level of client and each focus of care. Regardless of the level at which

Figure 5.1
Integrated model of community health promotion

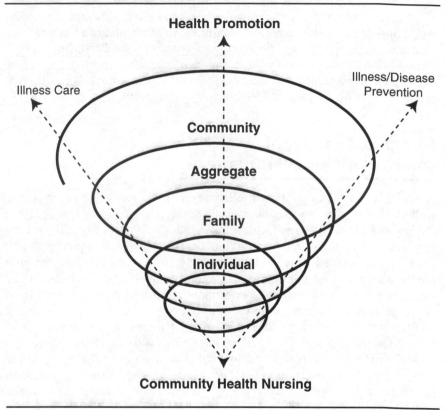

the nurse functions, the ultimate goal of community health nursing is promotion of optimal health of the community. Thus, health promotion is the central axis of the model, and community is the broadest circle, encompassing the other three levels in the client system.

The community includes its aggregates, families, and individuals, but has a unique identity and unique health needs. The community health nurse's roles may change from direct service provider, counsellor, or educator to advocate, social marketer, or community developer, as the system of care becomes more complex. At one extreme, the nurse may provide direct service to an individual client who is ill. At the other extreme, the nurse may participate with community leaders and citizens to develop health policies and resources for additional parks and recreation facilities to promote a healthier community.

The uniqueness of community health nurses lies in their ability to focus on individual clients within the context of their family, aggregate, and community, and also to focus on the community client with its own unique characteristics, while comprising aggregates, families, and individuals.

Two applications of the integrated model are described below. In the first application, illness care, preventive care, and health promotion care begin with an individual and move to the community (Table 5.1). In the second, the care begins with the community and moves to the individual (Table 5.2, p. 121). Examples are given of roles that a community health nurse may select for each level of client. You may suggest other nursing interventions and roles that are also appropriate for the situations described in these applications.

Application: Individual to community

Case Study

Mr. Jones, a 63-year-old man with chronic obstructive pulmonary disease (COPD), came to the attention of the community health nurse by a referral from a family member. As the community health nurse assessed Mr. Jones's responses to the chronic respiratory problems, she considered not only the impact on Mr. Jones, but also the impact on Mrs. Jones, the primary caregiver. The Joneses' oldest daughter, Mary, was widowed, had three children, and lived next door to her parents. Mary was employed but assisted with caregiving for her father and was a primary source of support to both her parents and her own children.

Illness care

As shown in Table 5.1, from an individual-as-client perspective, the nurse provided direct service by assessing Mr. Jones's breathing status, administering prescribed medications to ease his breathing, assessing his ability to cope with his disease, and assessing his home environment for factors that could affect his ability to cope. The nurse functioned as educator and counsellor by teaching Mr. Jones strategies that could ease his breathing and by supporting him to carry out his daily routine safely and comfortably. After several visits with the Jones family, the nurse evaluated the care to determine if there was improvement.

Working from a family-as-client perspective, the community health nurse provided direct service by assessing the level of family stress associated with Mr. Jones's illness-related needs. The nurse counselled the family, thereby reducing their stress level. She provided a list of community resources and made a referral for family counselling to reduce their stress and fear and to improve their coping skills. The nurse advocated for the family to obtain an earlier appointment with the community resource to which they had been referred.

Table 5.1
Individual to community: Respiratory care

Focus of Care	Individual	Family	Aggregate	Community
Illness care	• Administer medications to ease breathing • Teach measures to ease breathing	• Teach early detection of COPD among high-risk family members • Refer family for counselling for stress symptoms	• Assess prevalence of COPD in community • Develop a COPD support group	• Assess community for accessibility and adequacy of care providers for COPD patients
Illness/Disease/Injury prevention	• Teach beneficial effects of smoking cessation on morbidity, mortality • Assess home environment for respiratory hazards	• Teach deleterious effects of cigarette smoke on family health to prevent smoking in the home	• Develop classes on smoking risks for high-risk groups	• Incorporate community-wide multimedia education on health risks associated with tobacco use
Health promotion	• Empower individual to adopt a healthy lifestyle	• Plan with family to incorporate a healthy lifestyle	• Develop group education on benefits of clean air and healthy lifestyle	• Work with community leaders for clean air laws to maintain air quality

In addition, she assessed the family for knowledge of signs and symptoms of breathing problems and taught the early signs of bronchitis and emphysema.

From an aggregate-as-client perspective, the community health nurse was aware that individual and family health problems often reflect broader concerns in the community. Therefore, the prevalence of COPD in the community was assessed. The nurse identified a number of individuals with COPD and found many spouse caregivers in the community who were sharing similar experiences in caregiving, but who did not know one another.

Functioning as advocate, collaborator, and social marketer, the nurse participated with other community leaders and residents to develop a support program for persons with COPD and a program for an aggregate of caregivers. These groups provided participants with new information and skills. Members of aggregates experiencing common difficulties and successes were able to exchange support and assistance.

From a community-as-client perspective, the nurse assessed the community's level of services for lung disease. Assessing adequacy of services for COPD clients and environmental pollutants that might be associated with the rate of COPD and collaborating with other health care providers and consumers to develop facilities are examples of illness care at the community level. These activities reflect the roles of the nurse as community developer and policy formulator.

Prevention
The community health nurse strives to assess risk factors and institutes measures to alleviate risks prior to the diagnosis of any illness or disease. As shown in Table 5.1, to prevent lung disease, specific nursing care would include teaching an individual client the beneficial effects of smoking cessation; assessing a client's home for environmental hazards (individual as client); teaching the deleterious effects of smoking on the health of family members; recommending measures to prevent smoking in the home; providing information about community resources; and referring the family to a smoking cessation program (family as client). Preventive care for the aggregate as client would include collaborating with community leaders and residents to develop classes for high-risk groups about smoking risks and prevention. Preventive care for the community as client would include participating in community-wide multimedia education regarding community risks, such as reduced quality of air, and policy formulation regarding adoption of non-smoking rules in public buildings and restaurants.

Health promotion
Health promotion is the broadest and most complex focus of care and does not focus on a specific disease. It is provided by the community health nurse with each level of client. Examples of health promotion nursing care include

teaching individuals to adopt a healthy lifestyle (individual as client); planning healthy activities with a family or teaching well-balanced nutrition and physical activity to a young family (family as client); developing classes for an aggregate of workers about clean air and healthy lifestyle (aggregate as client); and participating with community leaders to establish clean air laws and develop recreation facilities (community as client). Thus, the roles are similar to those listed for prevention and illness care. However, as the nurse focusses on the aggregate and community, the roles of social marketing, community development, and policy formulation become more evident.

Application: Community to individual

Case Study

A community assessment was conducted by community health nursing baccalaureate students in collaboration with the health department. They discovered that the teen pregnancy rate had increased from six percent to 12 percent of the total number of pregnancies over a one-year period. Teens who said they were sexually active reported difficulty receiving services and lacked knowledge of family planning and of family planning services. The community assessment also revealed a strong sense of neighbourhood identity. Community leaders and residents expressed an interest in working together to improve the community.

Teen pregnancy is associated with physiological risks, such as malnutrition, toxemia, pre-eclampsia, anemia, and premature birth; psychological risks, such as isolation, lowered self-esteem, powerlessness, and depression; and social risks, such as lack of education, unemployment, and poverty (Alpers, 1998). The children of teen mothers also experience difficulties during infancy, school, and adulthood (see also Chapter 13). Thus, the costs of teen pregnancy can be seen at all levels of client. Table 5.2 illustrates how the integrated model can direct care at the four client levels. Can you identify some nursing roles that would be appropriate for each client level in this application to teen pregnancy?

Illness care

At the community-as-client level, the assessment of the community indicated increased numbers of pregnant teens and lack of available and acceptable prenatal and postnatal services for teens. A report of the findings was sent to the major clinics and the local health department, with a recommendation for increased services for the community. From an aggregate-as-client perspective, the students participated with the school nurses to explore the feasibility of developing a peer counselling program for pregnant teens and teen parents.

Table 5.2
Community to individual: Teen pregnancy

Focus of Care	Community	Aggregate	Family	Individual
Illness care	• Assess community for prevalence of pregnant teens	• Develop prenatal classes for pregnant teens	• Support family in making plans for pregnancy and delivery	• Encourage regular prenatal care
Illness/Disease prevention	• Conduct a targeted community assessment regarding beliefs and norms about family planning	• Participate with parent–teacher associations and schools regarding prevention of teen pregnancy	• Support family in anticipatory guidance regarding child and adolescent development and sexuality	• Assist teens to anticipate and deal with uncertainties regarding dating
Health promotion	• Hold discussions with leaders and residents regarding their wishes and hopes for the health of their community	• Participate in development of healthy and culturally appropriate recreation programs for teens	• Assist families to plan for recreation that is acceptable to all family members	• During health contacts with teens, emphasize self-esteem

The students offered to teach content about healthy nutrition, physical activity, and the signs of normal pregnancy and complications. Family-as-client care encouraged and supported the teens' families in making plans for the pregnancy and delivery, and individually oriented care encouraged the teens to obtain regular prenatal care.

Prevention

An initial step at the community-as-client level is to assess beliefs and norms about sexuality and family planning among community leaders and residents. Pregnancy prevention interventions for this age group must be sensitive to, and congruent with, the norms and beliefs of the community, including its families, schools, and churches. Involving the community in planning ensures programs that are culturally acceptable.

Aggregate-as-client care could include working with parent–teacher associations to plan pregnancy prevention programs for the aggregate of teens in the school. Developing peer counselling programs in schools and churches can assist teens to discuss sexuality, pregnancy, and family planning and to explore solutions.

Families also benefit from anticipatory guidance with regard to their children's development and sexuality. Family interventions may include appropriate referrals for counselling in high-risk situations. An intervention that targeted individuals could include responding to teens' concerns, assisting them to anticipate and deal with their uncertainties, and responding honestly to their questions regarding sexuality and pregnancy.

Health promotion

Collaborating with community leaders and residents to develop programs is an example of a health promotion intervention with the community. Developing school-related and community programs that provide enjoyable recreation for teens and including teens in the planning and organizing of such programs can ensure activities that are acceptable. Encouraging family involvement in school and after-school programs and developing and publicizing activities that families can do together for relaxation and enjoyment are examples of family-oriented health promotion interventions. Individual health promotion would include treating teens with respect; emphasizing their worth and self-esteem; involving them in planning; and teaching good nutrition, physical activity, relaxation, and recreation.

Conclusion

Given the worldwide emphasis on Primary Health Care and the goal of achieving health for all, community health nurses must have a full understanding of the scope of their practice and must continue to make meaningful contributions. The scope of community health nursing practice is broad, and no one nurse can attend to all levels of client and all types of care at the same time. Therefore, community health nurses must possess skills in communication, delegation, collaboration, and multidisciplinary work; place greater emphasis on identifying aggregates and communities at risk for health problems; and assist them to develop services that alleviate the risks and enhance overall health. Promoting a healthy community is the ultimate aim of community health nurses. As Mahler (1988, p. 94) pointed out, "the world needs nurses who can diagnose community health problems and institute measures to protect, advance, and monitor the health of populations as a whole."

QUESTIONS

1. What are the four levels of client with which community health nurses are concerned in their practice?
2. Using Table 5.1 on page 118 as a guide, what are specific community health nursing interventions for each level of client and type of community health nursing care (illness care, illness/disease prevention, and health promotion) for:
    a. community violence
    b. diabetes mellitus
3. What are some of the high-risk aggregates in your community that might benefit from community health nursing care?
4. Why is providing care to individuals for specific illnesses and diseases not sufficient to achieve a healthier community?

REFERENCES

Alpers, R.R. (1998). The importance of the health education program environment for pregnant and parenting teens. *Public Health Nursing, 15*, 91-103.

Anderson, E.T., & McFarlane, J.M. (1996). *Community as partner: Theory and practice in nursing*. Philadelphia: J.B. Lippincott.

Archer, S.E. (1985). An introduction to community health nursing. In S.E. Archer & R.P. Fleshman (Eds.), *Community health nursing* (3rd ed.). Monterey, CA: Wadsworth Health Sciences.

Baldwin, J.H., Conger, C.O., Abegglen, J.C., & Hill, E.M. (1998). Population-focused and community-based nursing—moving toward clarification of concepts. *Public Health Nursing, 15*, 12–18.

Bridges, J.M., & Lynam, M.J. (1993). Informal care: A Marxist analysis of social, political, and economic forces underpinning the role. *Advances in Nursing Science, 15*(3), 33–48.

Buhler-Wilkerson, K. (1993). Bringing care to the people: Lillian Wald's legacy to public health nursing. *American Journal of Public Health, 83,* 1778–1786.

Carruth, A.K., Gilbert, K., & Lewis, B. (1997). Environmental health hazards: The impact on a southern community. *Public Health Nursing, 14,* 259–267.

Clemen-Stone, S., Eigsti, D.G., & McGuire, S.L. (1995). *Comprehensive community health nursing: Family, aggregate, & community practice* (4th ed.). St. Louis: Mosby.

Canadian Public Health Association. *Community health/public health nursing in Canada.* (1990). Ottawa: Author.

Erickson, G.P. (1996). To pauperize or empower: Public health nursing at the turn of the 20th and 21st centuries. *Public Health Nursing, 13,* 163–169.

Freeman, R.B., & Heinrich, J. (1981). *Community health nursing practice.* Philadelphia: W.B. Saunders.

Hanchett, E.S. (1988). *Nursing frameworks and community as client: Bridging the gap.* Norwalk, CT: Appleton & Lange.

Hanchett, E.S. (1998, May). *A model for primary health care.* Paper presented at the Spring Institute of the Association of Community Health Nursing Educators, Chicago.

Kulbok, P., Laffrey, S.C., & Goeppinger, J. (1996). Community health promotion: A multilevel framework for practice. In M. Stanhope & J. Lancaster (Eds.), *Community health nursing: Promoting health of aggregates, families, and individuals* (4th ed.) (pp. 265–285). St. Louis: Mosby.

Laffrey, S.C. (1994, December). *An integrated model of community health nursing.* Austin, TX: Community Health Nursing Institute.

Laffrey, S.C., & Kulbok, P. (1994, November). *A multilevel framework for community health nursing.* Paper presented at the Annual Conference of the American Public Health Association, Washington, DC.

Laffrey, S.C., & Kulbok, P. (1999). An integrative model for holistic community health nursing. *Journal of Holistic Nursing, 17*(1), 88–103.

Laffrey, S.C., & Pagé, G. (1989). Primary health care in public health nursing. *Journal of Advanced Nursing, 14,* 1044–1050.

Laffrey, S.C., Loveland-Cherry, C., & Winkler, S.J. (1986). Health behavior: Evolution of two models. *Public Health Nursing, 3,* 92–100.

Laffrey, S.C., Dickenson, D., & Diem, E. (1997). Role identity and job satisfaction of community health nurses. *International Journal of Nursing Practice, 3,* 178–187.

McKnight, J., & Van Dover, L. (1994). Community as client: A challenge for nursing education. *Public Health Nursing, 11,* 12–16.

Mahler, H. (1988). Present status of WHO's initiative, "Health for All by the Year 2000." *Annual Review of Public Health, 6*(2), 92–102.

Nickel, J.T., Pituch, M.J., Holton, J., Didion, J., Perzynski, K., Wise, J., & McVey, B. (1995). Community nursing competencies: A comparison of educator, administrator, and student perspectives. *Public Health Nursing, 12,* 3–8.

Nightingale, F. (1860). *Notes on nursing: What it is and what it is not* (1969 ed.). New York: Dover.

Preston, D.B., & Bucher, J.A. (1996). The effects of community differences on health status, health stress, and helping networks in a sample of 900 elderly. *Public Health Nursing, 13,* 72–78.

Schultz, P.R. (1987). When client means more than one: Extending the foundational concept of person. *Advances in Nursing Science, 10*(1), 71–86.

Shuster, G.F., & Goeppinger, J. (1996). Community as client: Using the nursing process to promote health. In M. Stanhope & J. Lancaster (Eds.), *Community health nursing: Promoting health of aggregates, families, and individuals* (4th ed.) (pp. 289–314). St. Louis: Mosby.

Sills, G.M., & Goeppinger, J. (1985). The community as a field of inquiry in nursing. *Annual Review of Nursing Research, 3*, 3–24.

Stewart, M. (1985). Systematic community health assessment. In M. Stewart, J. Innes, S. Searl, & C. Smillie (Eds.), *Community health nursing in Canada* (pp. 363–377). Toronto: Gage.

Styles, M.M. (1994). Empowerment: A vision for nursing. *International Journal of Nursing Studies, 41*(3), 77–80.

Toronto Coalition Against Homelessness (1996). *One is too many: Findings and recommendations of the panel of the public inquiry into homelessness and street deaths in Toronto.* Toronto: Author.

Wallinder, J., White, C.M., & Salveson, C. (1996). New definitions [Editorial]. *Public Health Nursing, 13*, 81–82.

World Health Organization (WHO). (1978). *Primary Health Care. Report of the International Conference on Primary Health Care.* Geneva: Author.

Williams, C.A. (1996). Community-based population-focused practice: The foundation of specialization in public health nursing. In M. Stanhope & J. Lancaster (Eds.), *Community health nursing: Processes and practice for promoting health* (4th ed.) (pp. 21–33). St. Louis: Mosby.

Zerwekh, J. (1992). Community health nurses—a population at risk. *Public Health Nursing, 9*, 1.

Part 3
Health System Reform and Healthy Public Policy

This section depicts the current context of health system reform in Canada. Initially, the National Forum on Health's directions for a reformed health system are highlighted. Next, the importance of home care in a Primary Health Care system is exemplified by recent interest and initiatives. Finally, the pertinence of healthy public policy to a reformed system is stressed.

Noseworthy (Chapter 6) offers an exciting overview of the contributions of the National Forum on Health to health system reform in Canada. The Forum concentrated on values, striking a balance with determinants of health and evidence-based decision making. The Forum called for a rebalancing of investments in non-medical determinants of health, disease, and disability prevention, and a broad child and family strategy. The Forum, a policy think-tank, recommended support of community-based services, pharmacare, medicare, primary care, and home care.

In Chapter 7, MacWilliam probes the contributions of the home care initiatives in Canada. She offers an overview of trends, directions, and policy issues, and identifies relevant opportunities and challenges for community health nurses.

Glass and Hicks, in Chapter 8, contend that healthy public policy is a critical component in health system reform. As healthy public policy acknowledges the diverse determinants of health, it is necessarily multisectoral. Furthermore, it is founded on public participation and focusses on population health. Population health encompasses equity and multidisciplinary, intersectoral, and participatory elements—all Primary Health Care principles. The need for evaluation and research involving recipients and providers is stressed. The Canadian Nurses Association has contributed to health system policy development and emphasized healthy public policy. Community health nurses need to be cognizant of policy directions and the political process and to collaborate with other sectors in influencing healthy public policy.

C H A P T E R   6

Continuing to build on our legacy: National Forum on Health, 1994–1997

T.W. (Tom) Noseworthy

Health and health care are matters of national interest to Canadians. Accordingly, the Government of Canada established the National Forum on Health in October 1994. Its mandate was to involve and inform Canadians and advise the federal government of innovative ways to improve health and to ensure that Canada's health system will be equipped for the challenges of the future. Priorities for action called for by the Forum included maintaining the fundamentals of medicare and the single-payer, publicly funded system as the model upon which to build. Opportunities for improvement and innovation were seen to be appropriate and necessary as a means of preserving medicare in the areas of primary care, pharmacare, and home care. Beyond health care, the National Forum recommended tranforming knowledge about health into action, through a broader awareness of the fundamental determinants of health. Further, the Forum called on the federal Minister of Health to take a leadership role in the development of evidence-based culture and to establish a national health information structure as the fundamental basis upon which an evidence-based culture should rest.

LEARNING OBJECTIVES

In this chapter, you will learn:

- the complexity involved in aiming to improve public policy on health and health care
- that health care delivery is but one determinant of health, and that investments in health care must not exclude other important contributors to human health and well-being
- the necessity of public input on health policy and the health care system, which is an important social program that helps to unite Canada
- that future health systems must reflect the core values of the people to be served and must be driven by evidence directed at all decision makers, including politicians, health professionals, managers, researchers, and the public

128

Introduction

The last decade of the 20th century was characterized by a swirl of activities collectively referred to as health system reform and renewal. Canada's health care system is composed of 12 interlocking provincial pieces, with variable, defined, and shared responsibilities between the federal and provincial/territorial governments.

In October 1994, the newly elected government of Prime Minister Jean Chrétien established the National Forum on Health. This idea arose from pre-election commitments and later became a government initiative. The Forum was established as an advisory body to the federal government, with the Prime Minister as chair, the federal Minister of Health as vice-chair, and 24 voluntary members who contributed wide-ranging knowledge gained from the health system as professionals, academics, volunteers, and the public.

The National Forum on Health concluded its deliberations and tabled its report on February 4, 1997. This chapter describes the context, operation, and priorities for action of the National Forum and discusses the responses to date arising from the recommendations.

Context and conditions of the time

The health of Canadians and medicare continue to be matters of national interest. This was particularly true in the time leading up to and during the work of the Forum. In the early 1990s, it had become generally recognized that Canada's ballooning health care system had become unaffordable, needed improvements in efficiency and effectiveness, and lacked accountability. As most Canadians supported the notion of a public health care system, they were correspondingly concerned as fiscal realities took effect and resulted in substantial expenditure reductions to health care by the federal and provincial governments.

While much of health care reform was precipitated by fiscal restraint, many restructuring directions being introduced in Canada during this period were advocated by a series of provincial Royal Commissions and task forces during the 1980s. There was remarkable comparability of the findings of these bodies, which supported the notion that the system as a whole was fundamentally sound and adequately funded, but was in need of improvement.

Specifically, the problems identified included (a) unexplained variations in rates of surgical procedures and other interventions, (b) slow response to adopting practice patterns based on evidence of effectiveness, and (c) a substantial proportion of hospital days being used by people who did not require acute care. Within this context, newspaper headlines regularly proclaimed that the health care system was "in crisis." Media attention was often precipitated by salary reductions and lay-offs and by escalating conflicts among physicians, other health care professionals, providers, and governments. Hospitals were downsizing or closing, and public concern was developing with respect to waiting lists for surgery and high-tech diagnostic and therapeutic access.

With fewer and shorter hospital stays, families and friends, particularly women, were assuming more responsibility for care of the ill in the home. Across the care continuum, the private sector was pressing to gain greater access to new business opportunities in an industry that had hitherto been beyond reach. Critics of medicare asserted that Canada could no longer afford a universal, publicly funded health care system, and even supporters questioned whether or not the system would be there for their children.

Structure and process

The National Forum on Health was convened as a meeting of 24 Canadians who came from many perspectives and, for the most part, had never previously met. Not surprisingly, early discussions revealed widely divergent considerations as to the most important and critical issues for deliberation. It was recognized that, as the provinces were directly responsible for health care delivery, any recommendations made to the federal government had to support the directions of the provinces, in the context of maintaining a national system for all Canadians.

The National Forum on Health was not a Royal Commission. Rather, it was a policy think-tank attached to Health Canada through a secretariat and, while sensitive to the federal context, was committed to taking both a long-term and a national perspective on health and health care.

To perform its analytic work, the Forum formed four working groups, outlined in Table 6.1.

The working groups and staff secretariat addressed topics distilled from an original list of over 150 subjects that had been raised by members. Priority was given to issues of national interest and those with a long-term perspective. Particular attention was paid to broad inclusiveness of the determinants

Table 6.1
Working groups of the National Forum on Health

Values	Striking a Balance	Determinants	Evidence-Based Decision Making
Understanding the values Canadians hold about health and health care and ensuring these are reflected in a renewed health system	Considering how resources should be allocated within the health care system and between health care and other factors that enhance health	Determining what, beyond health care, makes and keeps people healthy in the first place (e.g., adequate income, employment, nurturance, childhood environment)	Using the best available and most up-to-date evidence in making decisions

of health, with the assumption that health care was but one of those determinants.

In-house research was complemented by commissioned research and works by respected experts in areas of interest (National Forum on Health, 1998). Thorough review of previous documentation, reports of Royal Commissions and provincial task forces, and an extensive reference collection was incorporated. Countless briefs, reports, and mailings from stakeholders and interested members of the public were received and included.

Public participation was central to the mandate of the National Forum on Health. The Forum undertook a major national consultation process with the public, involving 71 discussion groups in 34 communities across Canada. Most discussion groups involved about 25 participants, who represented the full range of living conditions in Canada and who voluntarily requested to be involved. The process was extended to include outreach consultations with Aboriginals, street youth, lone mothers, homeless men, and other disadvantaged or inaccessible groups. The national consultation was a community-based process that committed stakeholders to approximately 12 hours of intense exchange and discussion on key health issues upon which the Forum felt input was critical (see Table 6.2).

To supplement consultation with the public, working groups held multiple key-informant sessions around specific subjects. Additionally, there was engagement of health decision makers and stakeholders through national conferences, again using consultation workbooks, from which there was deliberation and feedback.

Toward the end of the National Forum's mandate, a second phase of joint public and stakeholder consultation took place, using large national conferences that included small group sessions, and addressing issues under three central and strategic directions (see Table 6.3).

In addition to the public and stakeholder consultations, further research was conducted on core values pertaining to health and health care, in April and May 1996. Eighteen focus groups distributed across Canada held detailed discussions on eight audiovisual scenarios, each of which illustrated

---

Table 6.2
Key topics in phase 1 consultations

- How to improve the health of Canadians
- How to maintain a fair and effective health care system
- How to ensure that decisions about health and health care are good decisions reflecting Canadian values and based on solid evidence
- How we move from research to action on the determinants of health

National Forum on Health (1996a).

Table 6.3
Key topics in phase 2 consultations

- Preserving the system by doing things differently
- Transforming into action our knowledge about what makes people healthy
- Using better evidence for better decisions

National Forum on Health (1996b).

---

an ethical issue or dilemma. These vignettes were used to clarify the core values of discussants, thereby elucidating those values most relevant to health and health care. Pre- and post-intervention surveys of focus group participants were conducted, as well as an attitude questionnaire administered to 800 participants, from centres in which focus groups were held. In addition, relevant information was gained from questions contained in the joint Canadian Policy Research Network/National Forum cross-Canada study of public opinion, supplemented by focus testing on values associated with social programs.

The findings from Canadians were voluminous. However, when considered within the context of other substantial input to the Forum, several key findings emerged, supported by the majority. There was strong reaffirmation of the basic tenets of a publicly financed and administered health care system, characterized by core values of equality of access and quality of care, in which there was a strong federal and provincial presence, and a demand for efficiency and effectiveness. While Canadians supported a fundamental investment in disease/injury prevention and health promotion as being critical, these were not seen as alternatives to necessary acute care and other health care services. Canadians recognized a growing interest in and use of alternative and complementary medicine, but limited their support on the basis of proven effectiveness.

There was a widespread view from Canadians that home care should be expanded without conscription and with adequate and sustained government funding. Furthermore, it was felt that decision making in health and health care could be improved, particularly through the exploitation of health information technology.

There was an unmistakable emphasis by Canadians that they did not accept a purely economic analysis of the issues associated with health care reform and renewal. While there were concerns that their health care system was deteriorating, Canadians appeared to hold a common view, which envisioned a flexible health care system that maintained the five principles of the *Canada Health Act*. They believed that the system's components should and could be better integrated, based on strong community action and driven by information.

The Forum's analytic, commissioned, and consultant works focussed on long-term and systemic issues, with the intention of providing advice appropriate to the development of national policies. Beyond the work on values, striking a balance, determinants of health, and evidence-based decision making, several other key areas were addressed, such as women's health, Aboriginal health, and pharmaceuticals.

The Forum's final report, *Canada Health Action* (1997a, 1997b), was addressed to governments and to the people of Canada. The recommendations and advice were intended to improve the health of Canadians and to ensure that Canada's health system would be equipped for the challenges of the future. The recommendations were meant to set a course for the future, and they were framed around actions in the three key areas shown in Table 6.3.

It was the intention of the National Forum on Health to call for action toward a health care system built on the key features of medicare and on the values that underlie it. The Forum envisioned a system that was much more fully integrated and in which care, not its location, would be funded.

Priorities for action

Values, an over-arching consideration

Exploring values is explicit acknowledgement of the need to be faithful to what people want, based on their core beliefs. Values are deeply rooted and relatively stable over time. Furthermore, they are imperfectly and indirectly revealed through the political process, because everyday thinking is so frequently influenced by opinions that are transitory and ever-changing. In recommending a course of action for Canada's health system, the National Forum on Health considered it essential that the foundations be consistent with the values held by the majority of the public. Accordingly, the Forum's consultations and discussion groups sought to elucidate core values and found that the basic principles of medicare accurately reflected people's values of equity, compassion, collective and individual responsibility, respect for others, efficiency, and effectiveness.

Medicare: The basics

Medicare was neither born overnight, nor was it the outcome of calm, reasoned debate. There have continued to be federal–provincial differences and confrontation. Nonetheless, after thorough consideration of 25 years' experience with medicare and recognition of many international perspectives, the Forum concluded that medicare should remain founded on the bedrock of a single-payer, publicly financed system. It was reasoned that this would ensure that Canadians would receive medical attention when they needed it, not only when they could pay for it. Publicly administered and financed, single-payer interlocking plans of the provinces reduce administrative costs and provide the potential for cost containment. Finally, the profit motive in financing health care was deemed to be inconsistent with the view of health as a public good, while at the same time leading to high administrative costs and inequities in both access and quality. In short, both from Canadian and international experience and evidence, it was judged that medicare should continue as a publicly financed model, as the best means of achieving fairness and value for money (National Forum on Health, 1995). However, it was nonetheless clear that medicare was in need of improvement. Ample evidence was available that resources could be used more efficiently and effectively.

Forum members felt that, at just over 10 percent of GDP, Canadians were spending enough through their taxes and private payments to support access to high-quality, needed health care. Notwithstanding that there could be reasonable debate about the relative share of public versus private funding, or the share of expenditures directed toward physicians, hospitals, pharmaceuticals, and so forth, simply doing more of what we had been doing with fewer resources was not seen to be a viable solution to the problems.

Typically, when public financing for health care is reduced, the system responds by offloading costs to others or doing less, instead of doing things differently. Accordingly, it is critical to focus on total system cost and value for money. The Forum's position was that increasing the scope of public expenditure could be the key to reducing total costs.

There was a recognized need to reorganize the system to ensure that medically necessary care was funded regardless of where it was delivered or by whom—not simply doing more with less but, rather, integrating the funding and delivery of health care services through primary care reform and other organizational changes. Forum members considered that this could be done while resisting the temptation to offload public costs onto private budgets, arbitrarily de-insuring people, or implementing user fees for medically necessary services.

The National Forum did not recommend changes to the *Canada Health Act*, although it realized that the Act had substantial limitations, given its focus on hospitals and physician services. Well-intended efforts to modernize or open the legislation to improve it could result in unforeseen and unintended consequences. Its inadequacies aside, the *Canada Health Act* has been a key legislative instrument in maintaining the single-payer, publicly financed system that Canadians know as medicare. The Forum felt that a continued and strengthened federal–provincial/territorial partnership was necessary to preserve and protect medicare and, furthermore, that existing federal cash contributions to medicare should not be permitted to decrease further (from $12.5 billion). The cash floor of the Canadian Health and Social Transfer was viewed as essential to preserving the real and symbolic leverage held by the federal government to maintain the *Canada Health Act* and national standards. Forum members were particularly concerned that further reductions in the cash transfer would adversely influence the rate, and perhaps the direction, of provincial reforms. Of particular importance, the Forum advocated $12.5 billion as a cash floor, not a ceiling; the federal government could not contribute less and expect to maintain either credible leadership or effective leverage.

While reassuring the government, and the public, that medicare was sustainable and built on sound foundations, aligned to Canadians' core values, the Forum nonetheless concluded that fundamental changes were necessary, specifically in the areas of primary care, home care, and pharmacare.

Primary care

The "store front" of the health care delivery system is primary care. While it may be traditional to think of primary care as the offices of general practitioners, the Forum saw it as being much more and requiring fundamental reform, removing the structural problems and inappropriate incentives that constitute barriers to achieving greater system effectiveness and efficiency. Primary care was defined as community-based, multidisciplinary collaborative practice including, but not limited to, primary care physicians. While a prescriptive model was not suggested, it was felt that alternative remunerative methods, other than fee-for-service, would serve such a system most appropriately. The Forum suggested that there should be encouragement to develop innovative strategies, approaches, and incentives to such primary care delivery.

Home care

The National Forum on Health recommended that home care should be an integral part of publicly funded health services in order to reduce the burden on informal caregivers, ensure commitment and standards of accessible home care services, and create incentives for cost-effective and sustainable health care. In short, Forum members felt that it was critical to fund the care, not the site or the provider. Accordingly, recommendations were made to broaden public financing of home care and implement and maintain national standards and accreditation. Special attention was directed toward informal caregivers, with any public policy taking into account the shifting burden of responsibility to them. In general, the objective was to enable individuals with major or minor limitations to continue to live at home or in supportive housing, thereby preventing, delaying, or substituting for acute or long-term institutional care. While detailed implementation issues were not developed, it was felt important to make this a universal system, yet to define comprehensiveness in terms of what should reasonably and normally be considered appropriate for public funding, taking into account necessary individual considerations. In general, the Forum suggested that provision of community-based services should be guided by best available evidence of appropriateness, namely, what works and what doesn't, delivered within the context of affordability. Nonetheless, broadening public coverage for community-based services needed to be aligned with the core values of universality and equality of access.

Pharmaceuticals

The National Forum on Health identified several key issues of relevance to pharmaceutical policy in Canada, including, but not limited to, accessibility, cost containment, appropriate prescribing, consumption, and usage. Pharmaceuticals attracted particular attention given their vital and increasing importance to health care and the approximate doubling of per capita cost from 1975 to 1994. Pharmaceutical costs by 1996 had amassed 14.4 percent of total health expenditures, or $75.2 billion. Costs increased as a consequence of price, volume, and new products, together with evidence of inappropriate prescribing, inappropriate use, and poor compliance.

The Forum studied the economic characteristics of pharmaceuticals and the pharmaceutical industry. Unlike medicare, in which two-thirds of costs are publicly financed, two-thirds of pharmaceutical costs are privately financed. Concern was expressed that rising costs may deter appropriate use for some and that insurance was least likely among the most vulnerable. As well as uneven insurance coverage, there were irrational patterns of coverage, with pharmaceuticals being free in hospital and, by-and-large, paid for by patients in the home. In general, pharmaceutical policies were recognized as being inconsistent across the country.

Given that pharmaceuticals are medically necessary and that public funding is the best way to promote universal access and to control costs, the Forum recommended that Canada should take steps to include drugs as part of the publicly funded health care system. Essential first steps, such as the development of pharmaceutical management information systems, were seen to be critical to improving management, prescription, use, and cost of pharmaceuticals.

The Forum cautioned against reliance on the pharmaceutical industry for research funding, as this practice has the potential to distort the Canadian health research agenda.

Innovation

The National Forum on Health recommended establishing a multi-year transition fund for pilot projects that would have a sound evaluation and research component. The intention was to create innovative solutions and results. Success stories could be disseminated and generalized so as to promote the implementation of best models, as determined by the evaluations.

Transforming our knowledge about health into action

To improve health status, the directions for change recommended by the National Forum on Health included serious attention to social and economic determinants of health, in particular investments in children, support for community action, and priority attention to the problems of unemployment, particularly in youth. In broad consideration of the non-medical determinants of health, the Forum indicated concern that investment was overly skewed toward health care services as the primary—indeed, almost the sole—strategy for improving population health. The Forum called for a rebalancing of investments, taking into account non-medical health determinants, disease and disability prevention, and injury control to produce greater returns than would otherwise come from money directed solely at health care delivery. Specific recommendations included a broad integrated child and family strategy for both programs and income support, with an integrated child benefit program, targeted community-based programs with home visiting components, better access to high-quality child care, and early childhood educational services (National Forum on Health, 1996c).

The Forum also recommended investment in knowledge infrastructure and the development of a foundation to strengthen community action that included the private sector. It recognized the substantial and specific needs of Aboriginal Canadians, and recommended an Aboriginal Health Institute, which would identify approaches to disease management that were culturally relevant and appropriate for the context in which Aboriginal people live. This Institute would perform and advocate health research, meet the needs of Aboriginal people, and share information within and outside Aboriginal communities. It would be a focal point for supporting Aboriginal workers and undertaking initiatives to increase advanced education for Aboriginal students in the health professions.

The Forum drew attention to how economic policies, particularly those related to employment, had significant health and social impacts. Accordingly, any strategy for maximizing the health of the population depended on achieving the lowest possible unemployment rates. The Forum felt that the problem of youth unemployment was particularly critical and accordingly suggested that priority be given to helping youths who are trying to enter the workforce.

Using better evidence to make decisions

Over the course of its mandate, the Forum recognized that opinions and propaganda, much more than facts and evidence, appeared to be governing

Canada's health care debates and undermining public confidence in medicare. It was recognized that the public often lacked objective information to understand or to counter claims or frightening anecdotes. In the Forum's view, Canada's health system was seriously underserved by inadequate capacity to measure performance, thereby leaving the public to judge the impact of change through subjective impressions and opinions, largely driven by the media. Accordingly, the Forum called on the federal Minister of Health to take leadership in the development of an evidence-based culture, in which decisions made by physicians and health care providers, administrators, policy makers, patients, and the public were based on appropriate, balanced, and high-quality evidence. In order to achieve this, the National Forum reaffirmed the critical requirement first cited by the National Task Force on Health Information in 1991, namely, a nationwide health information system. The National Health Infostructure would be a linkage of provincial and territorial information structures, based on privacy, confidentiality, security, high technical and data standards, and national funding for research and development. From this system, the provinces and territories could develop and maintain a standardized set of anonymous, longitudinal data on health status and health system performance.

In order to assist Canada in developing a broadening culture of evidence-based decision making, the Forum recommended that the National Population Health Institute be given a mandate to aggregate and analyze data, develop data standards and common definitions, and report to the public on national health status and health system performance. The Institute was envisioned as a resource for the development and evaluation of healthy public policy (see also Chapter 8).

Finally, the Forum recommended a comprehensive research agenda to advance the knowledge base and produce high-quality content for the health information system. It was suggested that research funding be shifted to create an appropriate balance between research on non-medical determinants and basic and clinical research. Furthermore, priority should be given to research on the impact of key determinants of health, such as gender and culture, with special attention to outcomes research.

Actions to date

Preserving the system by doing things differently

Although the National Forum on Health released *Canada Health Action: Building on the Legacy* in 1997, early assessment of outcomes is possible. This is best considered under the priorities for action, as outlined in the final report.

Support for the maintenance of the single-payer model has been widely endorsed. While the respective roles of federal and provincial governments continue to be a source of creative tension, there have been three federal–provincial conferences on home care, pharmacare, and health information structures. Each was directed to advancing the thinking of the Forum and to create action on the recommendations.

Following re-election of the Liberal government in 1997, the cash floor of $12.5 billion for the Canadian Health and Social Transfer was affirmed. Since then, subject to available revenue, there is every indication that this amount will be increased. Not surprisingly, the provinces have called for restoration to the original amount of some $18.5 billion. The federal government is now on record, as are the provincial premiers, that health and health care is the number one public program priority.

As a response to the request to foster innovation, the Health Transition Fund was put in place for three years at $50 million per year, with $30 million designated for national projects and $120 million for provincial initiatives. Since establishment, many Health Transition Fund projects have been announced and are under way across a variety of areas, including primary care, pharmaceuticals, and home- and community-based services. The extent to which these projects will provide sound, generalizable results for broader implementation remains to be determined. Nonetheless, the Health Transition Fund has shifted the focus of many researchers and evaluators, who are now more focussed on understanding the system and its elements: what works, what doesn't, and why.

While there has been a good deal of discussion, there has been no specific program or expenditure in the direction of broadening public financing for pharmaceuticals. Nonetheless, many provinces have moved to build or implement pharmaceutical management information systems.

There has been apparent attention to incorporating home care and community-based services within broader public financing. Health Canada has established an Assistant Deputy Minister portfolio for home care, and there has been substantial discussion and consultation with respect to developing home care services more broadly. This was a priority area for Health Canada and the 1999–2000 federal budget.

Transforming into action our knowledge about what makes people healthy

The federal and provincial governments have harmonized child tax and welfare benefits into the Child Tax Benefit, so as to make the tax system more equitable and advantageous to families with children. Emphasis has been placed on programs with a home visiting component, with continuing support by the federal government for community action programs for children and the Canada Prenatal Nutrition Program.

Discussion is underway in Health Canada toward the development of Aboriginal Health Institutes, but no firm direction is as yet established. Similarly, the National Population Health Institute is under active consideration as either a stand-alone entity or one linked with existing organizations. The Institute would bring together data collection and knowledge development, with elaboration of public policy options aimed at improving the health of Canadians.

Using better evidence to make better decisions

The federal and provincial governments have demonstrated leadership and support for the development and active dissemination of evidence-based decision making. Development of a Canadian health information structure is under way as a means of applying information technology to decision making associated with health and health care. At the provincial level, there is active development and investment in health information structures; at the national level, the Advisory Council on Health Infostructure has been established with a broad mandate to advise the federal Minister of Health regarding the essential needs, national priorities, challenges, and barriers involved in such an initiative. The Advisory Council has been asked to generate an effective agenda for action by stakeholders to enhance implementation of the most vital components of a health information structure (Advisory Council on Health Infostructure, 1998). The final report of the Advisory Council, *Canada Infoway: Paths to Better Health*, was released in February 1999. It contains wide-ranging recommendations for Canada's Information Highway.

Health Canada is currently working on several national initiatives, including a national health surveillance system meant to enable national and international surveillance of diseases and other potential risks or threats to health, allowing them to be dealt with on a timely basis. Such a system could greatly improve the capacity for disease prevention and health promotion, result in significant savings for Canada's health care system, and improve the health of Canadians. Health Canada is also developing the Canada Health Network as a means of consolidating public health and consumer information and resources, making them widely available. Such a network would provide Canadians with access to up-to-date and reliable information on health-related issues, enabling them to make informed health decisions.

Finally, Health Canada has done substantial developmental work and field implementation of the First Nations Health Information Systems, community-based, comprehensive computerized systems that would track information on a variety of issues relevant to Aboriginals. The intent is for the system to facilitate health program delivery, management, planning, and evaluation aimed at improving the health of the First Nations.

Finally, the federal government must increase Canada's capacity to carry out important world-class scientific research and technologic development, fundamental ingredients for a knowledge-based society. Responding to the advocacy of many, the federal government has established the Canadian

Foundation for Innovation to promote productive networks and collaboration among Canadian post-secondary educational institutions, research hospitals, and the private sector, seeking to accomplish national objectives in a regionally sensitive way. The details and characteristics of the Canadian Foundation for Innovation are being developed and will include a process for attracting matching funds from other sectors, which, together with federal funding, could provide substantial resources for the knowledge infrastructure necessary for education and research. Just as bridges and highways were the infrastructural elements of the industrial society, the Health Information Highway, which provides the best available information to decision makers, will be a key characteristic of the knowledge-based economy in Canada's health future.

Conclusion

In the face of aggressive health care delivery and restructuring by the provinces, and federal and provincial attempts to contain costs for health care, the National Forum on Health took a long-term and national view. Without any national framework or standards, Canada's provinces and territories would eventually see divergence of issues and solutions, and no national presence maintaining medicare.

While medicare is sustainable, it requires reaffirmation of the fundamental importance of the single-payer, publicly financed model. Sufficient federal cash transfers are required to maintain the national system. Necessary changes must ensue, focussed in the areas of primary care, home- and community-based care, and policy associated with pharmaceuticals.

The Forum has raised awareness and attention to the non-medical health determinants. While recognizing that health care is a critically important determinant of health for Canadians when they are ill, we must go beyond this to recognize the fundamental importance of socioeconomic and other health determinants, such as the effects of poverty, unemployment, and education.

The National Forum on Health set out to raise issues and broaden the quality of debate around health and health care. It saw Canada's health future as driven by the best available evidence and grounded on the solid underpinnings of core values held by Canadians. The Forum saw medicare as a legacy worth building upon—maintaining the fundamentals, while strengthening through change.

QUESTIONS

1. What are the arguments for a single-payer, publicly funded model of health care for Canada?

2. What is meant by the National Forum's recommendation to "fund the care, not the site or provider"?

3. Within the proposed culture of evidence-based decision making, at what levels did the National Forum on Health anticipate that it would affect decision makers, and for what purposes?

4. What does it mean to say that health care is one determinant of health, and not necessarily the most important, unless we are ill?

REFERENCES

Advisory Council on Health Infostructure. (1998). *Connecting for better health: Strategic issues. Interim Report*. Ottawa: Public Works & Government Services. (Cat. No. H49-118/1998)

National Forum on Health. (1995). *The public and private financing of Canada's health system*. Ottawa: Author.

National Forum on Health. (1996a). *Let's talk . . . about our health and health care*. Ottawa: Author.

National Forum on Health. (1996b). *Advancing the dialogue on health and health care: A consultation document*. Ottawa: Author. (Cat. No. H21-126/4-1996)

National Forum on Health. (1996c). *What determines health?* Ottawa: Author. (Cat. No. H21-126/3-1996E)

National Forum on Health. (1997a). *Canada health action: Building on the legacy. Final report* (Vol. 1). Ottawa: Health Canada. (Cat. No. H21-126/5-1-1997E)

National Forum on Health. (1997b). *Canada health action: Building on the legacy. Synthesis reports and issues papers* (Vol. 2). Ottawa: Health Canada. (Cat. No. H21-126/5-1-1997E)

National Forum on Health. (1998). *Canada health action: Building on a legacy*. Papers commissioned by the National Forum on Health include *Children and the young* (Vol. 1), *Adults and seniors* (Vol. 2), *Settings and issues* (Vol. 3), *Health care systems in Canada and elsewhere* (Vol. 4), and *Evidence and information* (Vol. 5). Ste-Foy, QC: Éditions Multi Mondes. (Cat. No. H21-126/6-[1-5]-1997E)

C H A P T E R   7

Home care: National perspectives and policies

Carol L. McWilliam

As a sequel to the 1997 National Forum on Health, the federal government of Canada identified three priorities for action: preserving the health care system by doing things differently, transforming knowledge about health into action, and using better evidence to make decisions. Home care was identified as one of three areas for action aimed at achieving these national priorities (National Forum on Health, 1997). The purpose of this chapter is to provide an overview of trends, directions, and policy issues related to the evolution of home care in Canada. The nursing opportunities and challenges that accompany development of this health care sector are elaborated and critical reflection is invited.

LEARNING OBJECTIVES

In this chapter, you will learn:

- the evolution of home care as a component of health system reform in Canada
- specific applications of Primary Health Care principles for in-home care
- the roles and responsibilities associated with the development of Canadian policy on home care

Introduction

Home care in Canada is often defined as "an array of services enabling Canadians, incapacitated in whole or in part, to live at home, often with the effect of preventing, delaying, or substituting for long-term care or acute care alternatives" (Health Canada Federal/Provincial/Territorial Working Group on Home Care, 1990). Generally, home care programs provide three functions: a *substitution* function for the services of hospitals and long-term care facilities; a *maintenance* function that allows clients to remain in their current environment rather than move to a new, and often more costly, venue; and a *preventive* function, which invests in client service and monitoring at additional short-run, but lower long-run, costs (Canadian Home Care Association [CHCA], 1998).

While the array and delivery of in-home services vary across Canada, about 90 percent of such services (Havens & Bray, 1995) are provided by publicly funded programs in every province and territory. Veterans Affairs Canada offers in-home services to clients with wartime or special-duty experience when home care is not available to them through provincial and territorial programs. As well, a limited home care program is offered jointly by the Department of Indian Affairs and Northern Development (DIAND) and Health Canada for on-reserve First Nations people.

As home care is not included in the *Canada Health Act*, home care services are not insured in the same way as hospital and physician services. Because health system reform has placed great emphasis on de-institutionalization, concerns about lack of universality have grown (Havens & Bray, 1995). Inconsistencies in provincial/territorial coverage of medications, equipment, supplies, and professional services create regional inequities in the comprehensiveness and accessibility of care available to Canadians. Furthermore, the mobility of Canadians requiring home care is restricted, as coverage of in-home needs is not portable from one province/territory to another. These contradictions of fundamental values espoused in the *Canada Health Act* currently constitute a federal health policy issue.

Increasingly, private organizations are providing services to those who are not eligible for publicly funded home care and to those who wish to complement public services, either through personal payment or private insurance (CHCA, 1998). This trend constitutes another dimension of this federal health policy issue, as it holds the potential for creating a system in which those with direct or indirect access to monetary resources have better care than those without.

While nurses may be employed by either public or private organizations, typically professional services such as nursing are provided free to the client through public funding. However, user fees based on income may apply to support services such as homemaking, personal care, house cleaning, and transportation. As well, clients may be charged for supplies, equipment, and the cost of their medications (CHCA, 1998).

The appropriateness and safety of the home setting determine eligibility for home care. One unique feature of home care arises from the fact that individual homes are not controlled environments, being greatly shaped by the family and client's lifestyle and their socioeconomic status, culture, and social support (i.e., determinants of health). Risk management, client-centredness, provider–client partnerships, interprofessional communication, and care coordination all present different challenges, opportunities, and policy issues for those who choose to work in this milieu. In particular, nurses have the opportunity to provide leadership in linking the principles of Primary Health Care to evolving in-home services. Emphasis on health promotion and preventive care through public participation and intersectoral collaboration to address the broader determinants of health will help to achieve optimal health system reform.

Growing demand and scope

In-home rehabilitative and long-term care for people with chronic medical conditions reflect growing health care needs. People over 65 years of age constitute the fastest growing sector of the Canadian population, with 3 934 000 (13.6 percent of the population) projected to be in this age cohort by 2001 and 7 781 800 (24.9 percent of the population) by 2031 (Statistics Canada, 1993). As 80 percent of this sector have chronic conditions (National Advisory Council on Aging, 1993), most users of home care, particularly chronic care, are older persons. Other at-risk groups of all ages, including the physically or mentally compromised or challenged, persons with AIDS, and the terminally ill, are also users of home care (Havens & Bray, 1995).

Changes in family structure, including diminishing nuclear and extended family supports (Beanlands & MacPherson, 1995), shifting employment patterns for women, and other social changes will continue to generate increasing demands for more formalized rehabilitative and chronic care services in the home. The spectrum of long-term care services in the home includes special palliative care programs, in-home respite services, homemaking, personal care, meal services, social assistance services, and social contact and security services. Additional services will appear as a consequence of consumer demands and provider innovation and entrepreneurship.

The broad spectrum of services spans all sectors of health and social service systems. For instance, in Ontario in 1993–94, those admitted to home care came from active treatment hospitals (57 percent), chronic hospitals (one percent), community services (34 percent), nursing homes (one percent), homes for the aged (one percent), rehabilitative services (two percent), and other places, including other home care programs (four percent) (Ontario Ministry of Health [OMH], 1995). In 1993–94, home care clients in Ontario received, on average, five nursing visits, nine hours of homemaking services, and one visit from another professional: physiotherapist, occupational therapist, speech language pathologist, social worker, or dietician. While comparable data on physician and hospital services are not available, clients also received support services: drugs (13 percent), dressings (39 percent), supportive equipment (38 percent), diagnostic/laboratory tests (18 percent), transportation services (five percent), meal services (0.07 percent), and oxygen (three percent).

Unquestionably, considerable time and knowledge are required to access and organize such services.

Public expenditure on home care totalled $2.096 billion in 1997–98, more than double what it was in 1990–91, with an average annual rate of increase of almost 11 percent (Health Canada, 1998). While interprovincial and territorial comparisons are not possible, the mix of services provided in Ontario affords a picture of the diversity of care needs. In 1993–94 admissions to home care per 1000 people were 13 for acute care, nine for chronic care, and 0.7 for school care; average lengths of stay for in-home care were 28, 140, and 335 days, respectively (OMH, 1995). Undoubtedly, health system restructuring across Canada will alter the numbers and proportions of clients in each category of service. Shorter lengths of hospital stay, downsizing of hospitals, de-institutionalization of clients requiring long-term care, demographic trends, and technological advances in treatment approaches and information management will increase the demand for in-home care.

Models for coordinating home care

Accessing, coordinating, and monitoring the multiple services and providers involved in care at home is complex. Potential duplication and fragmentation of service delivery can be averted by formalized case management. Community-based case management is defined as "a set of logical steps and a process of interaction within a service network which assure that a client receives needed services in a supportive, effective, and cost-efficient manner" (Weil & Karls, 1982). Case management mobilizes resources and coordinates services to individual clients.

Three generic models of case management prevail in Canada, reflecting three care management orientations (Rose, 1992a): the brokerage model, the integrated team model, and self-managed care.

Brokerage model

This model, the present approach in Ontario, provides an impartial, interorganizational approach to coordinating services, containing system costs, and preventing inappropriate client access and use of services (Kane, 1988). As the primary value of this system-driven model is cost effectiveness and cost reduction (Kane, 1988), this approach is also labelled a "service management model" (OMH, 1992). In this model, a professional nurse or social worker is designated full-time to the case management role (Zawadski & Eng, 1988), which includes determining client eligibility and needs, developing a care plan, organizing services, providing follow-up, reassessing the need for services, and monitoring client progress (Austin, 1983). Acutely ill, cognitively impaired, or socially isolated clients may find the dependence upon case managers appropriate, but those able and willing to manage their own home health care may resent the organizational control (OMH, 1992). Furthermore, the brokerage model may be inadequate when cases or caseloads reach a higher level of complexity. An interdisciplinary case management team may achieve more comprehensive (Roberts-DeGennaro, 1993) and continuous care (Bradley, Burke, Grant, & Robertson, 1994).

Integrated team model

An integrated team model is used in some provinces, for example, in the Extra-Mural Hospital in New Brunswick (Cormier-Daigle, Baker, Arseneault, & MacDonald, 1995; Ferguson, 1993). "Nurse coordinator" variations of this model exist in Québec (Birenbaum, 1990) and Alberta. In the fully integrated team model, one professional provider (physician, nurse, social worker, physiotherapist, or occupational therapist) on the team serves as the designated primary caregiver, with leadership responsibilities (Zawadski & Eng, 1988). The team model fosters continuity of care, thereby enhancing quality of care (McWilliam, Coderre, & Desai, 1995), comprehensive care assessment (Joshi & Pedlar, 1992), client–professional relationships, and professional autonomy and equality. According to this provider-driven model, health professionals share the goal of achieving client compliance with a care protocol reflecting their best professional judgement (Rose, 1992a). Negative system outcomes include conflicts of interest (Kane, 1988), duplication of services, and increased costs. Undesirable client outcomes, such as client dependence (Feldman, Olberding, Shortridge, Toole, & Zappin, 1993) and provider control over clients' care (McWilliam, Coderre, & Desai, 1995), are other limitations of this model.

Self-managed care

The third model, recently implemented in Vancouver's Home Care Program and piloted in Alberta (Alberta Ministry of Health, 1993) and in Manitoba (Manitoba Ministry of Health, 1994), emphasizes self-managed care. This client-driven model puts care management of personal and support services at a client-centred level. Clients are assessed as appropriate for self-managed care at time of intake, receive information on services, and select and coordinate needed resources within pre-established parameters. As of early 1995, approximately 50 percent of the clients of the Vancouver program required comprehensive case management, while the other 50 percent could manage their own care (CHCA, 1995). Evaluations of the pilot projects in Alberta and Manitoba revealed that clients reported more satisfaction and greater personal control over quality of care than in traditional service delivery (CHCA, 1995; Manitoba Ministry of Health, 1994). Client-driven models identify positive client outcomes of empowerment (Rose, 1992b), longer community tenure, increased independence in living arrangements, more involvement in meaningful and productive daily activities, and enhanced social networks (Rapp, 1986). However, real costs and care outcomes have not been rigorously evaluated. Informal caregivers often play a major role in managing care at home, absorbing indirect costs and sharing care responsibilities with a multitude of care providers.

Opportunities in home care

As acute in-home care expands, skilled practitioners will encounter new challenges and opportunities. Technological advances will continue to shorten hospital stays and expand ambulatory care, thereby increasing the complexity of care provided in the home and the demand for sophisticated technological skills (Health Canada Federal/Provincial/Territorial Subcommittee on Continuing Care, 1992). Home-based dialysis, infusion pumps, transparenteral nutrition, and other technologies have increased the units of service per client and the demand for more highly skilled professionals. De-institutionalization of technologically dependent children and adults and increasing survival rates achieved through technological advances will further expand the demands for these skills.

The opportunities for nurses to fulfil roles in primary, restorative, and supportive care are also growing, with accompanying demand for skills (Ballew & Mink, 1986). Given the vast array of in-home services, care management involves assessment of service needs and eligibility, development of trusting relationships, negotiation of expectations and roles, conflict resolution, facilitation of access to services, and coordination and monitoring of services provided by a multitude of professionals employed by many institutions. Because needs for health care are increasingly undifferentiated by institutional mandates, "transition care management" (i.e., planning, organizing, and coordinating care for individuals making the transition between services) has also become a part of care management.

Challenges of home care

Technological advances, complex service needs, comprehensive services, and increasing demand for services invite bureaucratization of in-home service delivery by governments and agencies focussed on cost-efficient health care. Health system restructuring threatens the power bases, resources, and sacred turfs of hospitals and medical specialists, thereby setting the stage for medically dominated and hospital-oriented approaches to be superimposed on in-home services. Bureaucratization and medicalization of in-home care create negative consequences for clients, informal caregivers, and quality of care.

The client's experience of fragmented, poorly coordinated, provider-centric services in the health/medical care system has been well documented (Donabedian, 1988; Naylor, 1990; Rachlis & Kushner, 1989; Thorne & Robinson, 1989). Professionally controlled, institutionally based, and medicalized care has seriously undermined personal health (i.e., the ability to realize aspirations, satisfy needs, and respond positively to one's environment and as a resource for everyday living [WHO, 1986]) and independence (McWilliam, 1992; McWilliam, Brown, Carmichael, & Lehman, 1994).

The orientation of the present health care delivery system toward institutionalization and professional control of care runs the risk of disenfranchising approximately 2.8 million informal caregivers who provide care in the home (Cranswick, 1997). In home providers traditionally have engaged in partnerships with informal caregivers, relying in part on caregivers to make informed decisions and to achieve quality and continuity in care. Imposition of a hierarchically controlled approach to care will undermine this invaluable informal resource and fail to meet consumer expectations for more informed involvement in care.

The potential impact on the quality of home care extends beyond fragmented, poorly coordinated, patronizing services that fail to engage care recipients and their informal care providers as partners. Services focussed primarily on cure undermine and devalue services aimed at holistic care for chronic or terminal illnesses and disabilities that cannot be "fixed." Bureaucratized services frequently fail to achieve quality of care and client satisfaction stemming from "continuity of relationship" with the provider (McWilliam, Stewart, Brown, Desai, & Coderre, 1996). Moreover, the division of labour associated with the traditional medical model of specialization fosters a "collusion of anonymity" among providers; accountability for overall quality of care is attributed to others. Continuous quality improvement and total quality assurance, therefore, remain elusive goals (McWilliam & Sangster, 1994).

Leadership strategies

Nurses are well positioned to provide leadership in evolution of approaches to home care. Nursing's long tradition of care in the community context, especially care provided in the home, has helped nurses to refine relevant professional skills. The holistic caring orientation of nursing focusses on clients as individuals within their larger life contexts (client-centredness). The community work context has afforded community nurses considerable autonomy for refinement of client-centred practice. Nurses must both demonstrate and justify through research the importance of client-centredness.

Community nursing also has a history of fostering partnership with clients, mutual aid in families and communities, and self-care. By virtue of their gender, minimized professional status in society, and experience in working with clients on their own "turf," nurses are well situated to empower clients and informal caregivers to be more equitable partners in care. The opportunity to develop (Stewart, MacPherson, Makrides, Hart, & Doble, 1993; Stewart, Ritchie, et al., 1994) and use new partnership resources (London Intercommunity Health Centre, 1997[1]) has never been greater.

While the acute care context has often focussed nursing education and work on health as "the absence of disease" and on health promotion as disease prevention or health education only (Hagan, O'Neill, & Dallaire, 1995; see also Chapter 16), nurses who have experience in the community setting continue to nurture health in its broadest sense. Opportunities to transform nursing knowledge about health into action and to promote valuing of health in society and in health system reform have never been greater. In particular, the potential for a more holistic, health-oriented approach to in-home care is high (McWilliam, Stewart, Brown, Desai, et al., 1996; McWilliam, Stewart, Brown, McNair, et al., 1997). Recent research suggests that nurses have the potential to make a major contribution to client health, independence, and quality of life (McWilliam, Stewart, Brown, McNair, et al., 1999), simultaneously reducing medical care costs and promoting health. Health promotion, a key Primary Health Care principle, is an integral component of home care.

While nurses have played a major role (McWilliam & Wong, 1994) in ensuring within-agency care coordination, the role of care coordinator for services extending across multiple disciplines and multiple agencies is more recent. The opportunity to play a leadership role in care coordination will take on increasing importance as the creation of an integrated health system is pursued. Nurses are already well positioned to lead the evolution of community care coordination, as the majority of executive positions in community-based health care organizations (other than hospitals) are nurses, and as the position of case manager is currently most frequently held by nurses. Nurses must maintain current knowledge of the vast array of services, technologies, and organizations. Linked data bases and information systems, which ensure interagency and interdisciplinary communication and access to client and service information, must be created. Nursing leaders will be challenged to find ways to integrate physician services without medicalizing in-home care. As well, nursing leaders must foster more flexible client-centred and health-oriented care coordination, building on the strengths of clients and their caregivers. Values regarding client-centredness, client empowerment, and partnerships among multiple providers, clients, and informal caregivers reflect Primary Health Care principles essential to positive health system reform.

With the shift to community-based care, the opportunities and challenges for nurses interested in home care have never been greater. If nurses take a leading role in championing client-centred, health-oriented care; partnerships with clients and informal caregivers; and client-centred, health-oriented care coordination, the challenges of bureaucratization and medicalization of in-home care may be minimized. To respond to the National Forum on Health's (1997) call to transform knowledge about health into action and to use evidence to plan programs and policies, nurses must lend their best critical reflection and leadership skills to evolving home care.

Policy implications

The shift of health care from hospitals to the community and the escalating demand for in-home care have heightened attention to relevant health care policy. The *Canada Health Act* (1970) ensures accessibility, portability, comprehensiveness, and universality of hospital and medical services. These characteristics are now important considerations in relation to home care. Establishing a coordinated system of health and social care with a single entry point and reallocating fiscal and human resources to parallel the shift of care from institutions to the community (Vowles, 1994) are pressing policy issues.

Program and policy planners will have to address the scope of coverage, program financing, quality of care, and models of care delivery with full consideration of both the *Canada Health Act* and the power wielded by existing organizations. Whether home care is spearheaded by hospitals or by community-based or private sector organizations will determine the services provided, who provides them, and the structure within which they are provided, with different outcomes in cost and comprehensiveness. Plans for health care reform and evolution of policy with respect to seniors currently espouse the values of independence, self-determination, security, and social integration (Béland & Shapiro, 1994). These values, along with the values of client-centred care delivery, including partnerships among clients, caregivers, and organizations, individualized care, provider accountability, flexibility of services, and a continuum of care (Béland & Shapiro, 1994), should be considered in developing policy for in-home care.

Other policy issues relate to the social, political, and economic impact of involvement of informal caregivers (Cranswick, 1997; Maritime Centre of Excellence for Women's Health, 1998; Rosenthal, 1994). The broader impact of informal caregiving on the social and economic welfare of Canadians should be considered. The costs in terms of accommodations in work patterns (Gignac, Kelloway, & Gottlieb, 1996; Keefe & Medjuck, 1997) and personal, career, and remuneration losses (e.g., diminished opportunities for advancement, supplementary benefits, and pension securities) (Barling, MacEwen, Kelloway, & Higginbottem, 1994; Gottlieb, Kelloway, & Fraboni, 1994) should be weighed, particularly in light of the disproportionate burden on women (Gilbert, 1991; Neysmith, 1994). Home care policy development should consider economic options such as tax credits and direct payment of informal caregivers, and mechanisms and financial options for consumer-managed care (Béland & Shapiro, 1994).

For too long, nurses have taken a low profile in developing and revising health care policy. The policy implications of the new emphasis on home care demand that nurses play a role in reforming health care. Nurses bring an appreciation of the broader notion of health to the health policy and programming arena. Indeed, active participation in policy and program development and revision constitutes a major challenge and opportunity for community health nurses.

Endnote
1. *Labour of Love* (1997) was produced by London Inter-Community Health Centre, 659 Dundas St., London, Ontario, 1997; *Caregivers video series* (1997) was produced by National Film Board of Canada; see also Happy, S. (1997), *Caregivers—A handbook for family caregivers*, London, Ontario: London Inter-Community Health Centre.

QUESTIONS

1. How can nurses help to develop home care as a component of positive health system reform?
2. How can nurses apply the principles of Primary Health Care to home care?
3. How might nurses help to minimize bureaucratization and medicalization of in-home care?
4. What nursing roles and responsibilities are associated with the development of Canadian policy on home care?

REFERENCES

Alberta Ministry of Health. (1993). *Self-managed care pilot project. Technical report.* Edmonton: Author.

Austin, C.D. (1983). Case management in long-term care: Options and opportunities. *Health and Social Work, 8*(1), 16–28.

Ballew, J.R., & Mink, G. (1986). *Case management in the human services.* Springfield, IL: Charles C. Thomas.

Barling, J., MacEwen, K., Kelloway K., & Higginbottem, S. (1994). Predictors and outcomes of eldercare-based inter-role conflict. *Psychology and Aging, 9*, 391–397.

Beanlands, H., & MacPherson, K. (1995). *Nova Scotia Health Survey: Caregiver support results*. Halifax: Nova Scotia Department of Health.

Béland, F. & Shapiro, E. (1994). Ten provinces in search of a long term care policy. In V. Marshall & B. McPherson (Eds.), *Aging: Canadian Perspectives* (pp. 245–261). Peterborough, ON: Broadview Press.

Birenbaum, R. (1990 Sept./Oct.). Despite achievements, home care crisis looms in Quebec. *Home Health Care* (p. 3).

Bradley, C., Burke, J., Grant, P., & Robertson, J. (1994). *Discussion paper on direct service provision integrated with case management.* Gloucester, Ontario: Regional Municipality of Ottawa–Carleton Health Department, Home Care Program.

Canadian Home Care Association (CHCA). (1995, Spring). *At Home: Official Newsletter of the Canadian Home Care Association.* Ottawa: Author.

Canadian Home Care Association (CHCA). (1998, March). *Portrait of Canada. An overview of Ottawa health/public home care programs.* Health Canada, background information prepared for the National Conference on Home Care.

Cormier-Daigle, M., Baker, C., Arseneault, A.M., & MacDonald, M. (1995). The Extra-Mural Hospital: A home health care initiative in New Brunswick. In M. Stewart (Ed.), *Community nursing: Promoting Canadians' health* (pp. 163–179). Toronto: W.B. Saunders.

Cranswick, K. (1997, Winter). Canada's caregivers. *Canadian Social Trends.* Ottawa: Statistics Canada.

Donabedian, A. (1988). The quality of medical care: A concept in search of a definition. *Journal of the American Medical Association, 260*, 1743.

Feldman, C., Olberding, L., Shortridge, L., Toole, K., & Zappin, P. (1993). Decision making in case management of home health care clients. *Journal of Nursing Administration, 23*(1), 33–38.

Ferguson, G. (1993). Designed to serve: The New Brunswick Extra-Mural Hospital. *Journal of Ambulatory Care Management, 16*(3), 40–50.

Gignac, M., Kelloway, K., & Gottlieb, B. (1996). The impact of caregiving on employment: A mediational model of work–family conflict. *Canadian Journal on Aging, 15*(4), 525–542.

Gilbert, N. (1991). Home care worker resignations: A study of the major contributing factors. *Home Health Care Services Quarterly, 12*, 69–83.

Gottlieb, B., Kelloway, K., & Fraboni, M. (1994). Aspects of eldercare that place employees at risk. *The Gerontologist, 34*, 815–821.

Hagan, L., O'Neill, M., & Dallaire, C. (1995). Linking health promotion and community health nursing: Conceptual and practical issues (Chapter 19). In M. Stewart (Ed.), *Community nursing: Promoting Canadians' health* (pp. 413–429). Toronto: W.B. Saunders.

Havens, B., & Bray, D. (1995). Long term care in Canada with specific reference to Manitoba. In J. Van Nostrand (Ed.), *International comparisons of long term care.* Hyattsville, MD: U.S. Department of Health & Human Services, National Center for Health Sciences.

Health Canada Federal/Provincial/Territorial Subcommittee on Continuing Care. (1992). *Future directions in continuing care.* Ottawa: Health Services and Promotion Branch, Health Canada.

Health Canada Federal/Provincial/Territorial Working Group on Home Care. (1990). *Report on home care* (p. 2). Ottawa: Health Services and Promotion Branch, Health Canada.

Health Canada Policy and Consultation Branch. (1998, March). *Public home care expenditures in Canada 1975–76 to 1997–98.* Ottawa: Health Canada.

Joshi, A., & Pedlar, D. (1992). Case managers for seniors: Educational needs and opportunities. *Educational Gerontology, 18,* 567–586.

Kane, R.A. (1988, May). Case management: Ethical pitfalls on the road to high quality managed care. *QRB: Quality Review Bulletin, 14,* 161–166.

Keefe, J., & Medjuck, S. (1997). Long term career costs as predictors of strain for employed female caregivers. *Journal of Women and Aging, 9*(3), 3–25.

Manitoba Ministry of Health. (1994). *Impact on self-managed care participants.* Technical report. Winnipeg: Author.

Maritime Centre of Excellence for Women's Health. (1998). *Home care and policy: Bringing gender into focus. Gender and Health Policy Discussion Series Paper No. 1.* Halifax: IWK Grace Health Centre, 5980 University Ave., P.O. Box/C.P. 3070, Halifax, NS, B3J 3G9.

McWilliam, C.L. (1992, Oct.). From hospital to home: The elderly patient's discharge experiences. *Family Medicine, 24*(6), 256–267.

McWilliam, C.L., Brown, J.B., Carmichael, J.L., & Lehman, J.M. (1994). A new perspective on threatened autonomy in elderly persons: The disempowering process. *Social Science & Medicine, 38*(2), 327–338.

McWilliam, C.L., Coderre, P., & Desai, K. (1995). Using action research to enhance geriatric case management. *Geriatric Care Management Journal, 5*(1), 13–19.

McWilliam, C.L., & Sangster, J.F. (1994). Managing patient discharge to home: The challenges of achieving quality of care. *International Journal for Quality in Health Care, 6*(2), 147–161.

McWilliam, C.L., Stewart, M., Brown, J.B., Desai, K., & Coderre, P. (1996). Creating health with chronic illness. *Advances in Nursing Science, 18*(3), 1–15.

McWilliam, C.L., Stewart, M., Brown, J.B., McNair, S., Desai, K., Patterson, M.L., Del Maestro, N., & Pittman, B.J. (1997). Creating empowering meaning: An interactive process of promoting health with chronically ill older Canadians. *Health Promotion International, 12*(2), 111–123.

McWilliam, C.L., Stewart, M., Brown, J.B., McNair, S., Donner, A., Desai, K., Coderre, P., & Galajda, J. (1999). Home-based health promotion for chronically ill older persons: A randomized controlled trial of a critical reflection approach. *Health Promotion International, 14*(1), 87–41.

McWilliam, C.L., & Wong, C. (1994). Keeping it secret: The costs and benefits of nursing's hidden work in discharging patients. *Journal of Advanced Nursing, 19,* 152–163.

National Advisory Council on Aging. (1993). Aging vignettes: A quick portrait. *Canadian Health and Seniors.* Ottawa.

National Forum on Health. (1997). *Canada health action: Building on the legacy. Final report* (Vol. 1). *Synthesis reports and issues papers* (Vol. 2). Ottawa: Health Canada. (Cat. No. H21-126/5-1-1997E)

Naylor, M. (1990). Comprehensive discharge planning for hospitalized elderly: A pilot study. *Nursing Resources, 39,* 156–161.

Neysmith, S. (1994). Working conditions in home care: A comparison of three groups of workers. *Canadian Journal on Aging, 13*(2), 169–186.

Ontario Ministry of Health (OMH). (Dec. 21, 1992). Debriefing note of the Ontario Ministry of Health and the Ontario Home Care Programs Association meeting. Toronto: Author.

Ontario Ministry of Health (OMH). (1995). *Ontario home care program: Interim statistical report for fiscal year 1993/1994.* Toronto: Author.

Rachlis, M., & Kushner, C. (1989). *Second opinion: What's wrong with Canada's health-care system and how to fix it.* Toronto: Collins.

Rapp, C.A. (1986, Spring). *The outcomes of case management services.* Unpublished presentation. Columbus, OH: Ohio Department of Mental Health.

Roberts-DeGennaro, M. (1993). Generalist model of case management practice. *Journal of Case Management, 2*(3), 106–111.

Rose, S.M. (Ed.). (1992a). *Case management and social work practice.* New York: Longman.

Rose, S.M. (1992b). Empowering case management clients. *Ageing International, 19*(3), 1–4.

Rosenthal, C.J. (1994). Long-term care reform and "family" care: A worrisome combination [Editorial]. *Canadian Journal on Aging, 13*(4), 419–427.

Statistics Canada. (1993). *Population projections for Canada, provinces and territories 1989–2031.* Ottawa: Author (Cat. No. 91-520)

Stewart, M., MacPherson, K., Makrides, L., Hart, G., & Doble, S. (1993). *Support-training intervention for family caregivers of seniors with stroke: Proposal.* Funded by the Heart and Stroke Foundation of Nova Scotia. (Report available from the Foundation)

Stewart, M., Ritchie, J.A., Ellerton, M.L., Salisbury, S., Sullivan, M., & Thompson, D. (1994). *Telephone support intervention for parents of young chronically ill children.* [Proposal funded by Canadian Children's Mental Health Unit]

Thorne, S.E., & Robinson, C.A. (1989). Guarded alliance: Health care relationships in chronic illness. *Image, 21,* 153–157.

Vowles, A. (1994, March). Home remedies: Home care network fills gaps in support system. *Health Economics,* 19–21.

Weil, M., & Karls, J.M. (1982). Historical origins and recent developments. In M. Weil & J.M. Karls (Eds.), *Case management in human service practice* (pp. 1–27). San Francisco: Jossey-Bass.

World Health Organization (WHO). (1986). *Health promotion. A discussion document on the concepts and principles.* Geneva: WHO Regional Office for Europe. [ICP/HSR 02]. Reprinted in *Health Promotion, 1,* 73–76.

Zawadski, R.T., & Eng, C. (1988). Case management in capitated long-term care. *Health Care Financing Review* (Annual Suppl.), 75–81.

C H A P T E R 8

Healthy public policy in health system reform

Helen Glass and Sue Hicks

There has been a shift in Canada in the last two decades from public health policy to healthy public policy. Based on population health and determinants of health, governments and communities are engaged in seeking comprehensive, intersectoral policies that enhance the health of individuals, families, and communities. The elements of healthy public policy are emerging, programs are being evaluated, and the knowledge gained is being applied to further policy development. This chapter provides an overview of the nature of healthy public policy development and of the role of community health nurses in policy making in system reform and renewal.

LEARNING OBJECTIVES

In this chapter, you will learn:

- the difference between public health policy and healthy public policy
- the relevance of healthy public policy in health system reform
- the skills needed for the development of healthy public policy in the community
- the significance of community involvement in the development of healthy public policy
- the impact of politics on the policy development process

Introduction

Healthy public policy is the policy direction of the future. It is a critical component in the move to shift health care from an illness-driven model to one that focusses on improving the health status of the population.

Traditionally in most Western countries, health has been defined within the context of the health care system, and institutional and professional arrangements have focussed on treatment of illness and chronic health problems. In Canada, introduction of hospital funding grants by the federal government in the late 1950s and of medical health insurance in the early 1960s greatly contributed to the growth in the number of hospitals and hospital beds in the system. The belief became prevalent that health depended upon the existence of these structures and services (see also Chapters 1, 2, and 24).

By the mid-1990s, with health services focussed mainly on hospital use and medical care, the health status of Canadians did not reflect the large amount of money spent on health care (Angus, 1991; Rachlis & Kushner, 1994). Canada's health expenditures stood fifth of all industrialized nations and the highest of all publicly funded universal health care systems globally (OECD, 1993a). Despite the amount of money spent on health care, Canada's current rank in health status, based on traditional measurements of life expectancy and infant mortality, is fourth in all industrialized nations globally (OECD, 1993b).

With the passing of the *Canada Health Act* in 1984, Canadians were assured of a universal, comprehensive, accessible, portable, and publicly administered health care system. It was assumed that by providing a quality system of health care, the health of Canadians would be protected. However, the focus was on the system, not on the health of the population. Health promotion was not a requisite, and there was no requirement to demonstrate scientifically that the system was appropriate in terms of health outcomes and cost effectiveness. Nor was there a requirement to demonstrate improvements in health status. As a result, demands on the system and costs of services have escalated with little evidence that they have contributed to improving the health status of Canadians.

It has become increasingly apparent that if the system is to focus on health status, much more than health care services will have an impact on the outcome. For example, populations that rank high on the socioeconomic risk index also have lower health status. Although the disparity in life expectancy between rich and poor is diminishing, the gap remains large. Similarly, although infant mortality has been cut in half since 1971, the rate among the poor remains almost double that among the rich (Saouab, 1993). This disparity can have a significant impact on the shaping of healthy public policy in the future (see also Chapter 9).

Simply increasing the resources allocated to the health care system will not improve health status. Improved health status has to come through economic growth, more equitable income distribution, social support, and education. All need to be incorporated into policy development.

The *Ottawa Charter for Health Promotion* lists, as the prerequisites for health, nine vital factors: peace, shelter, education, food, adequate income, a stable ecosystem (e.g., a stable interaction between humans and all aspects of their environment), sustainable resources, social justice, and equity (WHO, HWC, & CPHA, 1986). Recognition that population health is affected by a multiplicity of factors is essential for future policy development and program planning. Policy development must extend beyond the traditional realm of health care and begin to include those factors that truly influence health status. Unless Canadians approach policy development from this perspective, health system costs will continue to escalate, putting increasing pressure of higher taxation on Canadians, who continue to struggle with the national debt. If costs continue to escalate, Canadians may begin to see the dissolution of their health system and a decline of the health status of the population.

Nature of healthy public policy

Hancock (1982) conceived healthy public policy as "chiefly concerned with creating a healthy society" (p. 5) within an approach that would involve low technology and be holistic and future oriented. Healthy public policy differs from public health policy by being multisectoral; it explicitly recognizes the contributions made by sectors other than health (e.g., agriculture, education, transportation, energy, housing, and others) (HWC, 1988). Furthermore, healthy public policy is founded on public involvement in policy formulation and implementation. The surge to health promotion in the early 1990s brought about the establishment of many government health promotion branches and departments. By the end of the decade, health promotion tended to be subsumed, with issues related to population health, within the federal and provincial/territorial governments.

By the mid-1990s, a "healthy public policy" approach to health system planning was common. For example, the Manitoba health system reform process was developed around the premise of healthy public policy. Policy makers in Manitoba, including individuals at the grass-roots level, recognized that if health care was going to be reformed and reflect changes in health status, the community as a whole and many stakeholders would need to be involved in the entire process. In the late 1990s, the trend toward regionalization of health services provided a more manageable structure through which communities could become involved.

Healthy public policy is a process that cannot be developed in isolation. It requires a commitment to multisectoral collaboration among government departments, agencies, organizations, interest groups, and the community. Healthy public policy needs to focus on the development of policy and on allocation of scarce resources in a way intended to address the health needs of a specific population. For example, dollars spent on improving a community's water supply may have a greater impact on the health status of that population than building a new hospital or increasing the number of health professionals in the community. Thus, healthy public policy accepts the view that there are varied critical influences on health, many of which are beyond the control of individuals or the traditional health care system.

Characteristics of healthy public policy

The characteristics of healthy public policy include such determinants of health as environmental and socioeconomic factors, housing, support systems, and lifestyle choices. Healthy public policy focusses on population health with an emphasis on health status, equity, and multidisciplinary, intersectoral, and participatory elements, consistent with the principles of Primary Health Care (PHC). These principles are described in more detail below.

- *Determinants of health* typically fall outside the scope of the current health care system. For example, the relationship between health status and poverty has not been adequately addressed. To influence the broad determinants of the health of a population, health considerations need to be on the agenda of the public policy development process in every sector. For example, health should be considered in such areas as industrial development and environmental planning.
- *Population health* emphasizes health status of populations and health needs of communities. All determinants of health in a community must be taken into account. Factors favouring or deterring that community from achieving improved health are assessed. A community-health needs assessment identifies the strengths and needs of the community, enables the community-wide establishment of health priorities, and facilitates collaborative action directed at improving community health status and quality of life. Policy development should have a direct impact on improving the health status of the population.
- *Equity* is an underlying premise of health in any community. It means that there is a fair opportunity for individuals to attain their full potential. The notion of equity is embedded in a socioecological framework, an approach that recognizes the inextricable link between people and their environment. As a goal, equity drives many policy changes.
- *Multidisciplinary consideration* of determinants of health requires people with different skills and backgrounds to identify issues and develop implementation strategies in the process of formulating policy. Thus, health professionals, analysts, strategists, corporate and educational personnel, and other professionals are involved, depending on the composition of the community.
- *Intersectoral collaboration* recognizes that policy and strategy development must involve varied stakeholders. In a competitive society, stakeholders tend to protect their individual turf. In healthy public policy, each sector, including the health care system, has a contribution to make and is involved in decision making. A protective attitude does not lend itself to the policy process. Further, intersectoral action requires sectors to adjust their direction and to incorporate population health goals into

their mission statements. For example, in the development of highway infrastructures, not only do the cost and structure of a road need to be considered, but also such factors as potential impact on jobs in small towns, access to emergency resources, and locations of schools and hospitals.

- *Participatory* means involvement by all stakeholders. Traditionally, the usual stakeholders were health professionals, governments, institutions, and agencies, such as hospitals and community clinics. The broad-based approach in healthy public policy development includes groups and individuals in the community. Population health requires that people in the community identify their own needs and direct action to deal with those needs. This fosters a sense of ownership, which is essential if changes are to occur. Members of the community can be encouraged to participate on planning committees, become members of boards, or attend community meetings to express support or concern regarding issues. The people in the community should be involved from the outset of planning and policy making and continue through evaluation of health programs and policies.

- *Health systems* have traditionally been based on a medical care system. Today, data must reflect information on population health and health status outcomes. The technology is now available, but often is not structured into health information systems, which are important in defining population health needs and in supporting healthy public policy. The development of effective policies and strategies must be based on an objective analysis of relevant health information. This information must be drawn from such diverse sources as hospital utilization data, as well as socioeconomic, public health, epidemiological, and ecological data, to allow a comprehensive analysis of population health. The process of developing and analyzing health information must be integrated with policy development. Different structures for collecting and processing information are required at local, provincial, and national levels.

Values

Values provide a foundation for building goals, plans, and tactics, where things really happen and the world really changes (Kidder, 1994). Commitment to important values—such as leadership, facilitation, communication, consultation, conflict resolution, common ownership, and empowerment—guides the healthy public policy process.

- *Leadership*, not only from the top down but from the bottom up, facilitates the process of change. Whereas previously, governments have been seen as leaders in policy making, now it is essential that all strata of society be involved.

- *Facilitators* can assist in this transition.
- *Communication* enables ideas to flourish and policies to emerge based on discussion and congruence. To communicate effectively, all participants need the latest information pertinent to the problem at hand. A strategy then needs to be developed to communicate the policy to various sectors of society. This demands skill and marketing tools.
- *Consultation* among partners regarding a shared vision to shape the direction of policy is paramount. Consultation can focus on whether the policy supports the dominant values of individualism, competition, and inequality or moves toward more humane values of collectivism, cooperation, and equality (McPherson, 1987).
- *Conflict resolution* mechanisms may be needed, including ombudspersons, appeal boards, or watchdog committees, on a range of such issues as system management, implementation of regionalization, and citizens' concerns.
- *Common ownership* of issues and concerns can be achieved by involving the stakeholders as early as possible in the process. Once there is a sense of ownership through involvement and commitment, planning and implementation can proceed at a much faster rate.
- *Empowerment* ensures that those affected by decisions have the resources and power to influence those decisions. Involvement, participation, and partnership are means of empowerment, so that people in the community take responsibility for decision making based on what they value about their health and believe that the weight of that decision is theirs.

Policy decisions should begin with these values and move to framing issues, shaping solutions, resolving conflicts, and, eventually, framing policy.

Reconceptualizing health policy

Ideally, health should be on the agenda of such sectors as education, justice, environment, and many others. If policies are intersectoral, programs should also reflect this approach. The funnel-type organization of government departments and the funding policies within government should be changed to accommodate this shift. The Ontario document *Health for All Ontarians* (1994) states that "today's government structures do little to strengthen communities. In many cases, governments have become a collection of vertical solitudes with walls, narrow mandates and incentives to pass the buck."

Development of common goals among the various sectors, identification of priorities, and consensus on allocation of resources are essential. In times when resources are limited, there is a willingness to collaborate with other sectors and share or contribute resources. In the late 1990s, resources for health care were being allocated to create efficiencies in the system. New collaborative approaches are timely. Although the motivation may be fiscal restraint, one outcome may be a more intersectoral approach. This does not negate the need to establish formal mechanisms to sustain this intersectoral planning. Major reorganization within governments and of their relationships to the private sector may be necessary.

In the past, health policy development involved a disproportionate number of health professionals who were highly motivated to protect their own interests, often at the expense of policies promoting the best interest of the public. Interjection of other sectors into the policy development process is not simple. Achieving a balance between constructive participation and extreme advocacy is difficult when many stakeholders vary substantially in their level of knowledge, organization, and financial stability.

Health system reform in Canada has been instrumental in coordinating the country's approach to healthy public policy development. Through efforts to restructure the health care system, healthy public policy has become a recognized essential component of reform if Canada is to contain health care costs and improve the health of the population. Although the term *healthy public policy* is not broadly used in all provinces, most have incorporated its essential characteristics in developing provincial goals and discussing a national strategic direction.

Policy design

The process of policy formulation and implementation is deliberate. Ingraham (1987) defines policy design "as a process in which causal links between problems and solutions are systematically explored . . . [and] analytical attention will be directed to cause and effect at an early point in formulation activities, and that it be informed and guided by a broad explanatory framework" (p. 625). The overall process must be designed so that it moves in the desired direction. Tensions or problems lead to a need for policy. This then requires problem identification and definition, goals that arise from the definition, and specific targets. This is the stage of policy development leading toward implementation.

The *policy analysis* stage includes identification of issues, analysis of options, and choice of an optimal policy. The issues arise out of population health needs and priorities and, ideally, should be identified by individuals and groups within the general population rather than just by professionals or governments (see Figure 8.1). The *policy design* stage concerns communication with all sectors, planning, problem identification, and a definitive statement of the policy. In *policy implementation*, the next stage, deliberation focusses on strategies and instruments that will incorporate the policy into the health care system and touch on funding models, legislation, and involvement of non-governmental organizations (NGOs). Finally, *evaluation* of the policy once it is in place must be carried out, an indispensable element in all policy design.

Policy analysis and design planning are central to the process of developing healthy public policy. Planning for implementation is itself a political process requiring resource allocation, negotiation, and compromise.

Figure 8.1
Stages in the policy process for healthy public policy

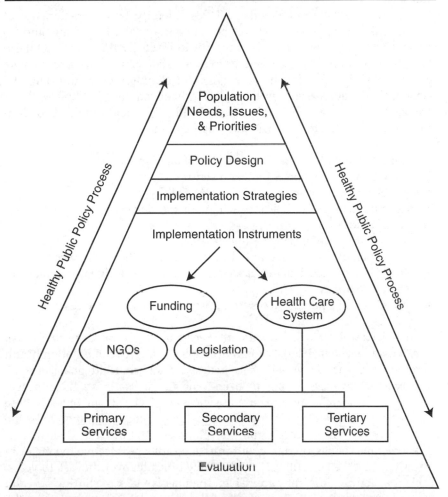

Adapted from Manitoba Health, Healthy Public Policy Division (1993).
Unpublished discussion paper.

Strategies are selected to enable implementation. The framework for health promotion (Epp, 1986) includes strategies and specific actions, such as fostering public participation, strengthening community health services, and coordinating healthy public policy. Many of these strategies have been adopted by provincial governments in Canada.

Problem definition develops as values, beliefs, and social attitudes toward a concern are delineated and the policy is defined (Cobb & Elder, 1983). Thus, policy problems tend to be socially constructed. Problems are redefined over time as the issues in human welfare take on changing public meanings. AIDS is a case in point, illustrating interrelatedness and changes in values, beliefs, and social attitudes.

Reeves, Bergwall, and Woodside (1984) identify two characteristics of health goals: they are (a) achievable both financially and technically and (b) responsive to the ideals of the community. In *Health for All Ontario* (Ontario Ministry of Health, 1987), goals refer to broad statements of desired change. In Manitoba, the goals for the new vision for community health (Manitoba Health, 1997) are based on the goals articulated in *Quality Health for Manitobans: The Action Plan* (Manitoba Health, 1992) and hundreds of consultations with Manitobans. The Manitoba goals include:

- improvement of general health status of all Manitobans
- reduction of inequalities in health status
- establishment of policies that promote health
- devolution of resources and action on the determinants of health to communities
- accountability to province-wide standards
- protection of basic community health and public health services
- changes in service delivery based on evidence of effectiveness and health status outcomes
- protection of equitable access to appropriate medical services

In the New Brunswick document *Report of the Commission on Selected Health Care Programs* (1989), "design principles to improve population health and the health care delivery system included: establish health goals, emphasize cost-effectiveness, orient to users, encourage health status improvements, emphasize community based services and focus on outcomes." These various principles and goals, identified by the provinces, continue to be the framework for policy and program development, but the shift is slow. This can sometimes be discouraging, but from a positive perspective the majority of provinces have been moving in the same direction over the last 10 years, each at a slightly different pace. Given the massive task of shifting a health system, progress is occurring, as evidenced in regular reports issued by the provinces.

Policy implementation

Implementation often occurs in an atmosphere of economic uncertainty. Conflicts may arise during this stage; some are inherent in the political process, such as resource allocation, negotiation, and compromise. Five factors shape the implementation of healthy public policy: (a) policy message, (b) multiplicity of perspectives, (c) multiplicity of ideologies, (d) availability of resources, and (e) political considerations (Hambleton, 1983). This stage involves top-down and bottom-up strategies.

The shift of health services from acute care settings to the community may be a sound policy, based on anticipated efficiencies, financial analysis, and research. However, the move challenges some entrenched values, such as the perceptions that hospital beds bring status to a community, that hospitals provide employment, and that the number of hospital beds affects the health of the community. A hospital closure or a bed reduction strategy cannot, therefore, just be announced. It requires extensive consultation with the stakeholders, development of strategies for alternative employment, and education within the community and about other health services within the existing physical structures of the hospital. For example, the conversion of hospitals into community health services could provide better use of facilities more closely related to the community's needs. This is a long, complex process, requiring skill, patience, and time.

A structure for implementation must be outlined clearly to ensure that a variety of stakeholders will understand it. Implementation strategies such as funding, program announcements, legislation, and taxation are some structural tools.

Policy evaluation

A feedback or monitoring process should be included from the beginning of any policy development. Feedback can provide information and lead to modifications and changes as needed. However, planned evaluation should be carried out at specified intervals throughout the process to monitor the impact of the policy (outcome evaluation) and to be certain that the policy deals with the identified needs, issues, and goals.

If the impact of policy design and implementation is to be measured, evaluation is essential. The healthy public policy process must include both providers and recipients of care in the evaluation. Evaluation must be clear, easily understood, and meaningful to those involved. Evaluation should not be considered a one-time activity but should be an integral, continuous component. It is the necessary link to research that keeps the theoretical base for policy design current and comprehensive.

The political system

The political system can be both intriguing and frustrating to those involved in policy and program development. The very nature of the Canadian democratic electoral system dictates short-term strategies. Priorities tend to be based on achievable short-term outcomes. This emphasis can be advantageous to the policy process, as it ensures that programs and policies are continually reviewed and changed. This in turn revitalizes the system. However, policies affecting social and attitudinal change cannot be dealt with in the short term. Therefore, strategies need to be built into the system to enable policies and programs focussing on social and attitudinal change to survive the political process.

The healthy public policy approach provides the framework to ensure that policies are well researched and have strong community support. It also enables partnerships with sectors outside government. Thus, ownership of the policies extends beyond government, making the policies less vulnerable to the political time-frame. Therefore, they are potentially more sustainable over a longer period of time.

Nurses need to be sensitive to the political process. Experience shows that positive results are most often obtained by working with the system, not against it. Working with the system, however, requires an understanding of the political process, the global perspective of the health system, and issues in the local community. If such knowledge is perceived to be irrelevant or intimidating, nurses and other professionals may avoid it and attempt to influence change only within the protected environment of their own profession. They then question why they appear to be powerless in effecting systemic change.

Community health nursing in healthy public policy

Within the infrastructure of healthy public policy, nurses have a responsibility to be knowledgeable about current policy directions, to be aware of the expected outcomes of community-developed programs and to participate in evaluation, and to recognize the significance of programs and policies in the context of the total health care system. Community health nurses should facilitate the development of programs that contribute to improving the health status of the population. They can play a significant role in ensuring measurable outcomes by participating in meaningful data collection and analysis. Community health nurses thus need community development skills, an understanding of the political process and its impact on health care, and an ability to function in an intersectoral environment.

Collaboration goes beyond participating in the traditional multidisciplinary team. Nurses need to function with ease among the many sectors influencing health and to facilitate their involvement in policy and program development. This can be achieved by sitting on community boards, participating in community activities, and developing an understanding of how other sectors develop policy and programs.

An organizational structure has evolved that fosters networking at all levels. Not only do governments "network" in relation to policy development, but the policy design process within non-governmental organizations enables shared contributions toward policy development.

Nursing's involvement in healthy public policy development is occurring nationally, provincially, and locally. Nursing, as a profession, on the international front, has been in the forefront of policy development in many countries. The World Health Organization (WHO) has been most influential in policy design. The national member states enunciated Health for All by the Year 2000 through Primary Health Care (PHC) (see also Chapter 2). Much of the thrust of PHC was generated by concerns of countries about the state of their health care. The International Council of Nurses (ICN) convened a workshop to determine policy for health care and directions for nursing both in formulating policy and in changing nursing services, education, and administration to improve the health of the population. ICN then presented a statement supporting the principles of PHC (see also Chapter 3) and reaffirming the commitment of nurses to effect necessary changes in education, practice, and management. Implicit in this statement were broadened responsibilities for nurses, including participation in health planning, decision making, and provisions of leadership (ICN & WHO, 1979).

Nationally, the Canadian Nurses Association (CNA) has been active in policy making over the decades. Outstanding leadership was shown by the CNA in the publication of *Putting Health into Health Care* (CNA, 1980), a response to a Health Services Review on health care in Canada (Hall, 1980). The CNA response was circulated worldwide as the policies in support of PHC were recognized by national nurses' associations and governments in other countries. In 1982, a Social Policy Committee was established by the CNA's board of directors. Numerous documents on specific areas of health care and policy continue to be developed by the CNA. (See Chapter 2.)

Most recently, there is a move to introduce healthy public policy into the CNA's agenda and to work with counterpart organizations and associations, such as the Canadian Public Health Association, the Canadian Hospital Association, and others through the Health Action Lobby known as HEAL (1994). HEAL addresses healthy public policy from the joint perspective of its member associations. HEAL acts in the political arena. The professional disciplines cooperate to design policy, define problems, seek solutions, implement programs, and evaluate the results of strategies that they support or resist based on their values and goals for healthy public policy directions.

Provincially, professional disciplines such as nursing may be guided by national and international directions in healthy public policy or may analyze and suggest alternatives to formulated policies. Locally, within interest groups, a similar process occurs. A shift in direction is clearly developing as the participation of all stakeholders is directed at collaborating toward common policy goals and outcomes.

As governments frame their healthy public policy, as organized bodies do the same, and as changes in health care reform occur, community health nurses are increasingly seen as a mainstay to the process. Hence, it is incumbent on nurses in the community—and, indeed, all nurses—to accept the challenge of a role alteration that concentrates on communities as the focal point for wellness care, long-term care, health promotion, and prevention of illness and disability. It means working closely with all partners. The mechanisms to do this are found in healthy public policy design.

Given that such a shift will identify gaps in skills, not only of nurses but of all health professionals and the public, it is important that gaps are identified in a spirit of cooperation and collaboration. For example, if nurses are to work intersectorally, they will need to examine their values and determine what values they share with other groups and with the public.

A number of skills will be needed, such as community development, education, and involvement. In many instances, communities know their needs and the types of programs they require. Strategies to assist communities to move toward their goals and to evaluate outcomes will be important. Working intersectorally with the public, governments, industry, and other community sectors requires yet another set of skills. There will need to be a shift from proactive and reactive to "preactive" strategies, which recognize challenges and opportunities and expedite the healthy public policy process in communities.

Governments are consulting with communities, and communities are developing their own policies with the help of governments as facilitators. This is the true healthy public policy approach. Community health nurses are key partners in the changing healthy public policy process.

Conclusion

Health reform in Canada has served to coordinate the country's approach to healthy public policy development, and a component of that reform has been to contain costs while improving the health of the population. The inclusion of all sectors of society is crucial to successful movement in a desired preconceived direction as healthy public policy takes shape.

It is essential for community health nurses to be knowledgeable about current policy directions, to be aware of the expected outcomes of community development programs, and to participate in the development of policy in the many sectors influencing health. Nursing as a profession will increasingly be in the forefront of policy development—internationally, nationally, and provincially—and will influence the direction of healthy public policy.

QUESTIONS

1. What are the main differences between public health policy development in the past and the healthy public policy process of the late 20th and early 21st centuries?
2. What are the key stages in the healthy public policy process?
3. What groups in your community are collaborating in the development of healthy public policy?
4. What evidence have you noted in your community that politics influences policy development?
5. What new skills will community health nurses need to bring to the development of healthy public policy in the community?

REFERENCES

Angus, E.E. (1991). *Review of significant health care commissions and task forces in Canada since 1983–84.* Ottawa: Canadian Hospital Association.

Canadian Nurses Association (CNA). (1980). *Putting health into health care: Submission to the Health Services Review '79.* Ottawa: Author.

Cobb, R.W., & Elder, C.D. (1983). *Participation in American politics: The dynamic of agenda building* (2nd ed.). Baltimore: Johns Hopkins University Press.

Epp, J. (1986). *Achieving health for all: A framework for health promotion.* Ottawa: Ministry of Supply & Services Canada.

Hall, E.M. (1980). *A commitment for renewal: Canada's national–provincial health program for the 1980s.* Ottawa: Health & Welfare Canada.

Hambleton, R. (1983). Planning systems and policy implementation. *Journal of Public Policy, 3*(4), 397–418.

Hancock, T. (1982). Beyone health care. *The Futurist, 26*(4), 4–13.

HEAL. (1994). *The Health Action Lobby: Getting it together.* Discussion paper. Ottawa: Author.

Health & Welfare Canada, Health Services & Promotion Branch (1988). *Coordinating healthy public policy: An analytic literature review and bibliography.* Ottawa: Author.

Ingraham, P.W. (1987). Toward a more systematic consideration of policy design. *Policy Studies Journal, 15*(4), 611–628.

International Council of Nurses (ICN) & World Health Organization (WHO). (1979,

October 1). *Report of the workshop on the role of nursing in Primary Health Care held in Nairobi, Kenya*. Geneva: Author.

Kidder, R.M. (1994). Universal human values. *The Futurist, 28*(4), 8–11.

Manitoba Health. (1992). *Quality health for Manitobans: The action plan. A strategy to assure the future of Manitoba's Health Services System*. Winnipeg: Government of Manitoba.

Manitoba Health. (1996). *Next steps: Pathways to a healthy Manitoba*. Winnipeg, MB: Author.

Manitoba Health. (1997). *Community health needs assessment guidelines*. Winnipeg: Government of Manitoba.

Manitoba Health, Healthy Public Policy Division. (1993). Discussion paper. Unpublished report.

McPherson, K.I. (1987). Health care policy, values and nursing. *Advances in Nursing Science, 9*(3), 1–11.

New Brunswick. (1989, July). *Report of the Commission on Selected Health Care Programs* (p. 43). Fredericton, NB: Author.

Ontario Ministry of Health. (1987). *Health for all Ontario: Ontario report*. Toronto: Government of Ontario.

Ontario Ministry of Health. (1994). *Health for all Ontarians: A provincial dialogue on the determinants of health*. Toronto: Government of Ontario.

Organisation for Economic Co-operation and Development (OECD). (1995a). *Health spending, major industrialized countries 1989*. OECD health data: Comparative analysis of health systems [Computer file]. Paris: CREDES.

Organisation for Economic Co-operation and Development (OECD). (1995b). *Life expectancy and infant mortality: OECD/World Health Organization data 1987–88*. OECD health data: Comparative analysis of health systems [Computer file]. Paris: CREDES.

Rachlis, M., & Kushner, C. (1994). *Strong medicine: How to save Canada's health care system*. Toronto: HarperCollins.

Reeves, P.N., Bergwall, D.F., & Woodside, N.B. (1984). *Introduction to health planning*. Arlington, VA: Information Resource Press.

Saouab, A. (1993). *Health policy in Canada: Report of the Political and Social Affairs Division, Research Branch*. Ottawa: Government of Canada.

World Health Organization (WHO), Health & Welfare Canada (HWC), & Canadian Public Health Association (CPHA). (1986). *Ottawa charter for health promotion*. Ottawa: CPHA.

Part 4
Nursing Practice in the Community

The principles of Primary Health Care should guide community health nursing practice. The impact of socioeconomic status on health status, health behaviour, and health services use is discussed in Reutter's in-depth investigation in Chapter 9. The role of the community health nurse in reducing inequities is stressed by Reutter in relation to the poor and by Kulig (Chapter 10) in relation to culturally diverse communities. Kulig pays particular attention to the immigrant population of Canada to and culturally appropriate assessment and intervention. These chapters emphasize that nurses need to promote accessibility for vulnerable and disadvantaged groups.

Another key principle is health promotion and illness prevention for clients representing varied cultures and ages. Burke and colleagues (Chapter 11) describe preventive interventions for children with chronic illness and their parents. The next two chapters delineate prevention and promotion issues pertinent to adolescents. Gillis (Chapter 12) discusses promotion of adolescent health and acknowledges the need for nurses to work with diverse disciplines—another principle. DiCenso and Van Dover (Chapter 13) examine community health nurses' role in preventing adolescent pregnancy and explore relevant research. Health promotion and injury prevention with older adults are discussed in the next two chapters. Craig (Chapter 14) reviews the importance of public participation in seniors' health promotion programs, and Edwards (Chapter 15) tackles the important subject of programs that prevent falls by seniors. Community health nursing roles are emphasized in these overviews of the diversity of clients encountered in practice.

The second half of this section reviews some pertinent roles and skills. The key roles of health promotion and of illness and injury prevention are the focus of Chapters 16 and 17. In Chapter 16, Hagan, O'Neill, and Dallaire observe that community health nursing and health promotion are inextricably linked and draw examples from health education by nurses practising in community health centres in Québec. In Chapter 17, Linwood and Willis propose basic premises for community-based injury prevention and control *programs. Cradduck (Chapter 18) elucidates and offers examples of key Primary Health Care roles.*

Health promotion and illness/injury prevention programs are typically directed at aggregates (groups) and communities as clients. Therefore, it is important to review appropriate tools that can be used by community health nurses. In Chapter 19, Neufeld and Harrison delineate and exemplify nursing diagnosis for aggregates and examine the suitability of such diagnoses for vulnerable populations. Reilly (Chapter 20) offers guidelines for health promotion interventions directed at the community. English (Chapter 21) also focusses on the community as client, but he stresses another Primary Health Care role—community developer—and provides a case study. Community assessment and program planning are integral to community development. Edwards and Meyer (Chapter 22) suggest suitable strategies and approaches to assessment and planning at the community level. Community development also fosters public participation and empowerment. Thibaudeau and Denoncourt offer a case study of an empowering community-level intervention targeting vulnerable groups (Chapter 23). Hughes (Chapter 24) emphasizes empowering strategies appropriate for nurses' interactions with individuals and families, the other two levels of clientele. Hughes depicts the communication skills relevant to such roles as consultant, facilitator, enabler, advocate, and communicator.

Thus, this section reinforces the premise that Primary Health Care principles, roles, and skills should predominate in community health nursing practice with all clients and in all contexts.

C H A P T E R 9

Socioeconomic determinants of health

Linda I. Reutter

This chapter explores the effect of socioeconomic status (SES) on the health of Canadians and the implications for community health nursing. The effects of SES on morbidity and mortality are presented, followed by an exploration of possible reasons for the relationship between SES and health. Factors such as health care utilization, health behaviours, and stress are discussed as mediating variables between SES and health. The role of community health nurses in reducing inequities created by socioeconomic factors is discussed using a critical social theory approach.

LEARNING OBJECTIVES

In this chapter, you will learn:

- the effects of socioeconomic status on health, health behaviours, and health care utilization in Canada
- explanations of the relationship between poverty and health
- how community health nurses can work to decrease the effects of poverty on health

Introduction

The impetus for the World Health Organization (WHO) Health for All 2000 initiative grew out of a concern about inequities in health within and among nations. As we near the turn of the century, in spite of tremendous health gains overall, the number of people living in absolute poverty worldwide continues to grow. Accordingly, the WHO reaffirmed the continuing need to address poverty and growing inequities into the 21st century (WHO, 1997a). Almost 20 years following the Alma Ata Declaration, the Jakarta Declaration on Health Promotion, developed at the Fourth International Conference on Health Promotion in 1997, pronounced poverty as the greatest threat to health (WHO, 1997b).

In Canada, reducing inequities has assumed increasing priority for policy-influencing bodies (e.g., Advisory Committee on Population Health [ACPH],

1994, 1996; National Forum on Health, 1997; Canadian Public Health Association [CPHA], 1997) and health sectors of government (e.g., Alberta Health, 1993; B.C. Office of the Provincial Health Officer, 1995). This emphasis is due, in part, to rising poverty rates (National Council of Welfare, 1998) as well as to changing conceptualizations of health and health determinants. Since the Ottawa Charter's (WHO, 1986) inclusion of income as an important prerequisite for health, there has been an increased understanding of the effects of social determinants, such as income, social status, and income inequality, on health (ACPH, 1994, 1996; Evans, Barer, & Marmor, 1994, Wilkinson, 1996).

Reducing inequities relates to the Primary Health Care principle of accessibility. A socioenvironmental view of health, which contends that the health of a population is closely tied to the social structure of society (Labonte, 1993), expands the conventional meaning of accessibility to include access not only to health care services but also to the "prerequisites" for health (WHO, 1986, 1997b) or "determinants" of population health (ACPH, 1994, 1996). This acknowledges the interrelationship between health and social and economic development and signifies the importance of intersectoral collaboration (a Primary Health Care principle) for addressing health determinants, such as SES. The challenge of reducing socioeconomically produced health inequities has major implications for the role of health professionals.

The purpose of this chapter is to provide a context for examining the relevant role of community health nurses. The chapter begins with a brief demographic profile of the economically disadvantaged in Canada. Next, the discussion turns to Canadian evidence of the effects of SES on health. This will be followed by interpretations of the relationship or connection between SES and health. Finally, implications for community health nursing practice will be considered.

Who are the poor in Canada?

In 1996, 17.6 percent of all Canadians were living in poverty, measured by Statistics Canada Low Income Cutoffs (National Council of Welfare, 1998). The relationship between SES and other social variables becomes evident when identifying who is most at risk for being poor. The overall rate of poverty for unattached individuals (37 percent) is about 2.5 times that for families (14.8 percent). Women are disproportionately represented among the poor, particularly single-parent mothers (61.4 percent); single-parent women under 25 years are at greater risk (91.3 percent). Although about 18.9 percent of all seniors were living in poverty, the burden falls disproportionately to unattached senior women (45.4 percent). With deterioration in the job market, the risk of poverty among young people under 25 has increased significantly;

unattached people under 25 years have a poverty rate of 61 percent (National Council of Welfare, 1998). Given the mounting evidence of the effect of early childhood development on health (ACPH, 1996), there is growing concern about the increasing rate of child poverty in Canada. In 1996, 20.9 percent of Canadian children were poor (National Council of Welfare, 1998), the highest rate in 17 years. Ironically, in 1989 the Canadian Parliament unanimously resolved to eliminate child poverty by the year 2000. To summarize, the risk of being poor is fairly high for unattached individuals in general, high for older unattached women, and very high for female-headed families and their children and for young unattached adults.

Other groups that are disadvantaged in terms of income, education, and labour force status are racial and ethnic minorities, particularly the Aboriginal population. In 1995, 44 percent of Aboriginals living off reserves had incomes below the poverty line (Statistics Canada, 1998). In 1991, the Aboriginal unemployment rate was 25 percent, and in some communities the rate is as high as 90 percent. An average of 29 percent of all Aboriginal people receive social assistance (CPHA, 1997). Another group at risk for being poor are visible minorities, the largest proportion of whom are recent immigrants (Statistics Canada, 1998).

How does socioeconomic status influence health?

The relationship between SES and health has been consistent and persistent, regardless of the measure of health used—mortality, morbidity, or self-perceived health and well-being. This section provides Canadian evidence supporting the relationship between SES and health. The examples given are meant to be illustrative rather than an exhaustive summary of available data.

Measures of SES are based traditionally on occupation, education, income, or some combination of all three. Recently, however, there has been a move toward using income and/or education as indicators of SES because these variables can be addressed by education and social welfare policies (Najman, 1993). The level of income that constitutes poverty is the subject of considerable debate in Canada. Although there are no "official" poverty lines in Canada, the Statistics Canada low-income cut-offs are viewed as such by most social policy groups (National Council of Welfare, 1998).

Indicators of health also vary. The most readily available national Canadian health indicators are mortality and morbidity data. Measures of health and well-being are less accessible. Canadian studies that correlate measures of health with indicators of SES are rare. National health-related surveys such as the Canada Health Promotion Surveys (HPS) (1985 and 1990), the Canada General Social Surveys (1985 and 1991), the longitudinal

National Population Health Survey (begun in 1994–95), and the National Longitudinal Survey on Children and Youth provide useful information that can be analyzed to determine the socioeconomic influence on health status, health behaviours, and health services use. (See Kendall, Lipskie, & MacEachern [1997] for a comprehensive overview of recent Canadian health surveys.)

Effects of SES on morbidity and mortality

The relationship between SES and mortality is borne out by Canadian data. In a national study based on Canadians living in metropolitan areas, Wilkins (1995) found that the greater the proportion of low-income individuals in a neighbourhood, the shorter the life expectancy of its residents. About 50 percent of men living in the poorest neighbourhoods will live to age 75, compared with 70 percent of men from the richest areas. The same gradient is evident for women, although less marked. Infant mortality rates in poorest neighbourhoods (7.5 percent) are considerably higher than in the most affluent neighbourhoods (4.5 percent).

The economically disadvantaged not only die younger but also are less likely to be healthy. The 1994–95 National Population Health Survey found that 77 percent of men and 74 percent of women in the highest household income group reported excellent or very good health, compared with 52 percent of men and 51 percent of women in the lowest income group (Millar & Beaudet, 1996). Those with lower incomes are more likely to have health problems, particularly adults aged 45 to 64 (Roberge, Berthelot, & Wolfson, 1995). Most chronic health problems, sleep difficulties, problems with moderate or severe pain, functional and activity limitations, and disability days are more commonly experienced by low-income individuals (Statistics Canada, 1994). Emotional well-being is also related to financial well-being (Statistics Canada, 1994); family dysfunction and parental depression are higher in poor families (Canadian Council on Social Development [CCSD], 1997).

The harmful effects of poverty on children are well documented. The rate of prematurity and "small for age" babies is greater in poor families (National Council of Welfare, 1997). Poor children are more likely than their counterparts to experience a variety of chronic medical problems such as diabetes, bronchitis, asthma, anemia, and psychiatric disorders (CCSD, 1997; Ryerse, 1990). A national study found that poor children had twice the rate of mental and physical disabilities as children from high-income families (Standing Senate Committee, 1991, cited in Edmonton Social Planning Council, 1994) and are at greater risk for injuries (Canadian Institute of Child Health, 1994). Children from low-income families experience dental decay at an earlier age, have more dental caries (Charette, 1993), and are less likely to visit a dentist (CCSD, 1997). Beyond its effects on mental and physical health, poverty also adversely affects children's social health. Poor children are at greater risk for poor school performance and are less likely to pursue post-secondary education (Ryerse, 1990). The 1994 National Longitudinal Survey of Children and Youth found that poor children do not have the same scholastic and verbal skills entering school as their non-poor peers (CCSD, 1997), and higher SES is associated with higher levels of academic achievement in reading, writing, and math (Lipps & Frank, 1997).

Various Canadian studies report on the relationship between family income and physical wife abuse (Ratner, 1993; Smith, 1990). A national survey revealed that women with household incomes below $15 000 were twice as likely as women with higher family incomes to have been physically or sexually assaulted by their spouse (Rodgers, 1994). There are more reports of child abuse and neglect among low-income families (Ryerse, 1990; Vanier Institute of the Family, 1994). The health effects of family violence are beginning to be documented. Ratner (1993) found that physically and psychologically abused women had more somatic complaints, higher levels of anxiety and insomnia, greater social dysfunction, and more symptoms of depression than those who did not experience abuse.

In sum, the Canadian studies cited above illustrate the relationship between SES and health using a variety of health indicators. The national surveys and studies cited, however, perhaps hide the health inequities experienced by one particularly vulnerable group, the Aboriginal population of Canada. The high rates of poverty among Aboriginals is reflected in health status indicators that are significantly lower than the Canadian average. The infant mortality rate is almost twice that for Canada as a whole, and life expectancy is about seven years less than for Canadians as a whole (ACPH, 1996). Aboriginal people also have higher rates of disabilities and chronic conditions, such as arthritis/rheumatism, diabetes, and tuberculosis (CPHA, 1997).

Exploring the connection between SES and health

What are the mechanisms or connections through which SES influences health? Although specific explanations vary, they can usefully be classified into the four general types first highlighted in Britain's Black Report (Department of Health and Social Security, 1980).

The *measurement artifact* explanation maintains that the relationship between SES and health is merely the result of biases in measuring and recording. This explanation is inadequate in explaining the connection between SES and health (see Blane, 1985; Marmot, Kogevinas, & Elston, 1987; and Wilkinson, 1996, for a detailed discussion). The *natural or social selection hypothesis* (also called the drift explanation) suggests that people suffer from ill health first and then, owing to resultant disability and reduced employment, "drift" down in social position. The overall impact of ill health on downward mobility is considered to be very slight (Blane, 1985; Marmot, Kogevinas, & Elston, 1987; Wilkinson, 1996; Williams, 1990) and limited to certain age groups and parts of the social structure (Blane, 1985). The *behavioural/cultural explanation* contends that those in the lower social hierarchy have poorer health because they engage in more health-inhibiting behaviours, such as smoking, substance abuse, and inadequate nutritional and exercise practices, and make less effective use of health care services. This explanation implies that these behaviours are the result of individual free choice.

The *materialist/structuralist explanation* is concerned with the effects that social structures, rather than individual behaviours, have on health outcomes. This explanation emphasizes that poor health results from decreased access to the material conditions and resources that facilitate health, such as the prerequisites or determinants of health (outlined in the Ottawa Charter and the Jakarta declaration). Those individuals with less purchasing power are more likely to be exposed to the ill effects of inadequate housing, inadequate nutrition, unsafe neighbourhoods, and occupational hazards. Although poor health may result from unhealthy behaviours, these behaviours are embedded in environmental living and working conditions. Over and above its recognition of the effect of income *inadequacy* on health, a structural explanation is also consistent with the growing body of evidence on the effect of income *inequality* on health (Wilkinson, 1996). In short, a structural explanation, congruent with a socioenvironmental view of health promotion, contends that living and working conditions can have both a direct and an indirect effect on health.

Intervening variables that explain the indirect effect of SES on health include utilization of health care, health behaviours, and psychosocial factors such as social support, perceptions of control, and stress resulting from family, occupational, and residential factors (Williams, 1990). The following section provides Canadian evidence for these mediating variables, with particular emphasis on health care utilization, health behaviours, and stress.

Health care utilization

Given that Canada has a universal medical care insurance system and that the economically disadvantaged have lower health status, it is reasonable to expect that their use of medical care services would be greater. Low-income Canadians are more likely to contact general practitioners, medical specialists, nurses, and psychologists (Statistics Canada, 1994); are more likely to be hospitalized; and more frequently use emergency rooms (Roos & Mustard, 1997) and mental health services (Lin, Goering, Offord, Campbell, & Boyle, 1996).

Nevertheless, there is an increasing body of research that identifies financial, cultural, structural, and personal barriers to use of health care services.

Financial barriers are particularly evident for working low-income families without extended health care benefits (Crowe & Hardill, 1993; Family Services Association & Income Security Action Committee [FSA & ISAC], 1991; Williamson & Fast, 1998). A study of working low-income families revealed that more than half these families expressed concerns about the lack of coverage for prescriptions, eyeglasses, over-the-counter drugs, and dental care (FSA & ISAC, 1991). Williamson and Fast (1998) found that lack of extended health care benefits prevented working poor families from obtaining services such as medications and dental care. Several provinces have indicated that they will use the National Child Benefit to extend health benefits (dental, optical, and drugs) to low-income working families with children.

Although preventive health care may have a greater impact on health status than illness care, the economically disadvantaged are less likely to access preventive services (Williams, 1990). Low-income Canadians tend to underuse prenatal care (Mustard & Roos, 1994), breast and cervical cancer screening (Maxwell, Kozak, Desjardins-Denault, & Parboosingh, 1997; Snider, Beauvais, Levy, Villeneuve, & Pennock, 1996), and dental services (Millar & Beaudet, 1996; Statistics Canada, 1994). Other illness prevention and health promotion programs, many provided by community health nurses, also are not well accessed by the poor. Prenatal education classes, for example, are less likely to be attended by low-income women (Bell Woodard & Edouard, 1992; Edmonton Board of Health, 1994), even though these women are at greater risk for adverse pregnancy outcomes. Low-income women are also less likely to attend postnatal support groups (Planned Parenthood Association of Edmonton, 1993).

The potential positive impact of illness prevention and health promotion programs compels us to ask why these programs may not be accessed by low-income individuals. Stewart's (1990) model describes barriers to effective health care utilization for the socially and economically disadvantaged that illustrate the dimensions of accessibility—financial, geographical, functional, and cultural—envisioned in Primary Health Care (Canadian Nurses Association, 1988). Such barriers include discrimination related to ethnicity/race and poverty status (Crowe & Hardill, 1993; Gaede, 1993); cultural/language barriers (Anderson, Blue, Holbrook, & Ng, 1993; Gaede, 1993); an uncomfortable environment, including insensitivity of health care workers to clients' circumstances (Anderson et al., 1993; Crowe & Hardill, 1993; Gaede, 1993); negative past experiences with the health care system (Gaede, 1993); lack of awareness of available services (FSA & ISAC, 1991; Gaede, 1993); lack of transportation and child care (Gaede, 1993); and inability to get time off work for appointments (Anderson et al., 1993). Health issues may also be low priority in relation to other survival needs (Gaede, 1993). Community health nurses, whose mandate is illness prevention and health promotion, need to decrease these barriers if the Primary Health Care principle of increased emphasis on illness prevention and health promotion is to be realized.

Health behaviours

Recent Canadian surveys provide some evidence that those with limited incomes may be more likely to engage in health-inhibiting behaviours. For example, there is a negative inverse relationship between smoking and each of income, education, and labour-force status (Manga, 1993). The Canada General Social Survey found that smoking was more than twice as high for adults who had not completed high school as for university graduates (Millar & Stephens, 1993). One in three women living in households with incomes under $20 000 a year smokes, compared with one in four women in households with incomes of more than $40 000 (National Council of Welfare, 1997). There is also evidence that poor children are more likely than non-poor children to smoke and take drugs (CPHA, 1997).

Low-income individuals also are less likely to engage in leisure-time physical activity. Sport participation for both men and women increases with income (Corbeil, 1995). Nearly half of poor families in Canada cite cost as a barrier to their children's participation in physical activities (CCSD, 1997). Seventy-nine percent of Edmonton food bank users indicated that their children were not able to access recreational and leisure activities for financial reasons (Edmonton Social Planning Council, 1998).

Nutritional intake is also influenced by socioeconomic status. Food insecurity has become a major issue among the poor in Canada. The study of food bank users revealed that only 16 percent ate the recommended servings of fruits and vegetables, grain products, and milk products, while only 25 percent ate the recommended servings of meat/alternates. About half of children did not eat the recommended servings from these food groups (Edmonton Social Planning Council, 1998). An analysis of the nutrient intake patterns of households in 15 urban areas across Canada showed that the proportion of diets with inadequate amounts of seven micronutrients increased as income decreased (Campbell & Horton, 1991). Low-income single mothers reported low intakes of fresh fruits and vegetables and dairy products (Tarasuk & Maclean, 1990). Breastfeeding is more commonly practised among those with upper-middle incomes and the more educated (Craig, 1993; Williams, Innis, & Vogel, 1996).

Why is it that those of lower socioeconomic status engage in health-inhibiting behaviours? A purely behavioural/cultural explanation would suggest that the poor may have inadequate knowledge of the harmful effects of these practices or may lack the motivation or skills to engage in health-enhancing behaviours. Interventions based on a behavioural/cultural explanation would be directed primarily toward changing knowledge, attitude, and/or behaviour. A structural explanation, on the other hand, would focus on understanding the *social determinants* of individual behaviour by exploring these behaviours within the life experiences of the economically disadvantaged. In other words, there is a need to contextualize risk factors by asking what it is about people's life circumstances that shapes their exposure to such risk factors (Link & Phelan, 1995). This perspective suggests that health-inhibiting behaviours may actually be coping strategies to manage the stress induced by decreased access to resources engendered by living and working conditions.

Stress

Economically disadvantaged individuals are more likely to be exposed to environmental conditions that give rise to socioecological stresses (Williams, 1990). They are more likely to work in low-status and less-rewarding jobs that carry greater risks of unemployment, exposure to hazards, and psychosocial stress, and they are more likely to live in dangerous and polluted neighbourhoods and in crowded or inadequate housing (CPHA, 1997; Manga, 1993; Smith, Bartley, & Blane, 1990).

There is considerable research indicating that the economically disadvantaged may experience more psychological distress (Mirowsky & Ross, 1989). In an Edmonton study of working low-income families, about two-thirds reported a very high level of stress resulting from uncertainty about income security, marital strain, inability to provide time and material resources for children, lack of affordable day care, and limited time and material resources for recreation (FSA & ISAC, 1991). Among food bank users, over half (52 percent) rated their stress levels as high (Edmonton Social Planning Council, 1996) and described the pervasive influence of poverty on their self-esteem and family life. Stigma is an additional stressor for those in poverty (FSA & ISAC, 1991; Pesznecker, 1984).

Although stress is by no means confined to those who are economically disadvantaged, the poor may have fewer resources to cope with stress. Moreover, the coping strategies used to counter stress may themselves be harmful to health. For example, those with lower incomes are more likely to use alchohol to overcome stress and tend to use more tranquillizers and sleeping pills (Manga, 1993). Stewart et al. (1996) found that cigarette smoking was a way for low-income mothers to cope with the stresses and isolation encountered in their daily lives. Non-nutritious food consumption by low-income families may result from the need to meet energy (rather than nutrient) requirements, to spend food money for other less expendable items such as housing (Tarasuk & Maclean, 1990), or to avoid stress caused by family conflict over food choices (Blackburn, 1991a). Travers (1996) found that the ability to purchase low-cost groceries was limited by lack of access to inexpensive stores as well as by welfare policies that resulted frequently in lack of funds. These studies underscore the need for community health nurses to consider the *context* of health behaviours, rather than focussing solely on the behaviour itself. In other words, "to change behaviour it may be necessary to change more than behaviour" (Wilkinson, 1996, p. 64).

The association between stress and health may be modified by protective factors such as social support (Mirowsky & Ross, 1989; Stewart, 1993; Williams, 1990; Williams & House, 1991). There is some evidence that those of lower SES have smaller social networks and less social support, and therefore more isolation (Oakley & Rajan, 1991; Williams, 1990). The Canada HPS (1990) found that the proportion of people who receive help from friends or relatives for health problems is inversely related to income level (Manga, 1993). Low-income families may also be unaware of community resources that could provide them with additional support (FSA & ISAC, 1991; Gaede, 1993).

Another buffer to stress is a sense of control or mastery (Mirowsky & Ross, 1989; Williams, 1990; Williams & House, 1991). People of low SES are less likely to have a strong sense of personal control (Mirowsky & Ross, 1989). Wallerstein (1992) argues that powerlessness is the broad risk factor for disease that underlies more specific physical and social risk situations.

To summarize the connection between SES and health, it may be said that SES affects health status directly through its influence on accessibility to the conditions that are the prerequisites for health and indirectly through its influence on health behaviours, accessibility to health services, and psychosocial factors, such as social support and personal control. Where should community health nurses direct their efforts to improve accessibility to "health"? What frameworks can guide their interventions?

Implications for community health nursing

What is nursing's role in decreasing inequities in health resulting from socioeconomic factors? Traditionally, nurses have tended to help individuals to change health-inhibiting behaviours through educational strategies. Increasingly, however, nurses are being challenged to "think upstream" to the broader environmental contexts of individual behaviours and to attempt changes at the societal rather than the individual level solely (Anderson et al., 1993; Drevdahl, 1995; Stevens & Hall, 1992). This means working to change health-damaging living and working *conditions* rather than focussing primarily on health-damaging individual *behaviours*, which may themselves be coping strategies in response to structural conditions. The importance of both an individual and a structural approach is articulated by Labonte (1993): "If we focus only on the individual . . . we risk privatizing—rendering personal—the social and economic underpinnings to poverty and powerlessness . . . But if we only focus on the structural issues, we risk ignoring the immediate pains and personal woundings of the powerless and people in crisis" (p. 57). Thus, nurses should provide support to individual families in poverty and also attempt to change public policy (Blackburn, 1991b; Pesznecker, 1984; Reutter & Williamson, 1997).

These roles reflect the mandate of community health nursing. Canadian documents, outlining the role of community/public health nursing, describe population-based approaches directed toward the determinants of health (CPHA, 1990; Working Group, 1991). The CPHA (1990) document describes the advocate role as one of helping the socially disadvantaged to become aware of issues relevant to their health and promoting the development of resources that would result in "equal access to health and health-related services." This latter statement speaks clearly to the Primary Health Care principle of accessibility and to the community health nurse's role in reducing inequities created by SES.

Critical social theory

A theoretical perspective that may be particularly useful in guiding nurses' attempts to reduce inequities is critical social theory (Butterfield, 1990; Stevens & Hall, 1992). Critical social theory attempts to describe and explain oppressive social conditions that limit people from reaching their full potential. In relation to health, the ultimate goal of critical social theory is to liberate (emancipate) people from health-damaging environmental conditions (Stevens & Hall, 1992).

A critical social approach includes asking critical questions to expose inequities, facilitating community involvement by listening to community needs, and assisting in bringing about changes (Stevens & Hall, 1992). Rather than presenting solutions and directing lifestyle changes, the nurse's role is facilitative: assisting individuals and groups to reflect on the social and political factors that influence health, sharing expertise, and providing support. The strategies best suited to reducing inequities are collective rather than individual. They often include forming alliances and coalitions with other individuals, groups, and agencies to provide a strong base of support for structural change.

These strategies require that nurses have a broad understanding of the context of poverty in terms of the systemic forces that influence access to the prerequisites for health. Questions such as the following contribute to critical reflection: What are the trends in relation to poverty? Who are the groups most at risk for being poor, and what are the reasons for this? How do Canadian poverty rates compare with those of other countries, and what accounts for these differences? How do current policies and programs contribute to or diminish the occurrence and effects of poverty? In addition, nurses may need to evaluate critically their own attitudes toward the economically disadvantaged, particularly in relation to beliefs about the "causes" of poverty and the relationship between poverty and health.

Nursing strategies

A critical social perspective to reducing inequities in health would include empowering strategies at the personal, interpersonal (small group), community, and policy levels (Labonte, 1993). At the individual level, nurses have a role in providing services that minimize the effects of poverty. "Empowering" services should be offered in ways that respect individual autonomy, are culturally sensitive, understand the psychosocial and socio-environmental contexts of the individual's concerns and problems, and increase the capacity of individuals to act upon the symptoms and roots of their distress (Labonte, 1993). More specifically, an empowering approach means listening to the impoverished to understand their experiences, acknowledging not only their constraints but also their strengths, exploring realistic suggestions and alternatives, and advocating for and with clients to access resources. Home visiting affords excellent opportunities for personal empowerment (Reutter & Ford, 1997a; Zerwekh, 1991) and has health benefits, particularly for families with limited resources (Ciliska et al., 1994). Accordingly, the National Forum on Health (1997) has advocated home visiting programs for at-risk families.

Nurses can also be involved in empowering strategies through small-group development and community development. Small groups are important vehicles for empowerment because they promote connectedness. Groups can decrease the social isolation often accompanying poverty by mobilizing and augmenting social networks and can provide affirmational, informational, practical, and emotional support (House, 1981; Stewart, 1993). Self-help mutual aid groups can increase the self-efficacy of their members (Stewart, 1993). The bidirectional or reciprocal help that is the hallmark of self-help mutual aid groups may be particularly empowering.

In addition to increasing personal empowerment, small groups may foster community action (Labonte, 1993); such collective action is particularly significant in diminishing the effects of social conditions such as poverty. In a community development approach, community health nurses can support community groups in identifying important issues and in organizing collectively to plan and implement strategies to resolve these issues. Public participation in all phases of community programming, with the goal of increased community self-reliance, is the hallmark of community development approaches (Labonte, 1993) and an important principle of Primary Health Care. "Strengthening communities" has been identified as a priority area for health promotion (CPHA, 1996) and for community health nursing practice (CPHA, 1990; Working Group, 1991). Although this approach presents new challenges (Chalmers & Bramadet, 1996; Reutter & Ford, 1997b), there are excellent examples of nurses' work with low-income communities that exemplify the principles of community development (e.g., Rutherford & Campbell, 1993).

A critical social perspective also requires nurses to advocate for structural changes that prevent the effects of poverty and even poverty itself. Advocating healthy public policies is seen as an effective strategy for addressing social determinants of health and for health promotion in Canada (CPHA, 1996). Professionals as a group can become politically active in relation to health and public policy issues identified by individual clients or community groups ("advocacy for"). More ideally, professionals support community groups in their own advocacy to challenge the social and economic causes of poverty ("advocacy with") (Labonte, 1993).

Community health nurses are well positioned for social action. They are the largest group of community health professionals and are organized into professional organizations (an important element for effective advocacy) (Labelle, 1986). But most important, community health nurses have firsthand information about how living and working conditions influence family and community health because they interact with people in their own environments. They can, therefore, raise awareness among other professionals, the public, and government of the effect of poverty on health and of the health impacts of social and economic policies. Such "consciousness raising" may help to dispel the myths about individuals living in economically disadvantaged circumstances, thereby decreasing the stigma of poverty. An excellent example of advocacy work by community health nurses is the Street Health program in Toronto. Nurses lobbied health care organizations and provincial and civic authorities to decrease barriers to health services for the homeless (Crowe & Hardill, 1993). Nurses in this program also were instrumental in forming the Toronto Coalition Against Homelessness, which initiated a coroner's inquest into the deaths of three homeless men and subsequently worked to implement the recommendations arising from the inquest (Sibbald, 1996).

Nurses can serve on intersectoral boards and committees that influence public policy in such areas as housing, unemployment, income security, child care, and environmental health. Intersectoral collaboration may also involve participation with other agencies, neighbourhood associations, citizen groups, and advocacy groups such as anti-poverty organizations. Finally, nurses can use their professional strength to influence public policy through such associations as the Canadian Public Health Association (and its provincial affiliates), the provincial arms of the Community Health Nurses Association of Canada, and the political action committees of provincial nursing associations. To date, advocating healthy public policy has not been well incorporated into the community health nurses' role (Chambers et al., 1994; Reutter & Ford, 1997b). Recent initiatives, such as the workshops and resources available through the Ontario Public Health Association (1996), will help to increase community health practitioners' skills in policy advocacy.

The following case study illustrates the community health nurse's roles in working with low-income families.

Mary is a lone-parent mother with a five-year-old son, Tim. They live in an urban area in which many families have incomes below the poverty line. Jane, the community health nurse for the area, visits the family and finds that Mary is feeling isolated and concerned that her income from social assistance is not sufficient to provide adequately for her family's basic needs; hence, she feels that she is not a good mother.

Jane listens non-judgementally to Mary's concerns, acknowledging the difficulties she is experiencing with the recent cutbacks to social services. She provides information about services Mary might access, including low-cost or free recreational activities in the neighbourhood. Jane affirms Mary's efforts in parenting her son, pointing out the strengths in her interactions with Tim, and helps her develop alternative ways of managing his behaviour. Jane sets up a meeting with Tim's teacher at school so that Mary can express her concerns and work with the teacher to her son's benefit.

After many visits, a trusting relationship has developed with Mary. With Jane's encouragement and support, Mary decides to attend a neighbourhood centre that offers a variety of educational and support services for parents and their children. Mary attends the parenting support group and, over time, makes new friends whom she sees socially and with whom she exchanges child care services. She learns new ways to deal with her concerns and finds that she is not alone; others have similar problems. Best of all, she realizes that she is "doing a lot of things right."

Mary joins the collective kitchen project at the centre. Her love of gardening leads her to become involved in a community garden project. Jane works collaboratively with the neighbourhood centre in facilitating these projects. She also encourages the women to become involved in a poverty advocacy group that is currently advocating for an increase in the minimum wage and for more affordable housing for low-income families.

As a community health nurse, Jane is a member of the Canadian Public Health Association; the provincial arm is lobbying the provincial government for increased resources for families on social assistance. At the community level, Jane is involved in an intersectoral partnership comprising public health professionals, churches, private businesses, social service agencies, educational institutions, and community families, working to develop the capacity of their community. Their aim is to make it more cohesive, vibrant, and responsive to the needs of citizens. Because she works with so many low-income families on a day-to-day basis in homes, community projects, and public health centres, Jane's input about the effects of poverty on family life is highly valued by the other partnership members.

Nursing interventions that support individuals and families living in poverty and that facilitate community involvement and political advocacy to counter the ill effects of poverty have implications for the preparation of community health nurses. The importance of public participation in empowering the economically disadvantaged requires a shift from the traditional professional–client relationship to a partnership characterized by a sharing of experiential and professional knowledge (Courtney, Ballard, Fauver, Gariota, & Holland, 1996; Stewart, 1993). Reducing inequities requires knowledge of political processes and skills that will enable nurses to dialogue, negotiate, and collaborate with stakeholders from professional, private, and public sectors (Reutter & Williamson, 1997). If nurses are expected to influence structural factors that inhibit health, nursing education will require a greater emphasis on the social context of health and health behaviour (Butterfield, 1990; Kendall, 1992). Nursing curricula based on the principles of Primary Health Care could prepare nurses to work with the economically disadvantaged, provided that appropriate experiential learning opportunities are incorporated.

Conclusion

In summary, this chapter provides evidence that inequities in health based on SES persist in Canada. The Health for All movement is aimed at reducing inequities through Primary Health Care. Community health nurses are ideally situated to make a contribution to reducing inequities. A critical social perspective could guide community health nurses' interventions to reduce inequities. This perspective is congruent with the Primary Health Care principles of accessibility to health and health services, maximum individual and community participation, and intersectoral cooperation and collaboration. Working to reduce health inequities will be particularly challenging in the present context; we have convincing evidence of the relationship between SES and health, but are faced with rising poverty rates, a widening gap between rich and poor, and increasing threats to the social safety net. The goal of Achieving Health for All Canadians into the 21st century, however, is predicated on meeting this challenge.

QUESTIONS

1.   Discuss policies in your community that have a negative impact on the health of low-income families. What policies have the potential to reduce health inequities? How did these policies evolve? Which of the four explanations of the relationship between poverty and health do each of these policies reflect?

2. Explore the role of community health nurses in your community in relation to reducing inequities. What is being done by individual community health nurses, community health nursing groups, and interdisciplinary professional groups?
3. What thoughts come to mind when you anticipate working with low-income families in your community? What attitudes toward the poor have you encountered? What do you think contributes to these attitudes?

REFERENCES

Advisory Committee on Population Health (ACPH). (1994). Strategies for population health. *Investing in the health of Canadians*. Ottawa: Minister of Supply & Services Canada.

Advisory Committee on Population Health (ACPH). (1996). *Report on the health of Canadians*. Ottawa: Minister of Supply & Services Canada.

Alberta Health. (1993). *Health goals for Alberta: Progress report*. Edmonton: Author.

Anderson, J., Blue, C., Holbrook, A., & Ng, M. (1993). On chronic illness: Immigrant women in Canada's work force—a feminist perspective. *Canadian Journal of Nursing Research, 25*, 7–22.

B.C. Office of the Provincial Health Officer. (1995). *Health goals for British Columbia: Identifying priorities for a healthy population. A draft for discussion*. Victoria: Author.

Bell Woodard, G., & Edouard, L. (1992). Reaching out: A community initiative for disadvantaged pregnant women. *Canadian Journal of Public Health, 83*, 188–190.

Blackburn, C. (1991a). *Poverty and health: Working with families*. Philadelphia: Open University Press.

Blackburn, C. (1991b). Family poverty: What can health visitors do? *Health Visitor, 64*(11), 368–370.

Blane, D. (1985). An assessment of the Black report's explanation of health inequalities. *Sociology of Health and Illness, 7*, 423–445.

Butterfield, P. (1990). Thinking upstream: Nurturing a conceptual understanding of the societal context of health behavior. *Advances in Nursing Science, 12*(2), 1–8.

Campbell, C., & Horton, S. (1991). Apparent nutrient intakes of Canadians: Continuing nutritional challenges for public health professionals. *Canadian Journal of Public Health, 82*, 374–380.

Canadian Council on Social Development (CCSD). (1997). *The progress of Canada's children 1997*. Ottawa: Author.

Canadian Institute of Child Health. (1994). *The health of Canada's children* (2nd ed.). Ottawa: Author.

Canadian Nurses Association. (1988). *Health care for all Canadians: A call for health care reform*. Ottawa: Author.

Canadian Public Health Association (CPHA). (1990). *Community health/public health nursing in Canada: Preparation and practice*. Ottawa: Author.

Canadian Public Health Association (CPHA). (1996). *Action statement for health promotion in Canada*. Ottawa: Author.

Canadian Public Health Association (CPHA). (1997). *Health impacts of social and economic conditions: Implications for public policy*. Ottawa: Author.

Chalmers, K., & Bramadat, I. (1996). Community development: Theoretical and practical issues for community health nursing in Canada. *Journal of Advanced Nursing, 24,* 719–726.

Chambers, L., Underwood, J., Halbert, T., Woodward, C., Heale, J., & Isaacs, S. (1994). 1992 Ontario survey of public health nurses: Perceptions of roles and activities. *Canadian Journal of Public Health, 85,* 175–179.

Charette, A. (1993). Dental health. In Health & Welfare Canada, T. Stephens & D. Graham (Eds.), *Canada's health promotion survey 1990: Technical report* (pp. 211–222). Ottawa: Minister of Supply & Services Canada.

Ciliska, D., Hayward, S., Thomas, H., Mitchell, A., Dobbins, M., Underwood, J., Rafael, A., & Martin, E. (1994). *The effectiveness of home visiting as a delivery strategy for public health nursing interventions: A systematic overview.* Hamilton, ON: Quality of Nursing Worklife Research Unit (McMaster University, University of Toronto).

Corbeil, J. (1995, Spring). Sport participation in Canada. *Canadian Social Trends, 36,* 18–23.

Courtney, R., Ballard, E., Fauver, S., Gariota, M., & Holland, L. (1996). The partnership model: Working with individuals, families, and communities toward a new vision of health. *Public Health Nursing, 13,* 177–186.

Craig, C.L. (1993). Nutrition. In Health & Welfare Canada, T. Stephens & D. Graham (Eds.), *Canada's health promotion survey 1990: Technical report* (pp. 125–137). Ottawa: Minister of Supply & Services Canada.

Crowe, C., & Hardill, K. (1993). Nursing research and political change: The Street Health Report. *Canadian Nurse, 89*(1), 21–24.

Department of Health & Social Security. (1980). *Inequalities in health: Report of a research working group (The Black report).* London: Author.

Drevdahl, D. (1995). Coming to voice: The power of emancipatory community interventions. *Advances in Nursing Science, 18*(2), 13–24.

Edmonton Board of Health. (1994). *Progress report on Healthy Edmonton 2000: Increasing prenatal instruction.* Edmonton: Author.

Edmonton Social Planning Council. (1994, March). Poverty and illness—an unhealthy connection: The effects on infants and children. *Alberta Facts, 13.* Edmonton: Author.

Edmonton Social Planning Council/Edmonton Gleaners Association. (1996). *Two paycheques away: Social policy and hunger in Edmonton.* Edmonton: Author.

Edmonton Social Planning Council/Edmonton Gleaners Association. (1998). *A return look at two paycheques away: Social policy and hunger in Edmonton Update '97.* Edmonton: Author.

Evans, R.G., Barer, M.L., & Marmor, T.R. (Eds.). (1994). *Why are some people healthy and others not? The determinants of health of populations.* Hawthorne, NY: Aldine de Gruyter.

Family Service Association (FSA) & Income Security Action Committee (ISAC). (1991). *Working hard, living lean.* Edmonton: Author.

Gaede, L. (1993). *Agency perspectives of Native health in Edmonton's inner city.* Edmonton: Boyle McCauley Health Centre.

House, J.S. (1981). *Work, stress, and social support.* Menlo Park, CA: Addison-Wesley.

Kendall, J. (1992). Fighting back: Promoting emancipatory nursing actions. *Advances in Nursing Science, 15*(2), 1–15.

Kendall, O., Lipskie, T., & MacEachern, S. (1997). Canadian health surveys, 1950–1997. *Chronic Diseases in Canada, 18,* 70–90.

Labelle, H. (1986). Nurses as a social force. *Journal of Advanced Nursing, 11,* 247–253.

Labonte, R. (1993). *Health promotion and empowerment: Practice frameworks. Issues in Health Promotion Series #3.* Toronto: Centre of Health Promotion University of Toronto & ParticipAction.

Lin, E., Goering, P., Offord, D., Campbell, D., & Boyle, M. (1996). The use of mental health services in Ontario: Epidemiologic findings. *Canadian Journal of Psychiatry, 41,* 572–577.

Link, B.G., & Phelan, J. (1995). Social conditions as fundamental causes of disease. *Journal of Health and Social Behavior,* [Extra issue], 80–94.

Lipps, G., & Frank, J. (1997, Winter). The social context of school for young children. *Canadian Social Trends, 47,* 22–26.

Manga, P. (1993). Socio-economic inequalities. In Health & Welfare Canada, T. Stephens & D. Graham (Eds.), *Canada's health promotion survey 1990: Technical report* (pp. 263–274). Ottawa: Minister of Supply & Services Canada.

Marmot, M., Kogevinas, M., & Elston, M. (1987). Social/economic status and disease. *Annual Review of Public Health, 8,* 111–135.

Maxwell, C., Kozak, J., Desjardins-Denault, S., & Parboosingh, J. (1997). Factors important in promoting mammography screening among Canadian women. *Canadian Journal of Public Health, 88,* 346–350.

Millar, W., & Beaudet, M. (1996). Health facts from the 1994 National Population Health Survey. *Canadian Social Trends, 40,* 24–27.

Millar, W.J., & Stephens, T. (1993). Social status and health risks in Canadian adults: 1985 and 1991. *Health Reports, 5*(2), 143–156.

Mirowsky, J., & Ross, C. (1989). *Social causes of psychological distress.* New York: Aldine de Gruyter.

Mustard, C., & Roos, N. (1994). The relationship of prenatal and pregnancy complications to birthweight in Winnipeg, Canada. *American Journal of Public Health, 84,* 1450–1457.

Najman, J.M. (1993). Health and poverty: Past, present, and prospects for the future. *Social Science & Medicine, 36*(2), 137–166.

National Council of Welfare. (1997). *Healthy parents, healthy babies.* Ottawa: Minister of Public Works & Government Services Canada.

National Council of Welfare. (1998). *Poverty profile 1996.* Ottawa: Minister of Supply & Services Canada.

National Forum on Health. (1997). *Canada health action: Building on the legacy. Synthesis reports and issues papers* (Vol. 2). Ottawa: Author.

Oakley, A., & Rajan, L. (1991). Social class and social support: The same or different? *Sociology, 25,* 31–59.

Ontario Public Health Association. (1997). *Building capacity for policy change.* Toronto: Author.

Pesznecker, B. (1984). The poor: A population at risk. *Public Health Nursing, 1,* 237–249.

Planned Parenthood Association of Edmonton. (1993). *Person to person: Creating a forum for intimate discussion.* Edmonton: Author.

Ratner, P. (1993). The incidence of wife abuse and mental health status in abused wives in Edmonton, Alberta. *Canadian Journal of Public Health, 84,* 246–249.

Reutter, L., & Ford, J. (1997a). Enhancing client competence: Melding professional and client knowledge in public health nursing practice. *Public Health Nursing, 14,* 143–150.

Reutter, L., & Ford, J. (1997b). Public health nurses as Primary Health Care practitioners. *Proceedings of making a difference: Using community health nursing research toward 2000 and beyond. 2nd International Conference on Community Health Nursing Research, Edinburgh, Scotland.* [Abstract].

Reutter, L., & Williamson, D. (1997). *Advocating healthy public policy: Implications for baccalaureate nursing education.* Poster presented at CPHA Conference, Halifax, July 6–9, 1997.

Roberge, R., Berthelot, J., & Wolfson, M. (1995). Health and socio-economic inequalities. *Canadian Social Trends, 37,* 15–19.

Rodgers, K. (1994, Autumn). Wife assault in Canada. *Canadian Social Trends, 34,* 2–8.

Roos, N., & Mustard, C. (1997). Variation in health and health care use by socioeconomic status in Winnipeg, Canada: Does the system work well? Yes and no. *Milbank Quarterly, 75*(1), 89–111.

Rutherford, G., & Campbell, D. (1993). Helping people help themselves. *Canadian Nurse, 89*(10), 25–28.

Ryerse, C. (1990). *Thursday's child: Child poverty in Canada. A review of the effects of poverty on children.* Ottawa: National Youth in Care Network.

Sibbald, B. (1996). One is too many. *Canadian Nurse, 92*(9), 22–24.

Smith, G., Bartley, M., & Blane, D. (1990). The Black report on socioeconomic inequalities in health 10 years on. *British Medical Journal, 301,* 373–377.

Smith, M. (1990). Sociodemographic risk factors in wife abuse: Results from a survey of Toronto women. *Canadian Journal of Sociology, 15*(1), 39–58.

Snider, J., Beauvais, J., Levy, I., Villeneuve, P., & Pennock, J. (1996). Trends in mammography and Pap smear utilization in Canada. *Chronic Diseases in Canada, 17*(3–4), 108–117.

Statistics Canada. (1994). *Health status of Canadians. General Social Survey Analysis Series.* Ottawa: Minister of Supply & Services Canada.

Statistics Canada. (1998). 1996 Census: Sources of income, earnings and total income, and family income. (May 12, 1998). *The Daily* (Online: http://www.statcan.ca/Daily/English/980512)

Stevens, P., & Hall, J. (1992). Applying critical theories to nursing in communities. *Public Health Nursing, 9*(1), 2–9.

Stewart, M.J. (1990). Access to health care for economically disadvantaged Canadians: A model. *Canadian Journal of Public Health, 81,* 450–455.

Stewart, M.J. (1993). *Integrating social support in nursing.* Newbury Park, CA: Sage.

Stewart, M., Gillis, A., Brosky, G., Johnston, G., Kirkland, S., Leigh, G., Persaud, V., Rootman, I., Jackson, S., & Pawliw-Fry, B.A. (1996). Smoking among disadvantaged women: Causes and cessation. *Canadian Journal of Nursing Research, 28*(1), 41–60.

Tarasuk, V., & Maclean, H. (1990). The food problems of low-income single mothers: An ethnographic study. *Canadian Home Economics Journal, 40*(2), 76–82.

Travers, K. (1996). The social organization of nutritional inequities. *Social Science and Medicine, 43,* 543–553.

Vanier Institute of the Family. (1994). *Profiling Canada's families.* Ottawa: Author.

Wallerstein, N. (1992). Powerlessness, empowerment, and health: Implications for health promotion programs. *American Journal of Health Promotion, 6*(3), 197–205.

Wilkins, R. (1995). *Mortality by neighbourhood income in urban Canada, 1986–1991.* Poster presented at the Conference of the Canadian Society for Epidemiology and Biostatistics (CSEB), St. John's, Newfoundland.

Wilkinson, R. (1996). *Unhealthy societies: The afflictions of inequality.* London: Routledge.

Williams, D. (1990). Socioeconomic differentials in health: A review and redirection. *Social Psychology Quarterly, 53,* 81–99.

Williams, D., & House, J. (1991). Stress, social support, control and coping: A social epidemiological view. In B. Bandura & I. Kickbusch (Eds.), *Health promotion research* (pp. 147–172). Copenhagen: WHO.

Williams, P., Innis, S., & Vogel, A. (1996). Breastfeeding and weaning practices in Vancouver. *Canadian Journal of Public Health, 87,* 231–236.

Williamson, D., & Fast, J. (1998). Poverty and medical treatment: When public policy compromises accessibility. *Canadian Journal of Public Health, 89,* 120–124.

Working Group of Federal/Provincial/Territorial Nursing Consultants. (1991). *Report of the working group on the educational requirements of community health nurses.* Ottawa: Community Health Division, Health Services & Promotion Branch, Health & Welfare Canada.

World Health Organization (WHO). (1986). *Ottawa charter for health promotion.* Ottawa: Canadian Public Health Association.

World Health Organization (WHO). (1997a). *Health for all in the 21st century.* (Online: http://www.who.ch/hfa/policy)

World Health Organization (WHO). (1997b). *The Jakarta declaration on health promotion into the 21st century.* (Online: http://www.dnttm.ro/arspms/jakarta.html)

Zerwekh, J. (1991). A family caregiving model for public health nursing. *Nursing Outlook, 39,* 213–217.

C H A P T E R   1 0

Culturally diverse communities: The impact on the role of community health nurses

Judith C. Kulig

Culture, community health nursing, and Primary Health Care are interrelated. This chapter includes definitions of major concepts within cross-cultural nursing. Cultural assessments and their usage with individuals, families, and communities, are discussed; practical suggestions and examples of actual questions are offered. The implications of cultural diversity for community health nursing and the relationship to community development are described. Throughout the chapter, examples from a variety of cultures are given to clarify points and provide realistic issues for discussion.

LEARNING OBJECTIVES

In this chapter, you will learn:

- the definitions of culture, cultural assessment, and cultural brokering
- the major components of Canada's multiculturalism law
- the implications of the cultural makeup of Canada's population for community health nursing
- the advantages and disadvantages of conducting cultural assessments with individuals and families
- three strategies that community health nurses can use to ensure the cultural diversity of clients is addressed

Introduction

Katherine, one of the community health nurses in the inner-city area, has arrived at the apartment building commonly referred to as "Little Cambodia." It is a large brick structure on a busy street. Although it appears quiet from the outside, within it is full of activity.

Most of the 50 units are rented to Cambodian families. The front entrance contains notices and posters written in Khmer, the native language; these announce Cambodian community meetings, English classes, and baby clinics at the local health unit. In the hallways, the smells of Cambodian cuisine and the sounds of Cambodian music remind visitors of the different world that they are about to enter.

The apartments are furnished sparsely; many families still prefer to sit on mats on the floor for their meals and for visiting. Other families have bought Western-style dinette sets, sofas, and coffee tables. The apartments are full of evidence that these are Cambodian homes: incense is burned frequently in front of statues of Buddha; colourful curtains surround beds; and utensils and condiments displayed on kitchen counters suggest a menu that emphasizes noodles, fish paste, and chillies. Tiger Balm and herbal medicines are also visible on counter tops. Posters of Buddha and Cambodian movie heroes and heroines line the walls. The women dress in simple sarongs, a piece of floor-length fabric wrapped around the waist; children are dressed in t-shirts and shorts or nothing at all. Katherine has several families to see on this visit. Sareoun has just had a new baby; two-year-old Samphor has had anemia and dietary problems since arriving with her family two months ago; and Kong's children have missed school frequently because of respiratory illness. Vannac, the male Cambodian interpreter, has arrived and with Katherine completes all the visits. They are both approached by several other Cambodian families regarding health, school, or financial problems.

Katherine finds out that Sareoun is taking herbal medicines to restore her balance and that Kong has had one of the elders use "coining" (rubbing the skin of the anterior and posterior chest wall with a coin for the purpose of releasing heat and thereby restoring health) on all her children. Katherine reminds them, and the others she sees, about the forthcoming meeting of the Cambodian Women's Group, developed in cooperation with the Cambodian women, in two days at the nearby school. She encourages them to come with their children, as a babysitter will be available.

On the way out, Vannac gives Katherine an invitation to the Cambodian Coul Chnam (New Year) in three weeks. Vannac and Katherine have worked together for over a year and have had numerous discussions about Cambodian politics, the issues facing Cambodian refugees, and the yearly Cambodian events and celebrations.

Not all community health nurses (CHNs) work as intensely with culturally distinct clients as Katherine, but all are exposed to diverse cultural groups at some point within their work. When this happens, it is important to have the necessary knowledge and skills that lead to interactions that are beneficial for both the nurse and the community. The purpose of this chapter is to discuss the interrelationships among culture, community health nursing, and Primary Health Care. The specific goals are: (a) to discuss Canada's *Multiculturalism Act* and examine its implications; (b) to provide a demographic profile of Canada, including statistics on Aboriginal groups and immigrants; (c) to discuss and explain cultural assessments; and (d) to discuss the impact of culturally diverse communities on the community health nursing role by identifying specific examples and models of community programming and care.

Throughout this chapter, culture refers to a "set of learned values, behaviors, and beliefs that are characteristic of a particular society or population" (Ember & Ember, 1981, p. 527). Two key features of culture are that it is *shared* and *learned* within a group. Like a piece of luggage, it travels with you and comprises many different items. Culture includes rituals, customs, taboos, beliefs, and behaviours. These terms and additional concepts are defined in Table 10.1.

Multiculturalism within Canada

Canada is often heralded for its openness to culturally diverse groups (Fleras & Elliott, 1992). Most Canadians are aware that Canada has an official policy of multiculturalism; far fewer understand its history or the implications of such a policy. Multiculturalism is a complex issue. It has been defined as "An official doctrine and corresponding set of policies and practices in which ethno-racial differences are formally promoted and incorporated as an integral component of the political, social, and symbolic order" (Fleras & Elliott, 1992, p. 22). This definition views multiculturalism on a multidimensional level: (a) in a descriptive manner that recognizes and describes the diversity of society; (b) in a prescriptive manner that advocates the ideas and ideals of diversity; (c) within a political perspective that emphasizes policies about diversity; or (d) as intergroup dynamics, the process by which various ethnic groups interact.

One other way to consider multiculturalism is by examining it at individual, group, institutional, or societal levels. At the individual level, "multiculturalism is experienced as the confidence and ability to relate to others who are culturally different" (Fleras & Elliott, 1992, p. 23). The group level refers to the identification of cultural differences and the maintenance of a group's heritage. The institutional level refers to the restructuring of organizations so that they are receptive to, and representative of, diversity. Finally, at the societal level, there is a harmonious co-existence of cultural traditions (Fleras & Elliott, 1992).

Canada is the only country in the world to have a national multiculturalism law. In part, this political action on multiculturalism emerged because of the pressures and challenges of the historical ethnic diversity in this country. The presence of Aboriginal peoples and the subsequent colonization of Canada by the French and British, followed by the arrival of other racial and ethnic minorities, created the need to develop a mechanism that would allow harmonious diversity (Fleras & Elliott, 1992).

Table 10.1
Overview of terms

Term/Concept	Definition/Explanation	Example

Rituals	• are a form of repetitive behaviour that does not have a direct, overt technical effect (Helman, 1990, p. 192)
	
	• include symbols or standardized objects, clothing, movement, words, and song
	
	• can be public or private
	
	• can serve expressive or creative functions
	
	• comprise three types:
	
	  - *calendrical*: rituals related to changing seasons
	  - *social transition*: changes within the life cycle; such rituals provide psychological comfort and security during a time of change
	  - *misfortune*: rituals at times of unexpected crises (Helman, 1990)
		• saying grace before meals
		
		• *Coul Chnam* or Cambodian New Year, which is a religious event and community celebration
		
		• puberty rituals; Sun Dance among Plains Indians
		
		• funerals

Cultural Practices	• are behaviours or activities that are specifically related to one's culture	• among the Chinese, "doing the month" (Pillsbury, 1982), a postpartum cultural practice to restore heat lost during the delivery • Cambodian women may ingest wine-soaked herbal medicines for up to four months post-partum; these are drunk daily, usually half a cup two to three times per day (Kulig, 1990)
Ethnocentrism	• is viewing others by unconsciously applying the standards of one's own group	• "Other immigrants have come to this country and done well; what's the matter with X group?"

(continued)

Table 10.1 *(continued)*

Term/Concept	Definition/Explanation	Example
Stereotyping	• is making inferences about people because of their membership in some group	• "All Indians are drunks"; "All Latin American men beat their wives"
Custom	• is a usual practice or habit	• giving tobacco to Aboriginal elderly when visiting
Taboo	• is "a supernaturally sanctioned law" (Buckley & Gottlieb, 1988, p. 4) • is a prohibition that, if violated, will lead to punishment (Ember & Ember, 1981) • acts as a form of social control and results in cooperative individual behaviour	• prohibition against menstruating women's participation in healing ceremonies such as sweats (in some N.A. Aboriginal cultures, sweats include ceremonies that are conducted in a specially constructed, enclosed area where steam is produced from hot rocks; during the ceremony, chanting and prayers are conducted) • incest taboo
Belief	• is an opinion or doctrine	• foods classified according to hot or cold (Helman, 1990); the terms do not refer to temperature, but to the inherent elements or properties of the food; South Asians believe that garlic and onions are hot (Manderson, 1981); Chinese believe that chicken, sesame oil, and rice wine are hot (Pillsbury, 1982); and Vietnamese believe that ripe mangoes, coffee, and black pepper are hot (Manderson & Matthews, 1981); rice is most frequently thought of as being neutral • illnesses are also categorized as hot or cold and are treated with the appropriate remedy to counteract the imbalance

Canada had leaned toward a "melting pot" philosophy in which individual cultures were not emphasized. However, this ideology did not prevent interracial tensions. The 1971 multiculturalism policy emphasized that Canada had no official culture but recognized all ethnic backgrounds. However, this policy was not deemed adequate, as changing trends in immigration resulted in more individuals arriving from countries other than Europe. On July 21, 1988, a national multiculturalism law was passed to preserve and enhance multiculturalism in Canada and to reduce discrimination, enhance multicultural awareness, and promote institutional change that exemplifies cultural sensitivity at the federal level. Multiculturalism Canada, under the Secretary of State, developed guidelines that would provide direction in implementing the *Multiculturalism Act* (Fleras & Elliott, 1992).

With the passage of this Act, racial and cultural equality is now protected by law. The recognition of diversity has become a permanent aspect of Canadian society. Initially, Canadians saw multiculturalism in terms of the "3-D" approach (i.e., diet, dance, and dialect). It has become apparent that multiculturalism also refers to removal of barriers within institutions so that all citizens have equal access and opportunities and ensures that needs associated with cultural diversity are considered in decision-making processes and resource allocation (Fleras & Elliott, 1992).

Understandably, the challenges of implementing such a law in health care continue. Some authors note that the infrastructure and policies of agencies largely fit those who are in the mainstream of society (Lipsky, 1980, cited in Teram & White, 1993). However, there are positive workplace changes within some community health agencies to represent and manage diversity more effectively. For this process of change to be successful, there needs to be a greater understanding of cultural diversity reflected in decision making, communication styles, and expectations. For practising CHNs, addressing the cultural needs of individuals, families, and communities is desirable not only because this results in potentially more satisfying and relevant care, but also because there is a legal and ethical mandate to respect such differences.

Multiculturalism in Canada, however, has been criticized on the basis that it has not led to acceptance or true understanding, but merely to tolerance of other groups (Bissoondath, 1994). Furthermore, Bissoondath, an immigrant himself, believes that multiculturalism leads more to divisiveness because it emphasizes differences among groups and categorizes people's behaviour and ideas. In addition, individuals become dependent upon the government and its policies to help in the creation of a sense of self and community. Bissoondath suggests that multiculturalism be removed from the political realm to assist individuals and communities to develop their own ways of maintaining their diversity and, in so doing, develop a more unified country.

In summary, Canada's unique national multiculturalism law challenges each community health nurse to work with culturally diverse groups on an individual and societal level. This will be a continuing role as Canada becomes an increasingly diverse society.

Cultural profile of Canada

A quick glance around any town, city, or work setting will likely indicate how culturally diverse Canada has become. In the 1996 census, 18 million claimed single origins such as British (3.2 million, 11 percent), French (2.6 million, nine percent), or European (3.7 million, 13 percent) to describe their ethnicity. Over 4.5 million (16 percent) Canadians use a non-official language as their mother tongue (Minister of Industry, Science & Technology, 1998a). Slightly over 10 million Canadians claim a heritage of multiple ethnic origins, such as British and French or multiple European origins. For the first time, in the most recent census, "Canadian" could be chosen as an ethnic identity; over five million individuals chose this category to describe themselves.

Immigration continues to influence the cultural makeup of Canada's population. The top 10 birthplaces of immigrants to Canada in 1996 were Hong Kong; People's Republic of China; India; Philippines; Sri Lanka; Poland; Taiwan; Viet Nam; United States; and United Kingdom (Minister of Industry, Science & Technology, 1998a). Almost five million immigrants (17.4 percent) arrived in Canada between 1991 and 1996, the highest figures in more than 50 years (Minister of Industry, Science & Technology, 1998b). Moreover, there are significant changes in the makeup of this immigrant group; up to 1981, most immigrants were of European origin but now, 31 percent are from Asia and the Middle East. Canada's largest cities continue to experience the impact of immigration. Twenty-one percent of Toronto's total population is composed of immigrants who arrived in the last 15 years; Vancouver is the second highest, with 20 percent of its population composed of immigrants who arrived in the last 15 years. In addition, Toronto continues to have the highest proportion of immigrants of all Canadian cities; the 1996 census indicates that its immigrant population is 42 percent, an increase from 38 percent in 1991. Vancouver is the second highest with 35 percent of its population being immigrants, an increase of 5 percent from the 1991 census. Ontario attracted the highest number of immigrants (54 percent) during the most recent census, and British Columbia was the next favourite choice for new arrivals (21 percent). Both provinces also have the two highest total immigrant populations in Canada, respectively. Alberta, however, has the third highest proportion of immigrants of its total population (15 percent) (Statistics Canada, 1997).

One prediction is that by 2016, one out of every five Canadians and one of every four children will be a member of a visible minority group. By this date, the largest visible minority group in Canada will be the Chinese, whose population is expected to rise to almost two million people (Statistics

Canada, 1996). Visible minority groups, which include Chinese, Blacks, Southeast Asians, Koreans, and Latin Americans, to name a few, currently comprise over three million Canadians (11 percent) (Minister of Industry, Science & Technology, 1998a).

In the 1991 census, over three-quarters of a million people in Canada claimed single Aboriginal ancestry. Of this total, 529 040 (66.2 percent) stated they are of North American Indian ancestry. Inuit ancestry was reported by 40 220 (5 percent), and Métis ancestry was reported by 204 115 (25 percent) (Minister of Industry, Science & Technology, 1998a).

Cultural assessments

Cultural assessment guides can help CHNs to make a systematic appraisal of the major beliefs and practices of any cultural group with which they work, including the individuals and families seen in practice (see Giger & Davidhizer, 1991; Herberg, 1995; Rosenbaum, 1991). Cultural assessments allow nurses to identify the major values, beliefs, and practices of a particular group and to process the information to provide culturally appropriate care.

The advantages of cultural assessments are that they (a) provide a systematic strategy to guide practice; (b) show respect for and interest in the client's culture; (c) improve practice by making it more meaningful for the client; and (d) serve as an educational tool for the CHNs to understand cultural diversity and learn about various beliefs and practices. The cultural assessment guides, however, also have disadvantages. For example, some guides include sections that deal with the political organization of the culture. Such questions may make a person who has left a war-torn country uncomfortable, particularly if he or she fled the country because of political persecution. Another concern is that some guides could be too time consuming or burdensome. In these cases, some sections may need to be deleted. Thus guides can be altered to make them more appropriate for specific situations.

Although there are different cultural assessment guides that can be used with any cultural group, most guides include common topics to be discussed within the interview. For example, there are sections that address family organization, including roles and functions; interpersonal relationships; communication; religious beliefs and practices; and cultural beliefs and practices in relation to health (see Giger & Davidhizar, 1991; Herberg, 1995; Rosenbaum, 1991 for specific examples). When a CHN conducts a cultural assessment with a postpartum client, it would be particularly helpful to discuss family organization; cultural beliefs and practices regarding pregnancy, labour and delivery; and postpartum care of both the newborn and mother.

CHNs need to be familiar with the guides and use them in their work. The guides are sometimes accompanied with specific questions to be used in the assessment (see, for example, Andrews & Boyle, 1995; Rosenbaum, 1991). Regardless, it is helpful to begin the discussion with a general question, such as "I would like to learn more about your cultural background. Do you mind if I ask you a few questions?" This open-ended statement conveys the nurse's interest and respect and encourages an open exchange of ideas with the client. This also helps to ensure that services are based upon the client's beliefs and practices.

Because of the length of most cultural assessment guides, the nurse will need to choose the sections that are most appropriate to the client. For example, in Herberg's (1995) guide, there is reference to values regarding physical beauty. Questions related to this topic may be appropriate for a postpartum couple that has experienced the birth of a baby with physical anomalies, but not for a mother who has concerns about her child's reaction to immunization.

After choosing a cultural assessment guide and identifying the appropriate sections, the nurse will need to develop several open-ended questions to begin the discussion with the client. For example, if visiting a Chinese postpartum woman, it would be worthwhile to ask if there are any dietary or activity restrictions in the postpartum and, if so, what these are; who helps with the care of the baby; and what, if any, herbal medicines are being used. Depending upon the responses to the last question, the nurse can also ask what herbs the woman is taking, how these are prepared, how often they are taken, and why they are taken. This illustrates that additional questions are based upon the client's answers and cannot always be developed before the interview.

If the nurse is using an interpreter, special approaches should be taken. Short, simple sentences are best as they allow the interpreter the opportunity to translate each of the questions accurately. Medical jargon and colloquialisms are difficult to translate and should be avoided. The nurse also should not state the question in an indirect manner. For example, "Ask her (the client) about . . ." is an indirect and impersonal way of communicating. Instead, the CHN should maintain eye contact with the client, if that is culturally appropriate.

Consider the following example:

CHN (looking at Rosa): Rosa, can you tell me how many hours the baby is sleeping during the night?

Interpreter: ¿Rosa, quantas horas esta dormiendo el bebe en las noches?

Rosa: Quatro horas.

Interpreter (to the CHN): Four hours.

Throughout the interview, the CHN may discover that the client is not able to explain why she or he follows particular cultural traditions. This is not surprising given that detailed information about traditions and customs is often lost from one generation to another. This is another positive feature of cultural assessment guides: they can help cultural beliefs and practices to endure over time. For CHNs who work with many people within the same cultural group, a detailed cultural assessment with each client would not be necessary. However, because cultures are dynamic, and because there is intracultural variability (i.e., differences within the culture), questions seeking clarification are important. For example, the CHN may have gained knowledge about postpartum practices of Chinese women and will likely have identified common themes. Visits with other Chinese women can include such questions as "Other Chinese women I know use herbal medicines after their baby is born. Do you use them too?"

CHNs can also carry out family cultural assessments, although there is little difference between individual and family assessments. For example, customs related to religious or cultural events apply to both. The differences may be apparent when the spouses do not share the same cultural background. In such a case, questions need to be asked about the family's ability to blend customs. One example relates to diet; questions could be raised about which culturally related foods are eaten. Other queries might focus on which language is spoken in the home or what religion is practised.

A third type of cultural assessment is at the community level. In this instance, community leaders (e.g., presidents of ethnic organizations), key informants (e.g., individuals identified by community members as having expertise and knowledge), and community members can all be interviewed to develop an overview of their culture. This process is important if community projects are goals of the health agency and the community within which the CHN works. For example, if the health agency is interested in developing educational sessions about family planning, then information pertaining to cultural beliefs and practices about sexuality (including menstruation, ovulation, and conception), about health and illness, and about communication styles is important. In this instance, traditional healers, midwives, and women and men should be asked about their beliefs as well as their advice regarding the intervention. Information gained before the planning and implementation of the intervention will help ensure acceptability and congruence.

Cultural assessments are useful tools for learning about the cultural traditions of individuals, families, and communities. Existing cultural assessment guides can be adapted easily to fit the particular situation; the information generated can then be used in developing, implementing, and evaluating intervention strategies and community programs.

Implications for community health nursing

One way to work with culturally distinct populations is to use the cultural assessment tools that have already been discussed. Further discussion is needed, however, about community-based programs for culturally diverse groups. Five approaches that community health agencies can use to serve culturally diverse clients are parallel services, ethno-specific services, generic services, bridging services, and adapted or "multiculturalized" mainstream services (Stevens, 1993). Table 10.2 summarizes these five approaches. Most CHNs would agree that combinations of these approaches are used on a regular basis. However, more community health agencies now are "multiculturalizing" their services and restructuring programs to meet the needs of the multicultural community. In some instances, an individual is employed to assist the staff through this multiculturalizing process; in other institutions, staff members are assigned activities related to multiculturalism as part of their regular workload. Whatever approach is used, all staff members of the agency should feel a sense of ownership of proposed changes. In other words, the CHN should recognize and acknowledge the importance of addressing multicultural issues within the workplace. Without commitment, multiculturalizing attempts will not be successful. Three steps can ensure commitment. The first step involves clarification of personal values. CHNs need to examine their own cultural beliefs and ideas before working with culturally diverse groups (Bernal, 1993). For example, if the nurse values women and men equally yet must visit a postpartum mother who is rejecting her infant daughter because of her gender, then there may be a value conflict. Value conflicts can impede communication, understanding, and implementation of nursing strategies.

The second step involves developing cross-cultural awareness. Along with other health professionals, CHNs can participate in cross-cultural workshops and in-service educational programs, read about other cultures, and experience ethnic diversity through cultural events. Community health agencies, in turn, are responsible for providing in-service education, information, and opportunities for CHNs to become more culturally sensitive. Flavin (1997) describes a cross-cultural training program for home health care nurses that resulted in an increase in positive interactions between the nurses and the cultural groups with whom they worked. The nurse can also consider joining organizations, such as the Canadian Council on Multicultural Health, to develop cross-cultural awareness and can read summary chapters of various cultural groups in books that focus on cultural diversity (see, for example, Lipson, Dibble, & Minarik, 1996; Purnell & Paulanka, 1998; Spector, 1996). When reading such chapters, CHNs must remember that each cultural group is dynamic and contains variations; hence, the summaries may not be applicable to the family or individual with whom they are working.

The third step for CHNs is to be aware of the culturally diverse communities in which they work. This can be accomplished partly by conducting cultural assessments with clients and identifying and working with community

Table 10.2
Models in providing care to culturally diverse clients

Type of Service	Description
Generic Services (predominant model)	Mainstream agencies that provide services to all people with no attention to ethnic or cultural diversity (disadvantage: most newcomers feel alienated from such a service and underutilize it)
Parallel Services	Resettlement and immigrant service agencies that provide services dealing specifically with newcomers; such agencies offer, e.g., translation services, assistance in resettling, orientation to life in Canada, and social support; personnel from these agencies are often used by health care professionals
Ethno-specific Services	Ethnocultural associations that provide services for community members; such services are limited, and most are in large urban areas
Bridging Services	Services, such as interpreter services, that are available and can be contracted by the health agency to assist in serving culturally diverse groups; communication is the emphasis
"Multiculturalized" Services	Agencies that recognize the need for special programs for culturally diverse clients and help to develop such programs

Compiled from information in Stevens (1993), pp. 29–33.

leaders and key informants. It is important that the nurse build a network within culturally diverse communities. Resources in these communities, such as shops, folk healers, churches, and ethnic organizations, will assist the CHN to see the culturally diverse community as a unit (Bernal, 1993). The individual CHN's role as a political and cultural advocate is useful. Several authors have discussed "cultural brokering" (e.g., Jezewski, 1990, 1993, 1995). Cultural brokering refers to "the act of bridging, linking, or mediating between groups or persons of differing cultural systems for the purpose of reducing conflict or producing change" (Jezewski, 1995, p. 20). Jezewski's cultural brokering theory also addresses nursing interventions that the CHN can follow when working with clients from other cultural groups. The first stage is to perceive the need for brokering by identifying the issue. The second stage focusses on the intervention, which includes establishing rapport and addressing the issue through such actions as negotiating, advocating, or mediating. The third stage, or outcome, includes assessing the situation for resolution. The process is repeated until a satisfactory outcome results.

In general, another strategy for front-line CHNs and agency administrators is to serve on advisory committees to achieve multiculturalizing of services. The nurse would need to network with individuals working in resettlement and ethno-specific agencies. These individuals belong to the culturally distinct community and are familiar with the language, culture, and current situation, like Vannac in the introductory case study. For example, while working as a CHN, the author was referred by a school teacher to an eight-year-old Cambodian boy who stated that "there was a dead man" behind his house. The resettlement worker came and talked with the child. The boy had seen a Cambodian man murdered in the Thai refugee camp where he used to live. On this particular day, he had experienced a flashback to that incident.

For individual home visits and interactions during clinic visits, such as immunization appointments, the nurse may not have interpreter services and will have to rely on basic communication skills. Tools can be developed to facilitate these interactions. Some CHNs have used infant cereal boxes and infant formula to ask and teach about infant nutrition; binders of illustrations to ask about clothing in winter and activities; and a booklet of colours to ask about the colour of a child's bowel movements.

During postpartum and clinic visits, the nurse can use a cultural assessment guide to inquire about the client's culture. The information generated can be used to develop an intervention strategy. For example, if a mother states that immunization makes her child "hot," the CHNs can explain that antipyretics can counteract the heat and cause a balance in the baby's body.

Although work with Aboriginal peoples has not been addressed specifically in this chapter, the points raised can all be used within Aboriginal communities. CHNs who work in northern locations should examine their own cultural values and be prepared to learn about the Aboriginal culture within which they are working.

One important principle is that the CHN, while trying to meet the needs of culturally diverse clients, interacts with the community as a unit, as part of a total approach to Primary Health Care and community development. Community development is the process of involving a community in the identification and reinforcement of those aspects of everyday life, culture, and political activity that are conducive to health (Canadian Public Health Association, 1990, p. 19). Community development emphasizes participation by community members in determining their own needs and the best strategies to meet those needs (see Chapter 21). In this instance, the CHN is a facilitator and an enabler (Hickman, 1997). Networking and cultural assessments with community members and key informants are steps within the community development process and help identify community members' priorities. The remaining steps include working with the culturally distinct group in developing, implementing, and evaluating community programs. In this case, the term *community programs* refers not only to workshops and group teaching, but also to development of educational materials, such as audio-visual aids, posters, and pamphlets.

For example, Cambodian members of a U.S. community provided valuable impetus in the development of a videotape on family planning in Khmer, their language (Lukas & Kulig, 1985). The community members, following their resettlement, had identified a desire to learn more about family planning. For this project, information was generated about Cambodian beliefs and knowledge regarding sexuality. The setting for the video recording was chosen after discussion with the Cambodian families. The Cambodian women agreed to act. A tentative script was developed, then read and modified by the Cambodian community. Although the original script was written in English, the videotape is in Khmer. Music, titles, and illustrations all reflect the Cambodian culture (Lukas & Kulig, 1985). The process took many months to complete; however, the positive responses from the Cambodian community that produced it, as well as from Cambodians in other communities, have reinforced the importance of adhering to community development principles.

Conclusion

The following principles can underpin CHNs' work within culturally diverse communities:

- Working with culturally diverse groups takes time. Time is needed for the building of trust in any contact with clients in community settings, and this is particularly important when working with culturally diverse groups.
- Individuals from specific cultural backgrounds can provide information that could affect the success or failure of a program. For example, when an owl was used on immunization posters with the caption "Be wise—Immunize," an Aboriginal community member pointed out that the owl represents death to West Coast tribes and would therefore be inappropriate for this community.
- Community members can screen words or phrases that, while appropriate in English, may be unclear or have a different connotation in another language.

- Community members' perceptions of community health programs should be sought. This step can permit alterations or changes as necessary.
- Community members can help to evaluate the program. It may be more appropriate to conduct an oral rather than a written evaluation at the end of the workshop, or to ask about reception of the program through the CHN's network within the culturally diverse community.

The CHN in the case study demonstrated strategies emphasized throughout this chapter. These strategies include: (a) networking and working with Vannac, the resettlement worker; (b) being involved with the Cambodian community; (c) developing a Cambodian Women's Group in collaboration with the community; and (d) being culturally sensitive and responsive to the individual Cambodian families' needs.

The diversity of Canadian society challenges all nurses to examine their values and develop ways to communicate and work with a variety of groups. The CHN can play a pivotal role in working with culturally diverse individuals, families, and communities. Self-awareness, values clarification, networking with culturally diverse groups, and enacting community development principles are all important strategies for CHNs to employ.

QUESTIONS

1. What customs and cultural practices are maintained in your family?
2. What are the various cultural groups in your geographic area? Does this match the diverse cultural groups that the CHNs in your community health agency see? Explain.
3. What model(s) is (are) being used by your community health agency to deliver care to culturally diverse clients? Provide specific examples to support your claim. Is this model appropriate? Why or why not? If it is not, what can you as an individual CHN or student do to change it?

REFERENCES

Andrews, M.M., & Boyle, J.S. (1995). Transcultural nursing care. In M.M. Andrews et al. (Eds.), *Transcultural concepts in nursing care* (2nd ed.) (pp. 323–352). Philadelphia: Lippincott-Raven.

Bernal, H. (1993). A model for delivering culture-relevant care in the community. *Public Health Nursing, 10*(4), 228–232.

Bissoondath, N. (1994). *Selling illusions: The cult of multiculturalism in Canada.* Toronto: Penguin Books.

Buckley, T., & Gottlieb, A. (1988). A critical appraisal of theories of menstrual symbolism. In T. Buckley & A. Gottlieb (Eds.), *Blood magic: The anthropology of menstruation* (pp. 1–53). Berkeley: University of California Press.

Canadian Public Health Association. (1990). *Community health–public health nursing in Canada.* Ottawa: Author.

Ember, C., & Ember, M. (1981). *Anthropology* (3rd ed.). Englewood Cliffs, NJ: Prentice-Hall.

Flavin, C. (1997). Cross-cultural training for nurses: A research-based education project. *American Journal of Hospice & Palliative Care, 14*(3), 121–126.

Fleras, A., & Elliott, J.L. (1992). *Multiculturalism in Canada: The challenge of diversity.* Toronto: Nelson.

Giger, J., & Davidhizar, R. (1995). *Transcultural nursing: Assessment and intervention* (2nd ed.). Toronto: Mosby.

Helman, C. (1990). *Culture, health and illness* (2nd ed.). London: Wright.

Herberg, P. (1995). Theoretical foundations of transcultural nursing. In J. Boyle & M. Andrews (Eds.), *Transcultural concepts in nursing care* (2nd ed.) (pp. 3–47). Philadelphia: J.B. Lippincott.

Hickman, P. (1997). Community organization. In J. Swanson & M. Nies (Eds.), *Community health nursing: Promoting the health of aggregates* (pp. 137–153). Toronto: W.B. Saunders.

Jezewski, M.A. (1990). Culture brokering immigrant farm worker health care. *Western Journal of Nursing Research, 12*(4), 497–513.

Jezewski, M.A. (1993). Culture brokering as a model for advocacy. *Nursing and Health Care, 14*(2), 78–85.

Jezewski, M.A. (1995). Evolution of a grounded theory: Conflict resolution through culture brokering. *Advances in Nursing Science, 17*(3), 14–30.

Kulig, J. (1990). Childbearing beliefs among Cambodian refugee women. *Western Journal of Nursing Research, 12*(1), 108–118.

Lipson, J., Dibble, S., & Minarik, P. (Eds.). (1996). *Culture and nursing care: A pocket guide.* San Francisco: USCF Nursing Press.

Lukas, A., & Kulig, J. (1985). *Bridging the gap: Birth practices, birth control and sexuality among Cambodian and Vietnamese women.* WID Working Paper Series No. 10. Cambridge, MA: WID–Joint Harvard–MIT Group.

Manderson, L. (1981). Roasting, smoking and dieting in response to birth: Making confinement in cross-cultural perspective. *Social Science & Medicine, 15B*, 509–520.

Manderson, L., & Matthews, M. (1981). Vietnamese behavioral and dietary precautions during pregnancy. *Social Science & Medicine, 11*, 1–8.

Minister of Industry, Science & Technology. (1998a). *Immigration and citizenship: The nation.* Ottawa: Author.

Minister of Industry, Science & Technology. (1998b). *Ethnic origin: The nation.* Ottawa: Author.

Pillsbury, B. (1982). "Doing the month": Confinement and convalescence of Chinese women after childbirth. In M. Kay (Ed.), *Anthropology of human birth* (pp. 119–146). Philadelphia: F.A. Davis.

Purnell, L., & Paulanka, B. (1998). *Transcultural health care: A culturally competent approach.* Philadelphia: F.A. Davis.

Rosenbaum, J. (1991). A cultural assessment guide. *Canadian Nurse, 87*(4), 32–33.

Spector, R. (1996). *Cultural diversity in health and illness* (4th ed.). Stanford, CT: Appleton & Lange.

Statistics Canada (1996). Projections of visible minority groups, 1997 to 2016. *Canadian Social Trends, 41*, 3.

Statistics Canada. (1997, Nov. 4). *The Daily*. (Online: http://www.statcan.ca/Daily/ English/971104/d971004.htm)

Stevens, S. (1993). *Community based programs for a multicultural society: A guidebook for service providers*. Winnipeg: Planned Parenthood Manitoba.

Teram, E., & White, H. (1993). Strategies to address the bureaucratic disentitlement of clients from cultural minority groups. *Canadian Journal of Community Mental Health, 12*(2), 59–70.

C H A P T E R   1 1

Children with chronic conditions and their families in the community

Sharon Ogden Burke, Elizabeth Kauffmann, Nesta M.W. Wiskin, and Margaret B. Harrison

Community health nurses encounter families with children who have chronic conditions in many settings. Nurses' work can be guided by several principles. First, most of these families encounter a similar set of tasks and stresses over time, but usually only a few are of current concern. Second, the most effective interventions are those that focus on the stressors and tasks of current concern to the family. Third, community health nurses can rely on research-tested and time-honoured methods of working with these families. Examples of how nurses implement primary, secondary, and tertiary prevention illustrate these principles.

LEARNING OBJECTIVES

In this chapter, you will learn:

- key theoretical underpinnings of nursing families with a child who has a chronic condition
- the range and variable nature of issues for these families
- the value of evidence-based nursing assessments and interventions for nurses who work with families with a child with a chronic condition

Introduction

This chapter provides an introduction to the concerns, challenges, issues, and burdens of families with a child who has a chronic condition. To help nurses collaborate with these families in the community, the authors provide an overview of key theoretical underpinnings, such as the concept of chronicity and other frameworks, for example, child development and family theory. While the focus is on direct contact with families, examples of community- and population-based approaches are given. This chapter addresses evidence-based assessment and interventions for community health nurses in primary prevention of disability, handicap, and chronic illness among children.

Primary prevention is of particular concern within populations at higher risk for chronic conditions, such as children living at socioeconomic disadvantage. Secondary prevention involves early identification of chronic conditions and helping families cope at home with changing care needs of their growing children. Chronic conditions may be stable or changeable, or may cause a steady decline in the child's abilities. Community health nurses engage in tertiary prevention of psychosocial and physical problems for the child and the family. Contact points with these families and children often occur during crises, stressful periods, or transition points such as care at home after hospitalization, entry into school, relapse in the child's condition, or change from walking to a wheelchair. This chapter provides the background for perceptive, efficient assessments and timely interventions that consider the whole child and the wider family perspective.

Children with chronic conditions in the community

Community health nurses who come in contact with children must be sensitive to chronic conditions, since up to 31 percent could have such a condition (Newacheck & Taylor, 1992). For most children, such conditions are mild or not troublesome. Others (5–10 percent of children) may be affected by a severe or serious chronic health condition or a physical disability, and 99 percent of these children live at home (Offord, Boyle, & Szatmari, 1987; Statistics Canada, 1992a, 1992b). This means that an estimated 280 000 Canadian families are coping day to day with a child who has a serious chronic condition or disability (extrapolated from Statistics Canada, 1992a). It is this group that accounts for the heaviest use of health care resources, including community health nursing, which is the focus of this chapter (Newacheck & Taylor, 1992).

Children with severe conditions are likely to have musculoskeletal impairments, hearing and speech impairments, cerebral palsy, diabetes, asthma, epilepsy, or arthritis (Newacheck & Taylor, 1992). The prevalence of childhood chronic conditions is not decreasing despite advances in control of infectious diseases (e.g., polio and rheumatic fever). Several factors contribute to the continuing high prevalence of chronic conditions among children, including:

- longevity among children with conditions once considered to result in childhood death, e.g., a sevenfold increase in cystic fibrosis survival to age 21, and twofold increases in spina bifida, leukemia, and congenital heart disease survival (Newacheck & Taylor, 1992)
- more infants with severe problems surviving infancy
- increases in severe asthma (Newacheck & Taylor, 1992)
- more children contracting AIDS (Boyle, 1991).

Morbidity rates are higher among Aboriginal children and children living in economically disadvantaged conditions (Boyle, 1991; Thompson & Hupp, 1992).

The scope and nature of the families' concerns and of nurses' work with these families are shaped by associated problems. Children with severe chronic conditions have more secondary health problems, for example, pulmonary infections in the presence of cystic fibrosis (Newacheck & Taylor, 1992). They are disproportionately higher users of psychiatric and social services (Boyle, 1991; Cadman, Boyle, & Offord, 1988; Cadman, Boyle, Szatmari, & Offord, 1987), are more likely to face neglect and child abuse (Thompson & Hupp, 1992), and are more likely to have a learning or developmental difficulty (Burke, Harrison, Kauffmann, & Wong, 1999a).

The concept of chronicity

The concept of chronicity is broad and includes the pathophysiology as well as the psychosocial factors associated with the children, their families, and the communities in which they live. Narrowly defined, chronic conditions are impairments in function, development, or disease states that are irreversible or have a cumulative effect (modified from Lubkin, 1986). They are usually of more than one year's duration. Nevertheless, children with a chronic condition can have periods when the condition does not trouble them greatly.

Of the many overlapping ways to view chronicity—medical diagnoses, staging, number of systems involved, degree of disability, number of complications—the generic approach has the most utility in community health nursing. The generic view of chronic conditions and illness postulates that these children and their families have more issues in common (concerns, stresses, solutions, coping patterns) across medical diagnoses than issues that differ (Perrin et al., 1993). The authors' research has found no significant differences in issues or effects of nursing intervention when children are grouped by diagnosis (Burke, Costello, Handley-Derry, Kauffmann, & Dillon, 1997; Burke, Harrison, et al., 1999a).

A small set of chronic illness trajectories has been suggested as a more clinically meaningful alternative to biomedical diagnostic groupings (Burke, 1997; Burke, Kauffmann, LaSalle, Harrison, & Wong, 1999; Corbin & Strauss 1991; Rolland, 1987; White & Lubkin, 1995). The authors found that parents of children with severe chronic conditions view their children's conditions as predominately life threatening, declining, or stable (Burke, Kauffman, LaSalle, et al., 1999). The assumption is that, across diverse medical diagnoses, psychosocial issues have more commonalities within a particular trajectory than within a particular medical diagnosis. Parents often hold different views of their children's trajectory than professionals, who focus on the child's biomedical diagnosis and stage (Burke, Kauffman, LaSalle, et al., 1999; Thorne & Robinson, 1988).

Community health nurse success stories

The following vignettes illustrate successful community health nursing practice with children who have chronic conditions and their families. Note the stress points in each and the variety of settings within which the nurse and families contact each other. Note the long-term relationships implied between nurse and family. These are examples of ideal situations; things do not always work out this well! These are the types of stories that community health nurses will experience and that make the inevitable difficult times easier when nursing families with children who have chronic conditions.

A new school

A mother communicated her concerns about the facilities and attitudes of students and staff to a community health nurse, when a group of physically disabled children were to be moved to a new school. The nurse recognized the need to educate and gain the cooperation of teachers, principals, and the other students. They needed to know about the handicapping conditions and about the needs and the strengths of the children. The nurse talked to the staff about what they could expect. Then she met with groups of students. She made an audio-visual presentation, answered questions, and demonstrated equipment. One strategy, which involved letting the children try using a wheelchair, was a "big hit." The junior and kindergarten children were especially open and curious. Questions were straightforward and honest: "Can we catch what they've got?" "Can the kids come out and play with us at recess?" "What kinds of things are they interested in?" "Are they going to die soon?"

The move, and integration with the entire school, proceeded smoothly. The mother was grateful to the nurse for the extra time and effort she took to coordinate the move.

Bending the rules

Once a school has managed the problems and solutions around the care of a child with a chronic condition, it is much easier for other children. One primary school had a boy with muscular dystrophy in Grade 8. The child's condition was deteriorating rapidly. Everyone knew that the adjustment to a new secondary school would be difficult and disruptive. The mother mentioned her dilemma to the community health nurse at a meeting of parents of children with muscular dystrophy. A school conference was set up, options were discussed, and a plan was formulated. The child was allowed to remain in the same school for an extra year. His condition worsened and he had to have a suction machine available, as he choked easily. He also had to be lifted on and off the toilet. The nurse taught the staff and students to do these things. They all helped and encouraged their friend.

He continued to attend school until he passed away. He had been very happy to be part of this group of students. The wider community of the principal, teachers, and students were also enriched by his presence.

Relatives and friends

Community health nurses know that relatives and friends can be both a support and a source of great stress. One mother of a girl with cerebral palsy was having a particularly difficult time with her parents. Initially, they had been afraid to handle the child and seemed shocked that they could not be helpful. They seemed to ignore explanations about the girl's condition. They vacillated from expecting too much from the child to coddling her. They had difficulty understanding the need to foster the child's independent growth and development at her own pace and in her own way.

The community health nurse listened and shared the observation that friends and relatives can be a double jeopardy: they feel their own confusion and distress, and also suffer pain with the parents and child. If a relationship has been strained under normal circumstances, it can become even more strained in situations involving illness. The community health nurse observed that, in her experience, some friends and relatives have greater difficulty than others in being supportive and realistic about the child's progress and capabilities.

The mother and the nurse discussed other sources of support. In the end, the mother sought the help of her sister and brother-in-law, whom she believed were too busy to help. They became most understanding, key supporters for the child's parents. Their role modelling in turn helped the grandparents to be more consistent, understanding, and helpful.

Time alone together for parents

One family felt "burned out" after a particularly difficult hospitalization of their child, who had spina bifida. Tempers flared. The community health nurse identified the problem and was able to counsel the parents on their need to have some time of their own. They needed firm encouragement to be able to leave their child, even in competent hands, and go out to dinner, a movie, or just take a walk together. They began to talk and renew communication. A weekend away seemed to revive their strong relationship. They noted that "they were a couple before they became a family." This closeness helped them to cope with the many stresses experienced in raising a child with a chronic condition.

Health care services for families with children with chronic conditions

Health care and technological advances result in new demands and needs for families, acute and chronic care institutions, and community-based health care agencies. The challenges for families with a child with a chronic condition are compounded by societal changes: more frequent family relocations, more working mothers, smaller families, and more female-headed, low-income families (Avard & Hanvey, 1989).

Public, private, and voluntary services for these children are shifting, and some services are shrinking or disappearing as the Canadian health care system is being restructured. These new directions can compound the challenges for families. The trend continues toward home-based care for children who are more acutely ill and dependent on high technology (Donlevy & Pietruch, 1996; Health & Welfare Canada, 1990; Ontario Ministry of Health, 1993; Peters, 1989).

Community health nurses can play a central role in helping families find resources. There are numerous ways families of children with chronic conditions can access services and resources, including physicians' offices, hospital ambulatory services, special clinics, public health school programs, and nursing agencies. Nurses often provide Primary Health Care for such families within diverse and sometimes isolated settings, such as ambulatory clinics with community outreach services.

Nurses and families now locate and effectively use services through the Internet, e-mail, and chat lines. Skilled Internet use is becoming an essential skill for community health nurses and families with children who have chronic conditions. There are home pages for most government-sponsored programs and many private organizations.

The differences among hospital nursing, ambulatory nursing, and community health nursing are less distinct than they were in the past. The critical point is that all these nurses need community health nursing knowledge and skills. The family often views the community health nurse as a first contact in times of doubt or difficulty and an aid to "navigating the system." In this way, community health nurses improve accessibility to health care resources and contribute to Primary Health Care for children and family—for example, through outreach support, consultation, telephone follow-up, and home visiting.

Community health nurses are involved in promoting and maintaining the health of families with children who have chronic conditions in the following contexts, settings, and roles:

- hospital discharge planning
- school health programs
- ambulatory care clinic consulting
- high-risk newborn home visits and consultation to lay home visitors
- immunization programs
- early-discharge home nursing care
- parent organizations (e.g., as a consultation or ex officio member of an organization of parents of children with cystic fibrosis)
- board member for groups involving or serving such families
- Native health centres
- community outreach health centres, especially in economically disadvantaged areas.

Although the best setting for interventions with families is considered to be the home (Barnard, Snyder, & Spietz, 1991), good community-based alternatives to the home visit are private conferences in other settings, e-mail, letters, and telephone calls. While each family's need for number of services varies, the community health nurse has a long period of contact with the family and their child who has a chronic condition.

Theoretical bases for nursing practice

What are the best guidelines for community health nursing practices involving families with children having chronic conditions? The research and theory presented below are grounded in clinical experience and provide direction and structure for nursing practice. Table 11.1 provides an overview of the types of nursing actions that emerge from theory as well as research and clinical experience.

There is no single, generally accepted theoretical framework for work with families affected by chronic conditions. Theory usually emerges from clinical experience; key examples of experience-based nursing actions are shown in the final column of Table 11.1.

Child development and family theory applications

Since the 1970s, *developmental theory* has been a central conceptual framework for work with children who have disabilities, handicaps, and chronic conditions. Assessment and evaluation use developmental measures, and

Table 11.1
Nursing intervention strategies for families with a child with a chronic condition

Authors	Nursing Intervention Strategies	Development
Burke, Kauffmann, Harrison, & Wong, 1994	**Nursing Intervention Record (NIR) used with Stress-Point Intervention by Nurses (SPIN) Assessments** • Do a *family genogram* • Elicit *child information*—medical history, current health problems, & parent concerns about child's condition • Elicit *family data*—medical history, current health problems, & family concerns about child • Assess level of *parental knowledge* about child, condition, & degree of coping with current stressors & tasks • Assess level of *child's knowledge*—condition & degree of coping with current stressors & tasks • Listen for &/or ask about current, past, & anticipated *stress points* using Burke Assessment Guide (Figure 11.1, p. 229) **Planning—Initial & Ongoing** • Help parent to identify *past successful ways of coping* with stress points • Spend time *thinking* about possible new ways the family might try to cope • *Develop an intervention with the parent* for dealing with current stress points • *Write* to family to confirm impressions of their central stress points & coping plans • Read *SPIN* manual or other resources to help with planned interventions • *Review overall assessment* of potential stress points for child & family	This is a modification of the NIR developed by Burke & Kauffmann and elaborated with Harrison & Wong. Research shows it to be effective with families with children before, during, and after repeated hospitalizations (Burke, Costello, et al., 1997; Burke, Harrison, et al., 1999a & b).

(continued)

Table 11.1 (*continued*)

Authors	Nursing Intervention Strategies	Development
	Interventions	
	• *Consult* with other health care professionals as needed	
	• Initiate *referrals* if needed	
	• Regularly *express confidence* in family's abilities to cope	
	• Actively *involve family & child* in decision making	
	• Contact parent with *new or revised ideas* about coping with a stress point	
	• *Visit* family where & when stressors occur, e.g., in hospital at home, or in school	
	• Teach or reteach *procedure(s)* related to child's health problems	
	• Teach parents *early warning signs* of potential problems	
	• Provide new or review *information* with parent &/or child	
	• Tell family about *new features* of services, medical or surgical management, or child's changing condition that might be different from their earlier experiences	
	• Work with family to plan *longer-term care*	
	• Assist parent in *problem solving* health or family concerns	
	• Help family recognize & find a balance among the needs & stresses of *individual members*	
	• Assist family to plan services or activities to *reduce unnecessary stress*	
	• Assist family to *communicate* more effectively *with professional* &/or act as the child's &/or family's advocate	
	• Be available to the parents by *phone* (e-mail, voice mail) at scheduled times	
	• *Check in with family* for new stress points & coping strategies	

(*continued*)

Table 11.1 (*continued*)

Authors	Nursing Intervention Strategies	Development

Hymovich, 1987 (adapted)	• Aid in seeking information & resources
	• Aid in using resources
	• Aid in managing stressors
	  - child's physical needs
	  - parents' emotional responses
	• Support when making modification to family lifestyle, parent behaviour, expectations, & attitudes
	• Assist with/support parental anticipatory planning including that directed at the child, family members, community, including health care personnel
	• Support parent strategy of helping or supporting others (individuals, groups, organizations related to their child's condition)
	• Support cognitive/affective evaluations of child's condition & responses, related values, attitudes, & beliefs
		Hymovich includes nursing intervention in her model, but has not studied it directly. This list is extrapolated from a content analysis of coping strategies among 38 families with a child with cystic fibrosis.

Barnard, Snyder, & Spietz, 1991: NPACE (Nursing Parent and Child Environment)	**Nursing Support to Meet Mothers' Goals** • Self-disclosure—provide input regarding personal experiences; therapeutic use of self • Mutual sharing—easy give and take; dialogue focussed on parent • Social sharing—interaction emphasizing family members, activities not related to high-risk child, having coffee, etc. • Active listening—responding to emotional message, reflection, etc. • Information exchange—nurse and client exchange of information, problem solving	A research-tested intervention for high-risk infants. Methods included videotapes of mother, baby, nurse interactions.

(continued)

Table 11.1 (*continued*)

Authors	Nursing Intervention Strategies	Development
	• Sounding board—listening, being there • Validation—praise, support of parent actions • Information giving—pamphlets, anticipatory guidance, teaching, demonstration • Actions—demonstration of infant care skills, arranging other resources • Baby or mother touching	
Gottlieb, 1994	• Develop and maintains working relationship • Gather information • Restructure cognitions • Develops problem-solving/coping strategies • Create a supportive environment • Teach • Work the system • Intentionally do nothing, "wait and see"	Research-tested intervention based on the McGill family nursing model. Each category has subcategories. Used in conjunction with a family problem list. Effective in improving child and family outcomes with a significant problem.
Kruger, Shawver, & Jones, 1980	• Support • Guide • Teach • Do for the person • Provide an environment that promotes personal development	Based on interviews with 14 families with a child with cystic fibrosis. Parent-identified issues and problems were related to Orem's categories.

(*continued*)

Table 11.1 (continued)

Authors	Nursing Intervention Strategies	Development
Leahey & Wright, 1994	**Directed at Cognitive Family Functioning** • Supply information about chronic illness • Make suggestions about appropriate family responses to illness • Supply information about community resources • Help with decision making **Directed at Affective Family Functioning** • Modify intense emotions that may be blocking problem solving • Validate family members' emotional responses • Show that family processes are normally slowed down in response to chronic illness **Directed at Behavioural Family Functioning** • Assign tasks aimed at better interactions • Deal with instrumental issues before affective issues • Encourage not to take precipitous major changes in response to a crisis • Encourage respite	Family nursing systems based. Derived from and modified with extensive clinical and teaching experience with family interviews. The members with a chronic condition were primarily adults.
Mott, James, & Sperhac, 1990	• Health promotion, health management, e.g., facilitating compliance • Activity-exercise, e.g., consulting, educating, and problem solving with family, health care professionals, and teachers to maintain developmental levels for child • Cognitive–perceptual, e.g., empowering the family by sharing knowledge • Self-perception, self-concept, e.g., assisting families to acknowledge and talk about fears, assisting in management of painful procedures for child • Role-relationship pattern, e.g., supporting continuation of normal parenting & assisting to develop new networks of social support • Coping, stress-tolerance pattern, e.g., helping a family to grow stronger, steadier, & deeper from their experiences	Experience- and literature-based.

(continued)

Table 11.1 (continued)

Authors	Nursing Intervention Strategies	Development
Craig & Edwards, 1983	• Help individual and family to achieve a realistic (re)appraisal of situation • Help individual and family to identify appropriate and helpful adaptive tasks • Facilitate development & utilization of beneficial coping behaviour	Extrapolated from Lazarus's (1974) stress and coping model.
Russell, 1987 (adapted)	• Provide realistic information about child's disability • Model positive therapeutic caretaking behaviours for parents • Encourage parents to explain situation to friends, relatives (helps parents come to terms with situation) • Adjust agency or institutional routines to allow normal parent–child interactions • Progress at parents' pace • Emphasize communication, keeping family together & assisting & working with family	Based on clinical practice with families with a newborn with a genetic defect, such as Down's syndrome.
Fewell & Gelb, 1983	• Involve parents as team members every step of the way • Inform about community resources • Give copies of reports to parents • Avoid jargon in all communications • Be sure parents understand diagnosis is subject to change • Help parents think of life with this child in the same terms as life with their other children	Developed by special educators for moderately handicapped children and their families, based on experience.
Jackson & Saunders, 1993	• Teach • Provide psychosocial support • Support mother • Support father • Support well siblings	Experience and clinical and research literature synthesized to derive categories of nursing interventions.

interventions are grounded in the developmental stages (e.g., Erickson, 1976; Zelle & Coyner, 1983).

Applications of *family nursing theory* have focussed on the primary caregiver, usually the mother. Siblings (Burke & Henderson, 1999; Stoneman & Berman, 1993) and fathers (McKeever, 1981; Murphy, 1986) are also recognized as important.

Nursing theory applications

Nursing theory has been used to inform practice involving families with a child having a chronic condition. For example, the intervention categories in Orem (1980) directed Kruger, Shawver, and Jones (1980) in the development of nursing actions for families with a child who has cystic fibrosis (see Table 11.1). Mott, James, and Sperhac (1990) used nursing diagnoses to categorize nursing actions with families of children with chronic conditions (see Table 11.1).

Conceptual models of chronicity

The best-developed conceptual models, specific to these families, are the McCubbin, Cauble, and Patterson (1982) Family Adjustment and Adaptation Response model (also called the double ABCX model); the Hymovich model (1987); Barnard's (Barnard et al., 1991) Child Assessment Interaction model; and the Burke model (1987). Stress and coping comprise the most common concepts used in research with these families (Burke & Roberts, 1990). Models created by Burke (1987), Hymovich (1987), and McCubbin, Cauble, and Patterson (1982) all incorporate stress, coping, resilience, and competence concepts. Social support is also a common construct.

Research evidence-based practice with families and children

Building on theory-based interventions, experimental studies can demonstrate the effectiveness of nursing interventions for children with chronic conditions and their families. Table 11.1 illustrates the overlaps between experience, theory, and research-based nursing interventions.

Olds and Kitzman (1990) and Olds, Echenrode, et al. (1997) found that nurse home visiting at the prenatal and infancy periods resulted in improved birth weights and gestational age for infants of smokers and young mothers. Home visiting also improved children's developmental status and reduced behavioural problems.

Six studies have found significantly better parent adjustment or psychological status of children with chronic physical disorders among those receiving an experimental intervention by health professionals compared with those in the control condition (Barnard et al., 1991; Burke, Harrison, et al.,

1999a&b; Pless, Feeley, et al., 1994; Pless & Satterwhite, 1975; Stein & Jessop, 1984). Three (Pless, Feeley, et al.; Barnard et al.; Burke, Harrison, et al.) focussed on nursing interventions; others studied interventions implemented by other professionals. Common interventions include providing information, teaching, and assistance with problem solving and dealing with the health care system.

Successful research-tested interventions include these characteristics:

- strategies are directed primarily at parents and address psychosocial factors
- strategies are clearly described
- professionals receive training
- interactions occur between professional and parent during periods of potential or actual parent or child distress, e.g., diagnosis, repeated hospitalizations, pregnancy, infancy
- nurse–family contact is of sufficient frequency and duration for the formation of a therapeutic alliance
- interventions focus on parent-identified issues
- interventions vary in response to parents' current needs, individual nurses' experience and skill, and health care services available
- interventions are multifaceted and may include several strategies (e.g., home visits, telephone calls).

Research evidence-based assessment

It is essential that assessments be sensitive to the issues faced by families with children who have chronic conditions. There are a number of well-developed assessment tools. The evidence-based assessment tools the authors use are identified in Table 11.2. Barnard (1991), Hymovich (1987), and McCubbin, Cauble, and Patterson (1982) have created theory-based, research-tested assessment and evaluation tools.

In this chapter, evaluation is limited to effects of nursing actions on the family and child. Levels of specificity vary by clinical setting and family situation. Some assessments are based on therapeutic conversation, resulting in agreement that issues around a stressor are resolved, are managed in a more effective or satisfying way, or are better understood or accepted. At the next level of specificity, the nurse and the parent may have a written contract or objectives that can be used as a basis for evaluation. At the next level of specificity, there might be a need for more concrete family, child, and nurse description or documentation. Communication with other professionals is often required. When needed, more formal, objective measures of child and family status are useful.

Table 11.2
Selected assessment tools for children with chronic conditions and their families*

Focus	Dimension	Selected Measures	Clinical Notes
Family	Family functioning	Feetham Family Functioning Survey (Feetham & Humenick, 1982)	Very sensitive to family changes; repeat as needed.
	Family coping strategies	Parent Stress Index (PSI; Abidin, 1986); the parent domain section and life stresses section	Father and mother norms are available.
	Coping specific to chronic conditions	Coping Health Inventory for Parents (CHIP; McCubbin et al., 1983)	CHIP scales concern friends and self, family, and health care system.
	Family stressors and tasks	Burke Assessment Guide to stressors & tasks in families with a child with a chronic condition	See Figure 11.2 (p. 231)
Parent	Parenting stress	PSI, life stresses section: Questionnaire on Resources and Stress (QRS; Holroyd, 1983)	PSI includes a stressful life events scale for concurrent family crises. QRS measures burden, stress, and resources.
	Physical health	PSI, parent domain	Questions on sleep, general health, and energy can tap areas a parent might not otherwise mention.
	Emotion health	PSI, parent domain	Good questions on depression and exhaustion.
Siblings	Development	Scales of Independent Behavior (SIB; Bruininks et al., 1985)	Scales for motor, social, emotional, and cognitive development. Watch for accelerated development in self-care, child care, and other domestic tasks.
	Emotional health	Child Behavior Checklist (CBC; Achenbach & Edelbrock, 1983); PSI, child domain	CBC has good section on individualized competencies. Behaviour checklist in CBC for severe problems. PSI covers similar behaviours.

(continued)

Table 11.2 (continued)

Focus	Dimension	Selected Measures	Clinical Notes
Child with chronic condition	Development	SIB	Note variation in developmental age between scales. Compare parent or child concerns with actual delays. Document regressions after stressful period, e.g., hospitalization.
	Physical health and growth	Physical assessment, height, weight, etc.	Track growth charts; watch for changes in usual percentile for height and weight. Physical assessment as a baseline for later changes.
	Behaviour and emotional health	PSI, child domain; CBC, competencies and behaviour sections	Document parent concerns or behaviours observed as problematic.

* These measures have been used extensively by the authors. See each measure's manuals for training, ensuring reliability, indications, and clinical cautions. Others in wide use are those by Barnard (Barnard, Snyder, & Spitz, 1991) and Hymovich (Hymovich & Baker, 1991).

Some of the tested tools identify the impact of stressors, coping, and functional and behavioural changes (see Table 11.2). Although the measures selected for this chapter can be self-taught, the assistance of a skilled user who has formal training in the use of the tool is desirable.

Each tool in Table 11.2 can be used in the full standardized form or more informally, by selecting the sections or subscales that are most relevant to the family. However, changing the manner of administration means that the results will not be comparable with the norms listed in the tool manual. The authors have found that the most suitable measures are developed specifically for similar families or children with similar chronic conditions. Such tools tend to have superior sensitivity to critical issues and subtle changes in these families. The measures in Table 11.2 meet these criteria.

Documentation is implicit in all levels of evaluation of child and family outcomes. The nurse should not underestimate the value of documenting informal assessment, agreement on issues, interactions, interventions, and critical stressors with these families.

Research-tested, theory- and experience-based nursing intervention strategies

Community health nurses will draw on their experience; their network of skilled nurses, other professionals and experienced families; and the clinical and research literature to select intervention strategies to employ in work with families that have children with chronic conditions (see Table 11.1, p. 218).

Nursing strategies have been tested in research involving families with very specific types of children and circumstances. Burke and her colleagues (Burke, Harrison, et al., 1999a&b) and Kauffmann, Harrison, Burke, and Wong (1998a) have tested an intervention with repeatedly hospitalized children. Barnard and colleagues (1991) and Olds, Echenrode, et al. (1997) evaluated an intervention focussed on pregnant women and high-risk newborns in low-income environments. In Pless, Feeley, et al. (1994) and Burke, Harrison, et al. (1999a&b), nurses worked with the families of children who attended outpatient clinics.

Stress-Point Intervention by Nurses: A research-tested intervention

The authors developed a model for nursing practice for families and their children with chronic conditions called Stress-Point Intervention by Nurses (SPIN) (Burke, Costello, et al., 1997; Burke, Harrison, et al., 1999a; Kauffmann et al., 1998a). The intervention (SPIN) and its expected outcomes for the child and family are illustrated in Figure 11.1. Brief, specific interventions with parents, timed to coincide with the hospitalization of essentially healthy children, can reduce distress and psychological and physiological effects in their children during and following short, single hospitalizations (Skipper & Leonard, 1968; Skipper, Leonard, & Rhymes, 1968; Wolfer & Visintainer, 1979; Zastowny, Kirschenbaum, & Meng, 1986). Importantly, the intervention given to the parent in one setting was also effective when the parent worked with the child before a specific, anticipated stressor arising in another setting.

The authors developed SPIN for a common stressful situation—repeated hospitalizations, which are the second most stressful event for these families. The most stressful is diagnosis and rediagnosis (Burke, Handley-Derry, & Costello, 1989). We postulate that SPIN can be used for other stressors that these families and children encounter. A comprehensive list of stressors is discussed in the next section and presented in Figure 11.2.

The stress associated with repeated hospitalizations of children with chronic or disabling conditions is different and potentially more severe than that associated with single hospitalizations of essentially healthy children (Association for the Care of Children's Health, 1982; Burke, Handley-Derry, et al., 1989). It is also linked to long-term psychosocial and learning problems (Quinton & Rutter, 1976). Hospitalization is a community health nursing issue because preparation and post-discharge management most often occur in the community, and the coordination of care between hospital and community is important (Canadian Association of Paediatric Hospitals, 1990).

Figure 11.1
Model of Stress-Point Interventions by Nurses (SPIN) and expected outcomes for children and families

---

Identification of family and child stressors	Enhanced parent coping	Improved family functioning
+	+	+
Customized intervention strategies by nurse ⟶	Improved use of family, community, and health care resources ⟶	Better development progress and adjustment

Modified from Burke, Harrison, Kauffmann, & Wong (1992).

Further, when a child with a chronic condition is hospitalized, family life is usually altered and strained (Burke, Handley-Derry, et al., 1989).

The authors tested SPIN and found it resulted in better child and parent outcomes than for those having usual care (Burke, Harrison, et al., 1999a&b). Nurses trained to use SPIN report that it broadens their perspective on key issues and focusses their nursing interventions to the issues currently of parental concern. SPIN uses elements of the overlapping strategies of counselling, crisis management, teaching, and primary nursing (Johnson, 1986), and a family systems nursing approach (Wright & Leahey, 1994). The specific strategies a community health nurse uses can be selected from among those suggested in the next section or from Table 11.1 (p. 218).

Stressors and tasks

In today's health care system, crises, new or difficult tasks, and stressful assessments and procedures often precipitate a point of contact with the nurse. What are the stress points for these families? Burke's research-based assessment framework of predictable, recurring stressors and tasks unique to families with a child having a chronic condition is shown in Figure 11.2 (Burke, 1988; Burke, Kauffmann, Costello, Wislein, & Harrison, 1998; Burke, Kauffmann, Harrison, & Wislein, 1999).

Nurses use the Burke Assessment Guide to screen, assess, provide anticipatory guidance, focus on the particular stressors of concern to a family, and evaluate the effectiveness of their interventions. Figure 11.2 identifies 11 sets of stressors/tasks, such as (a) gaining experience to manage the child's condition, (b) monitoring and managing the health of other family members, (c) managing the burden of care, and (d) adapting beliefs and values regarding such factors as disability and/or sibling issues. Each of the 11 sets of stressors includes subissues; for example, rearing a child with a chronic condition may include unmet or modified developmental milestones, segregation versus integration, or maintaining developmental gains outside the home.

Compared with normal family and child developmental tasks, tasks and stressors for these families can be more complex, continuing, and recurring (Burke, Kauffmann, Costello, Harrison, & Wislein, 1994). These tasks and stressors do not all occur for every family, and there is not necessarily a predictable order of occurrence. Further, the tasks are not necessarily less stressful on reoccurrence. When testing a community-based intervention (SPIN) focussed on stressors within the context of a repeated hospitalization, the authors found broader, beneficial effects on family functioning and child development (Burke, Costello, et al., 1997). This suggests that families can generalize coping learned with one stressor to another and/or that effective, focussed (SPIN) interventions foster better development and adjustment in other areas of family and child life.

Figure 11.2
Burke Assessment Guide to stressors and tasks in families with a child with chronic condition

1. Gaining and interpreting **knowledge, skills, and experience** to manage a child's health problem

☐ Amount of help (too much/too little)

☐ Timing of help (too soon/too late)

☐ Conflicting advice or help

☐ Missed or wrong information or help

2. Acquiring and managing physical **resources and services** to manage child's health problem

☐ Home

☐ School

☐ Equipment or supplies

☐ Medications

☐ Hassles with people and institutions to obtain the above

3. Acquiring and managing **financial resources** to care for child's health problem

☐ Direct costs for care of child (specify expense _____)

☐ Indirect costs; check if a stress-producing expense (e.g., travel, meals, child care, housing) (specify _____)

☐ Hassles within family about how much and what to spend money on

☐ Hassles with people and/or institutions to get financial help

4. Establishing and maintaining effective **social support**

☐ Extended family

☐ Community

☐ Friends

☐ Parents with similar children

5. Rearing a **child with a chronic condition**

☐ Unmet development milestones

☐ Segregation, least restrictive environment, integration issues

☐ Aiding normal development

☐ Modifying development expectations

☐ Preparing for adolescent and adult roles

☐ Behaviour problems

☐ Child care, babysitters

☐ Maintaining development gains outside home (e.g., school, hospital, community)

6. Developing **beliefs, values,** and philosophy of life

☐ Incorporating the child's health problems and ways family copes

☐ Acknowledging feelings, reactions

☐ Trying out new ways of coping

☐ Giving meaning

(continued)

Figure 11.2 *(continued)*

7. **Managing the care** of the child

☐ Distribution of tasks/responsibility among family members and health care system

☐ Conflicts between child, sibling, parent, and family care needs

☐ Shifts in care load (heavier/lighter)

☐ Accepting or rejecting need for family sacrifice

8. Identifying and managing **sibling issues**

☐ Balancing amount of involvement in physical, emotional, and/or financial burdens

☐ Providing an environment for normal development

☐ Helping sibling with philosophical and emotional issues related to child with health problem

9. Maintaining spousal, parental, and nuclear **family relationships**

☐ Dealing with emotional issues in daily management and coping with small changes in child with health problem

☐ Planning for expected and long-term changes

☐ Maintaining relationships that provide social support

☐ Adjusting to crises related to child with health problem

☐ Satisfaction/dissatisfaction with lifestyle

10. Maintaining **health of other family members**

☐ Managing illness of other family members

☐ Exhaustion of primary caregiver (usually mother)

11. Maintaining effective relationships with **health care system** and other sources of care

☐ Rediagnosis

☐ Changing or conflicting advice in treatment regimens

☐ Changes in physician, clinic, or hospital

☐ Hospitalization

☐ Finding a satisfying role with health care professionals (specify _____)

☐ Collaboration with team as a parent

☐ Taking advice and/or accepting services

☐ Advocating to change system

☐ Examining and/or using alternative models of care for child with health problem

12. Other stressors or tasks

☐

☐

☐

Modified from Burke (1988); Burke, Kauffmann, Costello, Wiskin, & Harrison (1998); and Burke, Kauffmann, Harrison, & Wiskin (1999). Permission is granted to copy and use as described in this chapter and in Burke, Kauffman, Costello, Wiskin, & Harrison (1998) and Burke, Kauffmann, Harrison, & Wiskin (1999).

Examples of an application of SPIN

To illustrate how SPIN works and how it may be applied by community health nurses, consider the stressor of hospitalization. SPIN uses specific points of contact with families timed to coincide with preparation for hospitalization and post-discharge care at home. This results in sustained pro-active contact close to and following the period in hospital.

A strategy used throughout is circular questioning (Wright & Leahey, 1994). Two examples of this kind of question are: "Who in the family is most fearful of the hospitalization? What part of the hospitalization bothers you most?" Using this technique, the nurse draws out the perspective of family members in relation to the stressors they face.

It is important to give the family the time and permission to communicate their concerns. This is done in a deliberate way for families who are not used to expressing their questions or concerns openly. A specific question might be: "What do you see as being stressful or of concern to you in the hospitalization coming up?"

In addition to the family's perspective, nurses have skills and knowledge of events and circumstances that a family is apt to encounter before, throughout, and after the hospitalization. This knowledge could relate to the child's condition, a new treatment, variations on the surgical procedure, recuperation, or ways to manage discomfort. The assessment phase involves an interweaving of the experience and knowledge of both family and nurse. The Primary Health Care principle of public participation guides this process. These interactions and the known stressors/tasks (listed in Figure 11.2) lead to identification of stressors and intervention strategies for the particular family and child.

The nature of the family or child stressor often signals the need for a particular nursing strategy. The mutual decision regarding intervention is shaped by available resources; the nurse's skill, knowledge, and experience; and the particular needs, knowledge, and coping patterns of the family.

The community health nurse reviews the stressors. These are then validated or modified by the family. A business card, identifying the nurse's name, phone number, and available times for contact, is given to the family. The back of this card is used by the nurse to list the mutually identified stressors and the strategies discussed. In this sense, the card is "customized" for the family. The family is encouraged to contact the nurse if any uncertainties or new stressors arise. As follow-up and reinforcement, a letter confirming the stressors and strategies is sent to the family.

Following the initial contact, any number of contacts are possible. The parent might want to contact the nurse, perhaps to reflect on the family's plans and resources for coping. These contacts can be made by phone or by a home or clinic visit. At a minimum, the community health nurse contacts the family shortly before the hospitalization to reinforce the plan and determine whether there are new issues. The next planned contact by the nurse is made during hospitalization. This contact is critical, as unexpected stressors arise and family coping strategies often have to be revised (Burke, Kauffmann, Costello, & Dillon, 1991). A post-discharge contact by the nurse, usually a phone call, is made within two to three days. This is a time to evaluate the hospital stay and discuss and review any new or different experiences. Support is encompassed in whatever strategy is used. Some common strategies are described below.

Information giving. If information is needed about hospital procedures, routine care, or nursing procedures, this is supplied by the community health nurse using an individualized approach to standard pamphlets and materials. The nurse predetermines whether the content of these materials will supply the correct information in the depth required by these parents. Some parents are already well informed about hospital procedures, while others are not. Parents may be accustomed to the routines of their local hospital but feel unfamiliar with the routines and facilities of the larger centres. The nurse's knowledge of these practical matters is helpful and reassuring to parents.

Enhancing parent–health professional communication. Information and strategies for successful communication are discussed. Community health nurses can help parents determine who are the best sources for certain types of information and how they can be accessed. Parents may find it useful to make lists of concerns before conversations with health care professionals. Finding out times that doctors, physiotherapists, and other professionals make visits is helpful. Role playing and rehearsal may be used to illustrate the kinds of approaches and questions to use. When family–health professional meetings are planned, taped explanations and information can provide families with a permanent record. Although this is not a common practice, it has been used successfully when treatment regimes are complex and not all family members can be present. For families moving among a number of centres and professionals, keeping records of dates, results of tests, and other information has been helpful.

Parents find it beneficial to identify a specific nurse or health professional with whom they can form a helping relationship (Burke, Kauffman, Costello, & Dillon, 1991). Continuity can help in communicating information about the child's routines, likes, and dislikes and in negotiating "parents' rules" with health professionals. (Parents' rules are "the do's and don'ts" that parents have learned and incorporated into their expectations for care of their child.)

Preparing for and helping a child cope with hospitalization and recovery at home. If the child needs emotional, informational, or physical support before, during, and after hospitalization, the community health nurse works with the parents to choose a strategy that "fits" the child. The developmental level of the child may preclude use of the usual aids in preparation programs. These children often have previous experiences with hospitals that conjure up fear and anxiety. Thorough history and assessment with the help of the parent is necessary. Parents often find invasive procedures difficult to endure. In these cases, the nursing intervention is directed toward assisting the parent, as well as the child, to handle such procedures. Early discharge and increased out-patient surgery and day admissions mean more recovery time. Responsibility for follow-up resides with the community health nurse.

Supporting family routines. Alternative strategies and resources for maintaining family routines are discussed. The nurse can assist the parents to identify in advance who among the parents' friends and relatives can help during this period. These supporters can visit the child in hospital, keep things running smoothly at home, care for siblings, or offer respite to the parent who is staying with the hospitalized child on a constant basis.

Conclusion

There are three expectations for community health nurses working with families who have a child with a chronic condition. The first is to know the issues these families often face. The second is to identify the family's critical issues quickly and to work with them in dealing with these issues. The third is to devise a flexible set of nursing interventions that can fit the family's and child's current stressors and tasks. Community health nurses who work with these families and children bridge the gap between the traditional institutional and community sectors. As more severely affected children now live longer and at home, the role of the community health nurse in maintaining continuity of care for families who have a child with a chronic condition is important.

QUESTIONS

1. Reread the "success stories" at the beginning of the chapter.
    a. Identify the stressors and tasks for the family using the Burke Assessment Guide (Figure 11.2, p. 231).
    b. Identify three other interventions that you could use as a community health nurse (refer to Table 11.1, p. 218).
2. Estimates of the number of children with a chronic condition can vary depending on how chronic condition is defined. Which factors would result in a lower estimate? Which would produce a higher estimate?

3. If you were new to a community, how would you find the services and agencies currently available to families of children with chronic conditions? Consider key professionals; parents; lay, professional and government organizations; library and Internet resources.
4. What community resources are available to help families who must travel to larger centres for specialized care?

REFERENCES

Abidin, R.R. (1986). *Parenting stress index.* Charlottesville, VA: Pediatric Psychology Press.

Achenbach, T.M., & Edelbrock, C. (1983). *Child behavior checklist and revised child behavior profile.* Burlington, VT: Department of Psychiatry, University of Vermont.

Association for the Care of Children's Health. (1982). *Preparing your child for repeated or extended hospitalization.* Washington, DC: Author.

Avard, D., & Hanvey, L. (1989). *The health of Canada's children: A CICH profile.* Ottawa: Canadian Institute for Child Health.

Barnard, K.E., Snyder, C., & Spietz, A. (1991). Supportive measures for high-risk infants and families. In A.L. Whall & J. Fawcett (Eds.), *Family theory development in nursing: State of the science and art* (pp. 139–176). Philadelphia: F.A. Davis.

Boyle, M. (1991). Child health in Ontario. In R. Barnhorst & L.C. Johnson (Eds.), *The state of the child in Ontario* (pp. 92–116). Toronto: Oxford University Press.

Bruininks, R.H., Woodcock, R.W., Weatherman, R.F., & Hill, B.K. (1985). *Development and standardization of the Scales of Independent Behavior.* Allen, TX: DLM Teaching Resources.

Burke, S.O. (1987). Assessing single-parent families with physically disabled children. In L.M. Wright & M. Leahey (Eds.), *Families and chronic illness* (pp. 147–167). Springhouse, PA: Springhouse.

Burke, S.O. (1988). *Ongoing stressors/tasks for family care givers of children with chronic conditions.* Unpublished manuscript, Queen's University, Kingston, ON.

Burke, S.O. (1997). Trajectories and transferability: Building nursing knowledge about chronicity. *Canadian Journal of Nursing Research, 28,* 3–7 (English), 9–14 (French).

Burke, S.O., Costello, E.A., Handley-Derry, M., Kauffmann, E., & Dillon, M. (1997). Stress-point preparation for parents of repeatedly hospitalized children with chronic conditions. *Research in Nursing and Health, 20,* 475–485.

Burke, S.O., Handley-Derry, M., & Costello, E.A. (1989). Maternal stress and repeated hospitalizations of children who are physically disabled. *Children's Health Care, 18,* 82–90.

Burke, S.O., Harrison, M.B., Kauffmann, E., & Wong, C. (1992). *Effects of a preparation program for parents of repeatedly hospitalized children: A proposal for a clinical trial of a clinic-based nursing intervention.* Toronto: Ontario Ministry of Health.

Burke, S.O., Harrison, M.B., Kauffmann, E., & Wong, C. (1999a). *Developmental and behavior outcomes among repeatedly hospitalized children from a trial of stress-point intervention by nurses.* Manuscript submitted for publication.

Burke, S.O., Harrison, M.B., Kauffmann, E., & Wong, C. (1999b). *Family effects of a nursing intervention for parents of repeatedly hospitalized children with chronic conditions.* Manuscript submitted for publication.

Burke, S.O., & Henderson, J. (1999). *Fairness issues and processes among siblings of children with chronic conditions.* Manuscript submitted for publication.

Burke, S.O., Kauffmann, E., Costello, E.A., & Dillon, M.C. (1991). Hazardous secrets and reluctantly taking charge: Parenting a child with repeated hospitalizations. *Image: Journal of Nursing Scholarship, 23,* 39–45.

Burke, S.O., Kauffmann, E., Costello, E.A., Harrison, M.B., & Wiskin, N. (1994). Stressors and tasks particular to families with a child who has a chronic or life threatening condition: Grounded theory and assessment framework. *Proceedings of the Third International Family Nursing Conference* (p. 73). Montréal: School of Nursing, McGill University.

Burke, S.O., Kauffmann, E., Costello, E.A., Wiskin, N., & Harrison, M.B. (1998). Stressors in families with a child with a chronic condition: An analysis of qualitative studies and a framework. *Canadian Journal of Nursing Research, 30,* 71–95.

Burke, S.O., Kauffmann, E., Harrison, M.B., & Wiskin, N. (1999). Assessment of stressors in families with a child who has a chronic condition. *MCN: The Journal of Maternal Child Nursing, 24,* 98–106.

Burke, S.O., Kauffmann, E., LaSalle, J., Harrison, M.B., & Wong, C. (1999). *Chronic illness trajectories: A confirmatory factor analysis of parent's perceptions.* Manuscript submitted for publication.

Burke, S.O., & Roberts, C.A. (1990). Nursing research and the care of chronically ill and disabled children. *Journal of Pediatric Nursing, 5*(5), 316–327.

Cadman, D., Boyle, M., & Offord, D.R. (1988). The Ontario Child Health Study: Social adjustment and mental health of siblings of children with chronic health problems. *Developmental and Behavioral Pediatrics, 9*(3), 117–121.

Cadman, D., Boyle, M., Szatmari, P., & Offord, D.R. (1987). Chronic illness, disability, and mental and social well-being: Findings of the Ontario Child Health Study. *Pediatrics, 79,* 805–813.

Canadian Association of Paediatric Hospitals. (1990). *Paediatric long-term care in Canada.* Ottawa: Author.

Corbin, J.M., & Strauss, A. (1991). A nursing model for chronic illness management based upon the trajectory framework. *Scholarly Inquiry for Nursing Practice: An International Journal, 5,* 155–174.

Craig, H.M., & Edwards, J.E. (1983). Adaptation in chronic illness: An eclectic model for nurses. *Journal of Advanced Nursing, 8,* 397–404.

Donlevy, J., & Pietruch, B. (1996). The connection delivery model: Reengineering nursing to provide care across the continuum. *Nursing Administration Quarterly, 20*(3), 73–78.

Erickson, M.L. (1976). *Assessment and management of developmental changes in children.* Saint Louis: Mosby.

Feetham, S.L., & Humenick, S.S. (1982). The Feetham family functioning survey. In S.S. Humenick (Ed.), *Analysis of current assessment strategies in the health care of young children and childbearing families* (pp. 249–268). East Norwalk, CT: Appleton-Century-Crofts.

Fewell, R.R., & Gelb, S.A. (1983). Parenting moderately handicapped persons. In M. Seligman (Ed.), *The family with a handicapped child: Understanding and treatment.* New York: Grune & Stratton.

Gottlieb, L. (1994). Pathways towards improving psychosocial adjustment in children with a chronic physical disorder. *Proceedings of the Third International Family Nursing Conference* (p. 59). Montréal: School of Nursing, McGill University.

Health & Welfare Canada, Health Services & Promotion Branch. (1990). *Report on home care.* Ottawa, ON: Federal–Provincial–Territorial Working Group on Home Care. (Cat. No. H39-186/1990E)

Holroyd, J. (1987). *Questionnaire on resources and stress for families with chronically ill or handicapped members.* Brandon, VT: Clinical Psychology Publishing.

Hymovich, D.P. (1987). Assessing families of children with cystic fibrosis. In L.M. Wright & M. Leahey (Eds.), *Families and chronic illness* (pp. 133–146). Springhouse, PA: Springhouse.

Hymovich, D.P., & Baker C.D. (1991). The needs, concerns and coping of parents of children with cystic fibrosis. In A.L. Whall & J. Fawcett (Eds.), *Family theory development in nursing: State of the science and art* (pp. 375–387). Philadelphia: F.A. Davis.

Jackson, D.B., & Saunders, R.B. (1993). *Child health nursing.* Philadelphia: J.B. Lippincott.

Johnson, S.H. (1986). *Nursing assessment and strategies for the family at risk: High-risk parenting* (2nd ed.). Philadelphia: J.B. Lippincott.

Kauffmann, E., Harrison, M., Burke, S.O., & Wong, C. (1998a). Stress-point intervention for parents of children hospitalized with chronic conditions. *Pediatric Nursing, 24,* 362–366.

Kauffmann, E., Harrison, M., Burke, S.O., & Wong, C. (1998b). *Training manual for stress-point intervention.* Kingston, ON: Queen's University School of Nursing.

Kruger, S., Shawver, M., & Jones, L. (1980). Reactions of families to the child with cystic fibrosis. *Image: Journal of Nursing Scholarship, 12*(3), 67–80.

Lazarus, R.S. (1974). Psychological stress and coping in adaptation and illness. *International Journal of Psychiatry in Medicine, 5,* 321–333.

Leahey, M., & Wright, L.M. (1987). Families with chronic illness: Assumptions, assessment and intervention. In L.M. Wright & M. Leahey (Eds.), *Families and chronic illness* (pp. 55–76). Springhouse, PA: Springhouse.

Lubkin, I.M. (1986). *Chronic illness: Impact and interventions.* Boston: Jones & Bartlett.

McCubbin, H.I., Cauble, A.E., & Patterson, J.M. (Eds.). (1982). *Family stress, coping, and social support.* Springfield, IL: Charles C. Thomas.

McCubbin, H.I., McCubbin, M.A., Patterson, J.M., Cauble, A.E., Wilson, L.R., & Warwick, W. (1983, May). CHIP—Coping Health Inventory for Parents: An assessment of parental coping patterns in the care of the chronically ill child. *Journal of Marriage and the Family, 45,* 359–370.

McKeever, P.T. (1981). Fathering the chronically ill child. *American Journal of Maternal/Child Nursing, 6*(2), 124–128.

Mott, S.R., James, S.R., & Sperhac, A.M. (1990). *Nursing care of children and families* (2nd ed.). Redwood City, CA: Addison-Wesley.

Murphy, C.M. (1986). Assessment of fathering behaviors. In S.H. Johnson (Ed.), *Nursing assessment and strategies for the family at risk: High-risk parenting* (2nd ed.) (pp. 41–60). Philadelphia: J.B. Lippincott.

Newacheck, P.W., & Taylor, W.R. (1992). Childhood chronic illness: Prevalence, severity, and impact. *American Journal of Public Health, 82,* 364–371.

Offord, D.R., Boyle, M., Szatmari, P., Rae-Grant, N.I., Links, P.S., Cadman, D.T., Byles, J.A., Crawford, J.W., Blum, H.M., Byrne, C., et al. (1987). Ontario Child Health Study: II. Six-month prevalence of disorder and rates of service utilization. *Archives of General Psychiatry, 44*, 832–836.

Olds, D.L., Echenrode, J., Henderson, C.R., Kitzman, H., Powers, J., Cole, R., Sidora, K., Morris, P., Petitt, L.M., & Luckey, D. (1997). Long-term effects of home visitation on maternal life course and child abuse and neglect. *Journal of the American Medical Association, 276*, 637–643.

Olds, D.L., & Kitzman, H. (1990). Can home visitation improve the health of women and children at environmental risk? *Pediatrics, 86*, 108–116.

Ontario Ministry of Health. (1993). *A healthier Ontario: Progress in the '90s*. Toronto: Queen's Printer for Ontario. (Cat. No. 4225539)

Orem, D.E. (1980). *Nursing: Concepts of practice* (2nd ed.). New York: McGraw-Hill.

Perrin, E.C., Newacheck, P., Pless, I.B., Drotar, D., Gortmaker, S.L., Levanthal, J., Perrin, J.M., Stein, R.E.K., Walker, D.K., & Weitzman, M. (1993). Issues involved in the definition and classification of chronic health conditions. *Pediatrics, 91*, 787–793.

Peters, D.A. (1989). A concept of nursing discharge. *Holistic Nursing Practice, 3*(2), 18–25.

Pless, I.B., Feeley, N., Gottlieb, L., Rowat, K., Dougherty, G., & Willard, G. (1994). A randomization trial of a nursing intervention to promote the adjustment of children with chronic physical disorders. *Pediatrics, 94*(1), 70–75.

Pless, I.B., & Satterwhite, B. (1975). The family counsellor. In R.M. Haggerty, K.J. Roghmann, & I.B. Pless (Eds.), *Child health and the community*. New York: Wiley.

Rolland, J.S. (1987). Chronic illness and the family: An overview. In L.M. Wright & M. Leahey (Eds.), *Families and chronic illness* (pp. 33–54). Springhouse, PA: Springhouse.

Russell, F.F. (1987). Intervening with families of infants with Down's Syndrome. In L.M. Wright & M. Leahey (Eds.), *Families and chronic illness* (pp. 257–274). Springhouse, PA: Springhouse.

Skipper, J.K., & Leonard, R.C. (1968). Children, stress, and hospitalization: A field experiment. *Journal of Health and Social Behavior, 9*, 275–151.

Skipper, J.K., Leonard, R.C., & Rhymes, J. (1968). Child hospitalization and social interaction: An experimental study of mothers' feelings of stress, adaptation and satisfaction. *Medical Care, 6*, 496–506.

Statistics Canada. (1992a). *Families: Number, type and structure*. Ottawa: Ministry of Industry, Science & Technology. (Cat. No. 93-312)

Statistics Canada. (1992b). *Profile of census divisions & subdivisions in Ontario—Part A.* Ottawa: Ministry of Industry, Science & Technology. (Cat. No. 95-337)

Stein, R.E.K., & Jessop, D. (1984). Does pediatric home care make a difference for children with chronic illness? Findings from the Pediatric Ambulatory Care Treatment Study. *Pediatrics, 73*, 845–853.

Stoneman, Z., & Berman, P.W. (Eds.). (1993). *The effects of mental retardation, disability, and illness on sibling relationships: Research issues and challenges*. Baltimore: Paul H. Brookes.

Thompson, T., & Hupp, S.C. (Eds.). (1992). *Saving children at risk*. Newbury Park, CA: Sage.

Thorne, S.E., & Robinson, C.A. (1988). Health care relationships: The chronic illness perspective. *Research in Nursing and Health, 11*, 293–300.

White, N., & Lubkin, I.M. (1995). Illness trajectory. In I.M. Lubkin (Ed.), *Chronic illness: Impacts and interventions* (pp. 51–73). Boston: Jones & Bartlett.

Wolfer, J.A., & Visintainer, M.A. (1979). Prehospital psychological preparation for tonsillectomy patients: Effects on children's and parents' adjustment. *Pediatrics, 64*, 646–655.

Wright, L.M., & Leahey, M. (1994). *Nurses and families: A guide to family assessment and intervention* (2nd ed.). Philadelphia: F.A. Davis.

Zastowny, T.R., Kirschenbaum, D.S., & Meng, A.L. (1986). Coping skills training for children: Effects on distress before, during, and after hospitalization for surgery. *Health Psychology, 5*(3), 231–247.

Zelle, R.S., & Coyner, A.B. (1983). *Developmentally disabled infants and toddlers: Assessment and intervention*. Philadelphia: F.A. Davis.

C H A P T E R   1 2

Adolescent health promotion: An evolving opportunity for community health nurses

Angela J. Gillis

The purpose of this chapter is to promote discussion on the topic of adolescent health. The developmental and social context of the adolescent experience is explored, and practical goals for health promotion are identified. A coordinated, multicomponent, multidisciplinary approach is important. Principles for guiding adolescent health promotion efforts and practical strategies and roles for community health nurses are outlined.

LEARNING OBJECTIVES

In this chapter, you will learn:

- the concept of adolescent health promotion as seen from a holistic perspective
- the importance of identifying broad goals for adolescent health promotion
- developmentally appropriate strategies and principles for adolescent health promotion
- the role of community health nurses in promoting the health of adolescents

Introduction

Personal and social developmental characteristics of adolescence support experimentation with a wide range of behaviours that predispose adolescents to disease, injury, or negative social consequences. This chapter reviews the developmental experience of adolescents and the multiple changes that have implications for health promotion. Health promotion goals are identified, and key principles for successful health promotion programming are discussed. The chapter concludes by exploring future trends and directions in adolescent health promotion. The aim is to call attention to the need for new directions in community health nursing practice surrounding adolescent health promotion and to promote reflection on what these new directions ought to be.

Definition of terms and assumptions in adolescent health promotion

There are numerous studies that purport to define health from child, adolescent, and adult perspectives (Cobb, 1992; Rosenbaum & Carty, 1996; Weiler, 1997).

- Social scientists define adolescent health from the perspective of successful transition and as successful coping and well-being (Raphael, 1996).
- Health-related perspectives focus upon developing healthy lifestyles and avoiding risky behaviours (Pender, 1996; Yarcheski, Mahon, & Yarcheski, 1997).
- The personal perspective of adolescents indicates health has a variety of meanings and is often taken for granted. It is expressed in such ways as a sense of well-being, the absence of illness, the acceptance of responsibility, and the ability to solve problems and deal with stress and crisis (Rosenbaum & Carty, 1996).

Health promotion assumes incorporation of prevention efforts aimed at adolescent risk behaviours and inclusion of health-enhancing behaviours. Further, policies and programs must transcend the physical and expand to include situations and behaviours that influence social and mental health in adolescents. Health promotion includes goals related to individual behavioural change as well as a variety of other goals, including environmental, social, political, organizational, economic, and policy interventions. Appropriate intervention programs and promotion strategies can enhance health, help adolescents take responsibility for their health, and, in turn, change their lifestyle and health behaviours.

Health promotion and the adolescent experience

The many physical, emotional, and social changes occurring during adolescence produce varying expectations for adolescent health promotion

(Edelman & Mandle, 1994). Clearly, the majority of nurses view adolescence from an eclectic developmental perspective (Estes & Hart, 1993) that emphasizes all aspects of development (Rice, 1996).

Adolescence is not a unified, undifferentiated stage of life (Feldman & Elliott, 1990; Irwin, 1993). Redefining adolescence into distinct stages of development emphasizes that early adolescence differs from middle adolescence, which in turn differs from late adolescence (Cobb, 1992; Ingersoll, 1989). For example, rapid physical growth, intense conformity with peers, and the need to be accepted and to "fit in" mark early adolescence. Middle adolescence is characterized by the emergence of new cognitive skills. Middle adolescents are increasingly self-directed; they are concerned about what is right and proper behaviour, and they focus on acceptability by peers of the opposite sex. Late adolescence is concerned with establishing a personal identity and with setting vocational goals. During this stage, adolescents are independent of their parents in many ways, and the need for peer approval has diminished.

Although there are unique aspects to each stage of adolescence, there are also commonalities that cut across stages, including preoccupation with bodily changes associated with puberty, search for self-identity and autonomy, strong attachment to the peer group, and conflict with family (Cobb, 1992; Dangerfield & Shaffer, 1979). Each of these characteristics has implications for health promotion.

Preoccupation with bodily changes

The series of biological changes known as puberty marks the beginning of adolescent life. Adolescents' images of themselves are deeply embedded in the impressions they have of their own bodies. They tend to focus only on those ways in which they do not meet their ideal image. Girls usually express greater dissatisfaction with their appearance, as weight increases and changes in fat deposition conflict with the desirable goal of thinness (Bezner, Adams, & Steinhardt, 1997; Holmes & Silverman, 1992; Weiler, 1997). For boys, puberty leads to increased satisfaction associated with greater muscle development and improved social status (Dorn, Crockett, & Petersen, 1988).

Adolescents' preoccupation with bodily appearance can provide motivation for instruction regarding such health topics as nutrition, exercise, safe methods of weight control, puberty, and sexuality. Adolescents are extraordinarily receptive to information about themselves and their bodies. Special attention should be paid to the risks of pregnancy and of contracting HIV and other sexually transmitted diseases. The preoccupation with bodily appearance and sexual development enhances the readiness for learning. Community health nurses who work with youth are in a strategic position to capitalize on adolescents' natural curiosity and self-interest and to explore the advantages of engaging in health-enhancing behaviours.

Self-consciousness

The central theme of adolescence is "finding oneself." In early adolescence this involves gaining autonomy (becoming independent and taking responsibility for one's actions) (Cobb, 1992; Rice, 1996). In late adolescence, the task is one of identity formation (creation of an integrated self and consolidation of changes that accompany autonomy). The adolescent's self-consciousness comes from having to find a personal identity within oneself rather than as a member of a family or of a peer group. Changes in self-concept that enable development of an integrated identity should be encouraged (Harter, 1990).

The adolescent's search for identity has implications for health promotion. Interventions designed specifically to promote self-expression and the provision of varied role models increase the likelihood of adolescents' finding roles compatible with their interests and talents. Activities that promote self-efficacy, independent decision making, and autonomy should enhance self-esteem. Parents, teachers, coaches, school nurses, and peers can provide opportunities for adolescents to feel successful in such areas as sports, academics, drama, music, or community work. Feelings of competence and success are extremely important in supporting a healthy sense of self-esteem and identity.

Conflict with family

Relationships with parents undergo important transformations that support the development of autonomy. Adolescents must separate themselves from family. Research has shown that this does not lead to detachment from parents (Dornbusch, Petersen, & Hetherington, 1991). On the contrary, adolescents continue to feel close to their parents, rely on them, and share similar values and beliefs (Feldman & Elliott, 1990; Garrad, Smulyan, Powers, & Kilkenny, 1995; Gillis, 1994, 1998). Parents and adolescents agree on values and attitudes more than adolescents and their peers agree on the same issues (Jarvinen & Nichols, 1996; Spruijt-Metz, 1995; Taylor, 1996). Serious conflict with parents is therefore not an expected stage; rather, it ought to be considered a predictor of potential problems, such as pregnancy or drug use.

Health promotion programs aimed at enhancing healthy lifestyles should consider not only adolescents but also their parents and other family members (Gillis, 1994, 1998). Parents can play supportive, mentoring roles. They can provide environments that empower adolescents to make healthy choices and can reinforce the messages of health promotion programs by modelling healthy behaviours. Community health nurses planning for adolescent health promotion must attend to the whole family's health behaviours.

At the same time, community health nurses need to be aware of changing family patterns in Canada and of economic realities that mean fewer adults are available for continuous interaction with adolescents. Increasing divorce rates have resulted in 25 percent of Canadian youth living in single-parent families in which there may be less time for interaction between teen and parent (Carr, 1994). Currently there are over 1.1 million lone-parent families in Canada, an increase of 60 percent from 1981. In the past, most single-parent families were the result of death of a spouse; however, today divorce and separation are the major causes of lone parenthood. Of these lone-parent families, 86 percent are headed by females, and these families are more likely to experience poverty than those headed by males (Guy, 1997). Many adolescents are spending more unsupervised time (i.e., with no adult present) with peers, which may lead to engagement in such behaviours as smoking, drug and alcohol use, and sexual intercourse. The problems associated with unsupervised time are intensified for single-parent families, low-income families, and families in which both parents are employed outside the home.

The changing social context of adolescents' lives affects adolescent health promotion. Creative strategies need to be developed to increase positive adult–adolescent communication within a working parent's daily schedule. Community health nurses should assist adolescents to seek out other adults with whom they are comfortable. This intervention may prove beneficial to teens whose parents are not available to them.

Attachment to peers

Throughout adolescence, changes occur in the structure, size, and importance of the peer group. In early adolescence, there is a fierce preference for the same-sex peer group, which is replaced with an opposite-sex allegiance in mid- and late adolescence. Similarly, a wider geographic group eventually replaces the neighbourhood group. When young adolescents leave the confines of their neighbourhood schools and communities, they are immediately exposed to a broader selection of friendships. The task at this stage is to learn how to relate to, and get along with, many different people.

The intensity of peer relationships increases the potential for peer influence on adolescent behaviour. Little is known about the ways in which peers actually encourage or discourage one another from engaging in health-promoting or health-compromising behaviours. Adolescents themselves report that they do what they think or know their friends are doing (Cotterell, 1996; Hofferth & Hayes, 1987). Girls are more concerned with harmonious relations, social approval and acceptance, and living up to peer expectations than are members of male groups.

Susceptibility to peer pressure is highest in early adolescence (Rice, 1996), which suggests that this may be a period of increased vulnerability. Adolescents report that conventional forces exert more influence than pressure toward negative actions (Brown, Lohr, & McClenahan, 1986). This sharply deviates from prior views of a peer culture in adolescence characterized by adherence to unconventional social norms (Coleman, 1961; Cotterell, 1996). Furthermore, there is increasing evidence that the values of peer groups tend to reflect prevailing social values (Cobb, 1992; Feldman & Elliott, 1990; Pender, 1996). Caution is warranted, however, in those situations where teens have greater peer than parental identification, particularly if the peer group models such behaviours as drinking, drug use, or violence. A substantial body of research suggests that these teens are more prone to health-compromising behaviours than those with strong parental identification (Cotterell, 1996; Dolcini & Adler, 1994).

It appears that peers can be a support and resource to one another in promoting healthy lifestyles. Peer-directed health promotion programs offer an opportunity to build the positive social support that all youth need. By linking younger adolescents with peers who have healthy values and behaviours, community health nurses can assist those most vulnerable to peer pressure. Health promotion programs based on peer support encourage adolescents to make decisions, to solve problems, and to exert some control over their lives. This is essential to the development of identity and autonomy.

However, not all relationships within the social network of adolescents are positive and healthy. Peers who model risk-taking behaviours may influence the development of such behaviours (Wang, Fitzhugh, Eddy, Fu, & Turner, 1997; Whatley, 1991). The social networks of adolescents may be destructive or insignificant (Pender, 1996). Further, the supportive ties of a network are often not distinct from its non-supportive ties. Some network members may exert pressure to behave in an inconsistent manner (Cotterell, 1996).

The impact of social networks on adolescent health behaviour has important implications for community health nurses, who need sound knowledge of how and under what conditions social support influences health behaviour in this age group. Although there is extensive empirical evidence to indicate the generally positive effect of social support on individual health and functioning (Frey, 1989; Wang et al., 1997), there has been little investigation of social support in adolescents. The degree to which peers as well as parents affect adolescent lifestyle in positive and negative ways should be explored (Perry, Kelder, & Komro, 1993; Taylor, 1996). There is also a need to identify the diverse sources of social support available to adolescents and the sources of support perceived to be most beneficial to their well-being. Further, community health nurses should test ways in which to guide adolescents in developing interpersonal skills to deal with peer pressure.

Adolescent health promotion goals

It is beyond the scope of this chapter to identify specific goals for adolescent health promotion that reflect the multiple perspectives of community health nursing practice. However, some authors suggest that the overall goal should be to enhance positive growth and adjustment, while promoting health-enhancing behaviours and reducing or eliminating health-compromising behaviours (Edelman & Mandle, 1994; Perry & Jessor, 1985; Raphael, 1996).

Crockett and Petersen (1993, p. 31) suggest six broad health promotion goals that are appropriate for Canadian youth: (a) promotion of physical health and well-being through proper nutrition and exercise, development of a positive body image and healthy sexuality, and adoption of a healthy lifestyle; (b) promotion of cognitive maturity and autonomous decision making; (c) promotion of a positive sense of personal identity, including self-efficacy, social responsibility, self-esteem, and positive future goals; (d) promotion of supportive relationships with families, peers, and other significant adults; (e) provision of opportunities for educational and occupational success; and (f) avoidance of outcomes that would compromise future health and development.

Critical evaluation of these goals indicates that they are sensitive to the developmental level of adolescents and remain current and relevant to adolescents who prepare to face the challenges of the 21st century. The goals focus on important concerns of Canadian youth, such as physical maturation, body image, self-esteem, and positive self-identity. Further, they acknowledge the social context in which adolescent health promotion efforts are positioned—family, peers, school, workplace, and community. These goals are timely and appropriate given the current emphasis on intersectoral planning, mutual aid, and public participation in a reformed Canadian health system. In addition, they are congruent with four determinants of healthy child and youth development (Guy, 1997). These include:

- A web of protection. Adolescents should be guided toward responsibility and independence, and away from dangerous choices such as unprotected sex and alcohol use. Through participation in community life and involvement with positive role models and other caring adults adolescents can learn to make healthy choices.
- The ability to maintain mutually supportive relationships with others. Supportive relationships buffer adolescents against "the slings and arrows" of life and assist young people to become fulfilled and responsible adults.
- Hope and opportunity: to be heard, to practise responsible decision making, to participate in communities, and to learn from mistakes. Opportunities enable adolescents to build self-esteem, gain confidence, and instil hope.
- A sense of successful community that provides supportive environments for youth. Such environments create a sense of belonging and shared involvement and interest.

These determinants, like the goals for adolescent health promotion, will have far-reaching benefits if resources are expended.

The need for adolescent health promotion

There is ample evidence that all is not well with Canadian youth. Adolescents are engaging in many behaviours that place their health at risk. Indeed, adolescents spend little thought on health-related matters; most assume adolescence is a time of health and well-being. However, Canadian statistics on major causes of morbidity and mortality indicate that adolescents have high rates of motor vehicle accidents, suicides, substance abuse, unplanned pregnancies, sexually transmitted diseases, mental disorders, school drop-outs, and unemployment (Canadian Council on Social Development [CCSD], 1997; Canadian Institute of Child Health [CICH], 1994). Further, many are at risk for engaging in health-compromising behaviours because of poverty, unemployment, and the economic consequences of recession.

In Canada in the early 1990s, more than one million children and youth under the age of 18 lived in poverty. The number of poor children and youth grew from 1.36 million in 1994 to 1.47 million in 1995. Approximately one out of every five children under the age of 18 resides in a family with income far below the poverty line (CCSD, 1997). An estimated 225 000 Canadian youth rely on food banks for nutritional support (Covenant House, 1997). Thirty percent of Canadian youth drop out of school annually; it is projected that one million will have dropped out between 1994 and 2002 (Carr, 1994). School drop-outs earn 25 to 50 percent less and are twice as likely to be unemployed as high school graduates (Carr, 1994). Unemployment rates for youth with high school education or less are at least twice as high as the national average, leaving many adolescents without the material resources required for a meaningful existence (CCSD, 1997). These socioeconomic determinants of health are likely to affect the health of adolescents, as poverty makes it extremely difficult to make healthy choices.

The two primary causes of mortality for Canadian youth are motor vehicle accidents and suicide, often associated with alcohol consumption. Together, these are responsible for more than 73 percent of all adolescent deaths (CICH, 1994). Teen suicide has increased dramatically in the last 30 years and is now the second leading cause of death among teenagers (Guy, 1997).

Alcohol and drug abuse are rampant among Canadian adolescents and have significant implications for school performance, self-esteem, and establishment of adult behavioural patterns. Although recent evidence suggests a decline in use of non-medical drugs by adolescents (Smart, Adlaf, & Walsh, 1991), alcohol remains a serious problem in Canada. Early patterns of alcoholism are evident in the lifestyle of Canadian youth. By the time they reach age 15, 60 percent of adolescents have been drunk at least once, and 25 percent drink alcohol at least once a week (King & Cole, 1992). Regular heavy drinking is most common among males; young men aged 15 to 24 are 2.5 times more likely to indicate heavy drinking than Canadians overall (Statistics Canada, 1995).

Sexually transmitted diseases, including HIV/AIDS, present significant health risks to adolescents, often with devastating effects on future fertility. According to Health Canada, the incidence of HIV infections in youth is increasing. Between 1975 and 1985, the median age of HIV infection was 29.6 years; by 1990 it had dropped to 24.5 years, and this trend is predicted to continue (CCSD, 1997). Only one-half of sexually active 17-year-olds in Canada use condoms. This lack of "safe sex" behaviour contributes significantly to the problem of sexually transmitted diseases. National survey data suggest that almost 50 percent of adolescents have had sexual intercourse at least once in the year preceding the survey (CICH, 1994).

Unwanted teenage pregnancies are a complex and serious public health concern for Canadians. Each year approximately 38 000 adolescents become pregnant and, of those, approximately 24 000 carry the pregnancies to term (CICH, 1994). Despite innovative programs, adolescent pregnancy remains one of the most pressing problems in health care (Bobak & Jensen, 1991; Porter, Oakley, Ronis, & Neal, 1996). The pregnancy affects the mother, her infant, the infant's father, their extended families, and, ultimately, society. The consequences of such pregnancies are well documented (Hechtman, 1989; Krishnomont, 1992). (See also Chapter 13.)

Babies born to adolescents are at higher risk for prematurity and lifelong problems. Research indicates that teenage mothers and their infants are more likely to experience educational, economic, and social difficulties (O'Sullivan, Brooks-Gunn, & Schwarz, 1992). Risks to the mother include poverty, low academic achievement, dropping out of school, anemia, divorce, and unemployment (Furstenberg, Brooks-Gunn, & Morgan, 1987). Risks to the children of teenage mothers include lower academic achievement, more school behavioural problems, violence, and greater risk of becoming a teenage parent (Moore, 1986). The latter finding is challenged by Furstenberg et al. (1987), who conducted a 17-year follow-up study of adolescent mothers. A substantial majority completed high school and found regular employment; even those on welfare eventually escaped public assistance. The researchers suggest that while many teenage mothers broke out of the cycle of poverty, the majority did not succeed as well as they might have had they delayed parenthood.

Canadian adolescents are more physically active than adults, but adolescent females participate less in physical activities, consider themselves less fit, and are less likely to be active by age 20 than males (King & Cole, 1992).

This highlights the need to develop health promotion programs that encourage physical activity throughout life, especially for females.

Canadian girls are more likely than boys to experience loneliness as adolescents, and they tend to score less positively on self-esteem (CICH, 1994). Canadian youth tend to have more difficulty relating to their parents and report more disagreements with parents than do youth from other countries (King & Cole, 1992). This problem is more pronounced for females than for males and increases in intensity with age. The difficulties experienced by youth in their relationships with their parents may contribute to increased health risks associated with isolation, lack of social support, and absence of adult role models.

Adolescence is an important time to intervene with health promotion strategies aimed at establishing healthy behavioural patterns, before health-damaging ones become too resistant to change. Although an empirical link between adolescent practices and adult health outcomes is absent in the literature, it makes sense to intervene with health promotion strategies in the younger age group.

Key principles for adolescent health promotion

1. The most obvious principle to uphold is the provision of opportunities to develop autonomy, while reducing the risk of negative consequences. Risk can be minimized in several ways.
    *   A major method of risk reduction is to spend time with adolescents, discussing the consequences of various courses of action and ensuring that they are well informed about alternatives. Yet, discussion of health-related information, by itself, rarely alters adolescent health behaviour. Multifaceted strategies are needed.
    *   Another approach is to improve problem-solving and decision-making skills by providing practice in considering alternative perspectives.
    *   A third approach is to reduce youths' susceptibility to negative peer influence by enhancing self-confidence, improving peer resistance skills, and teaching peer pressure reversal techniques (Crockett & Petersen, 1993). Peer pressure reversal, described by Scott (1985), requires adolescents to master a three-step skill: (a) "checking out the scene" (that is, noticing and identifying troublesome situations in their environment), (b) understanding the likely consequences of such situations, and (c) taking appropriate and effective action to protect themselves from unhealthy consequences. Peer pressure reversal makes adolescents more responsible by teaching them to

increase their awareness and develop good judgement. It also extends their ability to direct their own actions constructively.

2. Successful health promotion efforts usually provide an opportunity to capitalize on the adolescent's desire for independence in decision making.
   • Health can be presented as a resource over which the adolescent has control and personal responsibility. During adolescence, teenagers are making health decisions for the first time independently of their parents and other significant adults.
   • Introducing health in the context of personal choice provides an opportunity for youth to exert their autonomy and independence by committing to such health-promoting patterns of behaviour as exercise and good nutrition. This should facilitate the adolescent's sense of independence and promote the adoption of healthy lifestyles.

3. Affective, personal meanings that adolescents attribute to their behaviours may overrule any health-related knowledge and values as determinants of health and risk behaviours.
   • While an abundance of health information is available to adolescents, it is often no match for salient, personal meanings (Gillis, 1998). Adolescent health promotion could benefit by research into the development and nature of associations between personal meanings and choice of health behaviour.
   • Community health can help adolescents make and break these associations through health education. Such meanings could be incorporated into health promotion sessions and educational materials. Nurses can work with adolescents to create effective health promotion materials for use in schools, clinics, and other community settings.

4. Adolescents should be actively involved in the planning and implementation of programs.
   • This requires modifying the philosophical beliefs of nurses and other health professionals who may view adolescents as problems rather than resources. It requires moving from a traditional "professional" model to a "consumer/prosumer" model (Riessman, 1990). This paradigm shift involves demystifying the professional expertise of the nurse and other professionals and empowering adolescents to help themselves and one another (Gottlieb, 1985; Guy, 1997; Israel & Antonucci, 1987).
   • Community health nurses can make adolescents full partners in health promotion programs. By attending to adolescents' viewpoints

and including them in discussions relevant to their lives, programs communicate to adolescents that they are valuable participants in health promotion efforts.

5.   Nurses must learn to play a new role when working with this age group.
   • Nurses need to move away from being providers of care and focus more on developing cooperative learning groups among adolescents, using the skills of peer tutoring, or helping groups to promote health and behavioural change. In essence, nurses must work with adolescents in school, homes, and community settings to create an ethos of cooperation, caring, mutual respect, and participation (Benard, 1991).

6.   There is a need to focus on the short-term effects of health behaviours.
   • This principle contrasts with health promotion efforts aimed at adults, which tend to focus on long-term goals. Millstein (1993) notes: "The degree to which we will be successful in promoting adolescent health is probably a function of how well we can utilize adolescents' short term goals to reach adults' long term goals" (p. 113). Programs need to address underlying causes of health behaviours, such as inadequate life skills or lack of social support, rather than focus only on the health-damaging behaviour itself.

Status of adolescent health promotion in Canada

The status of adolescent health promotion is disheartening. There is no national adolescent health policy to support youth in gaining control of their lives. Although a variety of stakeholders are involved in promoting adolescent health at the local, provincial, and regional levels, there is no comprehensive, coordinated national plan or policy. Community health nurses can be a powerful influence in working with adolescents to lobby for such a policy and for the establishment of appropriate health programs.

Adolescent health promotion projects involving community health nurses

The most common adolescent health promotion programs reported in the literature are those situated in community colleges and on university campuses to address the needs of older adolescents and young adults. The division of student services at St. Francis Xavier University, accommodating 3400 students, offers a health and counselling program. This consists of individual counselling, health education, community outreach, and special programs (e.g., related to sexual assault, sexually transmitted diseases, peer mediation and conflict resolution, and contraception), all of which are designed to achieve the goal of health promotion. Health-related issues such as motivation, depression, sexuality, stress, and academic and career counselling are discussed. The program is staffed by registered nurses who work full time at the university as members of a multidisciplinary student services team. Other members of the team include psychologists, counsellors, chaplaincy representatives, and undergraduate nursing students. The program presents an interesting opportunity for community health nurses working in the university system.

A similar project continues in the Faculty of Nursing at the University of Toronto. The project theme is to promote health through healthy lifestyles, healthy environments, and healthy public policies. It includes a variety of programs, such as the Festival of Health, which is a fair consisting of displays and activities designed to increase the community's awareness of available health promotion services. Smoking cessation, alcohol use, sexuality, and stress management programs are core services of the project. Evaluation of the first three years suggests that the project is providing a needed service on campus and clearly demonstrates nursing's role in health promotion.

A second major Canadian thrust in adolescent health promotion is occurring through comprehensive school-based health programs. A comprehensive approach implies that health education should be coordinated with school health services, within a healthful school and community environment. Although progress is being made, a recent survey of Canadian provincial and territorial health curriculum guidelines indicated that the comprehensive health approach is still far from a reality (Cameron, Mutter, & Hamilton, 1991). However, some provinces, such as Newfoundland, are making progress in developing health curricula, and others are optimistic that the trend toward a holistic view of health and greater interagency collaboration will yield a more global approach to school health.

Community health nurses are in an excellent position to be catalysts for promoting adolescent health through comprehensive school health programs. Bartfay (1994) proposes two main arguments for involvement of community health nurses in school-based health promotion efforts:

- School is the most efficient point of access to large numbers of children. In 1990, the total enrollment in all elementary and secondary Canadian schools was 5 084 000; therefore, school-based health promotion interventions have the potential to reach a significant number of youth (Statistics Canada, 1991).
- Schools govern a large portion of the adolescent's life and thus are socializing agents for youth. The school's influence is pervasive in major areas

of knowledge, attitude, and behaviour that contribute to the development of lifestyle habits. Community health nurses who have special preparation in health and lifestyle education and expertise in primary prevention and health promotion are in an excellent position to identify and respond to adolescents' needs for health promotion. Through their networking and visibility in the community, nurses have contact with individuals, groups, families, agencies, and institutions that affect the daily lives of adolescents. By using their skills in collaboration and coordination, nurses can be effective members of a health promotion team that will make comprehensive school health a national priority.

A compelling example of schools working together with community health nurses to promote the health of youth is the collaborative partnership involving the Ottawa–Carleton Health Department, the University of Ottawa School of Nursing, and the Corpus Christi School System. The partnership is designed to foster a lifelong commitment to optimal health in the Corpus Christi School Community. Specific goals of the project include: (a) engaging community members in healthy lifestyle practices, (b) enabling individuals to take personal responsibility for their health, (c) facilitating healthy growth and development of youth, (d) promoting healthy self-esteem and interpersonal relationships in the school district, (e) reducing existing health risks, and (f) enabling youth to optimize their school, home, and community life. A partnership committee consisting of youth, parents, community health nurses, teachers, and nursing faculty was formed. The committee develops an annual action plan and evaluates progress yearly. It is particularly interested in exploring ways to promote and establish healthy lifestyle patterns early in life. A variety of projects have emerged from this initiative, including a smoking cessation project involving peer teaching, an injury prevention project that focussed on reducing head injuries through bicycle helmet safety, and a community assessment. Involving youth themselves on the partnership committee and listening and responding to youth representatives have helped to encourage project activities that are meaningful and relevant, together with a high rate of participation by youth.

The Teens for Healthy Living project (sponsored by the Community Health Promotion Fund of the Nova Scotia Department of Health) is another example of a school-based health promotion project spearheaded by nursing faculty in collaboration with community health nurses, teachers, and school administration (Gillis, 1995). The project was carried out with adolescents 10 to 19 years of age in Guysborough County, a large rural school district in eastern Nova Scotia. The project began as an attempt to involve adolescents in healthy lifestyle decision making with respect to issues of importance to them. An underlying belief was the ability of teens to enter into helping relationships with one another to provide support, assist in decision making, and direct one another to alternative sources of help and information. A model of peer helping formed a central core of this project. Evaluation of the project indicates it has been successful in reaching many adolescents who benefited from peer counselling on various health-related topics. Many adolescents became positive role models for others, provided support and counselling to their peers, and referred situations that were beyond their scope of knowledge and experience to professional counsellors. This project suggests that the peer-helping model may be an effective one for community health nurses to employ with adolescents to engage them in health promotion.

Other accessible avenues for adolescent health promotion include street clinics, peer support groups and centres, and short-term crisis intervention centres. These are particularly useful for homeless or runaway youth, as they provide a substitute for the role that school-based services have played in providing information and support for health promotion with this population. Homelessness is emerging as a fundamental health problem for Canadians (Canadian Public Health Association, 1997). There is compelling evidence of substantial growth in the number of street youth, particularly in large urban centres.

There are many examples of street clinics providing health promotion sevices to Canadian adolescents. Some are Street Health, a community-based nursing service in Toronto; Covenant House, a Toronto crisis intervention shelter for runaway youth; Evergreen Centre for Street Youth, Toronto; and the Red Door Clinic in Kentville, Nova Scotia. Street clinics such as the Red Door are multiservice, community-based health centres that provide comprehensive care for youth on a drop-in basis. Nurses, physicians, and volunteers staff the centre, which offers health awareness and health promotion programs on a variety of health issues and provides a broad range of referral services.

Street workers are another option for community health nurses to consider in reaching adolescents who may not attend school-based or community health clinics. Outreach workers, who interact with adolescents wherever they congregate, are used successfully in major Canadian cities to combat health problems. On the Street Outreach Van is an example of one such program responding to the needs of thousands of runaway and homeless Canadian youth. The goal of this Toronto program is to connect with youth on the street to meet some of their basic needs and provide an oasis of safety and counselling regarding lifestyle options. The program is one of the many services of Covenant House and operates with a trained team of youth workers who cover the downtown area of Toronto. Adolescents who use the service come from across Canada and are often on the street because of family breakdown, neglect, or physical, sexual, or emotional abuse. The wide range of services include emergency shelter; counselling in physical, emotional, and spiritual well-being; disease prevention; and outreach and aftercare. These non-traditional sources of health care may be especially appropriate for community health nurses if they wish to reach high-risk adolescents and prevent them from engaging in health-compromising behaviours.

A final option for community health nurses to consider in planning health promotion programs involves the new communication and information technologies. Interactive technology is a promising medium for introducing youth to health initiatives. Many adolescents are highly skilled in computer applications and are engaged by this technology. Community health nurses can capitalize on this new form of information sharing by tailoring health information to the particular needs of youth, providing unlimited information to adolescents through the World Wide Web and the Internet, and fostering contact with other adolescents around the world.

Video games are an example of technology that can be used to reach young people who are not interested in learning about healthy lifestyles. They are an attractive leisure activity for youth. The video game format lends itself to health promotion because messages can be individualized to each player based on performance. The video games can represent role-model characters, provide scenarios involving health decisions and self-care activities, and portray realistic consequences of behaviours and actions. Research on video games and other interactive media suggests that technology can improve intervening factors that lead to better health outcomes for adolescents. Such technology promotes active processing of health promotion messages, motivation to learn about health promotion, perceived self-efficacy for health behaviours, and communication about health with others who can provide social support (Lieberman, 1997). Evidence suggests that community health nurses can make health promotion programs and interventions more engaging and personally relevant by integrating interactive media such as stand-alone and online video games into health interventions targeted at adolescents.

Future directions

Numerous challenges lie ahead for community health nurses and others who are interested in promoting adolescent health. The context of adolescents' lives will continue to undergo extensive changes that will have implications for adolescent health promotion. An increasing number of Canadian youth are being raised in poverty and in single-parent families (Epp, 1986), where there are fewer opportunities for healthy interaction with adult role models. Today's homes have televisions and cassette players that permit adolescents unlimited exposure to aggression, violence, alcohol and drug consumption, smoking, and sexual experiences void of responsibility or protection. Increasingly, peer groups and schools are expected to fulfil roles previously performed by families and significant adults. Recently, economic cutbacks have resulted in the slashing of social programs. Often the least-established initiatives, such as those concerned with healthy youth and healthy public policy, are the first to be cancelled. This changing social context calls for new initiatives in adolescent health promotion.

A multicomponent approach to health promotion may hold promise for the future of Canadian youth. Although the Canadian literature rarely reports successful comprehensive health promotion programs for adolescents, the American and European literatures provide evidence of programs that work. A major American report by Lavin, Shapiro, and Weill (1992) has potential for Canadians in creating an agenda for adolescent health promotion. It calls for people in both the public and private sectors to understand the extent of the adolescent health problem and the comprehensive nature of the required solutions. The report suggests that families, neighbourhoods, the health community, and the public and private sectors must forge new partnerships to address the interconnected health and education problems of youth. It indicates that this will take much time, many resources, and great political will.

Dryfoos (1991) reviewed 100 successful adolescent health programs and identified seven components that characterized success: (a) provision of individual attention and counselling; (b) presence of broad community-wide, multi-agency, multicomponent interventions; (c) availability of early intervention; (d) methods for strengthening parenting skills and for making up for lack of parental support; (e) value of teaching youth how to recognize and deal with peer pressure and peer influences; (f) improvement of life skills and social skills training; and (g) training, supervision, and preparation of staff working with youth. An example of the seven components in action is the new institutional form of "community schools" proposed by Dryfoos. The community school enables youth to receive high-quality education and provides family access to a wide range of services such as health care, child care, after-school recreation, cultural events, mental health services, family planning services, satellite welfare offices, and job preparation. Although institutional arrangements are being promulgated, much remains to be done to negotiate difficult turf issues among the various government departments to enable the community school vision to come to fruition.

Conclusion

In summary, this chapter suggests that community health nurses who are concerned with adolescent health promotion must consider the broad range of factors that affect adolescent health decisions and behaviours. Individual, family, and environmental factors must be considered, together with many structural and societal factors. These include economic resource allocation, employment opportunities, and health and social policy development and implementation. These may be the most difficult to change, but in the long term, they may hold the greatest promise for improving the health and well-being of adolescents.

Effective health promotion will require support by many individuals, professionals, non-professionals, institutions, agencies, and, most importantly, adolescents themselves. A widespread commitment to a coordinated health promotion strategy that targets adolescents is needed to protect and enhance the health of youth and the future citizens of Canada. This is not to minimize the individual efforts of any one component, but rather to suggest that small efforts become part of an overall, integrated health promotion strategy (Millstein, Petersen, & Nightingale, 1993). For example, a community health nurse who teaches adolescents about the effects of cigarette smoking on their health will have more impact if the message is reinforced by teachers and parents; if the community prohibits sale of cigarettes to youth and prosecutes merchants who violate the law; and if the school is declared a smoke-free environment. Further, these efforts would be enhanced if the adolescent peer group supported similar values and behaviours, and if significant role models (e.g., coaches, rock stars, media personalities) simultaneously admonished adolescents to abstain. All these efforts collectively reinforce this important theme. Together, they contribute to a comprehensive health promotion strategy for adolescents.

QUESTIONS

1. In assessing the needs and concerns of adolescents related to health promotion, should adolescents be consulted? Why? How might this be done?
2. How can community health nurses facilitate partnerships with adolescents to promote healthy outcomes?
3. What role do supportive environments, community action, and self-care play in promoting the health of adolescents?
4. In what ways can community health nurses incorporate the concept of self-care into health promotion planning and program delivery?
5. Are community health nurses in Canada adequately prepared to address issues of health promotion in adolescents? Discuss.

REFERENCES

Bartfay, W. (1994). Reading, writing and health. *Canadian Nurse, 90*(2), 29–33.
Benard, B. (1991). The case for peers. *Peer Facilitator Quarterly, 8*(4), 20–27.
Bezner, J.R., Adams, T.B., & Steinhardt, M. (1997). Relationship of body dissatisfaction to physical health and wellness. *American Journal of Health Behavior, 21*(2), 147–155.
Bobak, I.M., & Jensen, M.D. (1991). *Essentials of maternity nursing* (3rd ed.). Toronto: Mosby.

Brown, B., Lohr, M., & McClenahan, E. (1986). Early adolescents' perceptions of peer pressure. *Journal of Early Adolescence, 6,* 139–154.

Cameron, H., Mutter, G., & Hamilton, N. (1991). Comprehensive school health: Back to the basics in the '90s. *Health Promotion, 29*(4), 2–10.

Canadian Council on Social Development (CCSD). (1997). *The progress of Canada's children 1997.* Ottawa: Author.

Canadian Institute of Child Health (CICH). (1994). *The health of Canada's children: A CICH profile* (2nd ed.). Ottawa: Author.

Canadian Public Health Association. (1997). *Position paper on homelessness and health.* Ottawa: Author.

Carr, R. (1994). Editorial. *Peer Counsellor Journal, 11*(1), 1–2.

Cobb, N.J. (1992). *Adolescence: Continuity, change and diversity.* Mountain View, CA: Mayfield.

Coleman, J.S. (1961). *The adolescent society: The social life of the teenager and its impact on education.* New York: Free Press.

Cotterell, J. (1996). *Social networks and social influences in adolescence.* New York: Routledge.

Covenant House. (1997). *Youth service statistics.* Toronto: Author.

Crockett, L.J., & Petersen, A.C. (1993). Adolescent development: Health risks and opportunities. In S.G. Millstein, A.C. Petersen, & E.O. Nightingale (Eds.), *Promoting the health of adolescents: New directions for the twenty-first century* (pp. 13–38). New York: Oxford University Press.

Dangerfield, D.E., & Shaffer, M.H. (1979). *Aggressive adolescents.* Tulare, CA: Professional Training Associates.

Dolcini, M., & Adler, N.E. (1994). Perceived competencies, peer group affiliation, and risk behavior among early adolescents. *Health Psychology, 13,* 496–506.

Dorn, L.D., Crockett, L.J., & Petersen, A.C. (1988). The relations of pubertal status to intrapersonal changes in young adolescents. *Journal of Early Adolescence, 8,* 405–419.

Dornbusch, S.M., Petersen, A.C., & Hetherington, E.M. (1991). Projecting the future of research on adolescence. *Journal of Research on Adolescence, 1*(1), 7–19.

Dryfoos, J. (1991). Adolescents at risk: A summation of work in the field: Programs and policies. *Journal of Adolescent Health, 12,* 630–637.

Edelman, C.L., & Mandle, C.L. (1994). *Health promotion throughout the lifespan* (3rd ed.). St. Louis: Mosby.

Epp, J. (1986). *Achieving health for all: A framework for health promotion.* Ottawa: Health & Welfare Canada.

Estes, S.D., & Hart, M. (1993). A model for the development of the CNS role in adolescent health promotion and self-care. *Clinical Nurse Specialist, 7*(3), 111–115.

Feldman, S., & Elliott, G. (Eds.). (1990). *At the threshold: The developing adolescent.* Cambridge, MA: Harvard University Press.

Frey, M.A. (1989). Social support and health: A theoretical formulation derived from King's conceptual framework. *Nursing Science Quarterly, 2,* 138–148.

Furstenberg, F.F., Brooks-Gunn, J., & Morgan, S.P. (1987). *Adolescent mothers in later life.* Cambridge, MA: Cambridge University Press.

Garrad, A., Smulyan, L., Powers, S., & Kilkenny, R. (1995). *Adolescent portraits* (2nd ed.). Boston: Allyn & Bacon.

Gillis, A.J. (1994). Determinants of health-promoting lifestyle in adolescent females. *Canadian Journal of Nursing Research, 26*(2), 13–29.

Gillis, A.J. (1995). *The development and evaluation of the Teens for Healthy Living project. Report of a Community Health Promotion Project.* Halifax: Nova Scotia Department of Health.

Gillis, A.J. (1998). *Lessons learned from listening: The meaning of adolescent lifestyle choices.* Presentation at the 4th Qualitative Health Research Conference, Vancouver, BC.

Gottlieb, B. (1985). Social networks and social support. *Health Education Quarterly, 1,* 5–22.

Guy, K.A. (1997). *Our promise to children.* Ottawa: Health Canada.

Harter, S. (1990). Self and identity development. In S. Feldman & G. Elliott (Eds.), *At the threshold: The developing adolescent* (pp. 431–457). Cambridge, MA: Harvard University Press.

Hechtman, L. (1989). Teenage mothers and their children: Risks and problems: A review. *Canadian Journal of Psychiatry, 34,* 569–575.

Hofferth, S.L., & Hayes, C.D. (Eds.). (1987). *Risking the future: Adolescent sexuality, pregnancy, and childbearing* (Vol. 2). Washington, DC: National Academy of Sciences Press.

Holmes, J., & Silverman, E.I. (1992). *We're here, listen to us: A survey of young women in Canada.* Ottawa: Canadian Advisory Council on the Status of Women.

Ingersoll, G.M. (1989). *Adolescents* (2nd ed.). Englewood Cliffs, NJ: Prentice-Hall

Irwin, C.E. (1993). The adolescent, health, and society: From the perspective of the physician. In S.G. Millstein, A.C. Petersen, & E.O. Nightingale (Eds.), *Promoting the health of adolescents: New directions for the twenty-first century* (pp. 146–150). New York: Oxford University Press.

Israel, B., & Antonucci, T. (1987). Social network characteristics and psychological well-being: A replication and extension. *Health Education Quarterly, 14*(4), 461–481.

Jarvinen, D.W., & Nichols, J.G. (1996). Adolescent's social goals, beliefs about the causes of social success, and satisfaction in peer relations. *Developmental Psychology, 32*(3), 435–441.

King, A.J., & Cole, B. (1992). *The health of Canada's youth.* Ottawa: Health & Welfare Canada.

Krishnomont, D. (1992). Pregnant teens: How can we help them cope? *Canadian Nurse, 88*(3), 20–22.

Lavin, A.T., Shapiro, G.R., & Weill, K.S. (1992). Creating an agenda for school-based health promotion: A review of 25 selected reports. *Journal of School Health, 62*(6), 212–227.

Liebermann, D.A. (1997). Interactive video games for health promotion. In R. Street, W. Gold, & T. Manning (Eds.), *Health promotion and interactive technology* (pp. 103–119). Mahway, NJ: Lawrence Erlbaum Associates.

Millstein, S.G. (1993). A view of health from the adolescent's perspective. In S.G. Millstein, A.C. Petersen, & E.O. Nightingale (Eds.), *Promoting the health of adolescents: New directions for the twenty-first century* (pp. 97–118). New York: Oxford University Press.

Moore, K.A. (1986). *Children of teen parents: Heterogeneity of outcomes.* Report to the National Institute of Child Health and Human Development. Washington, DC: Child Trends.

O'Sullivan, A., Brooks-Gunn, J., & Schwarz, D. (1992). Adolescents: Improving life chances. In L. Aiken & C. Fagin (Eds.), *Charting nursing's future* (pp. 340–362). Philadelphia: J.B. Lippincott.

Pender, N.J. (1996). *Health promotion in nursing practice* (3rd ed.). Stamford, CT: Appleton & Lange.

Perry, C.L., & Jessor, R. (1985). The concept of health promotion and the prevention of adolescent drug abuse. *Health Education Quarterly, 12*, 169–184.

Perry, C.L., Kelder, S.H., & Komro, K.A. (1993). The social world of adolescents: Families, peers, schools, and the community. In S.G. Millstein, A.C. Petersen, & E.O. Nightingale (Eds.), *Promoting the health of adolescents: New directions for the twenty-first century* (pp. 73–96). New York: Oxford University Press.

Porter, C., Oakley, D., Ronis, D., & Neal, R. (1996). Pathways of influence on 5th and 8th graders' reports about having had sexual intercourse. *Research in Nursing and Health, 19*, 193–204.

Raphael, D. (1996). Determinants of health of North American adolescents: Evolving definitions, recent findings, and proposed research agenda. *Journal of Adolescent Health, 19*, 6–16.

Rice, F.P. (1996). *The adolescent: Development, relationship, and culture* (8th ed.). Boston: Allyn & Bacon.

Riessman, F. (1990). Restructuring help: A human services paradigm for the 1990s. *American Journal of Community Psychology, 18*(2), 221–230.

Rosenbaum, J.N., & Carty, L. (1996). The subculture of adolescence: Beliefs about care, health and individuation within Leininger's theory. *Journal of Advanced Nursing, 23*, 741–746.

Scott, S. (1985). *Peer pressure reversal: An adult guide to developing a responsible child.* Amherst, MA: Human Resources Development Press.

Smart, R.G., Adlaf, E.M., & Walsh, G. (1991). *The Ontario student drug use survey.* Toronto: Addiction Research Foundation.

Spruijt-Metz, D. (1995). *On everyday health-related behavior in adolescence.* Doctoral dissertation, Vrije Universiteit, Amsterdam.

Statistics Canada (1991). *Elementary–secondary school enrolment 1989–90.* Ottawa: Minister of Industry, Science & Technology. (Cat. No. 81-210)

Statistics Canada (1995). *National population health survey, 1994–1995.* Original analysis.

Taylor, R.D. (1996). Adolescents' perceptions of kinship support and family management practices: Association with adolescent adjustment in African American families. *Developmental Psychology, 32*(4), 684–695.

Wang, M., Fitzhugh, E.C., Eddy, J.M., Fu, Q., & Turner, L. (1997). Social influences on adolescents' smoking progress: A longitudinal analysis. *American Journal of Health Behavior, 21*(2), 111–117.

Weiler, R. (1997). Adolescents' perceptions of health concerns: An exploratory study among rural midwestern youth. *Health Education and Behavior, 24*(3), 287–299.

Whatley, J.H. (1991). Effects of health locus of control and social network on adolescent risk taking. *Pediatric Nursing, 17*(2), 145–148.

Yarcheski, A., Mahon, N.E., & Yarcheski, T.J. (1997). Alternate models of positive health practices in adolescents. *Nursing Research, 46*(2), 85–92.

C H A P T E R   1 3

Prevention of adolescent pregnancy

Alba DiCenso and Leslie J. Van Dover

Adolescent pregnancy and its consequences present difficulties for the individual, family, and community and embody a growing health and social problem. In this chapter, recent data concerning trends in incidence are presented, and approaches to prevention are explored through review of theoretical models and findings from research. Several roles of the community health nurse/public health nurse in preventing adolescent pregnancy are briefly examined.

LEARNING OBJECTIVES

In this chapter, you will learn:

- the incidence of adolescent pregnancy in Canada
- the consequences of adolescent pregnancy for the individual, family, and community
- risk factors that increase or decrease the likelihood that adolescents will engage in early sexual behaviour
- features of prevention programs that have been rigorously evaluated
- implications for the community health nurse in preventing adolescent pregnancy

Introduction

Prevention of pregnancy in adolescents is a key area for health promotion because the consequences of early childbearing are serious for the individual, family, and community. In theory, adolescent pregnancy and its consequences are preventable. In fact, the situation is complex. Human sexual behaviour is determined through a dynamic interaction among physical, psychological, social, and spiritual factors and developmental processes. The powerful mechanisms of human reproduction are at its root.

Historically, conception of children by unmarried women was considered a moral offence in Western society (Chilman, 1980, p. 199). Serious social consequences accompanied the breaking of taboos against premarital sexual intercourse and pregnancy. Until this century, it was customary for adolescents to marry and to have an early pregnancy. The negative consequences of early marriage, however, became more pronounced as the years of formal schooling required to obtain secure employment increased; yet, at the same time, improved nutritional status of young women has accelerated sexual development and fertility.

Adolescent pregnancy often poses serious health risks to both mothers and infants. Young adolescents (particularly those under age 15) experience a maternal death rate 2.5 times greater than that of mothers aged 20 to 24 (Morris, Warren, & Aral, 1993). Common medical problems among adolescent mothers include poor weight gain, pregnancy-induced hypertension, anemia, sexually transmitted diseases, and cephalopelvic disproportion (Stevens-Simon & White, 1991). Infants born to mothers younger than 15 years of age are more than twice as likely to weigh less than 2.5 kg at birth and three times more likely to die in the first 28 days of life than infants born to older mothers (McAnarney & Hendee, 1989). After figures are controlled for birth weight, the post-neonatal mortality rate is approximately twice as high for infants born to mothers under 17 years of age as for infants born to older women. The incidence of sudden infant death syndrome is higher among infants of adolescents, and these infants also experience higher rates of illness and injuries (Morris et al., 1993). Many of these health risks are related to lifestyle and environmental factors (e.g., poor diet; tobacco, alcohol, drug use during pregnancy; inadequate prenatal care; poverty; insufficient supervision of infants) rather than to physiological immaturity or age.

Because of their fewer years of schooling, larger families, and lower likelihood of being married, teenage mothers acquire less work experience, have lower wages and earnings, and are substantially more likely to live in poverty (Brown & Eisenberg, 1995). Bonham et al. (1987) estimated the 20-year cost for providing support to new single-parent families created by first births to teenage mothers in the province of Alberta in 1985 to be $443 million.

Early pregnancy leads to premature parenting, which may create emotional and social problems for parents and children. The adolescent mother, who has not had adequate time to resolve her own developmental issues, is faced with the responsibility of meeting the needs of an infant or young child. Trying to meet her own and the child's needs simultaneously leads to stress (Baydar & Grady, 1993). The young mother often calls on her family of origin (if available) for support, particularly in the form of child care. This can strain the relationship between the young mother and her family.

If the pregnant adolescent elects to terminate her pregnancy by therapeutic abortion, she exposes herself to the short- and long-term physical and emotional hazards associated with the procedure (Gold, 1990; Statistics Canada, 1992, 1993a). Complications known to be directly related to the procedure include hemorrhage, uterine perforation, cervical injury, and infection, which is often due to incomplete abortion. The risk of all complications increases with increasing gestational age, being lowest for women obtaining abortions at or before eight weeks of gestation and increasing two to 10 times for procedures after 12 weeks of gestation (Brown & Eisenberg, 1995). A recent study by Millar, Wadhera, and Henshaw (1997) found that the repeat abortion rate among Canadian teenagers was four times the rate of first abortions (81 per 1000 vs. 19 per 1000).

Single women experience the vast majority of adolescent pregnancies. The burden of early pregnancy falls disproportionately on the young woman and her children, placing them at risk for future difficulties. For this reason, adolescent pregnancy is also a feminist issue.

Extent of the problem

Table 13.1 shows summary data on births, therapeutic abortions, and total documented pregnancies for 1981, 1987, 1991, and 1994 (Statistics Canada, 1991, 1993a, 1993b, 1998). The figures are conservative. The actual numbers, which would include spontaneous and "other" abortions (illegal, unspecified, attempted, performed outside Canada), are higher. If the estimated 20 percent of teen pregnancies that end in spontaneous abortion (Scott, 1990, p. 209) were included, this would add at least 8900 to the 1994 total, giving an estimated total of 53 600 teen pregnancies. In 1994, 53 percent of the pregnancies resulted in live births and 47 percent in abortions.

Through the early 1980s, the number of pregnancies experienced by women in their teens gradually declined. Since then, the total number of pregnancies has increased. In 1987, there were 41.1 pregnancies per 1000 Canadian women aged 15 to 19. By 1994, this rate had increased to 48.8 per 1000 (Statistics Canada, 1998). The steady increase in teen pregnancy rates in

Table 13.1
Births, therapeutic abortions, and total number of pregnancies to Canadian teenagers in 1981, 1987, 1991, and 1994

Year	Births	Abortions	Total
1981	29 330	18 406	47 736
1987	21 216	14 028	35 244
1991	24 445	13 833	38 278
1994	23 700	21 000	44 700

Canada is an alarming development and poses a significant community health problem across the country.

Populations at risk

Many studies have been conducted to identify the factors that influence whether an adolescent will engage in early sexual activity, will be an inconsistent user of birth control, or will become pregnant. Knowledge of these determinants can assist the design and implementation of prevention programs in two ways. First, the prevention program may be designed to modify factors that increase the chances of early sexual behaviour. Second, those adolescents who have the factors that place them at higher risk of early sexual behaviour can be targeted to receive the prevention program earlier or to receive a more intense program.

Many studies that seek to identify factors important to adolescent sexual behaviour use cross-sectional designs. In a cross-sectional study, data about the risk factor and about the outcome are collected at the same time. For example, in a sample of female adolescents, data about their self-esteem and their pregnancy status are collected; because the data are collected at the same time, it is difficult to establish whether poor self-esteem led to the pregnancy or whether experiencing a pregnancy lowered self-esteem. At best, with a cross-sectional design, one can establish an association between two variables, but no clear indication about whether the risk factor preceded the outcome. A stronger design for establishing a relationship between a risk factor and an outcome is a longitudinal study, in which individuals are assessed for the risk factor and then followed over time to determine whether they experience the outcome. For example, data related to self-esteem are collected from female adolescents who have not experienced a pregnancy, and they are then followed over time to identify those who experience a pregnancy. A statistical comparison can then determine if those who had lower self-esteem were more likely to become pregnant.

The first author (DiCenso, 1995) summarized longitudinal studies that examined the relationship between risk factors and sexual behaviour, using a systematic review and meta-analysis. A systematic review is a comprehensive consolidation of the literature. A meta-analysis is the statistical combination of the results of more than one study to provide a more precise estimate of the relationship between a risk factor and an outcome. DiCenso found a number of risk factors that independently influenced sexual behaviour; however, the strength of the relationship, while statistically significant, was often weak. For this reason, only the factors that most strongly influenced sexual behaviour will be presented here. The four factors that influenced early initiation of sexual intercourse in females were earlier pubertal development, the belief that the benefits of sexual intercourse exceeded the costs, the fact that the adolescent's mother had been pregnant as a teen, and non-coital sexual activity. The three factors that influenced consistent use of birth control in females were parent awareness of sexual behaviour, high autonomy, and payment for the birth control appointment through a federally funded insurance plan (e.g., Medicaid). The four risk factors that influenced whether or not a female adolescent became pregnant were African-American ethnic origin, delinquency, previous referral to counselling, and low educational goals. Very few studies examined the factors associated with male sexual behaviour. With respect to initiation of sexual intercourse in males, the two factors that influenced early initiation were intention to have sexual intercourse and delinquent behaviour in the past year. No factors that influenced consistent birth control use in males were identified. The risk factors that influenced male involvement in an adolescent pregnancy were African-American ethnic origin and low educational goals. More longitudinal research to examine the factors associated with sexual behaviour in adolescents is needed, especially studies of male adolescents.

Approaches to prevention

Community health nurses across Canada deliver programs aimed at decreasing the rate of pregnancy in women 15 to 19 years of age. These include sexual health education programs in schools, and contraceptive counselling and provision of prescription and other contraceptives in clinics. As health care resources become scarcer, there is greater emphasis on the evaluation of interventions to ensure that practitioners deliver services that have been shown to be effective. The two most common designs for evaluating health care interventions are the randomized controlled trial (RCT) and the cohort analytic study. An RCT is a true experiment in which people are randomly allocated to receive a new intervention (experimental group) or to receive a conventional intervention or no intervention at all (control group). Each participant is assigned to one group or the other by chance. Investigators follow participants over time and then assess whether they have experienced a specific outcome. The two most important strengths of RCTs are the random allocation of patients to groups, which helps to ensure that the groups are similar in all respects except exposure to the intervention, and the longitudinal nature of the study, whereby exposure to the intervention precedes the development of the outcome. These two features ensure that any differences in outcome can be attributed to the intervention. While the cohort analytic study also compares study participants who receive and who do not receive the intervention, it differs from the RCT because it does not include random assignment to groups. To evaluate a new sex education program using an

RCT, 10 schools would be randomized, five to receive the new program and five to continue with the usual program; using a cohort analytic study, 10 schools would self-select to receive the new program or to continue with the usual program. Schools that decide to receive the new program may differ from those that choose not to receive it in ways that influence the outcome; for example, they may have more students who have high educational goals or who come from economically advantaged families. Therefore, the cohort analytic design is subject to biases, which may influence the study results.

DiCenso (1995) conducted a systematic review and meta-analysis of RCTs and cohort analytic studies designed to evaluate adolescent pregnancy prevention programs and found that cohort analytic studies were more likely to conclude that an intervention had a positive impact on adolescent sexual behaviour (Guyatt, DiCenso, Farewell, Willan, & Griffith, in press). However, in most of these studies, the two comparison groups differed at the beginning of the study. For this reason, this chapter will focus on studies that used the RCT design only.

The programs evaluated in the RCTs include school-based sex education, abstinence programs, multifaceted community-wide programs (focussed on work experience, life skills, volunteer service, decision making, and communication skills), and education and counselling provided through family planning clinics. The three behavioural outcomes studied in RCTs of adolescent pregnancy prevention interventions are initiation of sexual intercourse, consistent use of birth control, and pregnancy. While trials using these outcomes will be summarized in the text, we have incorporated only the trials that include pregnancy as an outcome in Table 13.2. Studies that measure only knowledge and attitudes are not included in this review, because improvements in knowledge and attitudes, while important, do not necessarily result in changes in behaviour (Green & Kreuter, 1991).

Twelve RCTs have been conducted to evaluate interventions to delay the initiation of intercourse (Baker, 1990; Eisen, Zellman, & McAlister, 1990; Grossman & Sipe, 1992; Handler, 1987; Jorgensen, Potts, & Camp, 1993; Kirby, Korpi, Adivi, & Weissman, 1997a; Kirby, Korpi, Barth, & Cagampang, 1997b; Kvalem, Sundet, Rivo, Eilertsen, & Bakketeig, 1996; Mitchell-DiCenso et al., 1997; Slade, 1989; Smith, 1994). Thirteen RCTs have been conducted to evaluate interventions to improve consistent use of birth control (Baker, 1990; Eisen et al., 1990; Grossman & Sipe, 1992; Hanna, 1990; Herceg Baron, Furstenberg, Shea, & Harris, 1986; Jay, DuRant, Shoffitt, Linder, & Litt, 1984; Kirby et al., 1997a; Kvalem et al., 1996; Mitchell-DiCenso et al., 1997; Schinke, Blythe, & Gilchrist, 1981; Slade, 1989; Smith, 1994). Finally, 10 RCTs have been conducted to evaluate interventions to prevent pregnancy (Baker, 1990; Eisen et al., 1990; Grossman & Sipe, 1992; Handler, 1987; Herceg-Baron et al., 1986; Jay et al., 1984; Kirby et al., 1997a, 1997b; Mitchell-DiCenso et al., 1997; Philliber & Allen, 1992) (see Table 13.2). All these studies were conducted in

Table 13.2
Description of RCTs that include adolescent pregnancy as an outcome

Author, Year (Publication Type)	Setting	Sample Size/Characteristics	Theoretical Framework	Intervention	Outcome Variables	Results
School/Agency-based sex education						
Eisen et al., 1990 (published)	6 family planning service agencies & 1 school district in Texas & California, U.S.A.	1444 13- to 19-year olds (67% 15–17 years); 52% females; 53% Hispanic; 24% African-American; majority low-income, inner-city youth	health belief model; social learning theory	Intervention group: Teen Talk 12–15 hours: discussion re factual information, values, feelings, emotions, decision making, & responsibility for sexual behaviour Control group Usual sex education program, which varied among sites	initiation of intercourse; birth control use; pregnancy	36% of intervention group males initiated intercourse compared with 44% of control group males ($p<0.01$); no difference in initiation of intercourse in females, birth control use, pregnancy
Handler, 1987 (dissertation)	2 public schools in Chicago, Illinois, U.S.A.	63 7th-grade African-American females, mean age 13.3 years; majority in female-headed households and over half on public assistance	knowledge—access—empowerment	Intervention group: Peer Power Project One hour per week during school year to increase knowledge, enhance decision-making skills, improve self-concept, set goals, increase interpersonal communication skills, link with a supportive adult, visit clinics, establish career goals, participate in enrichment activities Control group No intervention	initiation of intercourse; birth control use; pregnancy	no difference in initiation of intercourse, birth control use, pregnancy

(continued)

Table 13.2 (continued)

Author, Year (Publication Type)	Setting	Sample Size/ Characteristics	Theoretical Framework	Intervention	Outcome Variables	Results
Kirby et al., 1997a (published)	6 schools with grade 7 in Los Angeles, California U.S.A.	1657 7th-grade students with a mean age of 12.3 years; 54% females; 64% Hispanics; 13% Asians; 9% African-Americans; low SES	health belief model, social learning theory	Intervention group: Project SNAPP 8 sessions over 2 weeks focussing on risks and consequences of teen sex; social influences, assertive communication and resistance skills; increasing participants' perceived susceptibility to pregnancy; identification of barriers to remaining abstinent and to using protection; contraceptive methods; medical and psychosocial resources in community; sessions led by trained peer educators. Control group: Standard curriculum	initiation of intercourse, birth control use, pregnancy	no difference in sexual or contraceptive behaviours
Mitchell-DiCenso et al., 1997 (published)	21 schools with grades 7 & 8 in Hamilton, Ontario, Canada	3289 grade 7 and 8 students with a mean age of 12.6 years; 52% females; majority white; range of income levels	cognitive–behavioural theory	Intervention group: McMaster Teen Program 10 sessions focussing on problem solving, decision making, puberty, male/female roles, media & peer pressure, responsibility in relationships, intimacy, teenage pregnancy, parenting. Control group: Standard curriculum	initiation of intercourse, birth control use, pregnancy	no difference in initiation of intercourse, birth control use, pregnancy

(continued)

Table 13.2 (*continued*)

Author, Year (Publication Type)	Setting	Sample Size/ Characteristics	Theoretical Framework	Intervention	Outcome Variables	Results
Abstinence programs						
Kirby et al., 1997b (published)	56 schools and 17 community-based agencies in California, U.S.A.	10 600 7th- and 8th-graders with a mean age of 12.8 years; 42–45% Hispanic, 30% white, 9% African-American, and 10% Asian	social influence theory	**Intervention group:** Education Now and Babies Later (ENABL) 5 sessions, each 45–60 minutes, delivered in classroom or small group settings, focussing on risks of early sexual involvement, resistance to social and peer pressures, assertiveness skills, and non-sexual ways to express feelings **Control group** Standard curriculum	initiation of intercourse pregnancy	no difference in initiation of intercourse or pregnancy
Multifaceted programs						
Grossman & Sipe, 1992 (unpublished)	5 U.S. cities: Boston, Massachusetts; Fresno, California; Portland, Oregon; San Diego, California; Seattle, Washington	3226 14- to 15-year-olds; economically & educationally disadvantaged; 51% females; 45% African-Americans; 18% Hispanicsx	not specified	**Intervention group:** Summer Training & Education Program (STEP) Mix of work experience, basic skills remediation, & life skills & opportunities instruction during 2 summers; sexuality component focussed on decision making & importance of responsible behaviour; 90 hours of work (half-time) at minimum wage, 90 hours of academic work; 5–15 hours of support during school years **Control group** Summer jobs	initiation of intercourse birth control use pregnancy	no difference in initiation of intercourse, birth control use, pregnancy rates

Table 13.2 (*continued*)

Author, Year (Publication Type)	Setting	Sample Size/ Characteristics	Theoretical Framework	Intervention	Outcome Variables	Results
Philliber & Allen, 1992 (published)	5 sites in U.S.A.	168 11- to 21-year-olds; 70% females; 40% African-Americans, 13% Hispanics, 40% whites	not specified	**Intervention group: Teen Outreach Program** School-based small-group discussions & involvement in volunteer service in the community; met once per week through school year to discuss values, communication skills, growth & development, parenting, family relationships, & community resources **Control group** Usual sex education	pregnancy	no difference in pregnancy rates

Education and counselling in family planning clinics

Author, Year (Publication Type)	Setting	Sample Size/ Characteristics	Theoretical Framework	Intervention	Outcome Variables	Results
Baker, 1990 (dissertation)	family planning clinic, Northeast New Jersey, U.S.A.	62 never-married, sexually active 15-18-year-old female first-time clinic attenders from minority racial groups living in female-headed households	cognitive–behavioural theory	**Intervention group: Self-efficacy training** One 5.5 hour session: 1 hour: factual information 1 hour: problem-solving skills 1 hour: modelling of verbal and non-verbal behaviours 2+ hours: role playing of problem solving and communication **Control group** Usual care	initiation of intercourse compliance with oral contraceptives pregnancy	no difference in initiation of sexual intercourse, compliance with oral contraceptives, or pregnancy rates

(continued)

Table 13.2 (continued)

Author, Year (Publication Type)	Setting	Sample Size/ Characteristics	Theoretical Framework	Intervention	Outcome Variables	Results
Herceg-Baron et al., 1986 (published)	9 family planning clinics in Philadelphia, Pennsylvania, U.S.A.	417 females <16–17 years; 53% African-Americans	not specified	**Intervention group:** **Supportive Care** Either promotion of greater family involvement through 6 weekly 50-minute counselling sessions or increased staff support through 2–6 telephone calls **Control group** No intervention	birth control compliance pregnancy	no difference in regularity of contraceptive use or pregnancy rates
Jay et al., 1984 (published)	adolescent gynecology clinic in Augusta, Georgia, U.S.A.	57 females aged 14–19 from lower SES on oral contraceptives; 96.5% African Americans	not specified	**Intervention group** Peer counselling on compliance with oral contraceptives **Control group** Nurse counselling on compliance with oral contraceptives	compliance with oral contraceptives pregnancy	no difference in compliance with oral contraceptives or pregnancy rates

the United States, with the exception of the one by Mitchell-DiCenso et al. (1997), which was conducted in Canada.

The length of time that study participants were followed after they received the intervention varied from six weeks to 54 months. An adolescent pregnancy prevention program should begin before adolescents initiate sexual activity and its evaluation should ensure the collection of sexual behaviour data from the study participants over a number of years to allow sufficient numbers of adolescents to experience the outcomes and to determine whether the program has a long-term impact. Once participants enter the study, it is important to follow as many as possible through to its completion. Adolescents who become pregnant and leave school may not be as easy to follow as those who are still in the school or agency in which the intervention was originally implemented. If tracking of participants is not maintained, data from those at highest risk of experiencing the outcome may not be included in the study findings.

Of all the RCTs, only one found a reduction in initiation of intercourse in males (Eisen et al., 1990), one found an improvement in use of birth control (Schinke et al., 1981), and none found a reduction in the number of pregnancies. Eisen et al. (1990) conducted an RCT involving 1444 adolescent males and females 13 to 19 years of age. Those randomized to the intervention received a 12- to 15-hour experimental curriculum, which included four components: factual information; group discussion of factual information; group discussion of values, feelings, and emotions; and group discussion of decision making and personal responsibility for sexual behaviour. The curriculum was delivered through a combination of lectures, simulations, leader-guided discussions, and role-playing. The intervention was based on both the health belief model and social learning theory. According to the health belief model (Rosenstock, Strecher, & Becker, 1988), the probability that an adolescent will undertake a particular preventive action is linked to perceived susceptibility to the problem, perceived seriousness of the problem, and perceived benefits and costs of undertaking the recommended preventive action. Bandura's (1977, 1986) social learning theory predicts that adolescents will be better able to avoid pregnancy if the intervention gives them a chance to observe both appropriate and inappropriate behaviours, participate in role-playing to learn ways of preventing pregnancy, and engage in guided practice with knowledgeable teachers. In the study by Eisen et al. (1990), males who had never had intercourse were more likely to maintain abstinence over the next year following the experimental program; there was no program effect, however, for females.

The study by Schinke et al. (1981) applied and evaluated the cognitive–behavioural model in pregnancy prevention programs. This model asserts that individuals need specific cognitive and social skills to resist pressures and to negotiate interpersonal encounters successfully. The experimental intervention consisted of 14 50-minute sessions focussed on contraceptive information and on problem-solving and communication skills. At six-month follow-up, both male and female high school students who participated in the experimental intervention were practising more effective contraception. The small sample size of 36 students and the lack of follow-up of students beyond six months were limitations of this study.

Those who oppose sexual health programs often make two claims: first, that these programs promote sexual activity in adolescents, and second, that the only programs that should be offered are those that focus solely on abstinence. The results of many scientifically rigorous RCTs (Table 13.2., p. 268) do not support the contention that pregnancy prevention programs promote sexual activity or promiscuity. The three RCTs that evaluate abstinence programs (Jorgensen et al., 1993; Kirby et al., 1997b; Miller et al., 1993) did not demonstrate any difference in initiation of intercourse or pregnancy. To illustrate, in the trial by Kirby et al. (1997b), over 10 000 seventh and eighth graders were randomized to the standard curriculum or to an abstinence program that focussed on risks of early sexual involvement, resistance to social and peer pressures, assertiveness skills, and non-sexual ways to express feelings. They found no difference between the two groups in initiation of sexual intercourse or pregnancy.

Why have the many pregnancy prevention programs evaluated to date using RCTs not been found to be effective? First, we seldom talk directly to the adolescents to learn more about the nature of the problem from their perspective and what they think a prevention program should include. Second, the programs offered to date have not reinforced learning over the school years. A study by Botvin et al. (1995) found significant reductions in drug use in adolescents who had received an intervention program consisting of 15 classes in seventh grade followed by 10 booster sessions in eighth grade and five boosters in ninth grade. Third, there have been no evaluations of a comprehensive program that includes both sex education and accessible, affordable, and confidential clinic services. In 1976, the Ontario Ministry of Health began funding sexual health clinic services and community outreach. Over the first five years of this program, there was a greater decline in adolescent pregnancy rates in localities that had established access to both school sexual health education, including contraception, and sexual health clinic services (Orton & Rosenblatt, 1993). Fourth, the experimental programs are often compared to conventional programs rather than to no program, making it more difficult to find a difference. It may be that conventional programs are providing the "bare essentials" and that no new programs evaluated to date have improved on these outcomes. At the very least, practitioners should continue offering the existing program until more effective programs are identified.

What can we learn from other countries? The Netherlands has one of the lowest adolescent pregnancy rates in the world. They attribute this to sex education in the schools, emphasis in the mass media (radio, television, popular youth magazines) on adolescent sexuality and preventive behaviour, positive public education campaigns (using the teenager's own language, popular images, humour), and few barriers to obtaining contraceptive services (e.g., confidential services by general practitioners, no minimum age limit for oral contraceptive prescription without parental consent, free contraceptives for those in lower income groups, no vaginal examinations before prescribing oral contraceptives, and access to family planning clinics heavily subsidized by the Ministry of Health) (Ketting & Visser, 1994).

Borthwick and colleagues (1998) recently completed a qualitative study in which 83 grade 9 and grade 11 students in Ontario were interviewed using 16 focus groups to hear their concerns about current sexual health services and their ideas for improving the delivery of such services. The adolescents revealed that they received "too little, too late" and that the information provided was not particularly useful. The participants had very limited knowledge of available services. Peers and media continue to be the main sources of information. The teens wanted to receive sexual health information from a confidential, reliable source. The socio-sexual climate in which adolescents negotiate their sexual health remains conservative and restrictive and continues to reinforce traditional gender roles. A substantial barrier to safe sexual health practices is adult refusal to accept and acknowledge adolescents as sexual beings. The findings of this study indicate that adolescents need sexual health services. Achieving the goal of effective sexual health services requires the coordination of boards of education and public health departments, and a curriculum that respects diversity of values, cultures, and sexual orientation.

Kirby (1997) has proposed nine characteristics of effective sexual health programs. They should (a) focus on reducing sexual behaviours that lead to unintended pregnancy; (b) include behavioural goals, teaching methods, and materials that are appropriate to the age, sexual experience, and culture of the students; (c) be based on theoretical approaches proven effective in influencing health-risk behaviours; (d) last a sufficient length of time to incorporate a wide range of activities; (e) employ a variety of teaching methods designed to involve the participants and personalize the information; (f) provide basic, accurate information about the risks of unprotected intercourse and about methods to prevent pregnancy and sexually transmitted diseases; (g) include activities that address social pressures on sexual behaviours; (h) provide modelling and practice in communication, negotiation, and refusal skills; and (i) include teachers or peers who believe in the program and have undergone training. Because few adolescents become abstinent once they initiate sexual intercourse, programs designed to delay the onset of intercourse should be implemented in grades seven and eight before the majority of youth initiate intercourse.

In summary, prevention of adolescent pregnancy is a challenge. Program developers should not focus naively on simplistic solutions, nor should they be unduly pessimistic and reduce their efforts. The high costs of adolescent pregnancy to adolescent mothers and fathers, their infants, and society demand that we give greater attention to risk factors that contribute to early sexual intercourse and to the continued exploration, development, and rigorous evaluation of promising prevention programs (Kirby, 1997).

Community health nursing roles and activities

Community health nurses (CHNs) have the potential to play a major role in the delivery of adolescent pregnancy prevention programs. The Canadian Public Health Association's (1990) guide to CHN roles and activities is used as a framework to identify and examine some contributions nurses can make to reduce the incidence of adolescent pregnancy in Canada.

Health promoter
The CHN has a major role to play in promoting reproductive health for individuals, groups, and the community. The healthiest outcome in Canadian communities is the avoidance of pregnancy until a young couple is sufficiently prepared developmentally, educationally, vocationally, and economically to care for themselves and their dependent children. The CHN's health promotion roles in preventing adolescent pregnancy require a substantial breadth and depth of expertise (see also Chapters 16 and 18).

Communicator
The CHN's role as a communicator is vital to enacting all the roles involved in assessing, planning, implementing, and evaluating programs directed toward prevention of adolescent pregnancy. Excellent skills in verbal and written communication are prerequisites for effective community work. The CHN must be comfortable discussing sexual behaviour clearly and explicitly with adolescents, asking difficult and sensitive questions of community leaders, and seeking opinions of people with a wide variety of values and viewpoints.

Planner
The planning role is central to the practice of nursing in community settings and will necessarily involve interdisciplinary teamwork. One of the most comprehensive and coherent planning models is the "precede–proceed model" for health promotion planning and evaluation (Green & Kreuter, 1991). Beginning with a careful consideration of desired outcomes, this model organizes

planning into nine phases, beginning with social diagnosis and ending with outcome evaluation. Adoption of this model can facilitate interdisciplinary communication and simplify planning of adolescent pregnancy prevention programs by clarifying which steps will be taken and in what order.

Care/service provider

As providers of direct nursing services to adolescents, CHNs who work in schools, clinics, and community sites assess the pregnancy prevention needs of individual clients as well as adolescent populations (e.g., school health classes, groups of street kids) served by the agency. Nurses and other health professionals plan and coordinate basic prevention and referral systems for these clients and change procedures and services as required for the populations served. Assessment of school and clinic populations should take into consideration the risk factors that have been identified as determinants of early sexual activity and pregnancy. CHNs should provide subgroups of the local population who are at greater risk with resources specifically tailored to meet their needs. Links with local hospitals and schools are an important prelude to appropriate preventive and follow-up care, focussed on prevention of second pregnancies, post-abortion counselling, and teaching of parenting skills. The teen's risk for repeat pregnancy may be reduced through careful teaching and counselling about effective behavioural and birth control measures.

Educator

Education plays a central role in most prevention-oriented activity. In an ideal scenario, parents begin preparing their children when they are very young for their roles as sexually active adults. CHNs can assist parents in preparing for these roles through assessment and intervention with prenatal couples, day-care and preschool staff, and parent–teacher associations. Instruction can include growth and development of the child as a sexual being, appropriate parental responses to child behaviour, and communication patterns that establish and maintain openness regarding sensitive subjects such as human sexuality.

Coordinated work between health and education sectors can ensure that children receive education informed by expertise from varied disciplines. Such multisectoral/multidisciplinary approaches are consistent with the principles of Primary Health Care. Many teachers who contribute to sex education within elementary and secondary schools have little preparation for these roles. CHNs can provide information about model sex education curricula and about community resources for pregnancy prevention. They can assist through presentation of instructional materials for subjects in which they are content specialists. CHNs can facilitate small-group discussion among teachers concerning their attitudes, values, feelings, and experiences in teaching sensitive sexual material to students; this can increase teacher comfort with such subjects and the effectiveness of instruction. If appropriate, CHNs may also participate in classroom teaching of sex education.

The nurse must find effective and efficient ways of providing information to adolescent clients, particularly those who are becoming sexually active. Unfortunately, much "education" often provides factual information solely. While this is important as a basis for effective planning, it is not sufficient to effect changes in behaviour. For example, many adolescent girls require direct, persuasive intervention from caring adults or friends to get them to a clinic where they can receive education, counselling, or a prescription method of birth control. Media and adolescent peer networks may direct youth to clinics where they can receive information and professional support. Peer tutors and counsellors are also able to provide support to encourage young women to use birth control.

Consultant

Some of the activities mentioned under "Educator" might also be considered part of the CHN's consultant role. In addition, the nurse's understanding of population statistics concerning adolescent pregnancy and ability to obtain and use local data will help the community to plan its programs. For example, a presentation to a local school board concerning the incidence and prevalence of adolescent pregnancy in the province and the local region could motivate people to examine the current sex education curriculum and explore strategies for change.

Local youth groups such as the Girl Guides, Boy Scouts, and those affiliated with churches or synagogues are natural settings within which to provide education to supplement that offered in schools. CHNs can offer training, educational resources, consultation, and referrals to enable these organizations to provide high-quality programming and to prepare their leaders.

Community developer

The care provider, communicator, educator, and consultant roles offer excellent preparation for a role in community development. Contact with youth in school and clinical settings develops understanding of adolescent problems, which prepares the nurse for advocacy. Connections with other health professionals, teachers, parents, school officials, and volunteers help the nurse to understand the varied values, attitudes, and concerns of the community. Moreover, genuine concern for adolescents, understanding of formal and informal political processes, and motivation to improve community health through collective action can lead the CHN to work in community development for pregnancy prevention. The CHN can raise the consciousness of community members concerning adolescent pregnancy, link interested individuals and groups, and encourage people to take action. Health departments can provide staff and infrastructure to assist community groups to begin work, which should eventually involve broad intersectoral communication, planning, and intervention.

Researcher/evaluator

The CHN who works with adolescents should become familiar with the research literature concerning adolescent sexual behaviour, teen use/non-use of birth control, and strategies to prevent pregnancy in this vulnerable group. A careful critical appraisal of published studies is necessary to identify factors or characteristics of adolescents that may predict desirable outcomes and of interventions that are research-based, effective, and relevant. It is not uncommon for clinical decisions to be made after asking "what is new?" rather than asking "what is effective?"

Nurses familiar with the clinical needs of clients should be actively involved in generating questions that can be answered through research. If a CHN wishes to adopt a new way of working with clients and no research evidence is available to support the approach, a study of outcomes could be initiated as part of the plan for implementation of a new intervention. If the necessary research expertise and support to design, conduct, and analyze study results are not available in the agency, CHNs can request research consultation and support from a university school of nursing or other source of research expertise within the province. Nurses and others who are studying for master's and doctoral degrees in the health and social sciences are sometimes able to offer time to such projects. Because graduate students are not paid for the time they spend working on their theses, such studies can be conducted more inexpensively than if the agency has to buy staff time to work on projects. Since the problem of small sample sizes plagues many quantitative research initiatives, it may be possible for staff from several regions to do research or evaluation studies by pooling clients from a number of schools or clinics.

To increase public participation in program planning and research, CHNs should involve representatives of their client populations (e.g., adolescent birth control clinic attenders). Teens can be helpful participants in focus group interviews, by generating ideas concerning the types and amounts of services desired by the client group. It may also be effective to involve teens in delivering peer-mediated interventions, after they have been appropriately trained.

Conclusion

Adolescent pregnancy remains a problem in Canadian society. Teens and their parents have important roles to play as key informants to the planning, education, and research needed to reduce adolescent pregnancy. Nurses, physicians, teachers, and others involved in schools, clinics, and youth-serving agencies have clinical, teaching, research, and consultant roles. Finally, the CHN has a key role in implementing the Primary Health Care principles—public participation, intersectoral collaboration, and prevention—with the adolescent population by involving various sectors of the community in planning, intervening using evidence-based strategies, and monitoring progress toward reduction of adolescent pregnancy.

QUESTIONS

1. Is the incidence of teenage pregnancy in your community increasing, decreasing, or remaining the same? How would a community health nurse find information on local statistics?
2. What kinds of programs are offered through the school system in your community that would affect adolescent pregnancy rates? (Check with a local junior high or high school.) Are community health nurses in your area involved in these school programs?
3. How might a community health nurse involve teenagers, parents, and teachers in the identification and implementation of adolescent pregnancy prevention programs?
4. Has research related to adolescent pregnancy been carried out in your community? Is any planned? Are local community health nurses involved?

REFERENCES

Baker, C. (1990). *Self-efficacy training: Its impact upon contraception and depression among a sample of urban adolescent females.* Doctoral dissertation, Seton Hall University.

Bandura, A. (1977). *Social learning theory.* Englewood Cliffs, NJ: Prentice-Hall.

Bandura, A. (1986). *Social foundations of thought and action.* Englewood Cliffs, NJ: Prentice-Hall.

Baydar, N., & Grady, W. (1993). *Predictors of birth planning status and its consequences for children.* Seattle, WA: Battelle Public Health Research & Evaluation Center.

Bonham, G., Clark, M., O'Malley, K., Nicholson, A., Ready, H., & Smith, L. (1987). *In trouble . . . a way out: A report on pregnancy and sexually transmitted diseases in Alberta teens.* Edmonton: Alberta Community Health System.

Borthwick, V., Busca, C., Creatura, C., DiCenso, A., Holmes, J., Kalagian, W., & Partington, B. (1998). *Completing the picture: Adolescents talk about what's missing in our sexual health services.* Ontario: Haldimand Norfolk & Niagara Regional Health Departments.

Botvin, G.J., Baker, E., Dusenbury, L., Botvin, E.M., & Diaz, T. (1995). Long-term follow-up results of a randomized drug abuse prevention trial in a white middle-class population. *Journal of the American Medical Association, 273*(14), 1106–1112.

Brown, S., & Eisenberg, L. (Eds.). (1995). *The best intentions: Unintended pregnancy and the well-being of children and families.* Washington, DC: National Academy Press.

Canadian Public Health Association. (1990). *Community health–public health nursing in Canada: Preparation and practice.* Ottawa: Author.

Chilman, C.S. (1980). *Adolescent sexuality in a changing American society: Social and psychological perspectives.* Washington, DC: Department of Health, Education & Welfare, U.S. Government Printing Office. (Pub. No. 79-1426)

DiCenso, A. (1995). *Systematic overviews of the prevention and predictors of adolescent pregnancy.* Doctoral dissertation, University of Waterloo, Waterloo, Ontario.

Eisen, M., Zellman, G.L., & McAlister, A.L. (1990). Evaluating the impact of a theory-based sexuality and contraceptive education program. *Family Planning Perspectives, 22*(6), 261–271.

Gold, R.B. (1990). *Abortion and women's health: A turning point for America.* New York: The Alan Guttmacher Institute.

Green, L.W., & Kreuter, M.W. (1991). *Health promotion planning: An educational and environmental approach.* Mountain View, CA: Mayfield.

Grossman, J.B., & Sipe, C.L. (1992). *Summer Training and Education Program (STEP): Report on long-term impacts.* Philadelphia: Public/Private Ventures.

Guyatt, G.H., DiCenso, A., Farewell, V., Willan, A., & Griffith, L. (in press). Randomized trial versus observational studies in adolescent pregnancy prevention. *Journal of Clinical Epidemiology.*

Handler, A.S. (1987). *An evaluation of a school-based adolescent pregnancy prevention program.* Doctoral dissertation, University of Illinois at Chicago.

Hanna, K.M. (1990). *Effect of nurse–client transaction on female adolescents' contraceptive perceptions and adherence.* Doctoral dissertation, University of Pittsburgh.

Herceg-Baron, R., Furstenberg, F.F., Shea, J., & Harris, K.M. (1986). Supporting teenagers' use of contraceptives: A comparison of clinic services. *Family Planning Perspectives, 18*(2), 61–66.

Jay, M.S., DuRant, R.H., Shoffitt, T., Linder, C.W., & Litt, I.F. (1984). Effect of peer counselors on adolescent compliance in use of oral contraceptives. *Pediatrics, 73*(2), 126–131.

Jorgensen, S.R., Potts, V., & Camp, B. (1993). Project Taking Charge: Six-month follow-up of a pregnancy prevention program for early adolescents. *Family Relations, 42,* 401–406.

Ketting, E., & Visser, A.P. (1994). Contraception in the Netherlands: The low abortion rate explained. *Patient Education and Counseling, 23,* 161–171.

Kirby, D. (1997). *No easy answers: Research findings on programs to reduce teen pregnancy.* Washington, DC: National Campaign to Prevent Teen Pregnancy.

Kirby, D., Korpi, M., Adivi, C., & Weissman, J. (1997a). An impact evaluation of project SNAPP: An AIDS and pregnancy prevention middle school program. *AIDS Education and Prevention, 9* (Suppl. A), 44–61.

Kirby, D., Korpi, M., Barth, R.P., & Cagampang, H.H. (1997b). The impact of the postponing sexual involvement curriculum among youths in California. *Family Planning Perspectives, 29*(3), 100–108.

Kvalem, I.L., Sundet, J.M., Rivo, K.I., Eilertsen, D.E., & Bakketeig, L.S. (1996). The effect of sex education on adolescents' use of condoms: Applying the Solomon four-group design. *Health Education Quarterly, 23*(1), 34–47.

McAnarney, E., & Hendee, W. (1989). Adolescent pregnancy and its consequences. *Journal of the American Medical Association, 262,* 74–77.

Millar, W.J., Wadhera, S., & Henshaw, S.K. (1997). Repeat abortions in Canada 1975–1993. *Family Planning Perspectives, 29*(1), 20–24.

Miller, B.C., Norton, M.C., Jenson, G.O., Lee, T.R., Christopherson, C., & King, P.K. (1993). Impact evaluation of facts and feelings: A home-based video sex education curriculum. *Family Relations, 42,* 392–400.

Mitchell-DiCenso, A., Thomas, B.H., Devlin, M.C., Goldsmith, C.H., Willan, A., Singer, J., Marks, S., Watters, D., & Hewson, S. (1997). Evaluation of an educational program to prevent adolescent pregnancy. *Health Education & Behavior, 24*(3), 300–312.

Morris, L., Warren, C., & Aral, S. (1993). Measuring adolescent sexual behaviors and related health outcomes. *Public Health Reports, 108* (Suppl. 1), 31–36.

Orton, M.J., & Rosenblatt, E. (1993). *Sexual health for youth: Creating a three-sector network in Ontario.* Toronto: Faculty of Social Work, University of Toronto.

Philliber, S., & Allen, J.P. (1992). Life options and community service: Teen outreach program. In B.C. Miller, J.J. Card, R.L. Paikoff, & J.L. Peterson (Eds.), *Preventing adolescent pregnancy: Model programs and evaluations* (pp. 139–155). Newbury Park, CA: Sage.

Rosenstock, I., Strecher, V., & Becker, M. (1988). Social learning theory and the health belief model. *Health Education Quarterly, 15*(2), 175–183.

Schinke, S.P., Blythe, B.J., & Gilchrist, L.D. (1981). Cognitive behavioral prevention of adolescent pregnancy. *Journal of Counseling Psychology, 28*(5), 451–454.

Scott, J.R. (1990). Spontaneous abortion. In J.R. Scott, P.J. DiSaia, C.B. Hammond, & W.N. Spellacy (Eds.), *Danforth's obstetrics and gynecology* (6th ed.). Philadelphia: J.B. Lippincott.

Slade, L.N. (1989). *Life-outcome perceptions and adolescent contraceptive use.* Doctoral dissertation, Emory University.

Smith, M.A.B. (1994). Teen incentives program: Evaluation of a health promotion model for adolescent pregnancy prevention. *Journal of Health Education, 25*(1), 24–29.

Statistics Canada. (1991). Therapeutic abortions 1990. *Health Reports* (Suppl. No. 9), 3(4). Ottawa: Author. (Cat. No. 82-003S9)

Statistics Canada. (1992). Hospital morbidity 1989–90. *Health Reports* (Suppl. No. 1), 4(1), 40. Ottawa: Author. (Cat. No. 82-003S1)

Statistics Canada. (1993a). *Therapeutic abortions 1991.* Ottawa: Author. (Cat. No. 82-219)

Statistics Canada. (1993b). *Births, 1991.* Ottawa: Author. (Cat. No. 84-210)

Statistics Canada. (1998). *Health Reports, Winter 1997, 9*(3). Ottawa: Author. (Cat. No. 82-003-XPB)

Stevens-Simon, C., & White, M. (1991). Adolescent pregnancy. *Pediatric Annals, 20,* 322–331.

C H A P T E R   1 4

Health promotion with older adults

Dorothy M. Craig

Health promotion programs for older adults have not been as prevalent as those for younger populations. There is growing evidence that health promotion for older adults has significant benefits. The Canadian health promotion framework (Epp, 1986) identifies strategies that increase coping skills of individuals with health problems and promote public participation and mutual aid. A skills training program developed by community health nurses, in partnership with older adults, illustrates the benefits of encouraging public participation and mobilizing mutual aid among older adults. Empowerment was a key concept in this health promotion project, as older adults were assisted to increase control over their lives. Implications for community health nursing practice are discussed.

LEARNING OBJECTIVES

In this chapter, you will learn:

- how older adults are a vulnerable population in terms of health
- that health promotion programs for older adults can be effective in maintaining/improving their health
- how the CHN role of facilitator, which supports the participation of older adults in defining their own needs and developing strategies to meet these needs, is empowering

Introduction

The Canadian population is aging. In 1995, approximately 12 percent of Canadians were age 65 or over. By the year 2016, 16 percent of the Canadian population will be age 65 or over (Statistics Canada, 1997). Contrary to popular belief, most of the elderly are community residents; only eight percent reside in institutions. Although only two percent of older adults between 65 and 69 are institutionalized, the overall percentage increases with age (Minister of Supply & Services Canada, 1993).

Health problems increase with age. In 1995, 81 percent of non-institutionalized Canadians 65 years of age and over reported a chronic health problem (Statistics Canada, 1997). Restrictions in activity, related to chronic health conditions, were reported by 39 percent of the non-institutionalized elderly (Statistics Canada, 1997). As health problems increase, the use of medications also increases. In Canada's Health Promotion Survey (Fowler & Graham, 1993), older adults reported greater use of sleeping pills and tranquillizers than younger adults (Penning & Chappel, 1993).

Many older adults also report that they experience stress in their lives. In the year prior to the Aging and Independence Survey (Minister of Supply & Services Canada, 1993), 46 percent of older adults reported that they experienced a stressful life event. Canada's Health Promotion Survey (1990) also noted that older adults described their lives as stressful, with women reporting greater levels of stress than men (Penning & Chappel, 1993).

In spite of these physical and emotional challenges, 73 percent of Canadians aged 65 and over reported that their health was good to excellent (Statistics Canada, 1997). This may reflect the perceptions of older adults that health is a resource for living, as defined in *Achieving Health for All: A Framework for Health Promotion* (Epp, 1986). As well, more older adults report positive lifestyle behaviours, such as smoking less than younger adults, eating breakfast, and engaging in frequent exercise (Penning & Chappel, 1993). In 1995, 38 percent of seniors living in private households reported that they were former regular smokers, and seven percent reported that they were former occasional smokers (Statistics Canada, 1997). These improved behaviours may be due to seniors' strategies to manage chronic illness or to a desire to attain or maintain good health.

Health promotion constraints and challenges

Although older adults reported that they were active and engaged in activities to protect and promote their health, some health promotion and protection activities that have received recent attention had not been integrated into their lives, such as breast self-examination, mammography, and avoidance of prescription drugs (Penning & Chappel, 1993). A 1995 Canadian survey revealed that 74 percent of non-institutionalized seniors had used prescription or over-the-counter medications in the two days preceding the survey (Statistics Canada, 1997). Older adults were less knowledgeable than younger adults about some health matters, such as heart disease, appropriate ways to lose weight, and prevention of sexually transmitted diseases (Penning & Chappel, 1993).

Perhaps these findings are not surprising. Early health promotion programs, which concentrated on behavioural change, targeted adolescent and young adult populations. Health professionals may perceive that the elderly are unlikely to change lifestyle behaviours or that the benefits of behavioural changes would be minimal: Young's (1996) study found that professionals believed that the elderly would not benefit from behavioural change. In contrast, 84 percent of the elderly reported doing something to maintain or enhance their health. Similarly, two other studies revealed that the elderly reported lifestyle changes (Ferrini, Edelstein, & Barrett-Connor, 1994), staying active, maintaining relationships, and attending to health practices that promoted their health (Frenn, 1996).

Recent health promotion programs have reported positive impacts on the health of older adults, including activity levels, stress management (Craig & Timmings, 1994), health knowledge levels (Benson et al., 1989; Simmons et al., 1989), energy levels, mood, self-confidence, life satisfaction (Emery & Blumenthal, 1990), and dietary changes (Rose, 1992). Programs that focussed on specific illnesses found that older adults gained knowledge and improved attitudes about arthritis (Bill-Harvey et al., 1989) and cancer risks (Keintz, Rimer, Fleisher, & Engstrom, 1988). Although health practices, psychological and spiritual well-being, and social integration were unchanged for participants in a health promotion program, post-test scores for health practices and well-being were lower among seniors who had not participated in the program (Ruffing-Rahal, 1994). The author suggests that health promotion groups for the elderly may have an important health maintenance function.

Community health nurses (CHNs) who worked with older adults traditionally used health education programs to provide information and support to individuals and small groups. Such information related to initiating or maintaining healthy lifestyle behaviours and managing responses to chronic or acute illness. The nurses functioned as "experts" or group leaders, imparting knowledge and skills to their clients. More recently, the premise of public participation in the Canadian health promotion framework (Epp, 1986) encouraged health professionals to discard traditional approaches. Professionals such as CHNs were challenged to increase their efforts to reduce health inequities, prevent disease and disability, and enhance people's ability to cope with these. As well, CHNs recognized the importance of the determinants of health as identified in the Canadian documents *Strategies for Population Health* (Minister of Supplies & Services Canada, 1994) and *Population Health Promotion* (Hamilton & Bhatti, 1996). The determinants of income and social status, social support networks, personal health practices, coping skills, and health services in particular were of concern to CHNs working with older adults. There was recognition that health promotion programs should address determinants of health and not concentrate exclusively on health behaviours. CHNs support the health promotion mechanisms of self-care and mutual aid (Epp, 1986) and recognize the need to monitor the impact of policy decisions on health.

Cairney (1996) found that income adequacy was the most consistent predictor of health status among the non-institutionalized elderly in Canada. The elderly with the highest incomes reported less heart disease, fewer respiratory problems, fewer sleeping problems, and more good health than those with less adequate incomes (Cairney, 1996). In Canada, 19 percent of people 65 years of age and over had incomes below Statistics Canada's low-income cut-offs. More women than men lived in poverty (26 percent and 11 percent, respectively). Women who were alone were the most deprived (53 percent compared with 32 percent of lone males) (Statistics Canada, 1997). One study, which examined the factors that influenced the financial status of women who had been employed at some time in their lives, found that widows were the most deprived of the financially deprived (McDonald, 1997).

Social support was positively associated with psychological well-being and negatively associated with anxiety and depression (Ploeg & Faux, 1989). Interpersonal resources and social support should be emphasized in health promotion strategies with the elderly. In studies with younger individuals, social support has been related to self-esteem and mastery (Hobfoll & Freedy, 1990) and to self-actualization (Ford & Procidano, 1990). Self-esteem and mastery are personal resources that may affect how individuals access and use social support (Hobfoll & Freedy, 1990). Interventions should aim to effect changes in self-concept and increase skills for accessing and using support. Similarly, self-actualization was positively related to social support (Ford & Procidano, 1990) and may influence how social support is accessed and used.

The strategy of public participation encourages people to assert control over factors that affect their health. Since this strategy is also a premise of Primary Health Care, CHNs have explored ways to incorporate public participation into their practice. As the aging population is most at risk for disease and disability, seniors are important participants in preventive efforts. Enhancing older adults' abilities to cope with health problems could decrease complications and increase quality of life. The health promotion framework's challenge, mechanisms, and strategies provide excellent guidelines for effective CHN practice.

CHNs recognize the need to work with the elderly in the everyday context of their lives and to work with aggregates and communities (see also Chapter 5). CHNs now function primarily in the roles of advocate, facilitator, consultant, and partner with older adults to enable them to move toward health (Canadian Public Health Association, 1990). This partnership recognizes that the experiential knowledge and skills of clients (Borkman, 1990) are as valuable as those of the nurse in attaining and maintaining clients' health. Thus, effective interventions can be developed that respect clients' rights and values and enable their participation.

Participatory health promotion project with seniors

Coinciding with the move of CHNs to work in partnership with their clients is the move by some researchers to collaborate with participants in participatory action research (Barnsley & Ellis, 1992) (see also Chapter 28). In contrast to other research, in which investigators are the experts who design and conduct studies without consultation with "subjects," in participatory action research the people who are experiencing the problem are the experts and become actively involved in the development and implementation of the research. This changes the power relationship between professionals and clients. Researchers, nurses in the community, and clients work in partnership to ensure that research studies involving seniors are not only scientifically sound but are also relevant.

For many Canadian provinces, this is a time of change and redirection of community health services (Hall, 1994). CHNs are faced with complex client situations in a health care system that is experiencing change and shrinking resources. A partnership of CHNs and researchers is timely. For example, the author has worked with a team of community health professionals, including nurses and researchers, in two research studies that were initiated because of the relevance of the research to clinical practice. Practitioners and researchers have learned to work together and participate jointly in all aspects of research.

An initial collaborative project was undertaken by the author, together with a student in a master's of nursing program and a nurse working in a seniors' recreation centre. The director of the seniors' centre supported this research endeavour. This project will be used to illustrate the benefits to community health nursing practice of researchers, practitioners, and older adults working in partnership. As well, it will demonstrate that public participation is invaluable in helping older adults to enhance their coping and self-care through mutual aid.

A needs assessment identified stress and loneliness as major concerns of older adults at an urban seniors' centre (Craig, 1991). The clients who participated in the needs assessment believed that a stress management program would be helpful. Thus, the older adults had identified both problems and desirable health promotion interventions. The professionals agreed with these clients, as poor physical and emotional health outcomes have been linked to stress (Bigbee, 1990; DeLongis, Folkman, & Lazarus, 1988) and loneliness (Lee & Ishii-Kuntz, 1987).

Initially, it seemed acceptable to the researchers to have the nursing student, who had a community health field placement with the seniors' centre, develop and offer a stress-coping program. However, it soon became evident that there was not enough information about specific stressors of these clients or the potential benefits of a stress-coping program. Consequently, older adults associated with the seniors' centre were invited to participate in developing and evaluating a stress-coping program. Instead of being passive recipients of a program developed for them by nurses, they were actively engaged in program development and the research process.

Before the older adults were recruited, the professionals identified the purposes of the project. They expected that the project would (a) identify the stressors specific to older adults, (b) develop guidelines for future stress-management programs to be offered to older adults at the seniors' centre, and (c) offer peer support to older adults.

Participants

The on-site nurse, who had developed a working relationship with many older adults who used the seniors' centre, posted flyers and contacted seniors to inform them of the proposed program. Many seniors had been exposed to health promotion sessions that focussed on nutrition and activity, which this nurse had offered previously. Thus, they had been participants in traditional group activities.

The older adults who became involved ranged in age from 60 to mid-70s. A core group of eight women attended all six weekly sessions, and two men and three women attended sporadically.

The role of participants in the group was introduced and fully discussed during the first session. Participants agreed to assist with decisions about the issues the program would address and the content and format of each weekly session. As well, they would evaluate the process and outcomes of each session.

Initial planning

The first session focussed on issues that emerged from the needs assessment, in which most older adults participated. They confirmed that coping with the stress in their lives was a central concern. Therefore, they wanted to learn how to develop friendships and peer support that would help them cope with their stress and loneliness.

The three aims of the program changed slightly when the older adults became involved. Clients and professionals agreed that the three purposes of the project would include identifying the life stressors of older adults, identifying strategies to manage these stressors, and discussing ways to develop friendships.

The facilitators (the nursing student and the on-site nurse) and the older adults decided that six weekly workshops would be held and that the content would be identified by the seniors. At the end of each session, plans were made for the next week.

Workshop content

The first three workshops focussed on identifying participants' stressful experiences. The facilitators introduced materials that would promote discussion and encourage sharing and support among group members. The hassles/uplifts scale (DeLongis, Folkman, & Lazarus, 1988) was used to facilitate discussion about daily events and life situations that created stress, anxiety, or pleasure. This scale was chosen because daily hassles are more strongly associated with health problems (DeLongis, Coyne, Dakof, Folkman, & Lazarus, 1982) and health status (Weinberger, Hiner, & Tierney, 1987) than stressful life events.

Throughout the workshops, the seniors identified factors that contributed to their stress, including unwanted intrusions, such as computer-generated telephone calls, market research calls, and sales calls. As well, the changing patterns within their neighbourhoods were considered threatening. They feared for their personal safety and limited their activities outside the home to social events held during the day.

Estate planning was another stressor. Several seniors shared their concerns that individuals whom they had chosen as executors for their estates were too intrusive and wanted too much information with regard to their assets. This left seniors feeling vulnerable. The facilitators recognized a need for expert consultation and located a resource that group members could use if they wished.

One stressful event that group members considered most threatening was an illness that resulted in hospitalization. This stressful situation, similar to estate planning and safety, was associated with a sense of vulnerability.

Once the older adults had identified their major stressors, they wanted to work on solving these problems. The facilitators suggested a simple problem-solving model to help focus the problems, identify alternative strategies for coping, and assess the strengths and limitations of strategies. As the level of trust grew in the group, the discussions became more open, with members disclosing many personal problems.

The seniors also identified resources that helped them to cope with stress, such as spiritual beliefs. These beliefs were not linked necessarily to organized religion, and included hope, a positive outlook, and a source of pleasure.

The older adults described supportive relationships and friendships as being critical to their well-being. They reported that they were at a point in their lives characterized by transitions and network loss: friends were dying or moving away from neighbourhoods where they had lived for many years, thus resulting in the loss of stable long-term connections. Therefore, the fourth workshop focussed on cultivating new friendships. The nurse facilitators introduced information about communication and listening skills. This enabled the group to share ideas about the meaning of friendship, desirable qualities in friends, and mechanisms to establish new relationships.

During the fifth workshop, discussion focussed on some of the commonly held myths about aging that can create stress for older adults. The Palmore (1977) quiz, which lists myths, was used to facilitate discussion. Although the Palmore quiz scores typically with true/false answers, the seniors insisted that many of the answers were, "it depends." Group members were adamant that ideas about aging were not absolute, and that different factors contributed to different scenarios.

In the sixth and final workshop, the seniors discussed how food and activity were used for managing stress. These older adults had participated previously in sessions on basic nutrition and believed that most older adults would benefit from this type of information. However, they also wished to examine whether the foods they chose to eat when they were under stress were supportive of health. Similarly, they wanted to discuss how the activities they engaged in when they experienced stress promoted or detracted from their health.

Evaluation

Process evaluation was built into each workshop. Older adults, following each session and the end of the support program, provided verbal feedback on content, structure, and group process. As well, paper was provided at each workshop for participants to provide anonymous, written feedback. During the last half hour of the final workshop, seniors engaged in an interactive discussion to evaluate the total program. This discussion was guided by six open-ended questions to elicit feedback on content and group process. Each senior also provided a final written evaluation based on overall impressions of the total program.

Encouraging group members to participate fully and openly in the evaluation process was a challenge. One older adult interpreted the group's initial reticence by saying, "We were brought up at a time when it was not polite to be critical, so we find it hard." To be sensitive to the group's level of comfort with evaluation, the facilitators suggested that responses focus on what was helpful and enjoyable and what experiences they wanted repeated.

The older adults provided positive feedback about their experiences in the program. They found scales and handouts useful for initiating group discussion, and they valued sharing common problems and experiences with peers. The opportunities to use their own life experience to elicit supportive suggestions from the group were appreciated. Several seniors commented on the inclusive nature of the workshops' content and the active participation by everyone. These clients appreciated having the chance to learn something new that was "useful and practical."

Seniors also contributed to the development of guidelines for future programs with other older adults at the seniors' centre. Group members believed that the group experience had been helpful and wanted to continue to meet after the six-week program finished.

Although social support, self-esteem, and mastery were not measured, the older adults reported that they gained information that they could use to resolve some stressors. Self-esteem may also have been affected by the group process. For example, by the fourth session, participants felt comfortable enough to try an introductory exercise that they had found threatening and refused to do in the first workshop. The exercise required a participant to find out two things about the person sitting closest and to report this information back to the group. When they gained confidence, they found the exercise interesting and enjoyable.

Insights into health promotion with older adults

Working collaboratively with this group demonstrated that it is possible to help older adults engage actively in promoting their own health. The seniors reported that they enjoyed the activity, work, and cooperation and benefited from participation in this health promotion program. Allowing group members the opportunity to structure the program was essential.

Encouraging older adults to establish what they wished to learn, how they wished to learn, and at what pace respected the wealth of life experience that these clients brought to the group program. This project suggests that older adults enjoy interactive forms of learning and are able to exchange peer support and guidance.

As noted earlier in this chapter, friendship was identified as a critical element in these seniors' lives. These older adults had more leisure than before and, therefore, had more time for friends. However, because of losses in their lives, they needed to meet new people and to develop friendships. Thus, a social time was important, as it gave seniors an opportunity to get to know peers. As the level of trust grew, personal sharing increased.

These older adults expressed concerns about critical comments in evaluations. Practitioners could acknowledge that other older adults who are completing evaluation forms or participating in discussions may have similar concerns. It may be as important to the evaluation to determine what is not documented or discussed as to note what is included.

The reluctance of these older adults to score the common myths as true or false could have implications for the use of other instruments. Questionnaires that use true/false or yes/no choices may elicit inaccurate or no responses from older adults who wish to respond in light of the context of each situation. These findings suggest that older adults may respond more accurately to open-ended rather than forced-choice questions. Finally, for health promotion programs dependent on printed matter, large-print materials that are user-friendly are critical to success.

Implications for CHN practice

This project has implications for CHNs who work with older adults. The clients who participated in this study were eager to moderate their daily stressors through sharing problem-solving strategies. Stewart (1990) notes that peers have a range of stress-coping and mastery strategies that they can share in self-help mutual aid groups through role modelling, thus reducing the need for reliance on health professionals. According to Rootes and Aanes (1992), a self-help group is educational and supportive and provides opportunities for personal growth. Leadership comes from within the group. Nurses who facilitate groups of seniors in the community can encourage them to function like self-help groups. Groups may then become self-sustaining and provide long-term support. Thus, a CHN can work in partnership with group members.

These older adults noted that social support was important to their well-being. The literature on social support also recognizes the link between social support and health status (Lambert, Lambert, & Klipple, 1990) and mortality (Bloom, 1990; Cox, Spiro, & Sullivan, 1988). The social support available to older adults often diminishes because of morbidity and mortality. The seniors in this project admitted that it was difficult for them to make new friends. CHNs may have a significant impact on the health of older adults by helping them to increase their skills in accessing and using social support.

CHNs should also examine the relationships that they have with older adults and whether their expertise creates an imbalance of power. Maintaining professional superiority and control can be disempowering (Raeburn & Rootman, 1998). Egalitarian partnerships with older adults can yield significant gains for clients and for CHNs (Courtney, Ballard, Fauver, Gariota, & Holland, 1996). Empowerment was a key premise of this project; facilitators encouraged seniors to take power into their own hands. Gibson (1991) defines empowerment as "a social process recognizing, promoting and enhancing people's abilities to meet their own needs, solve their own problems and mobilize the necessary resources in order to feel in control of their lives" (p. 359). Rodwell (1996) notes that empowerment is not only a process but also an outcome of "sharing resources and opportunities to achieve change" (p. 308). Labonte (1994) proposes that people gain mastery over their lives through empowerment. The older adults in this project reported that they had learned practical skills and thus felt empowered. As well, a few seniors offered to facilitate future groups for older adults, provided that they had some professional support. They believed that nurses could assist them to obtain resources and to solve problems. In this way, the seniors perceived that they would have control. CHNs must learn to give up power in favour of older adults' increasing their own power.

Conclusion

This project assisted all who participated to gain new insights into health promotion strategies that can be effective with older adults. The expertise with which the facilitators carried out their roles was undoubtedly an important factor in the success of this project. However, the experiential knowledge of the older adults, which they were willing to share freely, was equally important.

There are ample opportunities for CHNs to provide health promotion programs to the growing population of older adults in Canada. For example, programs that encourage active lifestyles, breast self-examination, mammography, and management of prescription and over-the-counter medications could have a significant impact on the health of older adults. CHNs working in partnership with seniors can ensure that programs are not only relevant for clients but also effective and efficient.

Health promotion programs should encourage peer interaction and support. Positive lifestyle practices and effective coping strategies will be enhanced by peer support. Furthermore, peer support in self-help mutual aid groups can empower older adults to increase control over their lives. The CHN can act as a resource or consultant.

When environmental issues interfere with older adults' safety or health, the CHN may act as an advocate to promote changes in policy or to ensure equal access to resources. For example, knowing that many elderly persons live in poverty, the CHN could become involved in lobbying for adequate pensions. Health promotion with older adults is still in its infancy. Innovative approaches should be tested for their impact on health and well-being.

QUESTIONS

1. A group of older adults has approached a CHN to help them to become more active. They live in a high-rise apartment building at the intersection of two heavily travelled roads. In winter, sidewalks are not always cleared of ice and snow. How would you, as the CHN, help?
2. Although a CHN is offering a series of classes on health promotion for older adults, attendance is poor. What strategies to enhance participation should the CHN consider before ending the sessions?
3. Loneliness is a major problem for many older adults. Should a CHN do anything about this problem? If yes, discuss appropriate intervention strategies.

REFERENCES

Barnsley, J., & Ellis, D. (1992). *Research for change: Participatory action research for community groups.* Vancouver: The Woman's Research Centre.

Benson, L., Nelson, E.C., Napps, S.E., Roberts, E., Kane-Williams, E., & Salisbury, Z.T. (1989). Evaluation of the Staying Healthy After Fifty educational program: Impact on course participants. *Health Education Quarterly, 16*(4), 485–508.

Bigbee, J.L. (1990). Stressful life events and illness occurrence in rural versus urban women. *Journal of Community Health Nursing, 7*(2), 105–113.

Bill-Harvey, D., Rippey, R., Abeles, M., Donald, M.J., Downing, D., Ingenito, F., & Pfeiffer, C.A. (1989). Outcome of an osteoarthritis education program for low-literacy patients taught by indigenous instructors. *Patient Education and Counselling, 13,* 133–132.

Bloom, J.R. (1990). The relationship of social support and health. *Social Science & Medicine, 30*(5), 635–637.

Borkman, T.C. (1990). Self-help groups at the turning point: Emerging egalitarian alliances with the formal health care system? *American Journal of Community Psychology, 18*(2), 321–335.

Cairney, J. (1996) Social class, health and aging: Socioeconomic determinants of self reported morbidity among non-institutionalized elderly in Canada. *Canadian Journal of Public Health, 87*(3), 199–203.

Canadian Public Health Association. (1990). *Community health–public health nursing in Canada.* Ottawa: Department of National Health & Welfare Canada.

Courtney, R., Ballard, E., Fauver, S., Gariota, M., & Holland, L. (1996). The partnership model: Working with individuals, families, and communities toward a new vision of health. *Public Health Nursing, 13*(3), 177–186.

Cox, C.L., Spiro, M., & Sullivan, J.A. (1988). Social risk factors: Impact on elders' perceived health status. *Journal of Community Health Nursing, 5*(1), 59–73.

Craig, D. (1991). *Senior citizens' perceptions of needs and services in the community.* Unpublished report.

Craig, D., & Timmings, C. (1994). Evaluation of the "Living Well" health promotion program for older adults. In G.M. Gutman & A.V. Wister (Eds.), *Health promotion for older Canadians: Knowledge gaps and research needs* (pp. 99–123). Vancouver: Gerontology Research Centre, Simon Fraser University.

DeLongis, A., Coyne, J.C., Dakof, G., Folkman, S., & Lazarus, R.S. (1982). Relationship of daily hassles, uplifts, and major life events to health status. *Health Psychology, 7*(2), 119–136.

DeLongis, A., Folkman, S., & Lazarus, R.S. (1988). The impact of daily stress on health and mood. *Journal of Personality and Social Psychology, 54*(3), 486–495.

Emery, C.F., & Blumenthal, J.A. (1990). Perceived change among participants in an exercise program for older adults. *The Gerontologist, 30*(4), 516–521.

Epp, J. (1986). *Achieving health for all: A framework for health promotion.* Ottawa: Ministry of Supply & Services Canada.

Ferrini, R., Edelstein, S., & Barrett-Connor, E. (1994). Factors associated with health behavior change among residents 50 to 96 years of age in Rancho Bernardo, California. *American Journal of Preventive Medicine, 10*(1), 26–30.

Ford, G.G., & Procidano, M.E. (1990). The relationship of self-actualization to social support, life stress, and adjustment. *Social Behavior and Personality, 18*(1), 14–51.

Fowler, S.T., & Graham, D. (Eds.). (1993). *Canada's health promotion survey 1990: Technical report.* Ottawa: Ministry of Supply & Services Canada.

Frenn, M. (1996). Older adults' experience of health promotion: A theory for nursing practice. *Public Health Nursing, 13*(1), 65–71.

Gibson, C. (1991). A concept analysis of empowerment. *Journal of Advanced Nursing, 16,* 354–361.

Hall, N. (1994). Health promotion research for older Canadians: Priorities from a community health unit perspective. In G.M. Gutman & A.V. Wister (Eds.), *Health promotion for older Canadians: Knowledge gaps and research needs* (pp. 77–97). Vancouver: Simon Fraser University.

Hamilton, N., & Bhatti, T. (1996). *Population health promotion: An integrated model of health and health promotion.* Ottawa: Health Promotion Development Division.

Hobfoll, S.E., & Freedy, J.R. (1990). The availability and effective use of social support. *Journal of Social and Clinical Psychology, 9*(1), 91–103.

Keintz, M.K., Rimer, B., Fleisher, L., & Engstrom, P. (1988). Educating older adults about their increased cancer risk. *The Gerontologist, 28*(4), 487–490.

Labonte, R. (1994). Health promotion and empowerment: Reflections on professional practice. *Health Education Quarterly, 21*(2), 253–268.

Lambert, V.A., Lambert, C.E., & Klipple, G.L. (1990). Relationships among hardiness, social support, severity of illness, and psychological well-being in women with rheumatoid arthritis. *Health Care for Women International, 11,* 159–173.

Lee, G.R., & Ishii-Kuntz, M. (1987). Social interaction, loneliness and emotional well being among the elderly. *Research on Aging, 9*(4), 459–482.

McDonald, L. (1997). The invisible poor: Canada's retired widows. *Canadian Journal on Aging, 16*(3), 553–583.

Minister of Supply & Services Canada. (1993). *Aging and independence.* Ottawa: Author.

Minister of Supply & Services Canada. (1994). *Strategies for population health.* Ottawa: Author.

Palmore, E. (1977). Facts on aging: A short quiz. *The Gerontologist, 17,* 315–320.

Penning, M.J., & Chappel, N.L. (1993). Age-related differences. In S.T. Fowler & D. Graham (Eds.), *Canada's health promotion survey 1990: Technical report* (pp. 247–261). Ottawa: Minister of Supply & Services.

Ploeg, J., & Faux, S. (1989). The relationship between social support, lifestyle behaviours, coping and health in the elderly. *Canadian Journal of Nursing Research, 21*(2), 53–65.

Raeburn, J., & Rootman, I. (1998). *People-centred health promotion.* Toronto: Wiley.

Rodwell, C. (1996). An analysis of the concept of empowerment. *Journal of Advanced Nursing, 23,* 305–313.

Rose, M.A. (1992). Evaluation of a peer-education program on heart disease prevention with older adults. *Public Health Nursing, 9*(4), 242–247.

Rootes, L.E., & Aanes, D.L. (1992). A conceptual framework for understanding self-help groups. *Hospital and Community Psychiatry, 43*(4), 379–381.

Ruffing-Rahal, M.A. (1994). Evaluation of group health promotion with community-dwelling older women. *Public Health Nursing, 11*(1), 38–48.

Simmons, J.J., Nelson, E.C., Roberts, E., Salisbury, Z.T., Kane-Williams, E., & Benson, L. (1989). A health promotion program: Staying healthy after fifty. *Health Education Quarterly, 16*(4), 461–471.

Statistics Canada. (1997). *A portrait of seniors in Canada.* Ottawa: Minister of Industry.

Stewart, M.J. (1990). Expanding theoretical conceptualizations of self-help groups. *Social Science & Medicine, 31*(9), 1057–1066.

Weinberger, M., Hiner, S.L., & Tierney, W.M. (1987). In support of hassles as a measure of stress in predicting health outcomes. *Journal of Behavioral Medicine, 10*(1), 19–30.

Young, K. (1996). Health, health promotion and the elderly. *Journal of Clinical Nursing, 5,* 241–248.

C H A P T E R   1 5

Prevention of falls among seniors in the community

Nancy C. Edwards

The importance of injury prevention is embodied in the principles of Primary Health Care (health promotion and injury/illness prevention). Community health nurses can play an important role in the design and implementation of programs to prevent injuries. In this chapter, fall prevention among seniors living in the community is used as an example. Fall prevention presents some important challenges to community health nurses who must assess a complex set of risk factors that contribute to falls, use a strong theoretical base to guide interventions, and apply health promotion strategies to tackle this health problem effectively.

LEARNING OBJECTIVES

In this chapter, you will learn:

- a theoretical base for fall prevention among seniors
- to view the problem of falls among the elderly from the perspectives of both health professionals and seniors
- the key differences between risk reduction and collective action approaches to fall prevention
- indicators that can be used to monitor the implementation of fall prevention programs

Introduction

Falls are leading causes of acute and chronic morbidity, premature institutionalization, and mortality among seniors (Alexander, Rivara, & Wolf, 1992; Riley, 1992; Scott & Gallagher, 1997). In addition to their obvious human toll, falls contribute to the high costs associated with health care. In Canada, the cost of falls among seniors was estimated to be $2.8 billion in 1994 (Ashe, Gallagher, & Coyle, 1999).

One in three older persons falls each year (Graafmans et al., 1996; Kellogg International Work Group on the Prevention of Falls by Elderly, 1987; Luukinen, Koski, Hiltunen, & Kivela, 1994), with an increase to 40 percent for those over age 80 (Sattin et al., 1990, Svensson, Rundgren, & Landahl, 1992). About five percent of falls among seniors result in soft tissue injuries requiring hospitalization or immobilization for an extended period, and a similar percentage result in fractures (Cwikel, 1992; Nevitt, Cummings, & Hudes, 1991; Nevitt, Cummings, Kidd, & Black, 1989; Speechley & Tinetti, 1991; Tinetti, Doucette, Claus, & Marottoli, 1995). By the time they reach age 90, one-third of women and one-sixth of men will have fractured a hip (Melton, Ilstrup, Riggs, & Bechenbaugh, 1982). The vast majority (over 90 percent) of these hip fractures will have resulted from a fall (Grisso et al., 1991).

The elderly accounted for 40 percent of 19 907 fall-related hospitalizations annually (O'Loughlin & Robitaille, 1991) according to hospital separation data in Québec for the years 1987 and 1988. The average length of hospital stay for fall-related injuries was four times higher for seniors aged 65 years or older than for those who are younger (8.4 days versus 33.8 days, respectively).

In Canada, falls are the sixth leading cause of death (Raina & Torrance, 1995). For people aged 75 years and older, falls are the major cause of fatal injuries and account for twice as many deaths as motor vehicle accidents (O'Loughlin & Robitaille, 1991; Raina & Torrance, 1995).

Forty percent of all admissions to nursing homes are attributable to serious falls (Smallegan, 1983), reflecting the potentially profound social impact of falls. It is estimated that 25 percent of falls cause people to limit their normal activities, because of either injury or fear of a repeated fall (Arfken, Lach, Birge, & Miller, 1994; Nevitt, Cummings, Kidd, & Black, 1989; Tinetti, Speechley, & Ginter, 1988). Only one in 13 falls is reported (Sorock, 1988). Seniors may be concerned that informing a health professional of a fall will lead the service provider to conclude that the senior cannot manage to live independently in the community. Given these statistics, it becomes obvious that community health nurses have an important role to play in fall prevention programs for seniors.

Risk factors for falls

In the last decade, community-based epidemiological studies have led to increased understanding of modifiable risk factors for falls. Risk factors are commonly categorized as intrinsic (those within the senior) and extrinsic (those outside the senior). Intrinsic factors most commonly implicated include impaired musculoskeletal function (e.g., weak muscular strength, gait problems, poor balance); cognitive impairment; polypharmacy and the use of certain medications such as benzodiazepine sedatives; and a history of falls within the past year (Campbell, Borrie, & Spears, 1989; Cummings et al., 1991; Graafmans et al., 1996; Luukinen, Koski, Laippala, & Kivela, 1995; Nevitt, Cummings, Kidd, et al., 1989; O'Loughlin, Robitaille, Boivin, & Suissa, 1993; Oster, Huse, Abrams, Imbibo, & Russel, 1990; Sorock & Labiner, 1992; Tinetti, Doucette, et al., 1995; Tinetti, Speechley, et al., 1988; Vellas, Bocquet, dePemille, & Albarede, 1987; Wickham, Cooper, Margetts, & Barker, 1989). Many other intrinsic risk factors have been investigated, including visual problems, hearing impairment, dizziness, and alcohol use (Arfken, Lach, McGee, Birge, & Miller, 1994; Felson et al., 1989; Lord & Webster, 1990; Nickens, 1985; Tobis et al., 1990). However, current evidence supporting a relationship among these risk factors and falls is inconclusive.

Extrinsic risk factors include various environmental hazards both in the senior's home and in public places (Archea, 1985; O'Loughlin & Robitaille, 1991). According to the 1994 National Population Health Survey, seniors are more likely to experience an injury in the home or surrounding area than in any other location (Health Canada, 1994). It has been estimated that environmental factors contribute to at least one-third of all falls (Lord, Ward, Williams, & Anstey, 1993; Tinetti, Speechley, et al., 1988). In O'Loughlin's study (1991), seniors' self-reports of reasons for falling indicated that, overall, 43 percent of falls were related to the environment, and environmental causes were attributed to 27 percent of indoor and 65 percent of outdoor falls.

O'Loughlin's study (1991) also provided detailed descriptions of the location of falls. Of the 197 falls reported by 417 community-dwelling seniors over a 48-week period, 59 percent were indoor and 41 percent were outdoor falls. Indoor falls most often occurred in the subject's own home, while streets, parking lots, and sidewalks were the most frequently reported locations of outdoor falls. Risk factors for indoor and outdoor falls differ substantially, and fall prevention programs may need to be targeted accordingly (O'Loughlin, Boivin, Robitaille, & Suissa, 1994).

Seniors' perspectives on risk factors

Designing fall prevention programs for seniors requires an understanding of fall events from the perspectives of both researchers and seniors. Data on seniors' perspectives come from studies that have used in-depth interviews and focus groups (Aminzadeh & Edwards, 1998a, 1998b; Borkan, Quirk, & Sullivan, 1991; Edwards, 1993; Edwards, 1994; O'Loughlin, 1991; Orlando, 1988). Several aspects of seniors' views of falls are germane to this discussion, including (a) why they fall, (b) what constitutes a fall, (c) risk factors for falls, and (d) social norms relevant to fall prevention.

In O'Loughlin's study (1991), seniors were asked to identify the causes of their falls. Content analysis revealed that seniors frequently described tripping or slipping as the key cause (about 25 percent in each category). Edwards, Birkett, Murphy, Nair, and Coristine (1993) have shown that some seniors think of slips or trips and falls as discrete events. Thus, seniors may fail to report events they categorize as slips or trips when asked about falls during history taking.

During focus group interviews (Aminzadeh & Edwards, 1998a; Edwards, 1994), carelessness, inattention, and distraction were often cited as factors contributing to falls. Seniors believed that falls were inevitable and thus could not be prevented. This fatalistic attitude can have a powerful influence on seniors' choices about becoming involved in fall prevention activities or modifying their own risk factors for falls.

Finally, discussions with seniors can highlight their perceptions of fall-related social norms. Recent community-based studies indicate that social stigma attached to aging, disability, and assistive device use may exert powerful influences on older persons' decisions to use assistive devices (Aminzadeh, 1997; Aminzadeh & Edwards, 1997; Aminzadeh & Edwards, 1998a).

Selecting a theoretical base for program design

The choice of a suitable theoretical base for health promotion and injury prevention programs must take into account the nature of the problem, the target population, and the type of intervention strategy that is expected to be effective. Nursing theories such as those proposed by Neuman (1982) and Archer (1985) provide a useful overall framework for program design and will help define the role of the nurse in program implementation. However, application of social–psychological theories is also essential to refine assessment protocols and delineate effective intervention strategies. Three relevant social–psychological models will be outlined briefly: the transtheoretical model, Bandura's social learning theory, and Rogers's information diffusion theory.

Transtheoretical model
The transtheoretical model (Prochaska, Velicer, et al., 1994) is an integrative model of behavioural change that has been used to interpret across a variety of health behaviours, including exercise (Marcus, Rakowski, & Rossi, 1992; Marcus, Rossi, Selby, Niaura, & Abrams, 1992), smoking (DiClemente et al., 1991), and mammography screening (Rakowski et al., 1992). The core constructs of the model are the stages and processes of change. The model proposes that changes in health behaviour progress through five stages:

precontemplation, contemplation, preparation, action, and maintenance. These stages reflect a person's readiness to change. The processes of change describe the differing activities and coping strategies used by individuals to modify behaviour, affect, cognitions, or relationships (Prochaska, Velicer, et al., 1994). The frequency and intensity of these processes differ within and between stages (Prochaska, 1991; Prochaska, Redding, & Evers, 1997;). Table 15.1 illustrates the application of these stages to the adoption of an exercise program to improve strength and balance.

Bandura's social learning theory

The construct of self-efficacy, which also can assist in plans for program implementation, comes from Bandura's social learning theory (Bandura, 1977, 1997). Self-efficacy concerns an individual's assessment of his or her confidence to be able to carry out a particular behaviour successfully under a specific set of circumstances (Bandura, 1992) (e.g., confidence that one can use a cane correctly when walking down stairs in one's own home). The second major dimension of Bandura's theory is outcome expectancy—the belief that implementing the behaviour would have positive health consequences. For example, outcome expectancy for the functional and safety benefits of cane use would likely increase as a senior developed skills to cope with the social and pragmatic inconveniences of cane use (Aminzadeh, 1997).

There are several powerful strategies that help to build self-efficacy (Bandura, 1992; Gecas, 1989). These include performance mastery (learning through personal experience, such as successfully negotiating a medication change with one's doctor) and modelling and vicarious experience (seeing others, particularly peers, successfully perform activities such as daily exercise). Less effective but useful intervention strategies include verbal persuasion (being encouraged to change your behaviour) and emotional arousal (receiving information about the consequences of fall risks and the benefits of change).

To improve outcome expectancy, the community health nurse guides the senior in making the connection between the behaviour and outcome(s). This involves exploring the potential advantages between changing behaviour (e.g., using an assistive device) and decreasing the risk of undesirable outcomes (e.g., loss of independence or institutionalization as the result of a fall).

Of particular relevance to community action programs is the concept of collective efficacy (Bandura, 1997). Two levels of collective efficacy are important—confidence in one's abilities to engage in collective activities and confidence in one's abilities to initiate collective action. Examples of the former might include seniors participating in a discussion about safety changes for a community centre or a meeting with store managers to identify environmental hazards in a shopping mall. Initiating collective action presumes efficacy for such behaviours as lobbying public transportation authorities to provide seating at bus stops.

Table 15.1
The transtheoretical model: Stages of change and their application to adoption of an exercise routine

Stages of Change	Illustrations
Precontemplation	Sedentary seniors not thinking about and not interested in adopting an exercise regime. Not thinking about risks of sedentary lifestyle.
Contemplation	Sedentary seniors thinking about adopting an exercise regime within the foreseeable future. No concrete plans to implement regime. Pros of exercise do not outweigh cons.
Preparation	Sedentary seniors are formulating plans for exercise regime, incorporating information about past experience. Pros of exercise outweigh cons.
Action	A six-month period in which the senior follows an exercise regime, faces challenges associated with continuing to follow progress, and revises plans as needed. Focussed on pros of exercise.
Maintenance	Senior has continued to exercise for at least six months. Most of the challenges have been faced. In behaviours such as those that involve developing new habits (e.g., putting mat in bathtub for bathing), may reach a point where there is no chance of relapse.
Relapse	Senior slips back at least one stage in the exercise program (e.g., stops exercising within first month and goes back to thinking about starting again within foreseeable future). A normative event; most people cycle through stages a number of times before reaching maintenance.

Compiled based on information from Prochaska, Velicer, et al. (1994).

Strategies that strengthen self-efficacy are also keys to improving collective efficacy. For example, using performance mastery techniques, a nurse might work with community organizers to help them collect data on environmental hazards, articulate a case for hazard reduction, and present the findings to a building manager. These activities would help to boost collective efficacy.

Rogers's diffusion innovation theory

Rogers's diffusion innovation theory (see Table 15.2) also has implications for implementing fall prevention programs for seniors. An innovation can be an idea (e.g., falls are preventable), a practice (e.g., use of canes), or an object (e.g., grab bars for bathrooms) that an individual perceives as new or as a new use for an old object. Seniors who are among the first to buy the product or implement a new behaviour (e.g., mall walking) are termed innovators. They are followed by the early adopters, who are more apt to take risks than the late adopters or laggards (those who are slowest to adopt the innovation). Rogers (1995) described five attributes of innovation: relative advantage, compatibility, complexity, trialability, and observability. Each of these may affect the "diffusion" rate of fall prevention programs for seniors, that is, how quickly program elements influence the fall-related knowledge, attitudes, and behaviour of the target population.

Innovations may be adopted as promoted or may be modified by the adopters. If modifications by early adopters render the innovation ineffective, the innovation diffused by these seniors will not reduce the incidence of falls. In the worst-case scenario, an innovation that does more harm than good may be diffused. For example, if early adopters were to suggest that seniors use towel racks as an alternative to grab bars to support them in rising from the bathtub, a harmful innovation would be diffused.

A set of innovations with similar characteristics has been termed a technology cluster (Rogers, 1995). Belief that one element of a cluster is closely connected to another may lead to the adoption of a series of related ideas. For example, it would be more difficult to get seniors to make three independent changes in behaviour—such as adopting the use of grab bars, a bath seat, and a bath mat—if each of these were seen as unrelated innovations. If, on the other hand, seniors perceive these innovations to be interconnected, it may be possible to encourage them to adopt all three as a group.

The mass media may be particularly useful in creating an awareness of a new product. However, interpersonal channels are more effective in persuading seniors to adopt new ideas, particularly when the innovation can be modelled by early adopters.

Intervention strategies

Two fundamentally different, but complementary, fall prevention interventions will be described: (a) a multifaceted risk abatement strategy that focusses on the individual and family and (b) a community action approach that involves working with seniors to strengthen their potential for collective action. Before describing these two types of interventions, several common issues that reflect Primary Health Care principles will be highlighted.

Table 15.2
Rogers's diffusion innovation theory: Attributes of innovation decisional categories and application to fall prevention

Attributes of Innovation and Definition	Examples
Relative Advantage The extent to which an innovation is perceived as better than the idea it replaces	Economics (lower cost); social networks (allows seniors to join their friends); improved function (increased independence); health (fewer falls)
Compatibility Consistency of intervention with existing norms, values, past experiences, or needs	An Able Walker meets seniors' needs for mobility and satisfies the desire to be perceived as independent
Complexity Difficulty in understanding or using an innovation	Senior has trouble installing grab bars due to complicated installation instructions or the need to obtain paid help
Trialability The option to experiment with an innovation before making a final choice about its use	Providing a lending cupboard allows seniors to borrow and try out assistive devices
Observability Extent to which innovation results are visible to others	Scheduling walking program at a time when other seniors are likely to see it

(continued)

Table 15.2 (*continued*)

Attributes of Innovation and Definition	Examples
Optional Choices an individual makes about adopting or rejecting an innovation that are independent of decisions by others	A senior's choice to take prescribed sedatives or get rid of scatter rugs
Collective Choices to adopt or reject an innovation made by consensus among members of a system	Seniors voting on whether to install grab bars in all units located in a cooperative apartment building
Authority Decisions made by a few individuals because they possess power, status, or technical expertise; individuals have little or no influence over innovation decision, but are responsible for implementation	Municipality passes by-law that requires all restaurants to have stair edges marked with yellow paint; restaurant owners responsible for implementation
Contingent Choices to adopt or reject an innovation are contingent on prior innovation decisions	A senior living in rental housing cannot act on a decision to install grab bars until regulations are put in place that allow grab bar installation

Compiled based on information from Rogers (1995).

To help ensure equitable program coverage and *accessible interventions*, the target population must be well defined and methods to reach this population clearly delineated. For example, if an intervention has been designed to prevent falls among active seniors, targeting clients who are receiving home care would be inappropriate. Furthermore, the intervention must be carefully matched to the client's level of risk. Frail, high-risk seniors require a more intense intervention than lower-risk seniors.

Fall prevention initiatives lend themselves to *intersectoral collaboration* that goes well beyond the traditional health professional team (Harris, Wise, Hawe, Finlay, & Nutbeam, 1995). Linkages among disciplines and sectors must be fostered actively (Aminzadeh & Edwards, 1997, 1998a). Fall prevention coalitions provide a forum for intersectoral activities (Aminzadeh, 1996; Butterfoss, Goodman, & Wandersman, 1993; Gallagher & Scott, 1995). The following examples illustrate important contributions that other disciplines might offer. The input of an architect may be vital to planning appropriate structural modifications to buildings (Pauls, 1998). Civil engineers may assist with reviewing building codes or redesigning pedestrian crosswalks. Physiotherapy input can be helpful in designing exercise programs that maximize gains in muscle strength, while pharmacists can reinforce advice about risks associated with sedative use. Communications experts can help plan a community awareness campaign and orchestrate timing of media releases to maximize information diffusion. To help overcome stigma associated with assistive device use, manufacturers can design devices (e.g., canes, walkers, bath seats) that are safe, convenient, and fashionable.

Finally, *active participation* of seniors is important in the design and implementation of relevant fall prevention programs. This involvement can be encouraged through such activities as membership on advisory committees and providing input on the role for volunteers in program delivery. Behavioural changes at both individual and collective levels are difficult to initiate and maintain. Use of reinforcement to help sustain behavioural change is important and should be built right into an intervention program. This might take the form of phone calls to seniors to reinforce successful behavioural change or public recognition for seniors who have worked as community organizers.

Individual action for fall prevention

Many fall prevention programs have adopted individual risk reduction strategies. These programs typically involve a thorough assessment of individual risk factors conducted during home visits or fall clinics, followed by multifaceted intervention strategies targeting high-risk individuals. Interventions commonly used include home safety inspection and modification, medication counselling, referral for medical conditions, instructions about safe mobility and transfer, and recommendations for exercise

(Edwards, Birkett, et al., 1993; Ploeg et al., 1994; Tideiksaar, 1997; Tinetti, Baker, et al., 1994; Wagner et al., 1994). Research examining the effectiveness of these programs indicates that many fall risk factors are potentially modifiable with appropriate interventions of sufficient intensity and duration (Moyer, Aminzadeh, & Edwards, 1998).

Nurses must be aware of two potential caveats in the design of risk-reduction programs. First, a weak element of many lifestyle programs is an implicit expectation that individuals in the program are prepared to take action to modify their behaviour (Hotz, Allston, Birkett, Baskerville, & Dunkley, 1995). Integrating theories such as the transtheoretical model or Bandura's social learning theory in program design will help ensure that interventions are appropriately tailored to fit a client's readiness to make decisions and take preventive action. Second, individually targeted risk modification approaches too often ignore contextual factors that discourage seniors from changing their behaviour (Kirscht, 1989). For example, a senior living on a fixed income below the poverty level will have to weigh carefully choices that involve finance. A decision to purchase a bath bench may have consequences such as being without grocery money for several weeks. A frail widow with poor mobility may choose not to have grab bars installed if she requires the permission of her landlord to do so.

Risk factors for assessment and subsequent intervention must be carefully chosen based on evidence of causation. As new research findings are constantly being generated, it is imperative that procedures be established to integrate new knowledge into risk assessment protocols. There are two objectives of risk assessment: identifying those at risk for falls and targeting client characteristics for risk reduction. Tools to assess the risk of falls for seniors have been developed for use in physicians' offices (Tinetti, Williams, & Mayewski, 1986), fall prevention clinics (Edwards, Céré, & LeBlond, 1993), and institutional settings (Heslin et al., 1992; Morse, Morse, & Tylko, 1989; Spellbring, 1992).

When skilfully used, a risk assessment tool may help to move a senior along the stages of change. When a senior's risk profile has been assessed and the nurse has established whether the senior might benefit from a more intense fall prevention initiative, the venue for follow-up visits needs to be decided. Visiting seniors in their homes offers a number of advantages over seeing them in a clinical setting. These include opportunities to (a) assess environmental hazards in the home, (b) verify information such as medication use, (c) obtain input of family members, and (d) identify barriers or supports that may influence choices about fall prevention behaviours. Determining clients' readiness for change and assessing their self-efficacy, outcome expectancy, knowledge, and attitudes toward fall prevention are complementary to a risk-factor profile that allows interventions to be tailored to clients.

During home visits, explicit contracting is an important strategy that helps the senior and nurse to establish mutually agreed-upon targets and time-frames for change (Bandura, 1997; Boehm, 1989; Wills, 1996). This behavioural intervention helps to ensure that goals are achievable and increases the likelihood that they will be acted upon. For example, while assessing a client's risk for falls, a community health nurse may identify the need for a senior to review current medications with a physician. From discussions with the client, the nurse learns that the senior is at the precontemplation stage, having been rebuffed previously by the physician for questioning medication orders. In this situation, the nurse might ask the client to begin weighing pros and cons associated with asking the physician to review the medications. Contracting with the client involves identifying a feasible increment of change, such as discussing advantages of a medication review with a friend. A time-frame for this step would be mutually agreed upon, and the nurse would reinforce the behaviour on the next visit.

A growing number of environmental hazard checklists are available for use with seniors (Health Canada, 1997; Tideiksaar, 1997). Community health nurses should be familiar with (a) the reading level required to use the tool, (b) prior testing of the tool with seniors, and (c) the basis for and accuracy of recommendations for corrective action (hazard reduction). Nurses should not automatically assume that a home hazard checklist that helps seniors identify risk factors will either get the seniors to do the assessment or prompt them to take corrective action. However, when properly selected and used, environmental hazard assessment checklists are helpful aids to guide seniors toward action.

Collective action for fall prevention

A second approach to fall prevention involves collective action, defined as intentional decision making and activity undertaken by an individual or group to create supportive environments for health and improve the quality of community life (Edwards, Murphy, Moyer, & Wright, 1995). Although community organization strategies for fall prevention are rare, their use is consistent with a growing trend to implement population-based programs that mobilize communities toward preventive health action (Flick, Given Reese, Rogers, Fletcher, & Sonn, 1994; Minkler, 1992; Thompson, Corbett, Barcht, & Pechacek, 1993). Community organization approaches can be used alone or in combination with individual fall prevention interventions.

A community mobilization phase is an essential starting point for a collective action intervention. This step engages seniors and community health nurses in a dialogue about falls and their prevention. This is a period when mutual learning takes place, relationships are formed, and partnerships are developed. It is a phase when the community health nurse establishes a presence in the community, gets known by seniors, and becomes associated with fall prevention activities. During this period, the community health nurse strives to "find the hooks," or entry points. Examples of potential hooks include (a) an individual's interests or skills (e.g., a handyman who likes to do carpentry work in a condominium), (b) personal experience (e.g., a senior who has recently had cataract surgery), (c) vicarious experience (e.g., a senior who recalls that a neighbour fell and fractured a hip after supporting himself with a towel rack that came off the wall), (d) concerns (e.g., difficulty obtaining the services of a homemaker), or (e) wants (e.g., desire for independence). Each of these represents a possible starting point to begin mobilizing seniors about fall prevention. A vital component of this early phase is identifying opportunities to make connections between fall prevention activities and "non-fall issues." For example, concerns about lack of heat in an apartment building may be the basis for (a) initiating dialogue about legal rights, (b) contacting community experts who can help with a dispute, or (c) becoming familiar with the process to follow in making requests to a building manager. Such activities may, in turn, be the basis for action on reducing environmental hazards in a building.

The community mobilization phase may be a period when a media blitz would be helpful in raising community awareness about an issue (Hastings & Haywood, 1991). Various messages and multiple approaches will be needed to connect with different population subgroups.

A variety of formal and informal networks operate within the community. Information about networks helps community health nurses identify key informants, possible community organizers, less visible segments of the target group (e.g., house-bound frail elderly), and potential supporters who might reinforce positive health behaviours and assist with environmental changes. Visual tools such as social network maps (Edwards, Goodick, LeBlond, Asselin, & Mooers, 1993) can be used with seniors to identify networks in each neighbourhood. This information can be used subsequently when developing an action plan.

Another important strategy commonly used in community action programs is the training of lay community organizers (Booker, Robinson, Kay, Najera, & Stewart, 1997; Eng & Parker, 1994; Lacey, Tukes, Manfredi, & Wanecke, 1991; Minkler, 1992). The use of lay community organizers multiplies the reach of professional staff into the community and ensures larger and more sustainable program impact (Lefebvre, Lasater, Carleton, & Peterson, 1987). Community organizers, particularly those with high visibility among other seniors, are effective role models because of the common characteristics they share with others of their generation. As credible early adopters of fall prevention innovations, community organizers promote the diffusion of health messages and shape community opinions (Earp et al., 1997; Love, Gardner, & Legion, 1997). Finally, by actively participating in planning and implementing fall prevention activities, lay organizers foster community control and ownership of the program (Brown, 1991; Minkler, 1992; Wells, DePue, Buehler, Lasater, & Carleton, 1990).

The training of community organizers should follow an experiential approach, consistent with social learning theory (Bandura, 1992; Wallerstein, 1993). There are two major categories of knowledge and skills that community organizers need for their role in a fall prevention program. The first concerns knowledge about risk factors and how to modify them. The second, but equally important, category includes the processes by which community organizers can initiate change among both their peers and those who have decision-making authority. Social marketing, lobbying, behavioural change strategies, and working with experts are examples of these processes.

Joint development of a fall prevention action plan results in a contract between the community health nurse and community organizers that summarizes the activities to be initiated. As is the case for individual contracting, the action plan is discussed explicitly and includes objectives, activities, time-frames, and designated person(s) responsible for each task. It is important that activities are mutually selected. When discussing alternatives, criteria may be used to help choose one activity over another (e.g., feasibility, visibility, cost, interest, likelihood that it will prevent falls, short- versus long-term impact).

Action plans should be prepared with the understanding that accomplishments will be reviewed at a predetermined time. This review (involving community organizers, other seniors, community health nurses, other collaborative team members) should include discussions of what activities took place (why or why not) and what did and did not seem to work. This sets the stage for planning further initiatives, thus helping to sustain fall prevention activities.

Evaluation

Increasingly, community health nurses are being asked to document that their interventions make a difference. It is important to measure process and outcome indicators, rather than relying exclusively on the more commonly used and readily measured structural indicators. Both qualitative and quantitative methods will be needed to assess a comprehensive range of indicators for program evaluation.

Structural indicators show whether or not program activities have actually occurred. Records of hours spent on home visits, numbers and characteristics of seniors attending fall prevention clinics, types of marketing campaigns mounted, and numbers of community organizers trained are all examples of structural indicators. Changes in knowledge, attitudes, and behaviours are frequently measured process indicators. The proportion of seniors moving from contemplation to action for targeted behaviours, the percentage of seniors who decide to review their medications routinely with their physician, changes in levels of collective efficacy among community organizers, the development of new social networks, and expressions of consumer satisfaction are all process indicators. Outcome indicators are generally measures of health status. These might include changes in some of the main indicators discussed at the beginning of this chapter, such as (a) incidence of falls, (b) percentage of falls resulting in injuries, (c) deaths resulting from falls, and (d) proportion of seniors reporting restrictions in daily activities due to fear of falling. Changes in these outcomes may take several years to appear.

When selecting indicators, both positive and negative outcomes that might arise from a fall prevention program should be considered. Examples of unintended results that might be important to measure include increased reports of fear of falling following a media campaign on the risk of falls, a rise in the number of injuries sustained during a mall-walking program, or reports of conflict in an apartment building where community organizers have been trained. Such data must be appropriately used to monitor and evaluate the impact of fall prevention programs and to modify existing or develop new programs.

Conclusion

Factors that lead to falls and influence the effectiveness of health promotion and fall prevention strategies require further study. Community health nurses working in fall prevention must develop ways to keep abreast of emerging data and to incorporate research findings in the design of programs and in the modification of their practice. With the aging of Canada's population, it can be expected that fall prevention will remain an important priority for community health nurses working with seniors for years to come.

QUESTIONS

1. What are the priority risk factors for falls in your community?
2. How would you interest and involve seniors in a fall prevention program if they do not perceive themselves to be at risk for falling?
3. How would you mobilize a coalition for fall prevention in your community? Whom would you invite to join the coalition?

REFERENCES

Alexander, B.H., Rivara, F.P., & Wolf, M.E. (1992). The cost and frequency of hospitalization for fall-related injuries in older adults. *American Journal of Public Health, 82*(7), 1020–1023.

Aminzadeh, F. (1996). *Stair falls among seniors: Hazards, safety recommendations, and building codes.* Community Health Research Unit, University of Ottawa. (Pub. No. DP96-2)

Aminzadeh, F. (1997). *Perceptions, attitudes, and subjective norms influencing seniors' decisions to accept or reject mobility aids in fall prevention: An application of the theory of planned behaviour.* Unpublished master's thesis, University of Ottawa, Ottawa.

Aminzadeh, F., & Edwards, N. (1997). *The use of assistive devices in fall prevention among community living seniors.* Ottawa: Community Health Research Unit. (Publication No. M97-1)

Aminzadeh, F., & Edwards, N. (1998a). Exploring seniors' views on the use of assistive devices in fall prevention. *Public Health Nursing, 15*(4), 297–304.

Aminzadeh, F., & Edwards, N. (1998b). *Perceptions, attitudes, and social norms influencing fall prevention behaviors: A comparison of English and Italian seniors.* Ottawa: Community Health Research Unit. (Pub. No. M98-3)

Aminzadeh, F., Plotnikoff, N., & Edwards, N. (1999). Development and evaluation of the cane use cognitive mediator instrument. *Nursing Research, 48*(5), 1–7.

Archea, J.C. (1985). Environmental factors associated with stair accidents by the elderly. *Clinics in Geriatric Medicine, 1*(3), 555–569.

Archer, S.E. (1985). *Community health nursing* (3rd ed.). Monterey, CA: Wadsworth Health Sciences.

Arfken, C.L., Lach, H.W., Birge, S.J., & Miller, J.P. (1994). The prevalence and correlates of fear of falling in elderly persons living in the community. *American Journal of Public Health, 84*(4), 565–570.

Arfken, C.L., Lach, H.W., McGee, S., Birge, S.J., & Miller, J.P. (1994). Visual acuity, visual disabilities and falling in the elderly. *Journal of Aging and Health, 6*(1), 38–50.

Ashe, C., Gallagher, E., & Coyte, P. (1999). *The cost of falls among older Canadians.* Manuscript submitted for publication.

Bandura, A. (1977). Self-efficacy: Toward a unifying theory of behavioural change. *Psychological Review, 84,* 191–215.

Bandura, A. (1992). Self-efficacy mechanisms in human agency. *American Psychologist, 37,* 122–147.

Bandura, A. (1997). *Self-efficacy: The exercise of control.* New York: W.H. Freeman & Company.

Boehm, S. (1989). Patient contracting. *Annual Review of Nursing Research, 7,* 143–153.

Booker, V.K., Robinson, J.G., Kay, B.J., Najera, L.G., & Stewart, G. (1997). Changes in empowerment: Effects of participation in a lay health promotion program. *Health Education & Behavior, 24*(4), 452–464.

Borkan, J.M., Quirk, M., & Sullivan, M. (1991). Finding meaning after the fall: Injury narratives from elderly hip fracture patients. *Social Science & Medicine, 22*(8), 947–957.

Brown, E.R. (1991). Community action for health promotion: A strategy to empower individuals and communities. *International Journal of Health Services, 21*(3), 441–456.

Butterfoss, F.D., Goodman, R.M., & Wandersman, A. (1993). Community coalitions for prevention and health promotion. *Health Education Research, 8*(3), 315–331.

Campbell, A.J., Borrie, M.J., & Spears, G.F. (1989). Risk factors for falls in a community-based prospective study of people 70 years and older. *Journal of Gerontology, 44,* M112–M117.

Cummings, R.G., Miller, J.P., Kelsey, J., Davis, P., Arfken, C.L., Birge, S.J., & Peck, W.A. (1991). Medications and multiple falls in the elderly: The St. Louis OASIS study. *Age and Aging, 20,* 455–461.

Cwikel, J. (1992). Falls among elderly people living at home: Medical and social factors in a national sample. *Israel Journal of Medical Science, 28*(7), 446–453.

DiClemente, C.C., Prochaska, J.O., Fairhurst, S., Velicer, W.F., Velasquez, M.M., & Rossi, J.S. (1991). The process of smoking cessation: An analysis of precontemplation, contemplation and preparation stages of change. *Journal of Consulting and Clinical Psychology, 59,* 295–304.

Earp, J.A., Viadro, C.I., Vincus, A.A., Altpeter, M., Flax, V., Mayne, L., & Eng, E. (1997). Lay health advisors: A strategy for getting the word out about breast cancer. *Health Education & Behavior, 24*(4), 432–451.

Edwards, N. (1993). Primary care research in the community. In M. Bass (Ed.), *Foundations of primary care research: Research in the practice setting* (pp. 233–244). Newbury Park, CA: Sage.

Edwards, N. (1994). *Population strategies for fall prevention.* Paper presented at the Public Health Branch, Ontario Ministry of Health, Eastern Ontario Health Units Health Elderly Workshop, Population Health: From Theory to Action, April 1994, Kingston, ON.

Edwards, N., Birkett, N., Murphy, M., Nair, R., & Coristine, M. (1993). *Fall prevention: Results of baseline interviews.* Paper presented at the Canadian Gerontology Conference, October 1993, Montréal.

Edwards, N., Céré, M., & LeBlond, D. (1993). A community-based intervention to prevent falls among seniors. *Family and Community Health, 15*(4), 57–65.

Edwards, N., Goodick, S., LeBlond, D., Asselin, G., & Mooers, W. (1993). *Social network mapping.* Paper presented at the International Conference of Community Health Nursing Research, September 1993, Edmonton.

Edwards, N., Murphy, M., Moyer, A., & Wright, A. (1995). *Building and sustaining collective health action: A framework for community health practitioners.* Ottawa: Community Health Research Unit. (Pub. No. GP95-1)

Eng, E., & Parker, E. (1994). Measuring community competence in the Mississipi Delta: The interface between program evaluation and empowerment. *Health Education Quarterly, 21*(2), 199–220.

Felson, D.T., Anderson, J.J., Hannan, M.T., Milton, R.C., Wilson, P.W., & Kiel, D.P. (1989). Impaired vision and hip fracture. *Journal of the American Geriatrics Society, 37,* 495–500.

Flick, L.H., Given Reese, C., Rogers, G., Fletcher, P., & Sonn, J. (1994). Building community for health: Lessons from a seven-year-old neighborhood/university partnership. *Health Education Quarterly, 21*(3), 369–380.

Gallagher, E.M., & Scott, V.J. (1995). *The STEPS Project: A project to reduce falls in public places among seniors and persons with disabilities.* University of Victoria, School of Nursing, Victoria.

Gecas, V. (1989). The social psychology of self-efficacy. *Annual Review of Sociology, 15,* 291–316.

Graafmans, W.C., Ooms, M.E., Hofstee, M.A., Bezemer, P.D., Bouter, L.M., & Lips, P. (1996). Falls in the elderly: A prospective study of risk factors and risk profiles. *American Journal of Epidemiology, 143*(11), 1129–1136.

Grisso, J.A., Kelsey, J.L., Strom, B.L., Chiu, G.Y., Maislin, G., O'Brien, L.A., Hoffman, S., Kaplan, F., & Northeast Hip Fracture Study Group. (1991). Risk factors for falls as a cause of hip fracture in women. *New England Journal of Medicine, 324,* 1326–1331.

Harris, E., Wise, M., Hawe, P., Finlay, P., & Nutbeam, D. (1995). *Working together: Intersectoral action for health.* Sydney: National Centre for Health Promotion.

Hastings, G., & Haywood, A. (1991). Social marketing and communication in health promotion. *Health Promotion International, 6*(2), 135–145.

Health Canada. (1994). *Injuries and seniors: The Canadian context.* Ottawa: Minister of Supply & Services Canada. (Cat. No. H49-89)

Health Canada. (1997). *The safe living guide: A guide to home safety for seniors.* Ottawa. Minister of Public Works & Government Services.

Heslin, K., Towers, J., Leckie, C., Thornton-Lawrence, H., Perkin, K., Jacques, M., Mullin, J., & Wick, L. (1992). Managing falls: Identifying population-specific risk factors and prevention strategies. In S.G. Funk, E.M. Tornquist, S. Hotz, J. Allston, N. Birkett, B. Baskerville, & G. Dunkley. (Eds.) (1995), Fat-related dietary behaviour: Behavioural science concepts for public health practice. *Canadian Journal of Public Health, 86*(2), 114–119.

Kellogg International Work Group on the Prevention of Falls by Elderly. (1987). The prevention of falls in later life. *Danish Medical Bulletin, 34* (Suppl. 4), 1–24.

Kirscht, J.P. (1989). Process and measurement issues in health risk appraisal. *American Journal of Public Health, 79,* 1598–1599.

Lacey, L., Tukes, S., Manfredi, C., & Wanecke, R.B. (1991). Use of lay health educators for smoking cessation in a hard-to-reach urban community. *Journal of Community Health, 16*(5), 269–282.

Lefebvre, R.C., Lasater, T.M., Carleton, R.A., & Peterson, G. (1987). Theory of delivery of health programming in the community: The Pawtucket Heart Health Program. *Preventive Medicine, 16,* 80–95.

Lord, S.R., Ward, J.A., Williams, P., & Anstey, K.J. (1993). An epidemiological study of falls in older community-dwelling women: The Randwick falls and fracture study. *Australian Journal of Public Health, 17*(3), 240–245.

Lord, S.R., & Webster, I.W. (1990). Visual field dependence in elderly fallers and non-fallers. *International Journal of Aging and Human Development, 31,* 267–277.

Love, M.B., Gardner, K., & Legion, V. (1997). Community health workers: Who they are and what they do. *Health Education & Behavior, 24*(4), 510–522.

Luukinen, H., Koski, K., Hiltunen, L., & Kivela, S.L. (1994). Incidence rate of falls in an aged population in Northern Finland. *Journal of Clinical Epidemiology, 47*(8), 843–850.

Luukinen, H., Koski, K., Laippala, P., & Kivela, S.L. (1995). Predictors of recurrent falls among the home dwelling elderly. *Scandinavian Journal of Primary Health Care, 13,* 294–299.

Marcus, B.H., Rakowski, W., & Rossi, J.S. (1992). Assessing motivational readiness and decision-making for exercise. *Health Psychology, 11*(4), 257–261.

Marcus, B.H., Rossi, J.S., Selby, V.C., Niaura, R.S., & Abrams, D.B. (1992). The stages and processes of exercise adoption and maintenance in a worksite sample. *Health Psychology, 11*(6), 386–395.

Melton, L.J., Ilstrup, D.M., Riggs, B.L., & Beckenbaugh, R.D. (1982). Fifty-year trend in hip fracture incidence. *Clinical Orthopedics, 162,* 144–149.

Minkler, M. (1992). Community organizing among the elderly poor in the United States: A case study. *International Journal of Health Services, 22*(2), 303–316.

Morse, J.M., Morse, R.M., & Tylko, S.J. (1989). Development of a scale to identify the fall-prone patient. *Canadian Journal on Aging, 8,* 366–377.

Moyer, A., Aminzadeh, F., & Edwards, N. (1998). *Falls in Later Life.* Ottawa: Community Health Research Unit. (Pub. No. M98-2)

Neuman, B. (1982). *The Neuman systems model.* Norwalk, CT: Appleton-Century-Crofts.

Nevitt, M.C., Cummings, S.R., & Hudes, E.S. (1991). Risk factors for injurious falls: A prospective study. *Journal of Gerontology, 46*(5), M164–M170.

Nevitt, M.C., Cummings, S.R., Kidd, S., & Black, D. (1989). Risk factors for recurrent nonsyncopal falls. *Journal of the American Medical Association, 261,* 2663–2668.

Nickens, H. (1985). Intrinsic factors in falling among the elderly. *Archives of Internal Medicine, 145,* 1089–1093.

O'Loughlin, J. (1991). *The incidence and risk factors for falls and fall-related injury among elderly persons living in the community.* Unpublished PhD dissertation, McGill University, Montréal.

O'Loughlin, J., Boivin, J.F., Robitaille, Y., & Suissa, S. (1994). Distinguishing risk factors for indoor and outdoor falls among the elderly: Implications for research designs. *Journal of Epidemiology & Community Health, 48,* 488–489

O'Loughlin, J., & Robitaille, Y. (1991). Les traumatismes dus aux chutes: Les chutes chez les personnes agées. In Gouvernement du Québec, *Les Traumatismes au Québec: Comprendre pour prévenir.* Québec: Les publications du Québec.

O'Loughlin, J., Robitaille, Y., Boivin, J.F., & Suissa, S. (1991). Incidence and risk factors for falls and injurious falls among the community living elderly. *American Journal of Epidemiology, 137,* 342–354.

Orlando, T.E. (1988). *The meaning of falling for elderly community-dwelling individuals.* Unpublished master's thesis, University of British Columbia.

Oster, G., Huse, D.M., Abrams, S.F., Imbimbo, J., & Russel, M.W. (1990). Benzodiazepine tranquilizers and the risk of accidental injury. *American Journal of Public Health, 80,* 1467–1470.

Pauls, J.L. (1998). Benefit–cost analysis and housing affordability: The case of stairway usability, safety, design and related requirements and guidelines for new and existing (pp. 21–38). *Proceedings of 1998 Pacific Rim Conference of Building Officials, Maui, Hawaii.*

Ploeg, J., Black, M.E., Hutchison, B.G., Walter, S.D., Scott, F., & Chambers, L.W. (1994). Personal, home and community safety promotion with community-dwelling elderly persons: Response to a public health nurse intervention. *Canadian Journal of Public Health, 85*(3), 188–191.

Prochaska, J.O. (1991). Assessing how people change. *Cancer, 67*(3), 805–807.

Prochaska, J.O., Redding, C.A., & Evers, K.E. (1997). The transtheoretical model and stages of change. In K. Glanz, F.M. Lewis, & B.K. Rimer (Eds.), *Health behavior and health education* (2nd ed.). San Francisco: Jossey-Bass.

Prochaska, J.O., Velicer, W.F., Rossi, J.S., Goldstein, M.G., Marcus, B.H., Rakowski, W., Fiore, C., Harlow, L.L., Redding, C.A., Rosenbloom, D., & Rossi, S.R. (1994). Stages of change and decisional balance for 12 problem behaviours. *Health Psychology, 13*(1), 39–46.

Rakowski, W., Dubé, C., Marcus, B.H., Prochaska, J.O., Velicer, W.F., & Abrams, D.B. (1992). Assessing elements of women's decisions about mammography. *Health Psychology, 11*, 111–118.

Raina, P., & Torrance, V. (1995). *Injury mortality and morbidity in Canadian seniors 1979–1991.* Unpublished Report, Division of Aging-Related Diseases, LCDC, Bureau of Cancer, Health Canada, Ottawa.

Riley, R. (1992). Accidental falls and injuries among seniors. *Health Reports* (Statistics Canada), 4(4), 341–354.

Rogers, E.M. (1995). *Diffusion of innovations* (4th ed). New York: The Free Press.

Sattin, R.W., Lambert Huber, D.A., DeVito, C.A., Rodriguez, J.G., Ros, A., Bacchelli, S., Stevens, J.A., & Waxweiler, R.J. (1990). The incidence of fall injury events among the elderly in a defined population. *American Journal of Epidemiology, 131*, 1028–1037.

Scott, V., & Gallagher, E. (1997). The epidemiology of fall-related injuries among older persons in British Columbia: Implications for prevention. *B.C. Health and Disease Surveillance, 6*(8/9), 94–106.

Smallegan, M. (1983). How families decide on nursing home admission. *Geriatric Consultant, 1*(5), 21–24.

Sorock, G.S. (1988). Falls among the elderly: Epidemiology and prevention. *American Journal of Preventive Medicine, 4*, 282–288.

Sorock, G.S., & Labiner, D.M. (1992). Peripheral neuromuscular dysfunction and falls in an elderly cohort. *American Journal of Epidemiology, 136*(5), 583–591.

Speechley, M., & Tinetti, M. (1991). Falls and injuries in frail and vigorous community elderly persons. *Journal of American Geriatrics Society, 39*(1), 46–52.

Spellbring, A.M. (1992). Assessing elderly patients at high risk for falls: A reliability study. *Journal of Nursing Care Quality, 6*(3), 30–35.

Svensson, M.L., Rundgren, A., & Landahl, S. (1992). Falls in 84- to 85-year-old people living at home. *Accident Analysis & Prevention, 24*(5), 527–537.

Thompson, B., Corbett, K., Barcht, N., & Pechacek, T. (1993). Community mobilization for smoking cessation: Lessons learned from COMMIT. *Health Promotion International, 8*(2), 69–83.

Tideiksaar, R. (1997). *Falling in old age: Prevention and management* (2nd ed.) New York: Springer.

Tinetti, M.E., Baker, D.I., McAvay, G., Claus, E.B., Garrett, P., Gottschalk, M., Koch, M.L., Trainor, K., & Horwitz, R.I. (1994). A multifactorial intervention to reduce the risk of falling among elderly people living in the community. *New England Journal of Medicine, 331*(13), 821–827.

Tinetti, M.E., Doucette, J., Claus, E., & Marottoli, R. (1995). Risk factors for serious injury during falls by older persons in the community. *Journal of American Geriatric Society, 43*(11), 1214–1221.

Tinetti, M.E., Speechley, M., & Ginter, S.F. (1988). Risk factors for falls among elderly persons living in the community. *New England Journal of Medicine, 319*(26), 1701–1707.

Tinetti, M.E., Williams, T.F., & Mayewski, R. (1986). Fall risk index for elderly patients based on number of chronic disabilities. *American Journal of Medicine, 80,* 429–434.

Tobis, J.S., Block, M., Steinhaus-Donham, C., Reinsch, S., Tamaru, K., & Weil, D. (1990). Falling among the sensorially impaired elderly. *Archives of Physical Medicine and Rehabilitation, 71,* 144–147.

Vellas, C.F., Bocquet, H., dePemille, F., & Albarede, J.L. (1987). Prospective study of restriction in activity in old people after falls. *Age and Ageing, 16,* 189–193.

Wagner, E.H., LaCroix, A.Z., Grothaus, L., Leveille, S.G., Hecht, J.A., Artz, K., Odle, K., & Buchner, D.M. (1994). Preventing disability and falls in older adults: A population-based randomized trial. *American Journal of Public Health, 84*(11), 1800–1806.

Wallerstein, N. (1993). Empowerment and health: The theory and practice of community change. *Community Development Journal, 28*(3), 218–227.

Wells, B.L., DePue, J.D., Buehler, C.J., Lasater, T.M., & Carleton, R.A. (1990). Characteristics of volunteers who deliver health education and promotion: A comparison with organization members and program participants. *Health Education Quarterly, 17*(1), 23–35.

Wickham, C., Cooper, C., Margetts, B.M., & Barker, D.J.P. (1989). Muscle strength, activity, housing and the risk of falls in elderly people. *Age and Ageing, 18,* 47–51.

Wills, E.M. (1996). Nurse–client alliance: A pattern at home health caring. *Home Healthcare Nurse, 14*(6), 455–459

CHAPTER 16

Linking health promotion and community health nursing: Conceptual and practical issues

Clémence Dallaire, Louise Hagan, and Michel O'Neill

In theory, community health nursing and health promotion seem inextricably intertwined, but in practice Canadian nurses have not been particularly involved in health promotion strategies. This chapter provides a brief overview of the evolution of health promotion in recent years and identifies some of its key concepts. As an example of health promotion, the practice of health education by community health nurses is described, drawing on an extensive study of nurses practising in Québec's Local Community Services Centres. The chapter concludes with an examination of why nursing has not been more influential in Canadian health promotion and of the challenges that need to be addressed.

LEARNING OBJECTIVES

In this chapter, you will learn:

- a brief overview of the evolution of health promotion in recent years
- some key concepts of health promotion
- how nursing and health promotion intertwine conceptually
- an example of the practice of health education by community health nurses, drawing on an extensive study of nurses practising in Québec's Local Community Services Centres
- why nursing has not been more influential in Canadian health promotion
- the challenges that need to be addressed

Introduction

Nursing, despite its potential to be a key player in health promotion (Meleis, 1990; Novak, 1988; Pender, 1990; Smith, 1990), has not taken an influential role in this movement (Gottlieb, 1992; O'Neill, 1997). Health promotion has evolved rapidly nationally and internationally, especially since the mid-1970s, and Canada has been at the forefront of this evolution. Canadian nurses, however, have not been extensively involved.

In this chapter, after a brief review of the history of the movement, we will address the link between nursing and health promotion in two ways. At the theoretical level, we explore how nursing and health promotion intertwine conceptually, examining how key nursing authors address some of the main concepts in health promotion. We then look at the practice of health education by community health nurses as an example of health promotion practice and refer to a specific study (Hagan, 1991) of Québec nurses practising in Centres locaux de services communautaires (CLSCs), the local community services centres that provide Primary Health Care services throughout the province of Québec. Finally, we explore why nursing has not been more influential in Canadian health promotion and discuss future challenges.

Historical turning points in health promotion

The recent history of health promotion, both internationally and in Canada, has been extensively explored elsewhere (Pederson, O'Neill, & Rootman, 1994). Health promotion emerged from two different streams. On the one hand, health education, focussing mainly on the voluntary alteration of individual health-related behaviours, was inspired mostly by American social psychologists beginning about the 1940s. On the other hand, the World Health Organization (WHO) Health for All movement, launched at the end of the 1970s by such ground-breaking events as the World Health Assembly's resolution on Health for All in 1977 and the Alma Ata conference in 1978, proposed a more social and political vision of health promotion than was promoted mainly by European and Canadian authors (O'Neill & Pederson, 1994).

Around the middle of the 1980s, these two streams merged and a new, widely disseminated vision of health promotion, in which individual and social change are intimately linked, resulted. Indeed, the watershed year is usually identified as 1986, when the first international conference on health promotion was held and the renowned *Ottawa Charter for Health Promotion* (World Health Organization [WHO], Health & Welfare Canada [HWC], & Canadian Public Health Association [CPHA], 1986) was adopted. It is not by chance that these events occurred in Canada, and that the Ottawa Charter is now internationally known and respected (Labonte, 1994; Raeburn, 1994).

The Lalonde report, released in 1974 under the title *A New Perspective on the Health of Canadians* (Lalonde, 1974), caused Canada to be seen internationally as the forerunner in health promotion and to be imitated by the rest of the world (Green & Kreuter, 1991; Kickbusch, 1986; Raeburn, 1994). Moreover, at the end of the Ottawa conference, another ground-breaking document was released by then federal minister of Health and Welfare Jake Epp (1986), which offered Canada a framework to put health promotion into practice.

Health promotion: The difficulty of definitions

In the second edition of their authoritative book, Green and Kreuter (1991) define health promotion as "any planned combination of educational, political, regulatory, and organizational supports for actions and conditions of living conducive to the health of individuals, groups, or communities" (p. 432). In the Ottawa Charter (WHO et al., 1986), it is defined as "the process of enabling people to increase control over, and to improve, their health" (p. 1). In this definition, health is seen in a positive way—as more than the absence of illness—and as a resource for functioning on a day-to-day basis. These two definitions, from among many others, have been cited here because they are probably the best known internationally and because they exemplify how the two streams mentioned earlier have converged into a consensus on what health promotion is.

However, even if there is now an agreement within the health promotion community, this consensus has not been successfully conveyed to others (O'Neill & Cardinal, 1994). Consequently, it is unclear whether health promotion will be part of the services provided by nurses or others in the various provincial health systems, which are undergoing significant reform under the pressures of cost containment. In general, health promotion has not gained acceptance beyond the rhetoric of community health professionals, politicians, academics, and policy makers because the concept covers two different and somewhat confusing realities.

On the one hand, health promotion is a philosophy or ideology about what health is and what creates or hinders it (O'Neill & Cardinal, 1994). This vision contends not only that health is a bio-psycho-socio-cultural-spiritual concept but also that it is produced or hindered by factors or determinants that go far beyond the provision of such health services as biology, lifestyles, and the environment (Lalonde, 1974). This vision has been championed by many, including nurses. Such a vision has inspired policies, charters, and declarations for decades and is reflected in documents such as the Lalonde (1974) report, the WHO (1984) health promotion document (often referred to as the Yellow Document), the Ottawa Charter (WHO et al., 1986), the Epp (1986) framework, and the Déclaration québécoise pour la promotion de la santé (Association pour la Santé Publique du Québec [ASPQ], 1993). It is also at the core of other recent statements to reform provincial health systems. Consequently, this vision has been referred to as the "new public health"

(Ashton & Seymour, 1988; Martin & McQueen, 1989; O'Neill & Cardinal, 1994), or the "ecological public health" (Kickbusch, 1989), to reflect the fact that the health issues at the end of the 20th century are different from those of earlier times.

On the other hand, the concept of health promotion also includes a series of strategies: health education, social marketing, mass communication, political action, community organization, and organizational development. These strategies aim at the planned change of human health-related behaviours of individuals or collectives, regardless of their health status (O'Neill & Cardinal, 1994).

The question, then, is: What position does nursing take toward health promotion?

Conceptual links between nursing and health promotion

The nurse is often considered "the most visible and the most strategically placed health professional to accomplish health promotion goals with clients" (Innes & Ciliska, 1985, p. 468). We will thus first explore how nursing authors have approached health promotion conceptually. We then will analyze how health promotion has been proposed as one of the key roles in the practice of community health nurses in Canada and provide a concrete illustration.

Nursing models that incorporate health promotion

The debate concerning nursing knowledge, the kind of knowledge needed for nursing practice, and thus the kind of knowledge that needs to be elaborated to organize the practice of nurses (Meleis, 1997; Mitchell, 1994) is still raging. However, it is clear that health promotion is often addressed in the theoretical propositions of nursing authors (Kulbok, Baldwin, Cox, & Duffy, 1997; Meleis, 1992; Reed, 1997; Smith, 1990). We will look first at one of the more general models, that of Dorothea Orem (1985), which has received wide acceptance in Canada and among community health nurses in Québec (Rocheleau & Hagan, 1993) and British Columbia. We will then deal with two that are more specifically labelled health promotion models, the McGill and Pender models.

Orem's self-care nursing model is congruent with health promotion in at least two respects. First, its definition of health refers, as health promotion does, to integrity and capacity to function in a multiplicity of dimensions: mental, psychological, physiological, and social (Orem, 1985, p. 214). Second, the partnership between nurse and client suggested by Orem goes hand in hand with the enabling, mediating, and advocating roles that the Ottawa Charter (WHO et al., 1986) identifies for health promoters.

In the model developed at McGill University in Montréal (Gottlieb & Rowat, 1987), the promotion of health is identified as the expected outcome of nursing interventions. In the McGill Model, health is interpreted as a learning process, and the role of nurses is interpreted as facilitator of this process to enable people to cope with various life crises and health problems. Moreover, the McGill Model is well known for its emphasis on the family as the client instead of the person.

The health promotion model developed by Nola Pender (1984, 1987, 1990) is the nursing model that focusses most explicitly on health promotion. In this model, health is defined as "a dynamic process inherent to the life experience of individuals, families and communities" (Pender, 1987, p. 34), and health-promoting behaviours are "continuing activities that must be an integral part of an individual's life style, . . . an expression of the actualizing tendency directed toward maximizing positive arousal such as increased self-awareness, self-satisfaction, enjoyment, and pleasure" (Pender, 1987, p. 59). Pender lists seven perceptions that determine human behaviour. These beliefs in turn are influenced by the demographic, biological, and environmental characteristics of the individual; by the opinion of significant people; and by the person's past experience with the behaviour. Pender's model has been used by many researchers among them Canadian nursing researchers such as Gillis (1993) and has been critically reviewed by such Canadian authors as Hilton (1986).

A perusal of general health promotion literature from the mid-1970s to 1998 revealed no references to any of these three nursing models nor to others. One notable exception is a paper by Rootman and Raeburn (1994). As we shall discuss later, there are legitimate reasons why nursing is not fully integrated into the general field of health promotion.

Critique of nursing theoretical efforts in health promotion

From the mid-1970s, the health education field began to criticize its theoretical foundations (O'Neill & Pederson, 1994); this was mostly related to a lack of success in implementation of its programs and interventions. Two pitfalls identified in this self-critical effort can be applied to theoretical efforts of nursing to define health promotion (Dallaire & O'Neill, 1991).

The first pitfall pertains to the belief that health-related behaviour is easily altered by applying educational strategies based on linear models, such as behavioural or psycho-cognitive models. For example, a number of nursing research projects used the health belief model (Kim, Horan, Gendler, & Patel, 1991; Kulbok, Earls, & Montgomery, 1988; Lauver, 1987; Yarchesi & Mahon, 1989). Later, however, Rosenstock (1990) mentioned several recurrent critiques of the validity, the predictive power, and the utility of the health belief model. It is clear that other forces also influence health actions, as discussed by Green and Kreuter (1991).

Much nursing research, influenced by the medical model, has focussed more on providing care to sick people than promoting health (Caraher, 1994; Gallagher & Kreidler, 1987; Greiner, 1987). Moreover, despite the importance of the Primary Health Care discourse in nursing, Meleis (1990) contends that nurses have not articulated their theories to the health-promoting dimension of Primary Health Care. Clarke, Beddome, and Whyte (1993) state that nurses should develop nursing frameworks consistent with the changing goals of the health system.

The second pitfall pertains to the ways in which the environment is defined and to whether or not it is included as a legitimate focus for health promotion intervention. Indeed, one of the most important elements of the evolution of the field of health education into the field of health promotion was the recognition that the sociopolitical environment is a key factor in personal behavioural choices (Milio, 1986). The trap of blaming people who do not adopt "appropriate" behaviours, despite inadequate environmental resources, has long been denounced as useless "victim blaming" (Allison, 1982). Nevertheless, nursing models usually tend to ascribe to individuals sole responsibility for their health (Clark, 1989; Katims, 1995; Meleis, 1990; Williams, 1989). In contrast, the McGill Model recognizes the family as a legitimate focus for intervention.

The broader definitions of the environment that characterize health promotion are thus almost totally absent from nursing models. According to such nursing authors as Duffy (1988), Stevens (1989), and Meleis (1990), a broader definition of the environment is completely compatible with the holistic vision of nursing. However, only a few nursing authors argue that nurses should develop the sociopolitical skills needed to become agents of social change in the environment (Barnes et al., 1995; Baumgart, 1995; Butterfield, 1990; Clarke et al., 1993; Hagan & Proulx, 1996; White, 1995; Williams, 1989), even if this has been an increasing concern for nursing in general.

Having dealt with the theoretical links between nursing and health promotion, we will now examine what nurses do about health promotion in their practice.

The practice of health promotion by community health nurses

Since 1979, nursing has clearly taken on the mission of promoting health, especially through the Primary Health Care philosophy that is reinforced in official statements of international, national (Canadian Nurses Association, 1989), and provincial nurses' associations. Moreover, the Canadian Public Health Association/Association canadienne pour la santé publique

(CPHA/ACSP) booklet that delineates the role of community health nursing in Canada (ACSP, 1990), the criteria defining the practice of community health nurses in Québec (Ordre des infirmières et infirmiers du Québec [OIIQ], 1986), the suggestions regarding the practice of community health nurses in CLSCs (Rocheleau & Hagan, 1993), and equivalent documents in other provinces explicate the status of health promotion. For example, the CPHA/ACSP document describes the focus of community health nursing practice as "mainly health promotion, illness and injury prevention, health maintenance and community development, regardless of the settings in which the nurses work" (ACSP, 1990, p. 20; free translation). The specific role of the community health nurse in health promotion is further described as:

assists communities, families and individuals to take responsibility for maintaining and/or improving their health by increasing their knowledge of, their control over and their influence on health determinants; facilitates and mediates to enhance community, group or individual strategies that assist society to anticipate, cope with and manage maturational changes and the environment; encourages communities', families' and individuals' ability to balance individual choices with social responsibility to create a healthier future; initiates/participates in health promotion activities in partnership with others, including the community, colleagues and other sectors. (ACSP, 1990, p. 7; free translation)

However, as everyone knows, what is written in official documents does not always find its way into the day-to-day practice of nurses. Indeed, a survey (Paul, Hagan, & Lambert, 1985) conducted in 1983 of a random sample of 954 nurses (2.5 percent of the total population of francophone Québec nurses) showed that nurses had the tendency to value health promotion concepts but were less frequently implementing health promotion in their professional practice. Perhaps this situation has changed somewhat over the past 10 years, but as mentioned earlier, health promotion has not been successfully accepted beyond the rhetoric of committed academics, policy makers, and politicians.

A look at the practice of health promotion by Québec nurses working in community health settings will illustrate this point.

The practice of health promotion by nurses in Québec CLSCs

CLSCs emerged from the thorough Castonguay-Nepveu reform of Health and Welfare services in the early 1970s. Their mission, as stated in article 80 of the provincial law on health and social services (Fédération des CLSC du

Québec, 1992), is to be the primary level of care by providing health and social services in prevention, treatment, and rehabilitation. Health promotion is still only implicit. In 1994, there were 161 CLSCs in Québec in which 3897 nurses were working (OIIQ, 1994). Those CLSCs cover the 18 "socio-sanitaires" regions of the entire province.

The health education roles and activities of nurses working in CLSCs were investigated in 1989 (Hagan, 1991). The network of CLSCs then comprised over 150 organizations; there were just over 3000 nurses working in those settings. Out of the 2917 French-speaking nurses registered to the Ordre des infirmières et infirmiers du Québec working in non-managerial positions, a random sample of 1000, stratified according to the level of the first nursing degree (university or college), was drawn. A questionnaire was sent by mail. After one recall, the response rate was 68 percent. The 631 questionnaires finally used in the analysis are a statistically representative sample of nurses in CLSCs.

The questionnaire focussed mostly on health education practice. As pointed out earlier in this chapter, health education is one health promotion strategy. From that viewpoint, the study explores the extent to which educational activities encompass the broad premises of health promotion by acting on individual and environmental determinants of health behaviours and by using active and participative approaches that enable people to enhance their health. Unfortunately, the data do not document other types of health promotion strategies in which CLSC nurses could be involved to effect planned change of health behaviours, such as social marketing, mass communication, political action, community development, or organizational development.

The vast majority (89 percent) of community health nurses working in CLSCs have a humanistic vision of health education, defined as "teaching and establishing a helping relationship aimed at facilitating individuals' choices of strategies to improve or maintain their global health" (Hagan, 1991, p. 278; free translation). In general, the health education interventions by nurses are planned activities. They focus more on groups than individuals. The themes on which the interventions are based include life cycles (growth and development) (39 percent); physical health (symptoms and treatment) (35 percent); lifestyles (nutrition, smoking and drinking habits, sexual activities, etc.) (19 percent); and mental health (developmental crises, relationships, etc.)(seven percent). Forty percent of the nurses in CLSCs spent more than half their weekly working time in health education activities. Nurses working in prenatal health and school health devoted more time to health education, whereas those in occupational health and home care gave less time to it. Neither the level of training nor the experience of the nurse were associated with the time devoted to health education as a health promotion strategy (Hagan, 1991, pp. 278–282).

When planning their health education activities and choosing priorities, experience and intuition are the predominant means utilized (41 percent), with theoretical models coming from nursing or elsewhere being primarily used in 35 percent of the situations. Experience is also the major resource (81 percent) utilized to design the intervention's objectives; literature and other pertinent documents were marginally used (33 percent), mostly by school health nurses. In general, the educational methods consist of dispensing written information (54 percent), formal lectures followed by discussion (48 percent), or informal discussion (40 percent). These nurses see their role mostly as counsellor (55 percent), expert (35 percent), sponsor (24 percent), and role model (four percent). Most of them (71 percent) involve partners in their interventions, the most frequent being (in descending order) nursing colleagues, professionals of other disciplines, community resources, and the client's family.

Half the nurses said they would like to undertake other actions to improve their teaching skills and to evaluate more thoroughly what they do; very few (seven percent) mentioned that they wanted to extend health education practices beyond what they already did. The reasons preventing them from undertaking other actions were lack of time, lack of cooperation from the organization or the client, and lack of resources. Personal reasons, such as poor time management and lack of experience or training, were also mentioned as barriers to health education and health promotion practice (Hagan, 1991, pp. 290–294).

Although most nurses perceived health education as a priority, they were less convinced that it had real impact on people's behaviour. They thought, moreover, that this type of intervention was not valued by the management of their organizations. Finally, they believed that they had little power to influence the orientations of CLSCs in a direction more favourable to health promotion (Hagan, 1991, pp. 294–295). In contrast, the factors facilitating nurses' role as health promoters were the length of their working experience in CLSCs; their training; the type of program in which they were involved; and the cooperation of colleagues and the organization.

Another study (Boudreau, 1994) examines health promotion practice by nurses. In this survey of 225 Québec nurses who declared "private practice" as their main occupation in 1992, health education was found to be the most prevalent type of services they perform. Health education was reported by 61 percent of these nurses, followed by 45 percent for other types of services such as massage therapy and acupuncture (45 percent), psychological support (45 percent), or health appraisal (44 percent) (Boudreau, 1994, p. 46). This author then goes on to argue that in Québec "nursing services offered in private practice tend to be close to community health services" (Boudreau, 1994, p. 46; free translation).

Discussion: The practice of health promotion by Québec nurses

Although these two Québec studies focus only on the practice of health education as a strategy of health promotion, they probably reflect the general practice of health promotion by community health nurses. In the CLSC study, it was surprising to see that most nurses spend less than half their working time in health education. Moreover, when performing health education tasks, nurses were acting more like traditional health educators, aiming at individual behaviours in the areas of physical problems (symptoms and treatment) and life crises (e.g., parental relationship with children and adolescents, mourning) rather than targeting the environment or the health of aggregates.

Other issues can be raised from this study. First, it is interesting to see that these nurses did not use a specific theoretical framework to guide their interventions. Is this because most conceptual frameworks are not adapted to community health nursing practice? The methods nurses used are rather traditional, passive, educational strategies. Are nurses working for, rather than with, people to solve their problems? Most nurses stated that they work in teams with other health professionals. Are nurses recognizing their role as agents for change involving community resources, such as families, school teachers, leaders of community groups, and politicians? This omission, we think, indicates that nurses involve more of their own environment in their professional practice than the client's environment (such as the family and other significant people). Further, it is disheartening to realize that even if most nurses value health education, they do not believe in its effectiveness and do not think that it is a priority of their organization. Moreover, they perceive themselves as having almost no power to influence the orientations of CLSCs toward more emphasis on health promotion.

This description is most likely a faithful reflection of 1989 reality, even if the way in which this research project was conducted underestimates other types of health promotion practices, including those aimed at the environment.

In June 1994, the OIIQ's report on the practice of 4000 nurses in 161 CLSCs (OIIQ, 1994) showed that more involvement of nurses in health promotion activities was not likely to occur unless nurses defined and affirmed more assertively their specific role in that area of community health nursing practice. Indeed, according to that report, CLSCs will prioritize services for target groups, such as families experiencing complex health and social problems and those socially and economically deprived. Most nurses interviewed believed that health promotion and primary prevention activities were not going to be their main role and that they will be increasingly limited to crisis interventions or curative roles in physical care.

Conclusion

We have seen that there is a theoretical link between community health nursing and health promotion, although some aspects of the link are still problematic. The practical link shows that community health nursing, in Québec CLSCs at least, tends to be mostly associated with one of the six strategies of health promotion: health education. To our knowledge, no study in Canada or Québec provides data concerning nurses' involvement in other health promotion strategies. This is not surprising, since most nursing theoretical frameworks used to guide practice are oriented toward the individual educational role of the nurse rather than toward a broader role, such as communicator, consultant, or political actor. Moreover, as we have discussed, in both theory and practice, the contemporary health promotion notion of emphasizing the environment over the narrowly focussed lifestyle orientation of health education has not permeated the nurses' world (Butterfield, 1990). Thus, most nurses seem to avoid the more political interventions in health promotion—those that involve collective action with clients to improve their quality of living.

Despite this, we should not forget that, in Canada, some nurses have played an important role in the field of public health. Many have served as president of the Canadian Public Health Association, are publishing in its journal, and have been co-authors of papers that have deeply influenced the field of health promotion (e.g., the "mandala of health" published by Hancock and Perkins [1985] and the Labonte and Penfold [1981] critique). This is less true in Québec, where nurses have not been as visible, leaving almost exclusively to physicians and others the redefinition and reorganization of public health and health promotion practices in the current reforms that are transforming the health system.

How can we explain the paucity of nursing involvement in general health promotion debates in Québec and elsewhere in Canada? During the past two decades, since the general debate on health promotion has accelerated, nurses have devoted much energy to defining their own role in health promotion (Guyon, 1988; Hagan, 1986, 1988; Hagan & Paul, 1988; Hagan & Proulx, 1996). However, even if this is an important and legitimate endeavour, an enlargement of nursing vision is now required, similar to the shift that occurred from health education to health promotion from the mid-1970s to the mid-1980s (Green & Kreuter, 1991; O'Neill & Pederson, 1994).

The tension between desirable internal reorganization of the profession and the participation of nursing as an important player in the more general interdisciplinary scene in health promotion, or within public/community health, is real. This tension was often present in the papers and debates during the First International Conference on Community Health Nursing Research held in Edmonton in 1993 (King, Stinson, & Mills, 1993), where the key themes were health promotion and illness/injury prevention. It is clear that nurses have something specific and important to say about health promotion; for example, they bring a broad vision of health and a wealth of practice in educating clients.

In general, however, they also need, as stated by Clarke, Beddome, and Whyte (1993), to develop nursing frameworks consistent with the system's changing goals and to articulate their vision of the future. To do so, they must increase their visibility and be official partners in the debates at the political level.

Canada is probably one of the countries in the world having the greatest potential to do so today. Nurses have always made a significant contribution to the practice of health promotion and should have a more important theoretical and political contribution to the health promotion movement in Canada. The real challenge thus lies ahead. The major issue is power, and how the relative position of nursing in society will affect nurses' actions (Dallaire, O'Neill, & Lessard, 1994).

QUESTIONS

1. What has been the position of Canada in the international development of health promotion?
2. Has nursing been a major player in the theoretical development of health promotion? Why or why not?
3. What are the six strategies in health promotion? In which one have nurses developed significant expertise?
4. Do you think that nurses, as suggested by the new health promotion rhetoric, should become more politically active in altering the environment? If so, how?

REFERENCES

Allison, K. (1982). Health education: Self responsibility vs. blaming the victim. *Health Education, 20*(3/4), 11–13.

Ashton, J., & Seymour, H. (1988). *The new public health.* Buckingham, UK: Open University Press.

Association canadienne pour la santé publique (ACSP). (1990). *Fonctions et compétences des infirmières et infirmiers de santé communautaire/santé publique.* Ottawa: Author.

Association pour la Santé Publique du Québec (ASPQ). (1993). *Déclaration québécoise pour la promotion de la santé.* Montréal: Author.

Barnes, D., Eribes, C., Juarbe, T., Nelson, M., Proctor, S., Sawyer, L., Shaul, M., & Meleis, A.I. (1995). Primary health care and primary care: A confusion of philosophies. *Nursing Outlook, 43,* 7–16.

Baumgart, A.J. (1995). Afterword. In M.J. Stewart (Ed.), *Community nursing: Promoting Canadians' health* (pp. 789–792). Toronto: W.B. Saunders.

Boudreau, M. (1994). *Portrait des infirmières exerçant en pratique privée au Québec.* Unpublished master's in nursing thesis, Université Laval, Québec.

Butterfield, P.G. (1990). Thinking upstream: Nurturing a conceptual understanding of the societal context of health behavior. *Advances in Nursing Science, 12*(2), 1–8.

Canadian Nurses Association. (1989). *Position statement on nurses' role in Primary Health Care.* Ottawa: Author.

Caraher, M. (1994). A sociological approach to health promotion for nurses in an institutional setting. *Journal of Advanced Nursing, 20,* 544–551.

Clark, P.G. (1989). The philosophical foundation of empowerment. *Journal of Aging and Health, 1*(3), 267–286.

Clarke, H.F., Beddome, G., & Whyte, N.B. (1993). Public health nurses' vision of their future reflects changing paradigms. *Image: Journal of Nursing Scholarship, 25*(4), 311–348.

Dallaire, C., & O'Neill, M. (1991). *Towards a wider approach to lifestyles research and increased participation of nursing in interdisciplinary health promotion research.* Paper presented at the Nursing Section of the Learned Societies Conference, Kingston, ON.

Dallaire, C., O'Neill, M., & Lessard, C. (1994). Les Enjeux pour la profession infirmière. In V. Lemieux, P. Bergeron, C. Bégin, & G. Bélanger (Eds.), *Le Système de santé au Québec: Organisations, acteurs, enjeux* (pp. 245–266). Québec: Presses de l'Université Laval.

Duffy, M.E. (1988). Health promotion in the family: Current findings and directives for nursing research. *Journal of Advanced Nursing, 13,* 109–117.

Epp, J. (1986). *La Santé pour tous: Plan d'ensemble pour la promotion de la santé.* Ottawa: Ministère de la santé nationale et du bien-être social.

Fédération des CLSC du Québec. (1992). *Les Services infirmiers en CLSC: Document de réflexion.* Montréal: Author.

Gallagher, L.P., & Kreidler, M.C. (1987). Nursing and health promotion. In L.P. Gallagher & M.C. Kreidler (Eds.), *Nursing and health: Maximizing human potential throughout the life cycle* (pp. 45–71). Norwalk, CT: Appleton & Lange.

Gillis, A.J. (1993). The relationship of definition of health, perceived health status, self-efficacy, parental health-promoting lifestyle, and selected demographics to health-promoting lifestyle in adolescent families. (Doctoral dissertation, University of Texas at Austin). *Dissertation Abstracts International, 54*(5), 2439–2449.

Gottlieb, L. (1992). Nurses not heard in the health promotion movement. *Canadian Journal of Nursing Research, 24*(4), 1–2.

Gottlieb, L., & Rowat, K. (1987). The McGill model of nursing: A practice derived model. *Advances in Nursing Science, 9*(4), 51–61.

Green, L.W., & Kreuter, M.W. (1991). *Health promotion planning: An educational and environmental approach.* Mountain View, CA: Mayfield.

Greiner, P.A. (1987). Nursing and worksite wellness: Missing the boat. *Holistic Nursing Practice, 2*(1), 53–60.

Guyon, L. (1988). Prévention et promotion de la santé: Les jeux sont-ils faits pour la profession infirmière? *Nursing Québec, 8*(1), 35–40.

Hagan, L. (1986). La Promotion de la santé: Á nous de jouer. *Nursing Québec, 6*(5), 6–12.

Hagan, L. (1988). L'Éducation pour la santé. *Santé et Société, 2,* 41–56.

Hagan, L. (1991). *Analyse de l'exercice de la fonction éducative des infirmiers et des infirmières des Centres locaux de services communautaires du Québec.* Unpublished doctoral dissertation, Faculty of Education Sciences, Université de Montréal.

Hagan, L., & Paul, D. (1988). La Promotion de la santé mentale: Du concept à l'action. *Nursing Québec, 8*(1), 13–18.

Hagan, L., & Proulx, S. (1996). L'Éducation pour la santé. Le temps d'agir. *L'Infirmière du Québec, 3*(3), 44–52.

Hancock, T., & Perkins, F. (1985). The mandala of health—A conceptual model and teaching tool. *Health Education, 24*(1), 8–10.

Hilton, A. (1986). Analysis of Pender's health-promotion behaviour model. *Nursing Papers/Perspectives en Nursing, 18*(1), 57–66.

Innes, J., & Ciliska, D. (1985). Health promotion strategies. In M. Stewart, J. Innes, S. Searl, & C. Smillie (Eds.), *Community health nursing in Canada* (pp. 462–495). Toronto: Gage.

Katims, I. (1995). The contrary ideals of individualism and nursing value of care. *Scholarly Inquiry for Nursing Practice, 9*(3), 231–244.

Kickbusch, I. (1986). Health promotion: A global perspective. *Canadian Journal of Public Health, 77,* 321–326.

Kickbusch, I. (1989). *Good planets are hard to find* (WHO Healthy Cities Papers No. 5). Copenhagen: FADL Publishers.

Kim, K.K., Horan, M.L., Gendler, P., & Patel, M.K. (1991). Development and evaluation of the osteoporosis health belief scale. *Research in Nursing & Health, 14,* 155–163.

King, M., Stinson, S., & Mills, K. (1993). *First international conference on community health nursing research: Health promotion, illness and injury prevention.* Edmonton: Edmonton Board of Health.

Kulbok, P.A., Baldwin, J.H., Cox, C.L., & Duffy, R. (1997). Advancing discourse on health promotion: Beyond mainstream thinking. *Advances in Nursing Sciences, 20*(1), 12–20.

Kulbok, P.P., Earls, F., & Montgomery, A.C. (1988). Lifestyle and patterns of health and social behavior in high-risk adolescents. *Advances in Nursing Science, 11*(1), 22–35.

Labonte, R. (1994). Death of program, birth of metaphor: The development of health promotion in Canada. In A.P. Pederson, M. O'Neill, & I. Rootman (Eds.), *Health promotion in Canada* (pp. 72–91). Toronto: W.B. Saunders.

Labonte, R., & Penfold, S. (1981, avril). Analyse critique des perspectives canadiennes en promotion de la santé. *Education Sanitaire,* 4–15.

Lalonde, M. (1974). *A new perspective on the health of Canadians.* Ottawa: Ministry of Supply & Services.

Lauver, D. (1987). Theoretical perspectives relevant to breast self-examination. *Advances in Nursing Science, 9*(4), 16–24.

Martin, C., & McQueen, D., (Eds.). (1989). *Readings for a new public health*. Edinburgh: University of Edinburgh Press.

Meleis, I.A. (1990). Being and becoming healthy: The core of nursing knowledge. *Nursing Science Quarterly, 3*(2), 107–114.

Meleis, I.A. (1992). Directions for nursing theory development in the 21st century. *Nursing Science Quarterly, 5*(3), 112–117.

Meleis, I.A. (1997). *Theoretical nursing: Development and progress* (3rd ed). Philadelphia: J.B. Lippincott.

Milio, N. (1986). *Promoting health through public policy* (2nd ed.). Ottawa: Canadian Public Health Association.

Mitchell, G. (1994). Discipline-specific inquiry: The hermeneutics of theory-guided nursing research. *Nursing Outlook, 42*, 224–228.

Novak, J.C. (1988). The social mandate and historical basis for nursing's role in health promotion. *Journal of Professional Nursing, 4*(2), 80–87.

O'Neill, M. (1997). Discourse. Health promotion: Issues for the year 2000. *Canadian Journal of Nursing Research, 29*(1), 71–77.

O'Neill, M., & Cardinal, L. (1994). Health promotion in Québec: Did it ever catch on? In A.P. Pederson, M. O'Neill, & I. Rootman (Eds.), *Health promotion in Canada* (pp 244–262). Toronto: W.B. Saunders.

O'Neill, M., & Pederson, A.P. (1994). Two analytic paths for understanding Canadian developments. In A.P. Pederson, M. O'Neill, & I. Rootman (Eds.), *Health promotion in Canada* (pp. 40–56). Toronto: W.B. Saunders.

Ordre des infirmières et infirmiers du Québec (OIIQ). (1986). *Normes et critères de compétence des infirmières et infirmiers en santé communautaire du Québec*. Montréal: Author.

Ordre des infirmières et infirmiers du Québec (OIIQ). (1994). *L'Exercice infirmier en CLSC: Constats et recommandations*. Montréal: Author.

Orem, D. (1985). *Nursing concepts and practice* (3rd ed.). New York: McGraw-Hill.

Paul, D., Hagan, L., & Lambert, J. (1985). *Étude descriptive des attitudes et comportements des infirmiers(ères) du Québec à l'égard de l'orientation globale de la santé et des facteurs associés à ces attitudes et comportements* (Rapport de recherche CQRS RS-655 582). Sherbrooke, Québec: Department des sciences infirmières, Université de Sherbrooke.

Pederson, A.P., O'Neill, M., & Rootman, I. (Eds.). (1994). *Health promotion in Canada: Provincial, national and international perspectives*. Toronto: W.B. Saunders.

Pender, N.J. (1984). Health promotion and illness prevention. *Annual Review of Nursing Research, 2*(2), 83–105.

Pender, N.J. (1987). *Health promotion in nursing practice* (2nd ed.). East Norwalk, CT: Appleton & Lange.

Pender, N.J. (1990). Expressing health through lifestyle patterns. *Nursing Science Quarterly, 3*(2), 115–122.

Raeburn, J.M. (1994). The view from down under: The impact of Canadian health promotion on developments in New Zealand. In A.P. Pederson, M. O'Neill, & I. Rootman (Eds.), *Health promotion in Canada* (pp. 327–334). Toronto: W.B. Saunders.

Reed, P.G. (1997). Nursing: The ontology of the discipline. *Nursing Science Quarterly, 10*(2), 76–79.

Rocheleau, L., & Hagan, L. (1993). Le point sur les orientations de la pratique des soins infirmiers en CLSC. *Nursing Québec, 13*(3), 40–46.

Rootman, I., & Raeburn, J.M. (1994). The concept of health. In A.P. Pederson, M. O'Neill, & I. Rootman (Eds.), *Health promotion in Canada* (pp. 56–71). Toronto: W.B. Saunders.

Rosenstock, I.A. (1990). The health belief model: Explaining health behavior through expectancies. In K. Mauz, F.M. Levis, & B.K. Rimer (Eds.), *Health behavior and health education: Theory, research and practice* (pp. 39–63). San Francisco: Jossey-Bass.

Smith, M.C. (1990). Nursing's unique focus on health promotion. *Nursing Science Quarterly, 3*(2), 105–106.

Stevens, P. (1989). A critical social reconceptualization of environment in nursing: Implications for methodology. *Advances in Nursing Science, 11*(4), 56–68.

White, J. (1995). Patterns of knowing: Review, critique, and update. *Advances in Nursing Science. 17*(4), 73–86.

Williams, D.M. (1989). Political theory and individualistic health promotion. *Advances in Nursing Science, 12*(1), 14–25.

World Health Organization (WHO). (1984). *Health promotion, a discussion document on the concept and principles.* Copenhagen: WHO Regional Office for Europe. (Document ICP/HSR 602 [no. 1])

World Health Organization (WHO), Health and Welfare Canada (HWC), & Canadian Public Health Association (CPHA). (1986). *Ottawa charter for health promotion.* Ottawa: Canadian Public Health Association.

Yarchesi, A., & Mahon, N.E. (1989). A causal model of positive health practices: The relationship between approach and replication. *Nursing Research, 38*(2), 88–93.

C H A P T E R   1 7

Role in injury prevention

Marjorie E. Linwood and Lucy D. Willis

*The Canadian community health nurse is becoming more aware of the critical prob-
lems evolving from injuries. While injuries have been a constant in society for hundreds of years, they have become more evident to the public through collection and
dissemination of statistics by the media. Community health nurses, collectively and
individually, play a major role in dealing with this problem. The historical development of injury control, a scientific basis for plans, and practical strategies for action
are discussed.*

LEARNING OBJECTIVES

In this chapter, you will learn:

- a brief history of injury prevention programs, internationally and in
  Canada
- how the principles of Primary Health Care and epidemiology guide the
  work of community health nurses in injury prevention
- an action plan for incorporating theoretical premises of injury prevention into community nursing practice

Introduction

Illness and injury prevention are important facets in the worldwide campaign of Health for All by the Year 2000. Prevention was identified as one
means of implementing Primary Health Care in 1978 (World Health
Organization [WHO], 1978) (see also Chapters 2 and 3). Historically, community health nurses have been committed to the principles of prevention
(Mosby, 1938).

Worldwide recognition of the problem has stimulated four international
conferences on injury control. The First World Conference on Accident and
Injury Prevention, held in Stockholm in September 1989, attracted about

400 registrants from around the world. At this conference, the following man-
ifesto was adopted:

The prevention of childhood injuries should receive priority emphasis in the development of programs to prevent and to control accidents and injuries. Childhood
injuries are closely related to stages of development and prevention strategies must
take into account these developmental stages. (Swedish National Child
Environmental Council, 1989, p. 67, addendum)

At the Second World Conference on Injury Prevention, held in Atlanta,
Georgia in 1993, over 1300 delegates from more than 70 countries again
brought to the world's attention the injury problem and the urgent need for
action. Injury control was by then recognized as a worldwide movement. At
the Atlanta conference, the International Society for Child and Adolescent
Injury Prevention (ISCAIP) was established. Membership is worldwide.
Through use of the Internet, members are able to communicate to discuss
common injury problems. In addition, members receive the *Injury Prevention
Journal*, which is published quarterly. This excellent international journal
reports on current research on reducing the number and severity of injuries
to children and adolescents. It is the only journal focussed entirely on injury
prevention and is both practical and useful for community health nurses.

Canada is the eighth highest among 18 industrialized countries in the rate
of occurrence of accidental deaths. Injuries are the leading cause of death of
Canadians in the first two decades of life. Injuries are the leading cause of
death of persons between one year and young adulthood (Statistics Canada,
1991a). The mortality rates and risks of injury are much higher for
Aboriginals (MacWilliam, Mao, Nicholls, & Wigle, 1987; Saskatchewan Vital
Statistics, 1988). The disabilities that result from injuries affect families,
employers, health care systems, and the immediate community. Overall, the
economic cost to Canadians is estimated at $11 billion per year (Wigle, Mao,
Wong, & Lane, 1991). In Canada, injuries account for more deaths than any
other cause up to the 44th year of life (WHO, 1991). This public health problem needs attention from the health system.

Health promotion should be a major focus of community health nurses,
who live and practise within the community setting (Kendrick, Marsh, &
Williams, 1995; Knox, 1994). The community health nurse will need to
involve the public in recognition and development of responsibility for self-
care with respect to injury control.

Despite extensive knowledge, tools, and access to the public through the
mass media, most efforts of health care workers and most health care dollars
are expended on curative rather than preventive interventions (Linwood &
Willis, 1988). Unfortunately, preventive measures do not attract media attention. Yet, preventive medicine and community health nursing have the
potential for serving large numbers of the population for a fraction of the cost

of curative care, with the added bonus of eventually reducing the need for many costly curative measures (Hellberg, 1988).

To understand injury control, community health nurses need to understand the history associated with this major public health problem. The development of a framework to guide community health nursing practice in injury prevention programs is essential. This chapter will look first at the development of injury prevention, internationally and in Canada. Then, the integration of two theoretical premises, based on Primary Health Care and epidemiologic principles (using Haddon's Matrix), together with their reflection in professional nursing roles, will be discussed. The chapter will conclude with a plan for action to show how community health nurses can combine theoretical premises within a practice framework.

International development of injury prevention programs

The World Health Organization, cognizant of the high worldwide death rates and illness from injuries, has investigated and promoted preventive programs around the world (WHO, 1986). European countries have proven to be the most efficacious in injury prevention. Sweden has experienced a marked reduction in child and youth injuries and deaths as a result of comprehensive collection of data on all injuries, identification of problem groups, planned interventions, and evaluation. It ranked first in a group of 18 industrialized nations in reducing childhood death through programs aimed at injury prevention (Schelp & Svanström, 1996; WHO, 1990). Other Nordic countries have emulated the Swedish model. The Finns, Norwegians, and Danes have successfully developed Child Accident Committees within their government departments. England and Wales have also had a major reduction in their accidental deaths (WHO, 1986).

Although ownership of injury control has been assured by governments of these countries, outstanding health professionals provided leadership. Ragmar Berfenstam, a pediatrician from Sweden, initiated and developed injury control in his country in the early 1950s and later provided his model programs for worldwide use through WHO (Berfenstam & Kohler, 1984). In Denmark, Thorsten Kruse, a pediatrician, developed prototype methods for injury data collection and shared his expertise with WHO (Kruse & Bentzen, 1993). Johan Lunde created the Norwegian Safe Communities programs (Hoff & Lunde, 1993). In the United Kingdom, Hugh Jackson (Jackson, 1993) and Michael Hayes provided leadership in the Child Accident Prevention Trust, directing the U.K. into an enviable decrease in children's deaths from injuries (Hayes & Pankhurst, 1993).

Leadership has not, until recently, been provided by community health nurses. However, the increased number registered for the Second World Conference in Injury Prevention in Atlanta, Georgia, in 1993 may reflect an increased interest in injury control by community health nurses.

The United States has developed a national plan for action (U.S. Department of Health & Human Services, 1992) to reduce injuries that has an element related to injuries that result from violence, a particular problem in that country (Novello, 1991; U.S. Department of Health & Human Services, 1992). In 1988, the Canadian homicide rate of 3.8 per 100 000 contrasted with the U.S. figure of 18 per 100 000 (WHO, 1990). Outstanding leadership in U.S. injury control has been provided by Susan Baker (Baker, 1992) and the late William Haddon (Haddon, 1980; Haddon, Suchman, & Klein, 1964).

Canadian action in injury prevention

Canada has a country-wide method of collating sound data on childhood injuries (Mackenzie, 1994). Health Canada has recognized injuries as a major health concern (Injury Awareness & Prevention Centre, 1991).

Sources of data

With the management of health care primarily in the hands of the provinces and territories, there are many similarities but some differences in provincial health care systems. One difference is in the various methods of data collection of morbidity and mortality resulting from injuries. *The International Classification of Diseases, Injuries and Causes of Death* (9th edition, 1975 revision), prepared by the World Health Organization, provides categories and subcategories of injuries (WHO, 1975). Researchers use this reference (usually referred to as the ICD document) to compare and contrast national with international data.

A major Canadian study in 1982, by the federal Department of Consumer and Corporate Affairs, Product Safety Division, Canadian Accident Injury Reporting and Evaluation (CAIRE), is an important initiation into comprehensive data collection in Canada, although it did not consistently subcategorize injuries. Since that time, the Children's Hospitals Injury Research and Prevention Program (CHIRPP) has initiated an ongoing epidemiological study (Senzilet, 1991). CHIRPP is building a computerized data bank, describing the how, when, where, and why of injuries to Canadian children, using a surveillance system of injuries reported to the emergency departments of various children's hospitals across Canada. Factors, products, or people contributing to injuries in children and youth are identified. Information is collected about safety devices, the nature of the injuries, and the outcome of treatments. This is the only Canadian source of this type of timely and valuable data. However, these data have limitations. As representative cases are recorded rather than all injuries, CHIRPP collects data only in hospital emergency departments. This practice excludes those who do not seek medical attention, those who attend a doctor's office or community clinic, those who die from injuries, those who are severely injured and bypass the emergency department, and those who receive the form but decline to complete it. Furthermore, the data come solely from the emergency departments of selected urban pediatric hospitals; anyone attending any other hospital is not counted. Accordingly, older teenagers and adults, Native peoples, and children in rural areas are excluded. As well, three provinces (New Brunswick, Prince Edward Island, and Saskatchewan) that do not have pediatric hospitals are not included in the data collection. The CHIRPP data collection strategy will soon change. All emergency departments at all hospitals within specified communities will participate. This information may facilitate identification of high-risk factors in different populations and environments, of interventions, and of appropriate evaluations (Laboratory Centre for Disease Control, Health Protection Branch, 1991; Sherman, 1994).

The Canadian Institute of Child Health (CICH), established in 1977, has focussed on improving the health of Canadian children. Their publications over the years, especially *The Health of Canada's Children: A CICH Profile*, have reported on children's health (CICH, 1989, 1994a). These profiles describe the demographics of pregnancy and birth, all child and youth age groups, Aboriginal children, and the impact of poverty. The 1994 edition also offers information on "AIDS, child sexual abuse, immunization status, life expectancy, low birth weight, low income groups, mental health, motor vehicle injuries, motor vehicle safety, newborn care, non-motor vehicle injuries, nutrition, STD, substance abuse, suicide, teenage pregnancy, weight and activity and smoking" (pp. iii–iv). For those who would like to study the data more fully, *The Health of Canada's Children: A Statistical Profile* is also available (CICH, 1994b). The statistical profile deals mostly with the shortcomings in children's health and, in addition, provides a basis for further study of injury control through the identification of particular causes of death from injuries.

Canadian plans for action

In 1991, the Injury Awareness and Prevention Centre of the University of Alberta Hospitals in Edmonton organized a national symposium to develop Injury Control Objectives for Canada for the Year 2000. The report on the symposium, *A Safer Canada: Year 2000 Injury Control Objectives for Canada* (Injury Awareness & Prevention Centre, 1991), identifies four recommendations, developed by consensus.

The first recommendation is that the federal government formally recognize that injuries are a major cause of death and disability requiring a national injury prevention strategy. The second recommendation states that six injury control goals should be adopted as a framework for a national strategy on injury prevention and control:

- *Goal 1:* reduce injury death and disability across Canada by using knowledge of what prevention interventions are most effective
- *Goal 2:* strengthen public policy regarding injury prevention by legislation that promotes a healthy, safe environment
- *Goal 3:* improve awareness and education programs in injury prevention and risk taking
- *Goal 4:* create safe environments
- *Goal 5:* decrease incidence of injuries related to alcohol and substance abuse
- *Goal 6:* improve systems of trauma care and rehabilitation

The third recommendation states that objectives developed at the national symposium be used to stimulate injury control initiatives throughout Canada at the local level. This would be achieved by awakening interest in the Injury Control Objectives for Canada by the Year 2000 by development of a National Advisory Committee on Injury Control that would guide federal, provincial/territorial, and local agencies in the implementation of strategies, and the development of provincial and territorial government committees to initiate and coordinate injury control initiatives.

The fourth recommendation states that a national surveillance system should be established to identify and to target trends.

Implementation of these recommendations has begun. In Alberta, this is being coordinated by the Injury Prevention Centre. Alberta and Saskatchewan have developed research-based injury reports to assist health workers to develop prevention strategies (Crue, 1993; Hader & Seliske, 1993; Saskatchewan Institute on Prevention of Handicaps, 1996). These data help workers to focus on specific high-risk populations in their communities. In Ontario and British Columbia, specific projects are being initiated. For example, the Child/Youth Injury Prevention Project in the Skeena Health Unit has produced its report, identifying injury, death, and hospitalization rates; patterns of injury occurrence; and increased knowledge about child and youth injuries in the northwest corner of British Columbia (Cerny & Tank, 1994).

The Aboriginal Nurses' Association of Canada and the Medical Services Branch of Health and Welfare Canada (1993) developed a curriculum for the education of community health personnel in injury prevention. This curriculum has been implemented in 14 Aboriginal communities across Canada. These three-day workshops encourage participants to share the unique characteristics of their communities. Common injury prevention strategies, modified to incorporate traditional Aboriginal beliefs, are emphasized (Campbell, 1994).

Nurses are presenting papers at conferences. For example, six papers focussed on injury control were presented at the First International Conference on Community Health Nursing Research in Edmonton in 1993. Subjects included injury surveillance, teaching injury control in academic curricula, reasons for injury, mobilization of a province in the reduction of injuries, health gains in injury prevention, and injury prevention in Aboriginal children (King, Stinson, & Mills, 1993). An exemplary paper by Ross (1993) highlighted the serious situation associated with injuries in the Canadian Aboriginal population.

In 1994, the Health Promotion Directorate of the federal government held a meeting of provincial/territorial representatives for a consultation on childhood injury prevention. Governments that identified injury prevention as a priority included British Columbia, Alberta, the Northwest Territories, Manitoba, Ontario, Québec, Newfoundland/Labrador, and Nova Scotia. A questionnaire completed by each jurisdiction elicited information on injury prevention activities. The results indicated that injury prevention is managed by a variety of governmental agencies and departments and that injury prevention plans generally focus on education, environment, and legislation.

These plans have resulted in the development and implementation of programs in collaboration with a variety of organizations and agencies. Committees coordinate the programs to reduce duplication and to identify risk areas requiring programming. In many provinces and territories, the relevant resources are clearly identified. Most have some type of evaluation process, such as a specific evaluation component for grants and for surveillance of mortality and morbidity data, or an evaluation format to be applied to all projects. Provincial funding is available in six provinces and one territory. Specific community organizations and their related injury prevention activities were noted.

Despite this increased vigilance, injuries remain the leading cause of Canadian deaths between the ages of one and 24. The years of potential life lost are phenomenal. The no-fault insurance plans for motor vehicles allow for some funding to support rehabilitation costs, such as in Ontario, Québec, Saskatchewan, and Alberta. For each fatality, there are another 45 injuries and 1300 emergency room visits ("Injury Prevention," 1989).

Theoretical premises

Theoretical premises pertinent to injury prevention provide a solid framework to guide the work of community health nurses. These are the principles of Primary Health Care (CNA, 1988; Stewart, 1992) and the epidemiologic principles (King-Collier, 1985), applied in Haddon's Matrix ("Injury

Prevention," 1989) and community health nursing roles (Linwood & Willis, 1988).

The principles of Primary Health Care that must be applied include the application of health promotion and illness and injury prevention; public participation; intersectoral and interdisciplinary collaboration; accessibility; and appropriate technology. These are discussed in other chapters of this book. Two further premises are discussed here in more detail.

Epidemiological principles

Epidemiologic principles (Kraus, 1987), applied in Haddon's Matrix, are the foundations upon which the scientific study of injury control is based. The basis of epidemiology requires a sound understanding of the history and prevention of injuries, including knowledge of the circumstances (how, when, where, and why) and conditions where they do or do not occur (see also Chapter 29). The following points represent four basic epidemiologic strategies for undertaking the study of injury control:

- observation and data collection demonstrating occurrence and distribution of risk groups
- correct interpretation and analysis of data
- rational explanation (hypothesis) leading to implementation and evaluation
- scientific construction explaining the problems.

William Haddon was the first researcher to apply scientific methods successfully to the problem of injury control ("Injury Prevention," 1989). He developed a matrix using the epidemiological approach (host, vector, physical environment, and socioeconomic environment; pre-event, event, and post-event) to study specific incidents (Table 17.1). Haddon's (1980) 10 countermeasures for injury prevention are discussed later in this chapter.

Community health nurses' resources and roles

Community health nurses require the ability to predict, a commitment to bring about change, and resources and roles that lend themselves to prevention (Linwood & Willis, 1988). Nurses need (a) to understand the illness and injury process sufficiently to be able to predict the probable outcome of certain events, (b) to become aware of sources of danger to health in the community, and (c) to learn to take steps to avoid undesirable outcomes by use of available data (Saskatchewan Vital Statistics, 1989; Statistics Canada, 1991b).

Table 17.1
Framework using the epidemiological and Haddon Matrix to assist in identification of specific links that require change

	Host (Human)	Vector	Physical Environment	Socioeconomic Environment
Pre-Event				
Event				
Post-Event				

Adapted from Haddon (1980).

Prevention is dependent on predicting injuries with certainty (Linwood & Willis, 1988). A systematic, organized approach to observation of the occurrence and distribution of injuries and identification of specific, high-risk populations or environments are essential (Linwood, Kasian, & Irvine, 1990). Community health nurses who ask questions related to injuries occurring in their communities and hypothesize answers have a sound basis for initiating and promoting injury control. Data for a particular community need to be located or collected, and the analysis should lead to an initial interpretation of the problem.

In 1994, the Family and Child Health Unit of Health Canada contracted the Injury Prevention Centre in Edmonton to prepare an annotated compendium of national and provincial/territorial sources relevant to childhood injury prevention programs. This compendium, called the *Routinely Collected Injury Data (RCID)*, provides detailed, non-technical information on the nature and availability of routinely collected data to persons who wish to develop injury prevention programs. This collection will be housed by the Injury Prevention Foundation of Toronto. It is expected to enhance the use of existing data (Family & Child Health Unit of Health Canada, 1994). As new knowledge is identified, new explanations and solutions should be developed and interventions initiated in tandem with evaluation strategies.

The Canadian federal government committed to the principle of prevention in the document *Achieving Health for All: A Framework for Health Promotion* (Epp, 1986). *Brighter Futures* is a federal action plan focussed on improving the overall status of Canadian children (Health & Welfare Canada, 1992). This action plan emerged from a 1990 World Summit for Children, where 71 countries produced strategies to improve the status of children worldwide. Children's safety is a major component of this well-funded federal plan.

The provincial/territorial governments have all recognized the need for a change of focus from hospital curative care to community health promotion. Major reviews of provincial/territorial health care systems have resulted in recommendations for change to a Primary Health Care (PHC) system (e.g., Alberta Health, 1993; Murray, 1990). Consistent with the PHC premise of intersectoral collaboration, community agencies are being encouraged to cooperate with one another to promote healthy environments and to trigger the individual's responsibility for health. For example, community health units, provincial and local safety councils, and various police forces have joined with school teachers and pupils in promotion of traffic safety.

The nursing profession emphasizes Primary Health Care premises of optimum self-care; health promotion, maintenance, and education; and promotion and preservation of the health of populations (WHO, 1978). Community health nurses, committed to injury control, can take direction from a variety of the Safer Canada Year 2000 recommendations (Injury Awareness & Prevention Centre, 1991). These recommendations can provide nurses with a basis for dealing with clients and collaborating with other health workers. The political climate now is more conducive to injury control development than at any other time in history.

Resources to assist practising community health nurses formulate, initiate, and implement the injury prevention role are becoming more accessible. The hallmark of Primary Health Care, and of any successful community venture, is public participation. Community organizations, such as national, provincial/territorial, and local safety councils, are composed of volunteers from communities. The divisions within safety councils are usually home, community, traffic, farm, and occupational. Community health nurses are becoming active participants within these divisions (Saskatchewan Safety Council, 1994).

Communities are more likely to become committed to a specific injury control venture because of some highly publicized tragedy or near tragedy, not because of well-founded statistics. A large-scale national example is the emergence of the Coalition for Gun Control, created in 1990 following the murders at l'École Polytechnique in Montréal. This coalition attempts to educate the public and sustain political pressure in favour of more regulated gun control ("Letters to Allan Rock," 1994).

Another active group that community health nurses should support is Mothers Against Drunk Driving (MADD). This is an international volunteer organization that lobbies governments to change and enforce more stringent drunk driving laws. Students Against Drunk Driving (SADD) is an active group in Canada that provides education for their peers. The Canada-wide program Prevent Alcohol and Risk-Related Trauma in Youth (PARTY) is a dynamic injury prevention program that targets students. The Safe Communities Foundation of Canada is committed to injury prevention (Kells, 1997), as is the Canadian Injury Prevention Foundation (Kingdon,

1995). Safe Kids Canada (Sidky, 1996) is a national program focussed on increasing the public's awareness of unintentional injuries. The impact of these initiatives is far-reaching to the community and to health care facilities.

Community health nurses should contribute to these voluntary groups involved in injury prevention activities. They can initiate prevention projects once needs are assessed. In collaboration with community groups and other professionals, community health nurses can identify a specific problem in the community and plan for prevention. They may examine local compendia of completed research or protocols that can be replicated (Bourgeouis, 1993; Feather, 1987; Raina, Hader, Sproat, & Feather, 1991). Insurance companies may be willing to be financial partners with volunteer groups.

Anna Lovasik, the manager of the Injury Prevention Centre, University of Alberta Hospitals, Edmonton, identified nine steps that can direct community health nurses in the development of an injury prevention program:

- Data are gathered and analyzed.
- Populations are selected and specific injuries are identified.
- Intervention strategies are selected and an intervention plan is developed.
- Community agencies, committed to injury control, implement the program.
- Protocols and materials are developed.
- Personnel are trained.
- Program is initiated.
- Program is supported and monitored.
- Program is evaluated and, if necessary, modified (Lovasik, 1994).

Other Canadian community health nurses are assuming leadership roles in injury prevention. For example, Naidene Thompson, an occupational health nurse who is the Health Services Coordinator at the head office of IPSCO Incorporated in Regina, was the 1995 chair of the Saskatchewan Safety Council. Ann Schulman, a community health nurse, is executive director of the Saskatchewan Institute on Prevention of Handicaps in Saskatoon. This organization vigorously promotes injury control and is noted for its production of injury prevention materials for the Aboriginal population (Cinépost Productions, 1990; Division of Audio Visual Services, 1994). Louise Hagel, an occupational health nurse, is a research associate and manager of the agricultural health and safety network in the College of Medicine, University of Saskatchewan, Saskatoon. She has an international reputation in agricultural safety (Hagel, 1998).

Community health nurses can be facilitators in lobbying governments to support injury control projects. Their leadership role is important for injury control interventions to be successful. Community health nurses who practise within the community setting have the advantage of direct access to clients. They will need to involve the members of the public in recognition and development of personal responsibilities for self-care. Self-care, a key component of health promotion (Epp, 1986), consists of the decisions and actions that people take to maintain or enhance their own health. Self-care can involve prevention of injuries.

Framework for a plan of action

The need for a plan of action was reinforced through the national development of the *Year 2000 Injury Control Objectives for Canada* (Injury Awareness & Prevention Centre, 1991). Community health nurses can provide the impetus to initiate local injury control programs, which should mesh with the national objectives. Data that identify high-risk groups who are likely to experience specific types of injuries should guide the community health nurse's plan of action. Any plan for injury control should be based on valid data. Although there remains a paucity of Canadian data, some sound data are available nationally, provincially/territorially, or locally. Community health and wellness clinics, local hospital records, and local coroners' and police records may provide valuable data. The data bases may be already established, such as CHIRPP and RCID, described earlier in this chapter.

The following section provides some guidelines to assist community health nurses in formulating plans for their own practices. Haddon's Matrix (see Table 17.1, page 341) and countermeasures will be used as the framework.

An injury prevention plan of action is focussed either at controlling the agent, the victim, or the environment. Controls directed at the environment are passive measures, while active measures are used to change human behaviour (Read, 1990).

Using the matrix

For every injury there is a pre-event, an event, and a post-event (see Table 17.1, p. 341).

In the *pre-event phase*, the community health nurse identifies a human (host) who may or may not demonstrate a characteristic that leads that person toward an injury. A common example in Canada is the drunk driver. This person driving a car (vector) may have a vehicle that has poor brakes or worn tires or may be speeding beyond the safe rate for driving conditions. The physical environment—for example, the road—may have many hazards, such as inadequate surfacing, poorly marked intersections, and insufficient signs. The socioeconomic environment may influence the driver's respect for speed laws, consumption of alcohol, or belief in personal risk invincibility (Health & Welfare Canada, 1990). Adolescents are particularly vulnerable to high-risk behaviours. To reduce injury in this group, the community health nurse needs to identify, assess, and teach individuals to reduce high-risk behaviours (Waxweiler, Harel, & O'Carroll, 1993).

In the *event phase*, the community health nurse would ask the police and road safety personnel if this person (host) was using a seat belt and about the presence of other safety devices. The vehicle's size and built-in safety devices could be studied. The physical environment, such as speed limits, barriers to prevent the car from going off the road, or light standards that break off easily at impact, should be evaluated. The socioeconomic environment includes support for the person's compliance or non-compliance with safety belts and adherence to the safety-belt law.

In the *post-event period*, the community health nurse identifies the age, stage of development, and general physical condition of the victim (host). The vehicle's (vector) condition following the event is evaluated. The pertinent physical environment includes the distance to travel to emergency treatment and the availability of recovery programs. The relevant socioeconomic environment involves the availability of emergency-trained personnel and the funding for health care facilities. The community health nurse may be expected to teach first aid and CPR to people in the local community. Community health nurses can lobby for well-trained rescue personnel to improve the outcome of the post-event phase.

Categorizing events or elements for any high-risk occurrence into this matrix will assist the community health nurse to identify weak links that could be altered to reduce injuries. This could include having speed limits reduced at sites where children cross a street near a school, having high fences erected along freeways, and training children to cross streets safely. Changes in environments, improved technologies, product changes, and enforceable laws are helping to prevent injuries.

Using the countermeasures

To prevent injuries, Haddon (1980) identified 10 countermeasures or strategies that may prove useful to the community health nurse:

- *Prevent the creation of a hazard.* This strategy was demonstrated recently in Canada with the passage of the law prohibiting the sale of baby walkers (Thein, Lee, Tay, & Ling, 1997). These devices had resulted in serious fall injuries. In addition, most municipalities have laws that require two-metre fences with locked gates surrounding swimming pools (Fisher & Balanda, 1997).
- *Reduce the amount of a hazard.* This countermeasure is evident in interventions reducing the capabilities of water heaters to heat water over 52°C and the installation of taps to produce temperate water that cannot cause scalding.
- *Prevent the release of a hazard that already exists.* Examples would include the safe storage of chemical wastes or application of a substance to bathtubs to make them less slippery.

- *Modify the rate or spatial distribution of the hazard.* This is illustrated by the Canadian law regarding the mandatory use of airbags in cars (Wilkins & Anderson, 1992). Other examples include the safe packaging of medications to prevent tampering and use of child car seats and seat belts.
- *Separate, in time or space, the hazard from that which is to be protected.* This strategy is used in the separation of parks from motor vehicle traffic routes, now considered the norm in most cities in Canada. Another application of this strategy is the development and use of special bicycle paths away from pedestrians and cars.
- *Separate the hazard from that which is to be protected.* Two illustrations of this strategy include covering electrical wiring with proper insulation and erecting proper barriers at excavation sites.
- *Modify relevant qualities of the hazard.* This is demonstrated in the Canadian law requiring crib slat spaces to be so narrow that no infant could get its head between the slats. Padding sharp corners on furniture or on dashboards of cars, adding handrails on stairways, and installing household nightlights in darkened traffic areas are other examples.
- *Make what is to be protected more resistant to damages from the hazard.* One application involves improving physical health and mental alertness through nutrition and exercise programs.
- *Begin to counter the damage already done by the hazard.* This strategy is reflected in improvements to rescue systems for injuries. Individuals involved with this approach may include the nurse teaching CPR and first aid to lay people.
- *Stabilize, repair, and rehabilitate the object of the damage.* This could include ensuring that acute and rehabilitative care are available to the injured person.

Basic principles

Eight principles, used in public health to control infectious diseases, can be applied to injury control by community health nurses (Read, 1990).

- *Identify the frequency and severity of injuries* that occur in a community, the risk groups, and the settings (who, when, where, why). The community health nurse can identify risk groups in the local community (Mowat, Wang, Pickett, & Brison, 1998).
- *Identify what caused the injury* and predict whether this situation is likely to happen again. The cause of the injury may be identified and research conducted to predict what, or whether, changes are required.
- *Develop and coordinate teams of people* with specific expertise regarding injury prevention. The collaboration of concerned citizens may require a facilitator. The community health nurse can perform this role, consistent

with the PHC premises of interdisciplinary collaboration and public participation.

- *Plan measures to reduce injuries.* Once the cause is identified, the collaborating agencies and individuals, including community health nurses, can intervene by altering circumstances (Health & Welfare Canada, 1990).
- *Implement measures to reduce injuries.* Community health nurses can help apply active or passive measures to alter a dangerous situation.
- *Evaluate the effectiveness of the measures* and alter if required. The evaluation process can be guided by the objectives of the project. For example, the outcome may involve reduction of injuries or changes in control measures (Green & Hart, 1998; Insurance Institute for Highway Safety, 1993).
- *Seek improvement of long-term nursing care.* The community health nurse has traditionally functioned as a facilitator, making suggestions to improve the client's family's situation through the use of community resources (Insurance Institute for Highway Safety, 1993). Teaching of injury control should be included along with other nursing measures (Kasian & Linwood, 1988).
- *Educate health workers in injury control.* Education of health workers in injury control is urgently required. Nursing educators are expanding curricula to include this significant health problem (Linwood, 1994; McLoughlin, 1997).

Conclusion

Injury control research involves identifying at-risk persons, the kinds of injuries they are likely to incur, and the most appropriate method of preventing these. Lack of up-to-date data is a barrier to the success of an injury prevention program. Well-tested interventions are rare. Research and conferences on injury control in Canada and networking of interested researchers and practitioners have increased markedly over the past decade. There is a Canadian infrastructure providing national direction; funding for injury research has increased; prevention programs are being initiated; and considerable success is reported in publications.

The need for interdisciplinary action in injury prevention and control is recognized. In this context, the number of persons trained in injury prevention needs to be increased. A wide variety of public service personnel, knowledgeable about injuries and their prevention, could collaborate in prevention projects. Community health nurses must be prepared to provide leadership in injury prevention.

QUESTIONS

1. Community health nurses need a variety of data to provide statistical information relevant to injury prevention programs. What are some sources of statistical information internationally, nationally, provincially, and locally?
2. What skills will the community health nurse require to carry out a local injury prevention project?
3. Over the past few decades the public seems to have become more aware of the serious problem of injury prevention. What factors can influence changes in people's attitudes and knowledge? Discuss the role of the community health nurse.

REFERENCES

Aboriginal Nurses' Association of Canada & Medical Services Branch of Health & Welfare Canada. (1993). *Education and training of community health personnel in injury prevention.* Ottawa: Queen's Printer.

Alberta Health. (1993). *Health goals for Alberta: Progress report.* Edmonton: Minister's Advisory Committee on Health Goals.

Baker, S. (1992). *Injury fact book* (2nd ed.). New York: Oxford University Press.

Berfenstam, R., & Kohler, L. (Eds.). (1984). *Methods and experience in planning for accident prevention.* Goteborg, Sweden: Nordic School of Public Health.

Bourgeouis, D. (1993). *Community health nursing research.* Ottawa: Health Canada.

Campbell, N. (1994, May). *Injury prevention education for community practitioners working with Aboriginal communities.* Poster and abstract presented at Injury V, Fifth Annual Injury in Alberta Conference, Edmonton.

Canadian Institute of Child Health (CICH). (1989, 1994a). *The health of Canada's children: A CICH profile.* Ottawa: Author.

Canadian Institute of Child Health (CICH). (1994b). *The health of Canada's children: A statistical profile.* Ottawa: Author.

Canadian Nurses Association (CNA). (1988). *Statement to the Special Committee of the Senate on Preventive Care.* Ottawa: Author.

Cerny, L., & Tank, S. (1994). *Child/youth injury prevention project.* Skeena, BC: Skeena Health Unit.

Cinépost Productions (Producer) & Campbell, M. (Director). (1990). *Mooshum's gift* (Videotape). Saskatoon: SGI Canada & Saskatchewan Institute on Prevention of Handicaps.

Crue, M. (1993). *Alberta data report.* Edmonton: Injury Prevention Centre.

Division of Audio Visual Services, University of Saskatchewan (Producer) & Holmlund, M. (Director). (1994). *Kookum's gift, the gift of fire* (Videotape). Saskatoon: SGI Canada & Saskatchewan Institute on Prevention of Handicaps.

Epp, J. (1986). *Achieving health for all: A framework for health promotion.* Ottawa: National Health & Welfare.

Family & Child Health Unit of Health Canada. (1994). *Routinely collected injury data (RCID)*. Ottawa: Queen's Printer.

Feather, J. (1987). *Northern Saskatchewan health research bibliography*. Saskatoon: Department of Social & Preventive Medicine, University of Saskatchewan.

Fisher, K.J., & Balanda, K.P. (1997). Caregiver factors and pool fencing: An exploratory analysis. *Injury Prevention, 3*(4), 257–261.

Green, J., & Hart, L. (1998). Children's views of accident risks and prevention: A qualitative study. *Injury Prevention, 4*(1), 14–21.

Haddon, W., Jr. (1980). Advances in the epidemiology of injuries as a basis for public policy. *Public Health Reports, 95*(5), 411–421.

Haddon, W., Jr., Suchman, E., & Klein, D. (1964). *Accident research methods and approaches*. New York: Harper & Row.

Hader, J.M., & Seliske, P. (1993). *Injuries in Saskatchewan*. Saskatoon: Department of Community Health & Epidemiology, University of Saskatchewan.

Hagel, L.M. (1998). *A descriptive study of non-fatal, unintentional injury in a rural population*. Unpublished master's thesis, University of Saskatchewan, Saskatoon.

Hayes, H.R.M., & Pankhurst, L. (1993). The safety of children in day care. In Centers for Disease Control and Prevention, *Proceedings of the Second World Conference on Injury Control* (pp. 206–207). Atlanta: Author.

Health & Welfare Canada. (1990). *The road to curb impaired driving*. Ottawa: Queen's Printer. (Cat. No. H49-41/1989E)

Health & Welfare Canada Communications Branch. (1992). *Brighter futures: Canada's action plan for children*. Ottawa: Minister of Supply & Services. (Cat. No. 74-47/1992E)

Hellberg, H. (1988, January/February). An evolving process. *World Health*, 5–9.

Hoff, S.A., & Lunde, J. (1993). A safer community handbook for local safetywork. In Centers for Disease Control and Prevention, *Proceedings of the Second World Conference on Injury Control* (p. 366). Atlanta: Author.

Injury Awareness & Prevention Centre. (1991). *A safer Canada: Year 2000 injury control objectives for Canada*. Proceedings of a symposium held in Edmonton May 21–22, 1991. Edmonton: Author.

Injury prevention: Meeting the challenge. (1989). *American Journal of Preventive Medicine, 5* (Suppl. 3), 3–303.

Insurance Institute for Highway Safety (Arlington, VA). (1993). North Carolina shows how: Belt use surges to 80 percent with enforcement. *Publicity, 28*, 14.

Jackson, H. (1993). Children at work. In Centers for Disease Control and Prevention, *Proceedings of the Second World Conference on Injury Control* (pp. 173–174). Atlanta: Author.

Kasian, G., & Linwood, M. (1988, July/August). Childproofing the home. *Contemporary Pediatrics*, 8–15.

Kells, P. (1997). A statistic of one. *Injury Prevention, 3*(4), 305–306.

Kendrick, D., Marsh, P., & Williams, E.I. (1995). How do practice nurses see their role in childhood injury prevention? *Injury Prevention, 1*(3), 159–163.

King, M., Stinson, S., & Mills, K. (1993). *Proceedings of the First International Conference on Community Health Nursing Research, Health Promotion, Illness and Injury Prevention*. Edmonton: Edmonton Board of Health.

King-Collier, M. (1985). Epidemiology: Definition and scope. In M. Stewart, J. Innes, S. Searl, & C. Smillie (Eds.), *Community health nursing in Canada*. Toronto: Gage.

Kingdon, C. (1995). Making injury prevention a top social issue: The Canadian Injury Prevention Foundation. *Injury Prevention, 1*(3), 202–203.

Knox, L.J. (1994). Demographic and epidemiological trends. In J.M. Hibberd & M.E. Kyle (Eds.), *Nursing management in Canada* (pp. 37–61). Toronto: W.B. Saunders.

Kraus, J. (1987). Epidemiology: An academic perspective. *Public Health Reports, 102*(6), 591–592.

Kruse, T., & Bentzen, I. (1993). Safety for children—Importing foreign ideas: It worked in Norway, will it work in Denmark? In Centers for Disease Control and Prevention, *Proceedings of the Second World Conference on Injury Control* (pp. 363–364). Atlanta: Author.

Laboratory Centre for Disease Control, Health Protection Branch. (1991). *Children's hospitals injury research and prevention program* (Technical Report #2). Ottawa: Queen's Printer.

Letters to Allan Rock. (1994, March). *Gun Control Today, 3.*

Linwood, M.E. (1994). *Syllabus and case book.* Saskatoon: University of Saskatchewan Printing.

Linwood, M.E., Kasian, G., & Irvine, J. (1990). Child and youth accidents in northern Native communities. *Canadian Journal of Public Health, 81*, 77–78.

Linwood, M.E., & Willis, L.D. (1988). An introduction to developments in prevention in nursing. In L.D. Willis & M.E. Linwood (Eds.), *Recent advances in nursing: Prevention and nursing* (pp. 1–10). Edinburgh: Churchill Livingstone.

Lovasik, A. (1994). *You can do it! A community guide for injury prevention.* Edmonton: Injury Awareness & Prevention Centre.

Mackenzie, S.G. (1994). Childhood injury: Deaths and hospitalizations in Canada. *CHIRPP News, 1*, 4–5. Ottawa: Health Canada.

MacWilliam, L., Mao, Y., Nicholls, E., & Wigle, D.J. (1987). Fatal accidental childhood injuries in Canada. *Canadian Journal of Public Health, 78*, 129–135.

McLoughlin, E. (1997). From educator to strategic activist for injury control. *Injury Prevention, 3*(4), 244–246.

Mosby, C.V. (1938). *A little journey to the home of Florence Nightingale.* St. Louis: Mosby.

Mowat, D.L., Wang, F., Pickett, W., & Brison, R.J. (1998). A case-control study of risk factors for playground injuries among children in Kingston and area. *Injury Prevention, 4*(1), 39–43.

Murray, R.G. (1990). *Future directions for health care in Saskatchewan.* Regina: Saskatchewan Commission on Directions in Health Care, Saskatchewan Department of Health.

Novello, A. (1991). Violence is a greater killer of children than disease. *Public Health Reports, 106*(3), 231–233.

Raina, P., Hader, J., Sproat, B., & Feather, J. (1991). *Injury research and prevention in Saskatchewan.* Saskatoon: Injury Research Network for Saskatchewan.

Read, J.H. (1990). Developing injury prevention strategies from infancy to teenage. In R. Berfenstam (Ed.), *Proceedings of the 1st International Conference of Child Accident Prevention* (pp. 12–17). Stockholm: Bohuslaningens Boktryckeri AB.

Ross, M. (1993, September). *Injury prevention in Aboriginal communities.* Paper presented at the International Conference on Community Health Nursing Research, Edmonton.

Saskatchewan Institute on Prevention of Handicaps. (1996, May). *Child injury in Saskatchewan 1989–1994.* Saskatoon: Author.

Saskatchewan Safety Council. (1994). *Link*. Regina: Author.

Saskatchewan Vital Statistics. (1988). *Indian deaths from injury and poisoning 1979–1986 Saskatchewan Region*. Regina: Queen's Printer.

Saskatchewan Vital Statistics. (1989). *Vital statistics by health region, 1989*. Regina: Queen's Printer.

Schelp, L., & Svanström, L. (1996). The Swedish National Safety Promotion Program. *Injury Prevention, 2*(3), 237–239.

Senzilet, L. (1991). *Children's hospitals injury research and prevention program (CHIRPP)* (Tech. Rep. No. 2). Ottawa: Laboratory Centre for Disease Control, Health & Welfare Canada.

Sherman, G. (1994, March). The Na ReS Project: A new dimension for CHIRPP. *CHIRPP News*, 1–2.

Sidky, M. (1996). Safe kids Canada. *Injury Prevention, 2*(1), 70–72.

Statistics Canada. (1991a). Mortality: Summary list of causes. *Health Reports 1989, 3*(1) (Suppl. 12). Ottawa: Queen's Printer.

Statistics Canada. (1991b). *Mortality and hospitalization*. Ottawa: Queen's Printer.

Stewart, M.J. (1992). Nursing education as preparation for primary health care partnership with lay persons. *Nurse Educator, 17*(2), 8, 15, 19.

Swedish National Child Environment Council. (1989). *Child accident prevention: Proceedings of a conference*. Stockholm: Author.

Thein, M.M., Lee, J., Tay, V., & Ling, S.L. (1997). Infant walker use, injuries, and motor development. *Injury Prevention, 3*(1), 63–66.

U.S. Department of Health & Human Services, Public Health Services, Centers for Disease Control. (1992). *Healthy people 2000: National health promotion and disease prevention objectives*. Atlanta: U.S. Government Printing Offices.

Waxweiler, R., Harel, Y., & O'Carroll, P. (1993). Measuring adolescent behaviors related to unintentional injuries. *Public Health Reports, 108*(Suppl. 1), 11–14.

Wigle, D.T., Mao, Y., Wong, G., & Lane, R. (1991). Economic burden of illness in Canada, 1986. In L.J. Anderson & K. Wilkins (Eds.), *Chronic diseases in Canada, 12*(3) (Suppl. May/June), 1–37.

Wilkins, K., & Anderson, L. (1992). Proceedings of the International Conference on Air Bags and Seat Belts: Evaluation and implications for public policy. *Chronic Disease in Canada, 14*(Suppl. 4), 1–138.

World Health Organization (WHO). (1975). *International classification of diseases, injuries and causes of death* (9th ed., 1975 rev.). Geneva: Author.

World Health Organization (WHO). (1978). *Primary Health Care: Report on the international conference on Primary Health Care, Alma Ata, USSR*. Geneva: Author.

World Health Organization (WHO). (1986). Accident mortality rates in selected countries. *World health statistics annual*. Geneva: Author.

World Health Organization (WHO). (1990). Homicide and injury purposely inflicted by other persons. *World health statistics annual*. Geneva: Author.

World Health Organization (WHO). (1991). Causes of death by sex and age in Canada 1989. *World health statistics annual*. Geneva: Author.

C H A P T E R   1 8

Primary Health Care practice

Geraldine R. Cradduck

The scope of practice of community health nursing has changed since the late 1980s in response to the principles and directions articulated in many landmark documents. To achieve Health for All, it is necessary for nurses to change from being mere providers of health care services to facilitators, consultants, and resources in partnership with the community. This chapter reviews past practice of community health nursing and discusses changes that are leading to an enhanced model of Primary Health Care practice for the next decade and beyond.

LEARNING OBJECTIVES

In this chapter, you will learn:

- the legacy of community health nursing practice, and how Primary Health Care provides the vehicle to reclaim this legacy and enhance the practice of community health nurses into the future
- the range of activities undertaken by community health nurses within their scope of practice
- the similarities between the concepts of health promotion and the principles of Primary Health Care
- the factors that affect the health of the individual, group, or community, and the strategies used by community health nurses in partnership with the individual, group, or community to enhance health status

Introduction

In Canada, public health nursing became a recognized area of practice in the early decades of the 1900s with the formation of departments of health by provinces and municipalities (see Chapter 1). The success of public health nursing led to the assimilation of the principles of disease prevention by the medically oriented curative system. The target of disease prevention was the individual, with the focus being the removal or avoidance of the causative agent (Stachenko, 1992). Public health practice adopted an epidemiological paradigm, which emphasized prevention and targeted high-risk populations and individuals. These prevention efforts aimed to modify high-risk lifestyles through health education. (See Chapter 16.)

Although this model of practice has been successful to some extent, it has had distinct limitations. Orientation to a medical model meant that public health nurses, along with other health care professionals, were socialized to be expert providers rather than equal partners, as is the case in Primary Health Care (Stewart, 1990). In this expert provider role, public health nurses tended to give advice and then expect clients to change their behaviour. This was done without the insight that environmental factors beyond the control of the individual often cause unhealthy behaviour; for example, a client may be knowledgeable about nutrition but have insufficient money to purchase nutritious food. Public health nurses also found themselves acting in the capacity of a safety net to fill the gaps in services in the community, thus attempting to be all things to all people.

The public health nursing sector of the Canadian Public Health Association (CPHA) has developed publications to articulate the role of community health nurses across Canada. The first two publications, *A Statement of Functions and Qualifications for the Practice of Public Health Nursing in Canada* (CPHA, 1966) and *The Nurse and Community Health: Functions and Qualifications for Practice in Canada* (CPHA, 1976), discussed the role of the nurse in the community. However, the emphasis for public health nursing practice was individuals and families. The 1966 edition discussed promotion of health, prevention of disease and disability, and provision of care to the non-hospitalized sick and disabled. The 1976 edition mentioned the health needs of the community and the impact of these needs on the individual and family. It should be noted that this edition was published two years after Lalonde's (1974) ground-breaking white paper, which described determinants of health such as lifestyle, environment, and economic factors; the white paper was not yet widely used in Canada by health care system policy makers (Kickbusch, 1994). The third publication, *Community Health/Public Health Nursing in Canada: Preparation and Practice* (CPHA, 1990) points to Primary Health Care as the vehicle for community health nursing practice and incorporates concepts from many major global health documents.

The landmark conference at Alma Alta in 1978, sponsored by the World Health Organization (WHO), which introduced the concept of Primary Health Care, influenced the practice of community health nursing in Canada (see also Chapter 2). Subsequent conferences and documents have also effected change in practice (WHO, 1978; WHO, Health & Welfare Canada [HWC], & CPHA, 1986). This chapter articulates the changed practice of community health nurses in Canada.

A changing perspective for community health nursing

Community health nursing is an art and a science that synthesizes knowledge from the public health sciences and professional nursing theories. Its goal is to promote and preserve the health of populations, and it is directed to communities, groups, families, and individuals across their lifespan, in a continuous rather than an episodic process. Community health nurses play a pivotal role in identifying, assessing, and responding to the health needs of given populations. They work in collaboration with, among others, communities, families, individuals, other professionals, voluntary organizations, self-help groups, informal health care providers, governments, and the private sector (CPHA, 1990).

The terms *community health nurse* and *public health nurse* are used synonymously in many jurisdictions. In this chapter, the terms will be used interchangeably; whichever term is used, it refers to a nurse whose practice focusses on health promotion, illness and injury prevention, and community development, and who uses Primary Health Care as the vehicle for practice.

Currently, health is seen as a resource for everyday life, not the objective of living; health is a positive concept emphasizing social and personal resources as well as physical capacity. This description acknowledges the interactive impact of many factors on health status and the need for collaborative action by many sectors in the community (Maglacas, 1988). The present focus of public health is community-wide approaches to promoting the health of populations and not merely an amelioration of individual risk factors (Chamberlin, 1988; Epp, 1986; Labonte, 1994).

It is interesting to note that by the late 1990s, with increasing research and focus toward healthy child development, the trend has reversed away from emphasizing population health toward interventions directed to individuals and families. This trend is particularly evident in Ontario with the funding of a new initiative, Healthy Babies, Healthy Children (Ontario Ministry of Health, 1997), to be administered by local public health units.

A review of the literature about health promotion and Primary Health Care reveals many similar themes and concepts that provide the foundation for the practice of community health nursing (Clarke, Beddome, & Whyte, 1993; Jones & Craig, 1988; Mills & Ready, 1988; WHO, 1978; WHO, HWC, & CPHA, 1986). The Alma Alta conference, which introduced the concept of Primary Health Care, also articulated its principles and components. The components include education about how to control and prevent local health problems; promotion of proper nutrition and an adequate food supply; basic sanitation and a supply of safe water; maternal and child care, including family planning and prenatal care; immunization against major infectious diseases; prevention and control of locally endemic diseases; treatment for common diseases and injuries; and promotion of positive mental health.

In developed countries such as Canada, it is sometimes thought that the components of Primary Health Care are simplistic and irrelevant. However, not everyone has adequate sanitation when raw sewage is still pouring into Canadian rivers and oceans; equal access to nutritious food remains a problem while food banks continue to assist in the fulfilment of community nutrition needs; and there are many other such examples.

Many of the concepts contained in *Achieving Health for All: A Framework for Health Promotion* (Epp, 1986) reflect the principles of Primary Health Care. Thus, one of the health challenges is to "increase prevention." Health promotion mechanisms include mutual aid and self-care, while an implementation strategy is to "foster public participation." These concepts reinforce the Primary Health Care principles of community participation and increased prevention and health promotion. Research and evaluation of health promotion strategies continues. Until the long-term effectiveness of health promotion is known, it is necessary to maintain individual, group, community, and inter sectoral strategies simultaneously (Maglacas, 1988; Mills & Ready, 1988; Registered Nurses Association of British Columbia, 1992). Primary Health Care provides the vehicle and health promotion the framework.

The roles of the community health nurse in Primary Health Care include direct care provider; teacher and educator, both of the public and of health care providers; supervisor and manager of Primary Health Care services; and researcher and evaluator of health care (Canadian Nurses Association [CNA], 1988). Rather than focus on the phrase "role of the community health nurse," which is somewhat prescriptive and restrictive, it is more efficacious to discuss the scope of practice of community health nursing. Scope of practice describes what a community health nurse actually does and the strategies and activities undertaken in practice (CNA, 1993; College of Nurses of Ontario, 1994). By taking this approach, it is possible to provide a general outline of activities that community health nurses in a variety of settings and situations might undertake, without expecting that every nurse will be able to accomplish all activities.

The client of a community health nurse can be a community, aggregate, group, family, or individual, depending on the expertise of the nurse and the context of the intervention (see Chapter 5). A model of empowering strategies described by the Registered Nurses Association of British Columbia (1992) depicts a continuum of strategies. The five points on the continuum include personal empowerment, small-group development, community organization, coalition advocacy, and political action. It is not expected that any one community health nurse within an agency will have the skills or energy to work at all points on the continuum; rather, it is a collaborative process.

Characteristics of community health nursing

The emphasis of community health nursing practice is on health promotion, illness and injury prevention (primary, secondary, and tertiary), and health protection. Community health nurses act as facilitators in partnership with the community, the family, and the individual. They are also leaders in the effort to promote health-enhancing public policy and the empowerment of communities. Community health nursing practice is unique in contributing to the health of the population or community, by facilitating the attainment of the goal of Health for All. In summary, Primary Health Care is the vehicle for practice (CPHA, 1990).

Primary Health Care practitioner

In a Primary Health Care model of practice, it is not possible to discuss every activity in which community health nurses might be involved. Therefore, general activities will be outlined with illustrative examples. Inherent in the practice of community health nursing is the belief that interventions involving communities, aggregates, families, and individuals contribute to the health of the total population. Thus, parenting classes to groups of economically disadvantaged single mothers are undertaken on the premise that these women and their children will benefit from the intervention and the health of this population will be enhanced.

Educator

The strength of community health nursing pertinent to the educator role is the broad knowledge base across age groups and health topics. The focus of education is not individual lifestyle change. Rather, education provides the appropriate information and allows the community, family, or individual to select the choice that is most suitable and acceptable. Education by community health nurses can include formal sessions with a set curriculum, such as prenatal or parenting classes, or informal, anecdotal teaching, such as answering questions at a health display. The expectation for the nurse teaching prenatal classes is that the health of infants in the community will be enhanced and that the parents will have a positive birth experience.

Since community health nurses provide education to a wide variety of age groups, they must be knowledgeable about teaching and learning principles and the behavioural sciences. Then, the nurse can tailor the teaching strategy to the learning needs of the clients. For example, when providing educational information to adolescents, a hands-on approach is much more effective than a lecture. Thus, a health fair with individual booths that include true/false buzzer boards, other interactive educational games, and nutritious cookies is an effective teaching strategy for that group.

Another educational strategy widely used in community health nursing is "train the trainer." The nurse as educator trains a group of lay facilitators to undertake the education of new groups. An example of this strategy is the Nobody's Perfect parenting program developed by Health and Welfare Canada (1986). Community health nurses will always have a new cohort of people needing training or updating.

The focus of all community health nursing education is health promotion and illness and injury prevention, one of the principles of Primary Health Care. Because community health nurses have contact with individuals and families when they are experiencing maturational and other transitions, such as birth, starting school, puberty, marriage, and death, anticipatory guidance is particularly important. An example of anticipatory guidance is the program developed by the Edmonton Board of Health for parents, entitled Talking With Your Child About Sexuality (Godard & Masson, 1993). The program was implemented by community health nurses in response to a needs assessment that recommended increased community involvement.

Consultant

The main principle of Primary Health Care is maximum public participation, which is predicated on informed involvement by the community (CNA, 1988, p. 6). The community health nurse is in a unique position to provide the necessary information to the community and to act as a consultant. With a broad base of knowledge in community health issues, the nurse is able to provide information to clients, lay helpers, professionals from other disciplines, community agencies, professional associations, and government. The community health nurse is adept at moving the community to what is called an "upstream" view of health (Butterfield, 1990); rather than focus on individual treatment care or individual lifestyle change, the upstream mode of thought focusses on prevention and social action to promote the health of the population. An exemplar of this type of activity involves the membership of a community health nurse on an interdisciplinary committee to plan a children's mental health program. The nurse might encourage the committee to develop a social skills and anti-violence program for all elementary school children in the community, rather than develop a treatment program that would benefit only a handful of hard-to-serve children.

Community health nurses, through their agencies, act as a clearinghouse for inquiries about appropriate community resources for particular needs and link those needing services to the resources. It is imperative that community health nurses acquire and maintain the necessary expertise and knowledge for the consultant role.

Community developer

There are a number of models of community development, ranging from the community's identification of health issues to community mobilization, where the professional encourages community members to be socially active on their own behalf (Chalmers & Kristjanson, 1989). Community health nurses can transfer their skills in individual and family assessment to the community. This allows nurses to undertake effective community assessment on which to base their practice and programs. In a Primary Health Care model, it is necessary to involve the community in decision making and ownership of constructive changes that promote the health of the community.

The new definition of health takes into account the multitude of factors that affect the health of the community. Thus, it is no longer possible for community health and social agencies to work in isolation and to focus on a narrow mandate. Community health nurses, with their broad view of community, are in a unique position to foster interagency linkages. One example is a support group for adolescents at risk for school failure, which is co-facilitated by three agencies and funded by a local interagency council for children and youth. Community health nurses were instrumental in having these agencies focus on prevention rather than treatment.

Facilitator

As facilitators, community health nurses use leadership, enabling, and advocacy skills. Many community health nurses use these skills with individuals and families. To move into a Primary Health Care model of practice and enhance community participation, nurses need to expand these skills to groups and communities. As a group facilitator, the nurse does not take the role as chairperson, but rather assists the group to reach consensus. The nurse helps group members to develop group rules and to express themselves, clarifies information, and assists the group to be effective.

Leader

The leadership area of practice is closely related to community development. Thus, nurses often act as an interim leader until the community can take over the role itself. This can be done by inviting all the community stakeholders to a meeting and assisting them to organize around the issue, such as organizing a local AIDS support committee or developing a proposal to bring a Health Centre to an underserviced community area. In a leadership capacity, the community health nurse needs current knowledge of professional, community, and political issues. If nurses are active in professional associations and special interest groups, community health nursing practice can remain vital and meet community needs. The nurse will also have the legitimacy to assume the leadership of community-based multidisciplinary teams.

There is considerable debate in the literature about the relationship between professionals and mutual aid/self-help groups and the appropriateness of the leader role for professionals (Cameron, Hayward, & Mamatis, 1992; Katz, 1993). Although it is important for mutual aid groups to have some involvement with professionals, it is most desirable for the professional to act in a referral or consultant capacity and encourage the members to take control of the group. In working with community groups, the community health nurse needs to be aware of the potential pitfalls in acting in even an interim leadership role. For example, a self-help/support group for young economically disadvantaged mothers and their children is co-facilitated by a community health nurse and a social worker from a child protection agency. After over a year of group development, there is still a problem with leadership and group ownership. Research by Lord and Farlow (1990) into personal empowerment concluded that health professionals should focus on the capacities of the individuals concerned and that people themselves are the best resource for community change.

Enabler

As an enabler, the community health nurse takes a more subtle approach than as a leader. Using group process and facilitation skills, the nurse encourages and supports the community to participate actively in identifying and taking ownership of health issues. The nurse acts as a catalyst to assist communities to resolve health issues and concerns. This may take the form of educating community members about the political process as it relates to community health issues. Thus, the nurse may assist in writing briefs and making a presentation to a local health planning body, municipal council, or provincial government. An enabler increases the awareness of community members that their experiential knowledge is their best resource.

Advocate

The community health nurse is often aware of disadvantaged individuals and groups. The individual or group may be disadvantaged because of socioeconomic status, isolation, culture, or lack of knowledge. In the role of advocate, the nurse is able to raise the awareness of the disadvantaged about issues of importance to their health. In an advocacy position, the nurse takes the Primary Health Care principles of equity and accessibility into account and actively promotes the development of needed resources for the disadvantaged.

For example, community health nurses have acted as advocates with seniors for walking clubs in local shopping malls in many communities. The malls provide an ideal climate-controlled location in which seniors may walk in safety. One example of a successful mall-walking program is held in the Mountainview Mall in Midland, Ontario. The local Parks and Recreation Department and a community health nurse worked together to advocate for the program (Joyce Fox, Assistant Director of Public Health Nursing, Simcoe County District Health Unit, personal communication, June 1994).

Communicator

Without the ability to communicate with individuals, groups, and the community, the community health nurse will have difficulty functioning effectively. It is an advantage for community health nurses to be able to hone their communication skills with individuals and groups before translating those skills to the larger community. The community health nurse establishes a helping relationship that assists clients to identify their options and to make positive choices regarding health needs.

Skill as a communicator is closely related to the community health nurse's skills as facilitator, leader, enabler, and advocate. As a communicator, the nurse uses negotiation, mediation, and contracting strategies to manage resource allocation and to facilitate interagency collaboration. For example, a community health nurse on a Healthy Communities steering committee communicated individually with other members, served on a small-group task force, and facilitated town hall meetings with community members. This activity incorporates the Primary Health Care principles of community participation, prevention and health promotion, and interdisciplinary and intersectoral cooperation.

Coordinator

In providing care to communities, groups, and individuals, the community health nurse involves participants in planning health services and in setting priorities for resource allocation. Community health nurses are integral to the allocation of human, financial, physical, or time resources. In a time of diminished resources, community health nurses are aware of where resources are needed and what resources are already available. As coordinator, the community health nurse shares information with the community about available resources. This activity of resource manager may be undertaken with an individual or with the community where the health agency is seen as an information source about community resources. Coordinating activities range from requests for information about the local food bank hours or about clubs for parents of twins to development of resources for victims of sexual assault.

Collaborator

Because Primary Health Care involves all community members and the most recent definition of health recognizes the impact of many factors on health, it is necessary for the community health nurse to foster collaboration by all players in the community. This collaboration goes beyond establishing linkages with other health disciplines to fostering linkages with other non-health disciplines, among community agencies, across different sectors, and with the general public.

An example of the success of linkages among the health sector and housing, economics, government, other sectors in the community, and community members is the Healthy Communities movement, in which community health nurses are integral players (Flynn, Rider, & Bailey, 1992). The Healthy Communities movement started in Toronto in 1984 at a conference entitled Beyond Health Care. A workshop at the conference, called Healthy Toronto 2000, brought together participants from varied interest groups and sectors to seek ways to make Toronto a healthier city. The Healthy Cities movement emerged. To avoid exclusion of the larger part of Canada that is rural, the movement throughout Canada was retitled Healthy Communities. This health promotion project embodies intersectoral involvement, community participation, healthy public policy, and local government commitment (Ontario Public Health Association, 1994). These premises are also embodied in a Primary Health Care model; thus, a community health nurse is an important member of the Healthy Communities team.

It is important in a collaborative approach that all members of the team be equal contributors. Thus, it is necessary for the community health nurse to use strategies that foster team building. Team players need to have honest relationships, respect each other's expertise, and be interested in enhancing the health of the community rather than furthering an agency or personal agenda.

Researcher

Community health nursing practice needs to be based on a thorough community assessment, involvement by community members in defining priority health issues, and a scientific research base. Epidemiology becomes the starting point for community health nursing practice and community assessment. However, it is necessary to reformulate the principles of epidemiology according to a nursing framework (Hanchett & Clarke, 1988). Nursing models focus on the interaction of the four concepts of person, health, nurse, and environment, while the focus of the epidemiological model is individual risk of illness and associated health beliefs and behaviours. (See Chapter 29.)

Health promotion provides the boundary for community health nursing practice. Thus, a community assessment that just focusses on morbidity and mortality statistics will not provide a complete picture of the health of the community. There is a need to assess community demographics and socioeconomic and other factors that determine health status to obtain a total view of the community and the context in which lifestyle choices are being made.

The community health nurse participates in research projects, allocates resources according to research findings, and shares research with colleagues and the community. The nurse also undertakes program evaluation to ensure that interventions are effective and to modify programs as appropriate. An example of research affecting community health nursing practice is the new data that link infant positioning to sudden infant death syndrome (Chance,

1994). Nurses involved in maternal/infant programs have changed their practice and ensured that this new information is incorporated into their teaching. Community health research is complex, because many phenomena are difficult to study. It is important to investigate processes and outcomes and to use findings to guide the practice of community health nursing.

Social marketer

Social marketing marries the techniques of commercial marketing with health promotion (Mintz, 1988/89). Innovative health promotion strategies and marketing skills and techniques are used to promote community health programs and healthy living. An example of the application of these techniques is in the Canada-wide Break Free campaign. In 1985, a national strategy to reduce tobacco use was launched, with a mission to produce a generation of non-smokers by the year 2000. By implementing a long-term program based on social marketing principles, Health and Welfare Canada reduced the number of Canadians who smoke (McElroy, 1990).

Community health nurses are also starting to use marketing techniques to foster the community's and health professionals' awareness of the activities undertaken by their specialty. Within the discipline of nursing, community health nurses have formed special interest groups in most provinces. These individual groups have formed a federation within Canada, the Community Health Nurses Association of Canada, which comes under the governance of the Canadian Nurses Association. These groups are active in responding to government discussion papers and promoting the practice of community health nursing provincially. For example, in Ontario the Community Health Nurses Interest Group (CHNIG) lobbied the Ontario government to have the words "the promotion of health" included in the scope-of-practice statement for nurses in the Regulated Health Professions Act (Chairperson's Report, 1991). At the local level, nurses promote the practice of community health nursing by writing articles for newspapers, developing public service announcements for radio stations, and organizing health displays at factories and shopping malls.

Policy formulator

To document community health nursing practice clearly at both the agency and the national level, community health nurses should develop a comprehensive nursing philosophy, policies, procedures, and standards that reflect current practice. As members of a multidisciplinary team, community health nurses should be involved in the establishment of clear program objectives with measurable outcomes. Policy formulation includes program planning so that programs are not developed in an ad hoc manner that does not meet community needs. Community health nurses at the staff level are best able to develop and monitor program implementation and evaluation.

In 1989, public health programs were documented for Ontario under four health goals: Healthy Growth and Development; Healthy Lifestyles; Communicable Disease Control; and Healthy Environments (Ontario Ministry of Health, 1989). Each program has an overall goal that relates to the provincial goals and several measurable objectives, such as decreasing the number of smokers or decreasing the number of low birth-weight babies by a certain date in a given area. These program objectives can then be customized by the public health agency depending on the local needs identified in community assessment (see also Chapter 21). Multidisciplinary program committees, with membership from all levels of agency staff, are charged with developing the program-specific operational plan. This gives community health nurses opportunities to be involved in the planning of program activities that reflect the strengths of nursing practice and of pertinent policies.

It is evident in this discussion of community health nursing practice that none of these activities happens in isolation. Thus, for example, communication skills are essential in the activities of community developer, consultant, or educator. This discussion has focussed on a Primary Health Care model of community health nursing. However, there has been no review of the practice of community health nurses in traditional areas, such as provision of direct care, communicable disease management, and the use of appropriate technology for follow-up of clients (CPHA, 1990, p. 7), all of which remain important and appropriate. The community health nurse's roles in health promotion and illness and injury prevention are covered in other chapters in this book (see Chapters 16 and 17).

Examples of Primary Health Care practice

There are innumerable examples of community health nursing across Canada that illustrate the changing scope of practice described in this chapter. Only a few will be highlighted here.

For example, the City of Winnipeg Health Department has a legislated mandate to protect, promote, and improve the health of the inner-city population. Public health nursing services are organized on a neighbourhood-based model of service delivery. Each public health nurse is assigned a geographic neighbourhood within the inner city, which enables the nurse to become familiar with the unique needs of the neighbourhood. Public health nurses work in many different community settings and in partnership with community service providers, groups, and inner-city families to address complex issues such as family violence, chemical dependency, and food and shelter concerns. The nurse is a health educator, counsellor, advocate, coordinator, and resource for the client. This neighbourhood model facilitates involvement in community development initiatives. Two examples of community development initiatives in the City of Winnipeg Health Department are described next.

The public health nurse in the Central Park neighbourhood, together with other members of the community, observed that many children are responsible for at least some food preparation at home but lack the skills and knowledge necessary to prepare nutritious meals safely. The Kid's Cooking Club for grade six pupils from the elementary school is funded by the local community church. It is facilitated by the public health nurse, nutritionist, church outreach worker, and volunteers. The main focus of the club is to provide opportunities for the children to have fun while tasting new foods, learning safe food preparation, acquiring cooking skills, and obtaining information about nutrition and health. At the end of each session, everyone enjoys a nutritious meal together.

The public health nurse assigned to the West Broadway neighbourhood, together with the staff from the neighbourhood school, recognized the increasing number of children coming to school hungry. During home visits, families in the community described rising food prices and difficulty affording proper nutrition. Initially, the nurse tried to provide nutrition education with foods donated by a local food bank. Then, the nurse and the school outreach worker began working with two families in the community to develop a Community Kitchen. Eventually, five families became involved, and now the enterprise functions independently, with only occasional assistance from the nurse or school outreach worker (Ursula Stelman, Director of Public Health Nursing, City of Winnipeg Health Department, personal communication, May 1994).

These are just two examples of community health nursing practice from the City of Winnipeg Health Department. However, the examples illustrate many of the activities discussed previously: educator, consultant, community developer, facilitator, communicator, team member, and social marketer.

Boards of Health throughout Alberta have also developed community kitchens under the name Collective Kitchens. The first collective kitchen was set up in Edmonton in 1989. There are now 34 throughout Alberta. The groups were supported initially by Health Department staff and volunteers but later become self-supporting. Funding assistance comes from a variety of community sources.

The Edmonton Board of Health has developed other programs in collaboration with inner city agencies. One example is the Health for Two program, which provides access to prenatal services for women who rarely use traditional health services. The women receive milk coupons to supplement their nutritional intake, easy-to-read health information, emotional support, and referral to other health services. The aim is to increase women's opportunities to make healthy, informed choices for themselves and their children, leading to the improved health of pregnant women, mothers, and infants.

Calgary Health Services are also working with community agencies to enhance the health of populations. Prenatal education is being provided to new Canadians in the context of an English as a Second Language (ESL) training program. The sessions are co-facilitated by a public health nurse and an ESL teacher. Recruitment to the program is facilitated through various community agencies, and funding is provided by Canada Employment and Immigration. Calgary Health Services, with the assistance of a community group and government agency, have also arranged to translate immunization information into Spanish and Vietnamese to enable informed consent by these immigrant populations. The information was put into both pamphlets and audio tapes to aid comprehension (Leanne Currie, Public Health Nurse, Edmonton Board of Health, personal communication, June 1994).

These three examples of community health nursing practice from Alberta demonstrate the Primary Health Care principle of accessibility.

The Simcoe County District Health Unit in Ontario promoted health in county schools by devising a Health Challenge project. They collaborated with three other local agencies, the public and separate school boards, and the Canadian Mental Health Association, and involved students in designing the project. Thus, they incorporated the Primary Health Care principles of interdisciplinary and intersectoral practice and involved the community in planning and implementing the project. Students were challenged to identify a health issue and to organize a project that would address it. Projects were intended to promote healthy change within the school and reach out to the community.

A key to the success of Health Challenge was recognition of the efforts of the students and schools. Some of the projects planned and carried out by students were walk-, run-, bike-, and ski-athons across the county; aerobics programs for kids by kids; milk and breakfast programs; healthy food concession booths at sporting events; and the change of pop machines to juice machines, the latter with assistance from the Parent's Association. The students have shown great creativity and responsibility.

The community health nurses demonstrated their leadership skills by acting as catalysts in the early stages of the project. They were also able to use skills of consultant, educator, community developer, facilitator, collaborator, and social marketer in working with the students, schools, and community partners on this initiative (Joyce Fox, Assistant Director of Public Health Nursing, Simcoe County District Health Unit, personal communication, June 1994).

Validation of a Primary Health Care model in community health nursing practice

Research was conducted in Ontario to examine public health nurses' perceptions of the CPHA's 1990 document in relation to public health nursing practice. A pilot study was undertaken by McLachlin (1992) and followed up by an Ontario-wide survey with funding from the Ontario Nursing Innovation Fund (Chambers, Underwood, & Woodward, 1994). The purpose of the survey was to determine whether the perceptions of practising public health nurses of their roles and activities concurred with the CPHA document, which describes the preparation and practice of community health nursing in Canada. The survey questionnaire was completed by 1849 public health nurses from all Ontario Health Units. This represented an 85 percent response rate.

The survey showed that public health nurses in all Ontario Health Units are engaged in all the activities outlined in the CPHA document. This does not mean that all public health nursing assignments include all activities, but that, collectively, roles cited in the CPHA document are apparently relevant to practice in Ontario. Most staff reported being active in the roles of educator, consultant, social marketer, facilitator, communicator, and collaborator. The activities of community developer, policy formulator, researcher, and coordinator were less frequently performed. The first category relates to activities undertaken with individuals or groups, while the last category relates to activities undertaken with communities.

Nurses have more experience and expertise working with individuals and groups. However, respondents stated they anticipated increased community-focussed activities in the future and that they would need further preparation to perform these activities. Two factors could account for these perceptions. Either nurses are not well prepared in their basic education for some Primary Health Care roles or the rapid changes taking place in public health nursing have undermined the confidence of nurses to carry out these roles, even though they have the necessary skills and knowledge.

Although this research was undertaken in only one province in Canada, it has important implications for the future education of community health nurses and the development of relevant curricula in faculties of nursing in Canadian universities. The research demonstrates that community health nurses are already following the Primary Health Care principles of equity, prevention, health promotion, and interdisciplinary practice. Community health nurses have the least experience and the most difficulty putting into practice the principles of maximum community participation and intersectoral functioning.

Conclusion

Nursing literature is dominated by descriptions of one-to-one relationships between nurse and client. Yet, people's cultural heritage, social roles, and economic situation have more influence on health and health behaviour than their individual interactions with health professionals. There is a need to "think upstream," not only to rescue the drowning, but to address the conditions causing individuals to fall into the river in the first place (Butterfield, 1990). It is necessary to view health both as an individual phenomenon and also from the broader perspective of societal change. Many of the early public health pioneers were also social reformers (Hancock, 1994). The unique scope of practice of community health nurses has the potential to influence health outcomes positively within a reformed health system (Mills & Relf, 1994).

The legacy of community health nursing is its multidimensional role, community orientation, and advocacy. Community health nurses were a leading force in social and health reform (Anderson, 1991; Erickson, 1987). In the move to a curative system, community health nurses lost sight of that legacy. The concepts of Primary Health Care will enable community health nurses to reclaim their legacy and to move forward into the 21st century with an enhanced model of practice.

QUESTIONS

1. How have the concepts and principles of Primary Health Care changed the practice of community health nursing? Discuss the most important skills required by community health nurses working within a Primary Health Care model of practice.
2. What are the strategies that can be used to promote community participation and involvement in health issues? Identify some of the barriers and limitations that might occur in this process.
3. What factors within the community environment determine health status? Discuss how interagency and intersectoral collaboration could be used to affect these factors.

REFERENCES

Anderson, F.T. (1991). A call for transformation. *Journal of Public Health Nursing, 8*(1), 1–2.

Butterfield, P.G. (1990). Thinking upstream: Nurturing a conceptual understanding of the societal context of health behaviour. *Advances in Nursing Science, 12*(2), 1–8.

Cameron, G., Hayward, K., & Mamatis, D. (1992). *Mutual aid and child welfare: The parent mutual aid organizations in child welfare demonstration project.* Waterloo, ON: Faculty of Social Work, Wilfrid Laurier University.

Canadian Nurses Association (CNA). (1988). *Health for all Canadians: A call for health care reform.* Ottawa: Author.

Canadian Nurses Association (CNA). (1993). *The scope of nursing practice: A review of issues and trends.* Ottawa: Author.

Canadian Public Health Association (CPHA). (1966). *A statement of functions and qualifications for the practice of public health nursing in Canada.* Ottawa: Author.

Canadian Public Health Association (CPHA). (1976). *The nurse and community health: Functions and qualifications for practice in Canada.* Ottawa: Author.

Canadian Public Health Association (CPHA). (1990). *Community health/public health nursing in Canada: Preparation and practice.* Ottawa. Author.

Chairperson's Report. (1991, Winter). *Community Health Nurses Interest Group Newsletter, 6.*

Chalmers, K., & Kristjanson, L. (1989). The theoretical basis for nursing at the community level: A comparison of three models. *Journal of Advanced Nursing, 14,* 569–574.

Chamberlin, R.W. (Ed.). (1988). *Beyond individual risk assessment: Community wide approaches to promoting the health and development of families and children* (Conference proceedings). Washington, DC: The National Centre for Education in Maternal & Child Health.

Chambers, L.W., Underwood, J., & Woodward, C.A. (1994). *Ontario survey on public health nurses: Preparation and practice.* Hamilton, ON: Hamilton–Wentworth Department of Public Health.

Chance, G.W. (1994). Sudden infant death syndrome: Preventive measures. *Ontario Medical Review, 61*(8), 33–35.

Clarke, H.F., Beddome, G., & Whyte, N.B. (1993). Public health nurses' vision of their future reflects changing paradigms. *Image, 25*(4), 305–310.

College of Nurses of Ontario. (1994, March). Scope of practice and controlled acts model. *Communiqué,* 9–10.

Epp, J. (1986). *Achieving health for all: A framework for health promotion.* Ottawa: Health & Welfare Canada.

Erickson, G.P. (1987). Public health nursing initiatives: Guide posts for future practice. *Public Health Nursing, 4,* 202–211.

Flynn, B.C., Rider, M.S., & Bailey, W.W. (1992). Developing community leadership in healthy cities: The Indiana model. *Nursing Outlook, 40*(3), 121–126.

Godard, L., & Masson, M. (1993). *Talking with your child about sexuality: Program evaluation.* Edmonton: Edmonton Board of Health.

Hanchett, E., & Clarke, P.K. (1988). Nursing theory and public health science: Is synthesis possible? *Public Health Nursing, 5*(1), 2–6.

Hancock, T. (1994). Health promotion in Canada: Did we win the battle but lose the war? In A. Pederson, M. O'Neill, & I. Rootman (Eds.), *Health promotion in Canada: Provincial, national and international perspectives* (pp. 350–373). Toronto: W.B. Saunders.

Health & Welfare Canada. (1986). *Nobody's perfect—Leaders' guide.* Ottawa: Author.

Jones, P., & Craig, D. (1988). Nursing practice in the community: Primary health care. In A. Baumgart & J. Larsen (Eds.), *Canadian nursing faces the future* (pp. 135–147). Toronto: Mosby.

Katz, A.H. (1993). *Self help in America.* New York: Twayne.

Kickbusch, I. (1994). Introduction: Tell me a story. In A. Pederson, M. O'Neill, & I. Rootman (Eds.), *Health promotion in Canada: Provincial, national and international perspectives* (pp. 8–17). Toronto: W.B. Saunders.

Labonte, R. (1994). Death of program, birth of metaphor: The development of health promotion in Canada. In A. Pederson, M. O'Neill, & I. Rootman (Eds.), *Health promotion in Canada* (pp. 72–90). Toronto: W.B. Saunders.

Lalonde, M. (1974). *A new perspective on the health of Canadians: A working document.* Ottawa: Government of Canada.

Lord, J., & Farlow, D. (1990, Fall). A study of personal empowerment: Implications for health promotion. *Health Promotion, 6,* 2–8.

Maglacas, A.M. (1988). Health for All: Nursing's role. *Nursing Outlook, 36*(2), 66–71.

McElroy, H. (1990). Break free: Towards a new generation of non-smokers. *Health Promotion, 28*(4), 2–5.

McLachlin, L. (1992). *Work perceptions and learning needs of practising public health nurses.* Unpublished master's thesis, University of Western Ontario, London ON.

Mills, K., & Ready, H.L. (1988). Health promotion in community nursing practice. In A. Baumgart & J. Larsen (Eds.), *Canadian nursing faces the future* (pp. 151–160). Toronto: Mosby.

Mills, K., & Relf, M. (1994). The changing practice of public health nurses. *Canadian Journal of Public Health, 85*(3), 153–154.

Mintz, J. (1988/89, Winter). Social marketing: New weapon in an old struggle. *Health Promotion, 4,* 37–43.

Ontario Ministry of Health. (1989). *Mandatory health programs and services guidelines.* Toronto: Author.

Ontario Ministry of Health & Ministry of Community & Social Services. (1997). *Implementation Guidelines for Healthy Babies, Healthy Children.* Toronto: Author.

Ontario Public Health Association. (1994). Ontario Healthy Communities coalition comes of age. *HealthBeat, 13*(3), 1, 4–5.

Registered Nurses Association of British Columbia. (1992). *Determinants of health: Empowering strategies for nursing practice. A background paper.* Vancouver: Author.

Stachenko, S. (1992). Towards a system for health, the Heart Health opportunity. *Health Promotion, 30*(4), 5–7, 41.

Stewart, M. (1990). From provider to partner: A conceptual framework for nursing education based on primary health care premises. *Advances in Nursing Science, 12*(2), 9–27.

World Health Organization (WHO). (1978). *Primary Health Care: Report of the International Conference on Primary Health Care.* Geneva: Author.

World Health Organization (WHO), Health & Welfare Canada (HWC), & Canadian Public Health Association (CPHA). (1986). *Ottawa charter for health promotion.* Ottawa: Author.

C H A P T E R   1 9

Nursing diagnosis for aggregates and groups

Anne Neufeld and Margaret J. Harrison

Community health nurses work within the context of Primary Health Care to pro-mote health and prevent illness among population groups and aggregates. There has been limited consideration of the utility of nursing diagnosis for this type of nursing practice. In this chapter, the authors define wellness and deficit diagnoses for aggre-gates and groups. We then discuss the use of nursing diagnosis within the context of Primary Health Care principles, including the blurred boundary between health pro-motion, health maintenance, and risk reduction; nursing's contribution in interdis-ciplinary and intersectoral collaboration; and work with vulnerable population groups. We recommend a format for nursing diagnosis with illustrations that address the range and complexity of three related issues: the inclusion of both well-ness and deficit diagnoses; the selection of the client group; and confirmation of the appropriateness of diagnoses. Nursing diagnosis is flexible enough to be employed in the context of Primary Health Care principles and community health nursing prac-tice with aggregates and groups.

LEARNING OBJECTIVES

In this chapter, you will learn:

- definitions of wellness and deficit nursing diagnoses for aggregates and groups
- how nursing diagnosis is used within the context of Primary Health Care principles
- key issues in formulating nursing diagnostic statements for aggregates and groups

Introduction

Community health nurses work within the context of Primary Health Care to promote health and prevent illness. Often this involves working collaboratively with community members and other professionals to achieve these goals with aggregates and groups. There has been limited consideration of the utility of nursing diagnosis for this type of nursing practice or the ways in which this may differ from use of nursing diagnosis with individuals.

This chapter discusses the use of nursing diagnosis with aggregates and groups within a Primary Health Care framework. First, a definition of nursing diagnosis is presented. Second, the authors examine the use of nursing diagnosis within the context of Primary Health Care principles. Finally, we outline a format for formulating nursing diagnostic statements and offer specific illustrations.

Background

Community health nursing practice encompasses the principles of Primary Health Care, which emphasize promotion of wellness and health of families, groups, aggregates, and communities. Community health nurses facilitate access to health care and encourage public participation in health care planning. In addition, nurses work in partnership with other health professionals and organizations within other sectors of society to address the determinants of health and to improve the health of the community (Canadian Public Health Association [CPHA], 1990).

In applying the nursing process (which is a decision-making process), community health nurses need to consider how to synthesize assessment data into statements about the health of the aggregate or group with whom they work. One method is the use of nursing diagnosis. A prominent approach to nursing diagnosis is that proposed by the North American Nursing Diagnosis Association (NANDA), which has developed a taxonomy of nursing diagnoses. Initially, the Association concentrated on nursing diagnoses for ill individuals in acute care settings. In 1990 both community-as-client and wellness diagnoses were incorporated (NANDA, 1990), but there has been limited application of these. Recent initiatives have encouraged use of the NANDA approach in Europe, although several challenges remain to be addressed (Hogston, 1997). Another approach to diagnostic summaries was developed for use in the community by the Omaha group (Martin & Scheet, 1992). Although they include a health promotion focus, their work addresses only individuals and families. In addition to use in North American settings, the Omaha system has been used successfully in an assessment of rural elderly in Iran (Maggs & Ali Abedi, 1997). Nevertheless, there continues to be little guidance available for applying nursing diagnosis to the planning of nursing interventions for aggregates and groups in community settings.

Nursing interventions in community health address goals of wellness and health promotion. Although some (e.g., Labonte, 1993) use the terms health and wellness synonymously, others (e.g., Popkess-Vawter, 1991) differentiate between these terms. The authors of this chapter distinguish between wellness, defined as a "pleasurable, purposeful, and balanced life-style in which individuals choose to reach optimal potential, regardless of presence or absence of disabling conditions" (Popkess-Vawter, 1991, p. 20), and health, which is "a state that is absent of disease and in which one can function well physically, mentally, and socially" (p. 20).

Health promotion may be viewed from varying perspectives in different countries. For a review of health and health promotion in a Canadian context, see Rootman and Raeburn (1994). Recently there has been renewed affirmation of health promotion, as well as support for the concept of population health. A population health perspective recognizes the influence of determinants of health and inequities in access to the resources essential for health (Federal, Provincial, & Territorial Advisory Committee on Population Health, 1994). The Canadian Population Health Promotion model integrates concepts of population health and health promotion (Hamilton & Bhatti, 1996). Principles of health promotion were affirmed in a recent position statement by the Canadian Public Health Association (1996) that also emphasized developing new knowledge and establishing strong alliances. The National Forum on Health (1997), which engaged in a process of extensive public consultation, recommended priorities for action that support health promotion and population health principles and the tenets of the Canadian health care system.

At the international level, a recent World Health Organization (WHO, 1997) conference advocated priorities for health promotion that included promoting social responsibility; increasing investment in health development; expanding partnerships; increasing community capacity and individual empowerment; and securing a local, national, and global infrastructure for health promotion. For the first time, private sector involvement in promoting health was included.

In the context of this growing emphasis on health promotion and population health, wellness diagnoses are an essential complement to deficit diagnoses (unhealthy client responses), particularly for those who work toward health promotion in communities. Wellness diagnoses can assist nurses working in the community to (a) facilitate maintenance of health promotion practices, (b) promote strengths to enhance wellness and contribute to positive long-term outcomes, and (c) document available resources and strengths for use in managing unhealthy responses (Neufeld & Harrison, 1990).

Definition of nursing diagnosis

The authors use a definition of nursing diagnosis (Mundinger & Jauron, 1975, p. 97) in which the term *client*, referring to any family, group, aggregate, or community, is substituted for the term *patient*. The term *aggregate* is here used to refer to a population whose members share some common health-related characteristics but are not part of an interdependent, interactive group (see Chapter 5). The term *population groups* refers to aggregates as well as to client groups in which there is interaction and combined effort to meet collective goals (Neufeld & Harrison, 1990; Schultz, 1987; Williams, 1977).

There is a need for two types of nursing diagnosis. The most common type addresses a deficit in health. A *deficit nursing diagnosis* is defined as the statement of a client's response that is actually or potentially unhealthy and that nursing intervention can help to change in the direction of health. The diagnosis should identify essential factors related to the unhealthy response. To meet the goals of health promotion, there is also a need for wellness diagnoses. A wellness diagnosis (Houldin, Saltstein, & Ganley, 1987) can be formulated by substituting a statement of the healthy response in lieu of the unhealthy response. A *wellness diagnosis* is thus defined as the statement of a client's healthy response, which nursing intervention can support or strengthen. It should identify essential factors related to the healthy response.

Primary Health Care and the use of nursing diagnosis

The principles of Primary Health Care include an emphasis on health promotion, interdisciplinary and intersectoral collaboration, access to resources essential for health, and community participation in addressing inequities. These principles need to be considered when integrating nursing diagnosis for groups and aggregates within community health nursing practice. A number of issues arise: the blurred boundaries between health promotion, health maintenance, and risk reduction; the nature of nursing's contribution to interdisciplinary collaboration; and the appropriate application of nursing diagnosis when working with vulnerable populations.

Blurred boundaries: Health promotion, health maintenance, and risk reduction

The blurred conceptual boundary between health promotion and risk reduction contributes to the difficulty of incorporating wellness diagnoses in community health nursing practice. Carlyon (1984) argues that health promotion for individuals is in reality risk reduction. Alternative views that support health promotion as more than risk reduction are incorporated into international statements from the World Health Organization (WHO, 1997), as well as Canadian documents on health (CPHA, 1996; Epp, 1986; Federal, Provincial, & Territorial Advisory Committee on Population Health, 1994;

Kickbusch, 1986; National Forum on Health, 1997). As stated in the Jakarta declaration (WHO, 1997), health promotion is the process of enabling people to improve their health by taking action to influence the determinants of health. Thus, health promotion is characterized by an emphasis on the social, cultural, political, and economic determinants of health and the policies and programs required to modify them.

Within a nursing context, distinctions have been made between the absence of disease and a more positive, growth-oriented state. For example, Tripp and Stachowiak (1992) argue that wellness is characterized by growth and realization of potential. This is distinct from a stable disease-free state in which there is neither differentiation nor growth. Popkess-Vawter's (1991) distinction between wellness and health is similar. A *health maintenance diagnosis*, therefore, focusses on the goal of protecting against illness and preserving or stabilizing health. Client attributes such as growth and the desire to achieve wellness or personal potential distinguish a *health promotion diagnosis*. The distinction is made on the basis of a combination of the client's characteristics and the nursing intervention. For example, in either case the nurse may assist the client to engage in aerobic exercise, but the client attributes may differ.

We suggest that a *risk diagnosis* be used when reliable information is available about a probable risk. To use an at-risk nursing diagnosis, several conditions must be met. First, a risk must be present. Second, only modifiable risk factors are included. Not all risk factors are a legitimate focus for community health nursing intervention. Some risk factors associated with increased probability of a disease, such as gender or family history, should be excluded from a nursing diagnosis as these are not amenable to nursing action. For example, all infants in day care have the potential to develop infectious diarrhea. They cannot be said to be at risk unless there is an outbreak of diarrhea in a specific day care and evidence of the conditions required for its transmission. In this example, the age of the child is a risk factor that is not amenable to nursing intervention. If there was evidence of inadequate handwashing and inappropriate methods for diaper disposal, the diagnosis could be stated as "infants in a day care are at risk for diarrhea related to lack of handwashing by staff and inappropriate disposal of soiled diapers."

It is important for community health nurses to clarify whether the focus of the diagnosis is risk reduction or health promotion. The focus that is chosen will reflect priorities. There may be tension between groups who favour distribution of resources for risk reduction and those who advocate a priority on health promotion activities. This tension may be particularly apparent within community agencies in times of economic constraint.

Nursing's contribution in interdisciplinary and intersectoral collaboration

In community health nursing, particularly within the context of Primary Health Care, not all the factors influencing the situation in which change is desired will be the focus of nursing intervention. Some factors will need to be addressed by other health disciplines or other sectors, often—but not always—in collaboration with nursing. The collaborative nature of community health nursing practice challenges the individualistic view of nursing diagnosis held by some such as Sanford (1987). Often, community health nursing practice with population groups must be differentiated from that of other disciplines within settings and programs in which there is considerable role flexibility and overlap. Nurses who work in advanced practice, such as pediatric nurse practitioners (Martin, 1995), also need to clarify their shared and unique contributions and that of physicians in community settings.

In community settings there are shared and interdependent contributions from many disciplines. This is particularly important in the development of nursing diagnoses regarding environmental health (Neufer, 1994). For example, given a diagnosis of risk for hearing loss related to exposure to noise and lack of use of protective devices, the nurse may collaborate with engineers to identify controls that reduce the noise level. In environmental health, as in many other situations, rigid disciplinary boundaries are inappropriate and ineffective in addressing identified concerns of population groups. Limiting nursing diagnosis to areas of independent nursing practice may restrict unnecessarily the nurse's scope of practice in a community-based interdisciplinary setting. There are few areas in which community health nurses function without collaboration and shared responsibility.

The identified issue may not be the unique concern of nursing, and some, but not all, of the factors related to the issue may be amenable to nursing intervention. The authors propose the development of diagnoses that require collaborative interdisciplinary intervention, with explication of the nursing contribution. Our approach, similar to that of Martin (1995), clarifies nursing's contribution to intervention, but does not require that these diagnoses be the exclusive domain of nursing.

Use of nursing diagnosis with vulnerable populations

Primary Health Care principles emphasize access to the determinants of health and health services and the importance of community participation. These principles are of primary importance when working with vulnerable populations, but challenge traditional perspectives on use of nursing diagnosis. An emphasis on social, economic, and political determinants of health expands the focus of nursing diagnoses beyond the more traditional nursing-specific action related to individuals. Community health nurses who recognize the broader context of vulnerable populations, such as those with low incomes, may place a priority on change in social, political, or health care systems rather than on individual behavioural change. This emphasis is beyond the usual scope of nursing diagnoses. For example, the community health nurse may work with clients to obtain new housing units rather than focus on accident-proofing inadequate homes. A community development approach is one way to facilitate community participation and enhance the control of vulnerable populations over the definition and resolution of their primary concerns (Chalmers & Bramadat, 1996; Wallerstein, 1992; WHO, 1997) (see Chapter 21). In this approach the community or group, not the nurse, determines the focus of action.

Working with marginalized, vulnerable groups also requires a focus on diversity (Hall, Stevens, & Meleis, 1994; Reutter, Neufeld, & Harrison, 1995; Walker, Martin, & Thompson, 1988; Wallerstein, 1992). This requirement challenges the implicit assumption that nursing diagnosis, as an "expert" nursing judgement, should be accorded more weight than the client's view. If this assumption is made, there is the risk that the use of nursing diagnosis will become another form of oppression that potentially negates the power of vulnerable client groups to define and control their own health. To avoid this risk, some argue that it is important to work with vulnerable populations from the perspective of critical social or feminist theory (Stevens & Hall, 1992; Walker et al., 1988). Principles based on this perspective include (a) recognizing the social, political, economic, and cultural context of the group as possible sources of oppression that threaten health; (b) establishing responsive, mutual interactions with group members that give priority to their perspectives; and (c) fostering collective actions of the group members themselves (Stevens & Hall, 1992). This reduces the risk of harm from inaccurate assumptions that are rooted in the nurse's culture and may lead to inappropriate nursing actions (Mitchell, 1991). For example, diagnoses such as "ineffective family coping" or "dysfunctional grieving," which are accepted NANDA diagnoses (NANDA, 1996), may be assigned on the basis of assumptions that are inaccurate for a particular cultural group. Consequently, inappropriate and potentially harmful nursing actions may result (Kelley & Frisch, 1990).

In working with vulnerable populations, it is important that the community health nurse function as a resource in relation to issues defined by the population group, rather than as an expert responsible for defining the issues of concern. Use of standardized nursing diagnostic statements with vulnerable groups may not acknowledge their unique and diverse social and political conditions and may preclude their ability to define their own concerns. The implicit assumption that nursing diagnosis, as an "expert" judgement, should be more influential than client perspectives diminishes the dignity and power of population groups and aggregates and contributes to ineffectual interventions. For these reasons, consistent with the Primary Health Care principle of community participation, the authors recommend collaborative generation of nursing diagnostic statements that are unique to the population group. Traditional nursing diagnosis labels may be irrelevant; unique statements generated and owned by the group may be more appropriate.

Developing nursing diagnoses for population groups

Although the authors propose the use of uniquely generated statements in some situations, these may be stated in a format similar to other diagnoses. The specific format we propose includes the name of the client aggregate or group, the healthy or the actually or potentially unhealthy response, and related factors. For example:

Adolescents in James High School are at risk for sexually transmitted disease related to a high percentage of the students who report being sexually active (70 percent) and reluctant to use condoms (50 percent).

The first clause names the group or aggregate (adolescents at James High School) and refers to the response identified (risk for acquiring a sexually transmitted disease). The second clause lists the factors that are related to the response (sexual activity and reluctance to use condoms). These factors may include characteristics of the group such as motivation, attitudes, knowledge, and skills, as well as physical, psychosocial, political, cultural, or environmental resources (e.g., income, environmental hazards, social support). Only factors that nursing or nursing in collaboration with others can influence for change are included. In this example the related factors, sexual activity and reluctance to use condoms, provide the focus for nursing interventions. The community health nurse may develop a peer education program to assist sexually active students to be assertive with partners in discussing the use of condoms.

Because the assessment of a group or aggregate is complex and includes considerable data, we suggest that a detailed preliminary nursing assessment be documented separate from the nursing diagnosis statement. However, a community health nurse could list the key characteristics that substantiate the diagnosis at the end of the statement by using the words "as manifested by" and listing the data. In this example, the data were based on a comprehensive survey of adolescent lifestyle and health practices.

In a preliminary study of the use of nursing diagnosis by community health nurses and undergraduate nursing students (Neufeld & Harrison, 1994), the authors identified three issues associated with application of nursing diagnosis to population groups. These issues were identification of the range and complexity of related factors, inclusion of both wellness and deficit diagnoses, selection of an appropriate client group, and confirmation of the diagnoses.

Range and complexity of related factors

One issue is the need for a comprehensive assessment that specifies the range and complexity of related factors to inform nursing intervention and selection of multidisciplinary partners. An example of a complex nursing diagnosis that includes several factors is the following:

Seniors in community X have potential for increased hypertension related to: lack of knowledge of cardiovascular function; use of fast foods high in fat and cholesterol; sedentary lifestyle; and possible misuse of medication. (Neufeld & Harrison, 1994, p. 167)

From our study we identified three common categories of related factors: characteristics of group members; characteristics of the physical and social environments of group members; and community resources. Characteristics of group members included self-esteem, development, role performance, social isolation, socioeconomic status, health behaviours, coping ability, or physiological characteristics such as anoxia or mobility. Interaction and relationships among group members are additional examples of group characteristics. Other factors were closely related to the social or physical environment of the group. For example, in occupational health settings, related factors included noise pollution, repetitive body motions, and exposure to other hazards related to the job. Community resources, such as wellness clinics or transportation services, were identified as additional related factors. These categories of related factors are similar to those reported by Lunney (1982) and similar to the signs and symptoms incorporated in the Omaha system (Martin & Scheet, 1992).

Inclusion of wellness and deficit diagnoses

Some (Houldin et al., 1987; Popkess-Vawter, 1991) have argued that wellness-oriented diagnoses are appropriate for both well and ill individuals. We agree with this argument as it is consistent with health promotion premises, but also argue that it needs to be extended to population groups as well as to individuals. The Omaha system (Martin & Scheet, 1992) uses a modifier, "health promotion," when the individual or family is interested in maintaining or enhancing wellness. NANDA (1996) has incorporated wellness diagnoses and suggested that they be one-part statements beginning with the phrase "potential for enhanced." We suggest that, when a wellness diagnosis is used, it is important to include the clause that focusses on related factors. If the related-factors clause is omitted in a wellness diagnosis, direction for intervention is not specified. For example, in the following diagnosis, which includes a related-factors clause, nursing intervention would focus on maintaining preschoolers' attendance at clinic, as well as parental education on the importance of immunization.

Preschoolers in Region X have a high immunity level related to regular clinic attendance for immunization and ongoing parental education about immunization. (Neufeld & Harrison, 1994, p. 169)

Are there common as well as unique categories of wellness diagnoses? Based on our earlier study, in which we identified many deficit and wellness diagnoses that were congruent with published categories of nursing diagnoses focussed on individuals (Houldin et al., 1987; NANDA, 1990), we contend that when similar issues are addressed, the same domain labels may be employed for both types of diagnoses. For example, diagnoses (NANDA, 1996) such as parenting or social isolation may be pertinent to community aggregates. This approach is also used in the Omaha system (Martin & Scheet, 1992).

We propose that generic statements that are supplemented by specific modifiers can be used for wellness and deficit diagnoses for population groups. To illustrate our approach, we include examples of generic statements. A generic format for a deficit diagnosis in an occupational health setting is:

Employees A are at risk for disease (injury) X related to exposure to W.

A generic format for a wellness diagnosis is:

Employees A have potential for improved (or maintenance of) Y related to Z.

An example of a deficit diagnosis in an occupational health setting is:

Employees in the poultry processing plant are at risk for back strain related to inappropriate use of devices for lifting and poor physical fitness.

A parallel example of a wellness statement in the same setting is:

Employees in the poultry processing plant have potential for improved physical fitness related to union interest in securing on-site exercise facilities and regularly scheduled work breaks.

Selection of appropriate client group
The selection of an appropriate client group as the focus for intervention is an important decision for nurses working in the community. One example pertains to children in day care who have inadequate nutrition. The nurse could work with different groups, such as the children, the day-care staff, or parents. Nursing diagnoses that address a specific issue may be stated in relation to either the focal client group (the children) or another group that directly or indirectly influences it. The decision about which group to select as the focus for intervention may be made after consideration of access to the group, the motivation of group members, resources available, and the nurse's own skills.

Alternatively, several diagnoses and related interventions could be developed to guide nursing action with all groups when the focus is nutrition of the children. If one group is more influential in relation to the identified health concerns, it would receive priority. Another view is that the diagnoses should be formulated for the focal client (e.g., the children in a day-care setting) regardless of the group(s) selected as the recipient(s) of nursing intervention. When there are multiple potential client groups, we suggest that the direction for intervention is clearer if the diagnosis is formulated in relation to the client group(s) selected as the focus for intervention. This approach indicates the priority for intervention and facilitates evaluation.

A community health nurse whose mandate is providing programs for a large population group or developing national health policy may formulate an assessment and diagnosis (including related factors) for an aggregate at a broad level. The emerging diagnoses and nursing interventions will differ from those of an occupational health nurse concerned with the health of a group of workers in one plant. For example, the community health nurse concerned with a large geographical jurisdiction might formulate a diagnosis such as the one submitted by a community health nurse in our earlier study:

English speaking women [in a geographical area] 20–65 years of age have potential for late diagnosis of breast cancer related to lack of knowledge about the importance of early detection, lack of skill regarding . . . breast self examination, lack of motivation regarding caring for [the] body, and perceived value of engaging in early detection practices—mammography and breast self examination. (Neufeld & Harrison, 1995, p. 88)

To be most useful, the level of client selected and the consequent nursing diagnoses and related factors must be appropriate to the mandate of the nurse's position, as well as to the scope of professional nursing practice. A potential difficulty, however, is employer constraint of the community health nursing role. This issue is one that might be faced by nurses whose employer is not supportive of intervention in relation to certain health issues or groups. Examples include occupational health nurses who may be concerned about health effects of an employer's policies or community health nurses who wish to develop programs for groups that are not considered a high priority by their employing agency.

Confirmation that the diagnosis is appropriate

The extent to which a diagnosis is shared by members of a population group should be considered in determining whether an aggregate-level diagnosis is appropriate. When the diagnosis is related to an individual risk behaviour, such as failure to use safety equipment in an occupational setting, it may be shared by most, but not all, members of the group. In other groups the diagnosis, such as potential for exposure to radiation, may be common to all group members, although the specific factors related to their exposure differ. It is possible that the relationship between related factors and the diagnosis is indirect. For example, low-income groups who lack access to sufficient economic resources may consequently live in hazardous environmental conditions. When diagnoses of risks are directly related to environmental characteristics, such as air pollution or substandard housing, it is more likely that a diagnosis will be pertinent to all group members.

Information from multiple sources, including epidemiological data, would assist the community health nurse to determine whether a group-level diagnosis is appropriate. Community health nursing diagnoses are often confirmed by obtaining information from individual members of a group, without consideration of group-appropriate methods of data collection (Neufeld & Harrison, 1994). Group-appropriate methods might include random sampling of group members, aggregate scores from group members, use of epidemiological data pertinent to the aggregate, focus groups, group interviews, or other systematic methods of collecting data about group characteristics.

A dilemma related to selecting individual behaviour or environmental change as the priority focus for a nursing diagnosis is illustrated in the following example from our earlier study:

There is the potential for permanent hearing loss in all laundry employees related to prolonged exposure to unsafe sound-intensity levels, lack of hearing protection devices in use, lack of knowledge about the effect of noise, and lack of motivation to employ [appropriate] safety devices. (Neufeld & Harrison, 1994, p. 170)

In this example, if the primary focus is on environmental characteristics, then the nursing intervention will be centred on the employer or policy issues. If priority is given to protective measures, intervention will involve workers' and employers' actions to ensure that mechanisms are in place to support use of protective equipment. The emphasis that is selected will vary depending on the nature of the specific setting, the mandate of the nurse's appointment, and the needs of the client. However, the full responsibility for protection from hazards that could be reduced by environmental modification should not be displaced onto workers. Unfortunately, as Brown (1991) and Labonte (1994) note, emphasis is often given to individual change in health behaviours rather than to environmental change, which may affect health status and health behaviours.

When variations are evident within an aggregate or group, it may be useful to define subgroups and formulate separate diagnoses for each. However, this variation among individuals within a population could be addressed by a range of alternative program components tailored to diverse individual characteristics. It may also be useful to develop a cluster of interventions that include both group and individual strategies. For example, in encouraging individuals to quit smoking, community health nurses could offer support groups, counsel individuals, develop self-help programs, and participate in community-wide media campaigns.

Conclusion

For community health nurses who work within a Primary Health Care context, nursing diagnosis is flexible enough to address issues related to health promotion as well as the prevention of illness or injury. Our preliminary research supports its potential for use with population groups and aggregates as well as individuals. In addition, nursing diagnosis can be used to identify nursing's contribution when community health nurses work with professionals from other sectors or with community groups. It is important that nursing diagnoses for population groups and aggregates be developed in a partnership of nurses and group members that promotes clients' participation. We advocate special caution in the use of nurse-initiated diagnoses for vulnerable groups such as the poor or members of a different culture and suggest that unique diagnostic statements be developed with input from group members.

Acknowledgement
Portions of this chapter were published in A. Neufeld & M.J. Harrison (1994), Use of nursing diagnosis with population groups, *Nursing Diagnosis*, 5(4), 165–171 and A. Neufeld & M.J. Harrison (1995), Integrating nursing diagnosis for population groups within community health nursing practice, *Nursing Diagnosis*, 6(1), 37–41.

QUESTIONS

You are working as a community health nurse in a rural area with high levels of unemployment and poverty. One of your responsibilities is to promote the health of pregnant women. You have noted that most of the women in the community smoke and delay seeking prenatal care when it is not the first pregnancy. A number of the women developed complications during pregnancy and had extended hospitalizations in a tertiary care hospital located in a large urban centre some distance from your community. Some of their infants have also been ill or premature. When the women return to your community, they tell you that they were depressed and very isolated from their families and other sources of support during their hospitalization. They had no idea what to expect on admission to the hospital and had little time to prepare their families for the separation or to make arrangements for care of their other children. They were anxious and uncertain about where to find help on return to the community with an infant whom they perceived as fragile and requiring extra care.

1. What are the strengths and limitations of using a nursing diagnosis when working with this group of women?
2. Which level of nursing diagnosis would you use:
   a. group diagnoses
   b. individual diagnoses
   c. a combination of both levels
   What is your rationale?
3. Which client group or groups form the appropriate focus for nursing diagnoses in this situation? Discuss which client focus is of highest priority and the rationale for your choice.
4. What wellness diagnoses would be appropriate for this group? What deficit diagnoses would be appropriate?
5. In your opinion, which other professional and/or community groups may be involved in this situation? Discuss the potential role of each in relation to each of the diagnoses formulated in response to question 4.

REFERENCES

Brown, E.R. (1991). Community action for health promotion: A strategy to empower individuals and communities. *International Journal of Health Services, 21*(3), 441–456.

Canadian Public Health Association (CPHA). (1990). *Community health–public health nursing in Canada.* Ottawa: Author.

Canadian Public Health Association (CPHA). (1996). *Action statement for health promotion in Canada.* Ottawa: Author.

Carlyon, W.H. (1984). Disease prevention/health promotion—bridging the gap to wellness. *Health Values: Achieving High Level Wellness, 8*(3), 27–30.

Chalmers, K.L., & Bramadat, I.J. (1996). Community development: Theoretical and practical issues for community health nursing in Canada. *Journal of Advanced Nursing, 24*(4), 719–726.

Epp, J. (1986). *Achieving health for all: A framework for health promotion.* Ottawa: Health & Welfare Canada.

Federal, Provincial, & Territorial Advisory Committee on Population Health. (1994). *Strategies for population health: Investing in the health of Canadians.* Ottawa: Health Canada.

Hall, J., Stevens, P., & Meleis, A. (1994). Marginalization: A guiding concept for valuing diversity in nursing knowledge development. *Advances in Nursing Science, 16*(40), 23–41.

Hamilton, N., & Bhatti, T. (1996). *Population health promotion: An integrated model of population health and health promotion.* Ottawa: Health Promotion Development Division, Health Canada.

Hogston, R. (1997). Nursing diagnosis and classification systems: A position paper. *Journal of Advanced Nursing, 26*, 496–500.

Houldin, A., Saltstein, S., & Ganley, K. (1987). *Nursing diagnoses for wellness.* Philadelphia: J.B. Lippincott.

Kelley, J., & Frisch, N. (1990). Use of selected nursing diagnoses: A transcultural comparison between Mexican and American nurses. *Journal of Transcultural Nursing, 2*(1), 16–22.

Kickbusch, I. (1986). Health promotion: A global perspective. *Canadian Journal of Public Health, 77*, 321–326.

Labonte, R. (1993). *Health promotion and empowerment: Practice frameworks.* Toronto: Centre for Health Promotion, University of Toronto & ParticipAction.

Labonte, R. (1994). Death of program, birth of metaphor: The development of health promotion in Canada. In A. Pederson, M. O'Neill, & I. Rootman (Eds.), *Health promotion in Canada: Provincial, national and international perspectives* (pp. 72–90). Toronto: W.B. Saunders.

Lunney, M. (1982). Nursing diagnosis: Refining the system. *American Journal of Nursing, 82*(3), 456–459.

Maggs, C., & Ali Abedi, H. (1997). Identifying the health needs of elderly people using the Omaha Classification Scheme. *Journal of Advanced Nursing, 26*, 698–703.

Martin, K. (1995). Nurse practitioners' use of nursing diagnosis. *Nursing Diagnosis, 6*(1), 9–15.

Martin, K., & Scheet, N. (1992). *The Omaha system: Applications for community health nursing.* Philadelphia: W.B. Saunders.

Mitchell, G. (1991). Nursing diagnosis: An ethical analysis. *Image: Journal of Nursing Scholarship, 23*(2), 99–103.

Mundinger, M., & Jauron, G. (1975). Developing a nursing diagnosis. *Nursing Outlook, 23*(2), 94–98.

National Forum on Health. (1997). *Canada health action: Building on the legacy.* Ottawa: Author.

Neufeld, A., & Harrison, M.J. (1990). The development of nursing diagnoses for aggregates and groups. *Public Health Nursing, 7*(4), 251–255.

Neufeld, A., & Harrison, M.J. (1994). Use of nursing diagnosis with population groups. *Nursing Diagnosis, 5*(4), 165–171.

Neufeld, A., & Harrison, M.J. (1995). Integrating nursing diagnosis for population groups within community health nursing practice. *Nursing Diagnosis, 6*(1), 37–41.

Neufer, L. (1994). The role of the community health nurse in environmental health. *Public Health Nursing, 11*(3), 155–162.

North American Nursing Diagnosis Association (NANDA). (1990). *Taxonomy I.* St. Louis: Author.

North American Nursing Diagnosis Association (NANDA). (1996). *Nursing diagnoses: Definition and classification 1997–1998.* Philadelphia: Author.

Popkess-Vawter, S. (1991). Wellness nursing diagnoses: To be or not to be? *Nursing Diagnosis, 2*(1), 19–25.

Reutter, L., Neufeld, A., & Harrison, M.J. (1995). Using critical feminist principles to analyze programs for low-income urban women. *Public Health Nursing, 12*(6), 424–431.

Rootman, I., & Raeburn, J. (1994). The concept of health. In A. Pederson, M. O'Neill, & I. Rootman (Eds.), *Health promotion in Canada: Provincial, national and international perspectives* (pp. 56–71). Toronto: W.B. Saunders.

Sanford, S. (1987). Administrative applications of nursing diagnosis. *Heart & Lung,* 16(6, Pt. 1), 600–605.

Schultz, P.R. (1987). When client means more than one: Extending the foundational concept of person. *Advances in Nursing Science, 10*(1), 71–86.

Stevens, P., & Hall, J. (1992). Applying critical theories to nursing in communities. *Public Health Nursing, 9*(1), 2–9.

Tripp, S., & Stachowiak, B. (1992). Health maintenance, health promotion: Is there a difference? *Public Health Nursing, 9*(3), 155–161.

Walker, A., Martin, S., & Thompson, L. (1988). Feminist programs for families. *Family Relations, 37,* 17–22.

Wallerstein, N. (1992). Powerlessness, empowerment, and health: Implications for health promotion programs. *American Journal of Health Promotion, 6,* 197–205.

Williams, C.A. (1977, April). Community health nursing—What is it? *Nursing Outlook, 25,* 250–254.

World Health Organization (WHO). (1997). *The Jakarta declaration on health promotion into the 21st century.* Jakarta: Author. (Online: http://www.dnttm.ro/arspms/jakarta.html)

C H A P T E R   2 0

A pragmatic approach to community health promotion

Sandra M. Reilly

This chapter provides a practical approach to community health promotion. Beginning with a fundamental question—"what is health promotion?"—it identifies the theoretical underpinnings to health promotion versus the traditional biomedical approach. Then discussion is focussed on the international and Canadian policies that have fostered community health promotion. Obstacles to community health promotion are considered before examining nursing's role in this new health endeavour. A brief discussion follows regarding the nature of communities in health promotion. In the final section, the Community Health Promotion Practice model is described.

LEARNING OBJECTIVES

In this chapter, you will learn:

- the differences between community health promotion and traditional approaches to community health
- the evolution of national and international health promotion policies
- obstacles to community health promotion
- the appropriateness of different strategies in community health promotion
- how to apply the Community Health Promotion Practice model in health promotion practice

Introduction

Nurses have a critical role in the implementation of community health promotion. Certainly, Mahler, director-general of the World Health Organization (WHO), encouraged nurses to move into the community, assume an active role in health promotion, and participate more fully on Primary Health Care teams (Mahler, 1985). However, nurses still do not assume a leadership role in community health promotion (O'Neill, 1997). Typically, they participate neither in conceptual (Gottlieb, 1992) nor in policy development (Williams, 1989). Instead, they focus on the practical aspects of their work (O'Neill, 1997).

Whatever the past practices, nursing leaders have begun to urge nurses to advocate politically on behalf of their clients. At the 1998 biennial conference of the Canadian Nurses Association, several speakers challenged nurses to step outside the culture of service, to become spokespersons in making health policies, and to work with clients (Coutts, 1998).

This chapter makes a similar statement on behalf of community health nursing. Nurses play a critical role in health promotion (Campbell, 1993) because nursing seeks to enable clients and to engage in client advocacy. As enablement and advocacy are central to health promotion, nurses need to implement these activities in public health practice.

What is community health promotion?

In an emerging discipline such as health promotion, individuals and organizations seldom agree on definitions (Rissel, 1994). For the sake of discussion, the author will use the WHO definition of health promotion endorsed by the internationally recognized Pan American Health Organization: *health promotion is the process of enabling individuals and communities to increase control over the determinants of health and thereby improve their health* (Pan American Health Organization, 1996, p. 344).

According to this definition, health promotion focusses on enabling individuals and communities to improve their health. Enablement is a complex process (McMillan, Florin, Stevenson, Kerman, & Mitchell, 1995). Enablement differs for individuals and communities. Individuals feel enabled when they exercise greater control over their lives, such as when they participate in collective political action. Communities feel enabled when individual members participating in political action accomplish their goals; and in health promotion, goals usually emphasize the social–economic determinants of health.

Community health promotion represents a shift in how most health workers think about health. This shift requires "a revolution in thinking and in knowledge" (Bunton & Macdonald, 1992, p. 231). Some researchers and practitioners cannot make the leap. They confuse health promotion with traditional biomedical notions of prevention and treatment (Wilkinson, 1997).

Biomedical notions of prevention and treatment differ from current ideas of health promotion in several important respects. *Prevention* focusses on averting problems or negative functioning. It visualizes individuals and communities as vulnerable and health workers as experts who alone can reduce the incidence or alleviate the consequences of a problem. In short, prevention aims to control a hostile environment. *Treatment* endeavours to alleviate the consequences of a problem or disease that has already occurred. Health workers again appear as experts who manage or counteract diseases and problems. Treatment begins with the notion of deficiency or deficit; disabled or weak individuals or communities become the objects of treatment. *Promotion* differs significantly from both prevention and treatment. The promotion model focusses on enhancement and on self- or collective efficacy (Bandura, 1995). By emphasizing individual or community control over life events, it takes a proactive approach. Competencies and capabilities become the focus of intervention. Healthy living becomes the criterion for evaluation.

In summary, prevention focusses on protection, treatment concentrates on correction, and promotion centres on competency. That is, prevention supposes susceptibility, treatment presumes deficiency, and promotion assumes capability.

What principles underlie health promotion?

Several documents provide direction to Canadian practitioners and researchers in community health promotion. As policy statements, these documents delineate the principles of health promotion (Labonte, 1993a; O'Neill, 1997; Pederson, O'Neill, & Rootman, 1994; Raeburn & Rootman, 1998).

In 1974, the Lalonde report argued for a "new perspective." Although it took a comprehensive view of the health field, the report focussed on finding ways to alter lifestyles as a health promotion strategy. Many believed that the Lalonde report's emphasis on lifestyles resulted in victim-blaming (Buck, 1985). For example, the focus on lifestyles fostered a belief that individuals who smoked and developed lung disease had only themselves to blame. The cultural, social, educational, and economic factors associated with such behaviour did not receive sufficient consideration. Yet, as Wilkinson (1997) writes, "social and physical environmental factors contributed more significantly to [the poor health of the economically disadvantaged] than did individual behaviour" (p. 195). To appreciate the effects of these socioeconomic determinants on health, consider the situation of status Indians in Canada. Often socially isolated and economically deprived, they have an incidence rate for tuberculosis of 81.3 per 100 000, compared with an incidence of 1.9 per 100 000 for non-Aboriginals born in Canada (Mitchell, 1994).

The determinants of health play a critical role in health promotion. The determinants-of-health perspective differs from a lifestyles approach or a "downstream strategy." For example, imagine that someone standing at a river's edge hears a cry for help coming from the water. Suppose that the person jumps in, brings the drowning victim ashore, and resuscitates him. Then, the rescuer hears another cry and successfully repeats the same strategy. This goes on for the rest of the day, though not always with the same success. The rescuer cannot save everyone; some die. Yet, at no time does the rescuer go upstream to find out why all these people have fallen into the river. Possibly the railing on a bridge is broken and only needs a minor repair or a sign warning pedestrians of the danger. The point is that a lifestyles or "downstream strategy" expends many resources and takes a narrow view of a situation by focussing on treatment. Alternatively, an "upstream strategy" takes a more comprehensive proactive approach that focusses on health promotion and the determinants of health.

The narrowness of the lifestyles approach to health promotion forced a change in thinking. The leadership came from WHO (1978), which proposed a Health for All strategy, with Primary Health Care as its basis. WHO specified that communities should initiate, plan, and implement decisions related to Primary Health Care. The Health for All movement takes a positive approach to health; it emphasizes the relationship between health and the social–environmental circumstances in which people live and promotes community ownership and responsibility for health. (For a discussion of Primary Health Care, see Chapters 2 and 3.)

WHO's positive approach to health ultimately finds expression in health promotion, a key principle of Primary Health Care. As the introduction to the *Ottawa Charter for Health Promotion* (WHO, Health & Welfare Canada [HWC], & Canadian Public Health Association [CPHA], 1986) states, "health is . . . a resource for everyday life, not the objective of living." As a resource, health provides the conditions whereby people develop socially, economically, and personally. In these circumstances, the health of individuals and actions to promote their health result from a mix of politics, economics, society, culture, the environment, and behavioural and biological factors. Consequently, the Ottawa Charter recommends that governments adopt five strategies for health promotion:

- Build healthy public policy by analyzing the consequences of all government decisions on health promotion.
- Create supportive environments by recognizing the inextricable connection between the health of people and their environment.
- Strengthen community action by promoting community participation as a means of strengthening public participation in health matters.
- Develop personal skills by supporting personal and social development through lifelong learning.
- Reorient health services by creating linkages between the health sector and the broader social, political, economic, and physical environmental sectors.

These strategies reinforce the notion of health as a resource that belongs to the people, who have the right to define its meaning for themselves. *Achieving Health for All: A Framework for Health Promotion* (Epp, 1986) specified three strategies for health promotion in Canada:

- fostering public participation in a national effort to achieve health
- strengthening community health services to include the public in accomplishing community objectives
- coordinating healthy public policy to provide all sectors of society with opportunities to participate in health choices.

These three strategies reinforce community action in health promotion, community identification of priority needs, use of local resources, and strengthened community affiliations.

The five strategies of the Ottawa Charter and the three strategies of the Epp framework appear similar because both emphasize a comprehensive approach to health. They differ with regard to the emphasis placed on the delivery of health services. Whereas the Ottawa Charter recommends the "implementation of new approaches" in the delivery of health services, the Epp framework advocates the allocation of resources to community-based services and less emphasis on institutional services. Both documents emphasize health promotion, accessibility, intersectoral collaboration, and public participation. Together, they emphasize four of the key principles of Primary Health Care.

In the years since the Ottawa Charter and the framework, WHO has held three more international conferences on health promotion. The second international conference on health promotion, held in 1988, focussed on public policy-produced papers on women's health, nutrition, and the environment. In general, the conference argued that equity demanded active government participation (WHO, 1988). The third international conference focussed on supportive environments for health (WHO, 1991) and linked health promotion with sustainable development. Conference handbooks proposed methods to promote public health and the physical, social, and economic environments. The fourth international conference on health promotion had an imposing agenda, *New Players for a New Era: Leading Health Promotion into the 21st Century* (WHO, 1997). It embarked on two themes: global changes to the determinants of health and the need to involve other sectors of society in health promotion. That is, globalization of trade and changes in communications, behaviour, and living conditions have affected the determinants of health. Health promotion strategies now require new resources from all sectors of society. Public and private sectors together have to "promote social responsibility for health" (p. 4) by assessing the impact of their policies and practices on health. Intersectoral cooperation has to "increase investment for health development" (p. 4), especially related to marginalized or disadvantaged groups. Furthermore, community health promotion demands that all sectors examine means "to consolidate and expand partnerships for health" (p. 4) that "increase community capacity and empower the individual" (p. 5).

Two more recent Canadian documents also focus on health promotion. The first, *Strategies for Population Health* (Minister of Supply & Services Canada, 1994), a discussion paper tabled at a meeting of federal, provincial, and territorial deputy ministers of health, conceived the future of population health or community health promotion in three ways. One, the public still requires education about the various determinants of health. Two, decision makers in the private and public sectors require education about the impact of their decisions on the health of the community. Three, to achieve the benefits of a population health focus, Canadians have to implement intersectoral population health initiatives. These recommendations are particularly noteworthy for two reasons. First, they represent acceptance by politicians of the premises associated with community health promotion. Second, the recommendations focus on strategies for implementation. The second document, *Action Statement for Health Promotion in Canada*, published in 1996 by the Canadian Public Health Association (CPHA), provides explicit strategies for the implementation of population health objectives. Under the heading "Enhance Knowledge and Skills," the CPHA document ties the future of population health to health-impact assessments and evaluation studies. Under another heading, "Build Alliances," the building of coalitions and partnerships across multiple sectors receives attention. The CPHA invites public and private sectors, non-governmental organizations, and vulnerable groups in the community to form coalitions that can effect broad changes to the determinants of health.

What are the challenges to health promotion?

Health promotion does not yet enjoy the popularity of curative medicine for several reasons. The first probably is the inertia of the professions in accepting a shift in thinking. Second, there is inherent confusion over the use of the term *health promotion* as both a goal of public health and a description of health promotional practices (O'Neill, 1997). Third, consumer capitalism emphasizes individual consumption and wants, not the collective needs of communities for healthy living. Among developing nations, affluence has an untoward effect on the health of individuals and communities. Politicians, lacking either the insight or the political will, do not realign limited resources in favour of health promotion because it rarely provides a "quick fix."

Results derived from health promotion endeavours take longer to produce and more often present themselves in less demonstrable qualitative terms. Researchers cannot draw causal relationships from such work, thereby failing to provide proof for an intervention's efficacy (Guldan, 1996). Finally, health promotion requires a longer commitment because it takes an ecological approach. It assumes a multisectoral (e.g., professional, governmental, and volunteer), multidisciplinary (e.g., nursing, medicine, and social work), and multifactorial (e.g., political, social, anthropological, and economic) approach. The coordination and mobilization of so many players and interests requires time and dedicated, qualified individuals. Partnering the right health practitioners with various communities is often complex.

How does the community participate?

As the WHO definition of health promotion makes clear, health promotion strategies and services relate directly to the political, social, and economic realities of communities. Unilateral planning by professionals, who often "parachute" into communities, has become problematic. It alienates communities from the sources of power and ultimately marginalizes the health of individuals.

Given the prominence of community participation in health promotion, an explicit definition of community seems in order (see Chapter 5). Documents such as the Ottawa Charter (1986) and the Alma Ata report (WHO, 1978) speak of communities as coherent units within specific localities, sharing similar characteristics. Adopting a utopian approach, they portray communities as homogeneous and complementary units within a larger nation. Practitioners and researchers in public health question the usefulness of such a definition (Jewkes & Murcott, 1996), which does not account for diversity within communities nor the variety of contemporary communities. For example, the definition does not apply to all sole-support mothers, nor to newsgroups whose members communicate over the Internet about specific diseases or health issues. Does each of these represent a community? In some respects, yes. Yet, none represents a homogeneous, geographically specific group of individuals.

One research study (Jewkes & Murcott, 1996) analyzes how community workers and community members describe a community. The two do not always agree. Those in the professional, governmental, and volunteer sectors typically characterize a community as a group of people working together with a spirit of oneness that differs only in context (i.e., where and when it takes place). Such a portrayal presumes that everyone shares the same characteristics. Alternatively, community members recognize the similarities but also the differences among themselves. They describe community in terms of people's sharing some characteristic(s) or coming together for some specific purpose. What does such research tell us?

Communities constitute heterogeneous groups that change depending on the issues. Consequently, community workers need to cooperate with established groups in the community. By doing so, workers accept diversities and avoid the mistake of assuming that all communities have the same agenda. Workers in health promotion have to recognize that communities do not subscribe to preconceived notions of membership. Communities come together on a "need-to" basis.

How can nurses participate in health promotion?

Of all health workers, nurses have unique opportunities to participate in health promotion. In clinics, community centres, and schools, among other places, nurses enjoy multiple points of entry into the community. Respected more than other health workers (Coutts, 1998), nurses have a unique opportunity for implementing the Canadian federal government's three strategies for health promotion: fostering public participation, strengthening community health services, and coordinating healthy public policy (Epp, 1986). To paraphrase the *Action Statement for Health Promotion in Canada* (CPHA, 1996), in these contexts community health nurses can join in the implementation of health-impact assessments as well as the development of coalitions and partnerships with communities.

As knowledge specialists, community health nurses have multiple competencies, which they can make available to communities that want to develop their own action plans. According to *Community Health–Public Health Nursing in Canada* (CPHA, 1990), communities accept nurses as direct care providers, teachers/educators, researchers/evaluators, consultants, community developers, communicators, resource managers, planners, coordinators, team members, collaborators, social marketers, policy formulators, and facilitators (CPHA, 1990). (See Chapter 18 for a discussion of the community health nurse's role as it relates to these Primary Health Care activities.)

Of all these roles, that of facilitator embodies the key principles underlying community health promotion. As the CPHA (1990) document makes clear, when community health nurses act as facilitators, they function as leaders, enablers, and advocates. In effect, nurses have an obligation to speak out on behalf of Primary Health Care, become politically active in support of the "new public health," change their focus from curative hospital care to community action, and participate more fully in decision making at the policy level (Stacy, Down, & Donaghue, 1987).

Although they possess the opportunity and means, nurses, like other health workers, exhibit a reluctance to participate fully in community health promotion endeavours. In addition to the challenges to health promotion described earlier, nurses seem hesitant for other reasons (Antrobus & Brown, 1997; Chalmers & Bramadat, 1996; Goodwin, 1992; Sutherland, 1996). They are overly cautious about articulating the significance of their work and appear unwilling to participate in decision-making and policy-making endeavours. Without nursing input, however, community health promotion cannot reach its strategic objectives.

Community health nurses need a conceptual framework for community health promotion (Chalmers & Kristjanson, 1989). As the Canadian Public Health Association (1990) maintains, "there is a need to more fully develop existing nursing models to reflect a community focus and a synthesis of nursing and public health theory" (p. 2). A first step in this process includes the adoption of a conceptual matrix that contains critical elements in the community health promotion process. In a practical sense, the Community Health Promotion Practice model (CHPPM) serves such a purpose (Figure 20.1).

An examination of the CHPPM shows a set of five concentric circles that contain the elements critical to health promotion as discussed in this chapter. In addition, the CHPPM locates a nursing framework in the process, demonstrating how traditional nursing practice fits in with the other elements in any health promotion strategy. Lastly, this model displays the interrelationship between the principles driving a health promotion strategy, from a nursing perspective, and the kinds of communities involved in community health promotion.

The outermost circle contains two essential elements in health promotion. The first, *community action research*, refers to the process whereby communities participate in problem solving or evaluation (University of British Columbia Institute of Health Promotion Research, 1995). That is, the process of action research proposes to break down the division between the producers and consumers of information (Sohng, 1996). Rather than leave control with the "experts," all participants share power and control of decision making and action. This process of critical inquiry typically focusses on the experiences and needs of vulnerable and marginalized people. It assumes mutual trust and acceptance by participants, who through a consultative process use the findings to produce practical changes. People become empowered, form communities, collectively reflect on their experiences, validate their ideas, and take political and social action. (See Chapter 28.) The other element in this outermost circle is *communitarian values*. A well-known Canadian activist, Ronald Labonte, contends that all public health practitioners are communitarians (Labonte, 1993b) who believe that participation in community affairs is essential to daily living (Buchanan, 1989). Communitarians define each person by his or her obligations and commitments to others. As such, communitarianism

Figure 20.1
Community Health Promotion Practice model

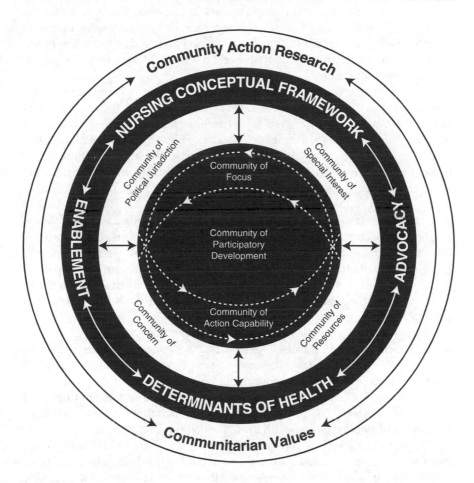

Determinants of Health
- Social
- Political
- Economic
- Biological

Reilly (1998, revised). Copyright by the author.

embodies the underlying logic of health promotion. Both share several assumptions: (a) every life has importance; (b) people, as social beings, gain from collective action; (c) mutual assistance is critical to the success of any society; (d) people have the right to expect justice and equitable treatment from government; and (e) the peaceful resolution of conflict benefits everyone (Smith, 1996). In summary, health action research, when driven by communitarianism, strives to create an equitable and harmonious society. These principles underlie community health promotion.

If the first concentric circle in Figure 20.1 represents the fundamental components of any health promotion enterprise, the second focusses on how nurses can participate. It contains four elements: besides a *nursing conceptual framework*, the circle also includes *determinants of health, enablement*, and *advocacy*. These last three are not exclusive to nursing and are important in any health promotion enterprise. Consequently, they directly inform any nursing approach in health promotion. Every nursing approach, however, begins with a nursing framework. Such a framework predisposes nurses to look at events in a certain manner, to collect certain kinds of data and information, and to approach situations with certain kinds of questions. In community health promotion, the nursing framework considers how social, economic, and political circumstances affect health and how nurses can participate in making structural changes. When nurses synthesize all these elements in their practice, they fully participate in the community health promotion process.

The remaining two circles in the CHPPM depict seven kinds of communities ordinarily found in society. Together, they serve as a comprehensive representation of communities; they do not represent a classification of all different kinds of communities, nor do they typify communities according to some theory. (See also Chapter 5.) These seven communities, defined and represented in Table 20.1, portray the diverse groups that can form coalitions in support of a community health initiative. When committed to community health promotion, nurses constitute a *community of action capability*. Their membership is conditional on their understanding and acceptance of communitarianism and action research, as well as on the possession of a nursing framework that incorporates enablement, advocacy, and the determinants of health. When they have met these conditions, nurses form a community ready to work with the public. However, a community of action capability has meaning only when it engages with a *community of focus*. Made up of members from the public, the community of focus organizes for some specific purpose. It often requires, because of the complexity of contemporary society, information about how the bureaucratic and political structures function and how to prepare formal documents or evaluations. In doing so, it benefits from the critical judgement of a sympathetic supporter. In this way, when the community of action capability and the community of focus come

Table 20.1
Definition and example for each of the seven communities in the Community Health Promotion Practice model

Community	Definition	Example
Community of Focus	A group of individuals with shared values who have identified their health goal(s) and want to to address them	Community of single mothers meets to discuss mutual interests, including day care, infant nutrition, and child safety
Community of Action Capability	Community health nurses who define health promotion from a social-environmental perspective and propose to enable communities to make choices and take actions	Community health nurse, on her own initiative, appears before a municipal government task force studying options to reduce family violence
Community of Participatory Development	Forms when the Community of Focus and Community of Action Capability collaborate in a social action process that addresses the goals of a community	Community of senior citizens meets with a group of public health nurses to prepare a proposal for government funding to assess bereavement needs in a rural community
Community of Special Interests	People who have a significant professional and/or economic interest in health services, who apply their expert skills on behalf of the Community of Participatory Development	Geriatric nurses, in a consultative practice, prepare a manual of safety protocols for a community group that provides transportation to frail seniors

(continued)

Table 20.1 (*continued*)

Community	Definition	Example
Community of Resources	People without significant economic interest in health services, who make available their knowledge of and access to actual and potential human and financial assets to a Community of Participatory Development	Group of executives develops a corporate fundraising campaign to support a local crisis nursery
Community of Concern	People without significant financial resources or economic interest in health services, who voluntarily participate in a community development endeavour to advance the public's health	Group of seniors in a lodge volunteer to sew quilts for a crisis nursery
Community of Political Jurisdiction	Individuals who have the power to influence political decisions, laws, and government policies, and who make their services available to the Community of Participatory Development	Municipal official offers to support a community proposal for the establishment of an outreach centre for single mothers who, while receiving social assistance, attend post-secondary school

Reilly (1998, revised). Copyright by the author.

together, they form a coalition and become a *community of participatory development*. It, more than any other community, embodies the principles of community action research, in which participants share power and control throughout the decision-making process. Such cooperation ensures that the community of focus never becomes the object of study, but remains a full participant in the evaluative process. This consultative *community of participatory development* forms alliances with other communities that possess the resources or skills required to implement change. Some are included in the four communities that orbit the innermost circle. The examples provided in Table 20.1 illustrate how these four communities play different, but indispensable, roles. Think how the *community of resources*, with access to philanthropic resources, can help a crisis nursery when government limits its financial assistance. Consider how the *community of political jurisdiction*, with its financial and human resources, can effect sweeping changes in the lives of sole-support mothers who require social assistance in order to finish high school. Similar, though possibly less dramatic, changes also accompany the interactions between the *community of special interest* or the *community of concern* with the community of participatory development. Together, all these communities can contribute to community health promotion.

Conclusion

This chapter has addressed the meaning and underlying principles of community health promotion and the challenges to its implementation. It has explored community participation and the role of nursing. More specifically, the Community Health Promotion Practice model has been used to describe the critical elements that constitute a community health nursing approach to health promotion.

This approach challenges practitioners to make a paradigm shift in thinking. That is, the community, no longer the professional, drives any health promotion enterprise, ultimately requiring multifactorial input from all sectors and disciplines. This "upstream strategy" in health promotion requires a comprehensive perspective that considers all the determinants of health.

QUESTIONS

1. What are the interrelationships between economic and social changes in a community and its health promotion needs? For example, if a key local industry (e.g., a fish processing plant, a pulp-and-paper plant, or a company that makes car parts) shuts down, what effects might this have on

the community's need for health promotion programs? What would the community health nurse's role be in community health promotion?

2.   Imagine that a women's organization in your community has proposed the development of a drop-in centre for teenagers. Should community health nurses become involved? If so, how? Use the Community Health Promotion Practice model to guide your response. Identify how each of the seven types of communities participate in the community action research process.

3.   In the example given for question 2, what other disciplines and/or groups (sectors) might be involved in the collaborative process? How would individual community health nurses become involved in health promotion initiatives with these disciplines and sectors? What constraints might inhibit such collaborative community health promotion initiatives?

REFERENCES

Antrobus, S., & Brown, S. (1997). The impact of the commissioning agenda upon nursing practice: A proactive approach to influencing health policy. *Journal of Advanced Nursing, 25,* 309–315.

Bandura, A. (1995). *Self-efficacy in changing societies.* New York: Cambridge University Press.

Buchanan, A.E. (1989). Assessing the communitarian critique of liberalism. *Ethics, 99,* 852–882.

Buck, C. (1985, May/June). Beyond Lalonde: Creating health. *Canadian Journal of Public Health, 76* (Suppl. 1).

Bunton, R., & Macdonald, G. (1992). *Health promotion: Disciplines and diversity.* London: Routledge.

Campbell, A.V. (1993). The ethics of health education. In J. Wilson-Barnett & J. Macleod Clark (Eds.), *Research in health promotion and nursing.* London: Macmillan.

Canadian Public Health Association (CPHA). (1990). *Community health–public health nursing in Canada: Preparation and practice.* Ottawa: Author.

Canadian Public Health Association (CPHA). (1996). *Action statement for health promotion in Canada.* Ottawa: Author.

Chalmers, K., & Bramadat, I.J. (1996). Community development: Theoretical and practical issues for community health nursing in Canada. *Journal of Advanced Nursing, 24,* 719–726.

Chalmers, K., & Kristjanson, L. (1989). The theoretical basis for nursing at the community level: A comparison of three models. *Journal of Advanced Nursing, 14,* 569–574.

Coutts, J. (1998, June 17). There's strength in numbers, nurses told. *Globe and Mail,* p. A6.

Epp, J. (1986). *Achieving health for all: A framework for health promotion.* Ottawa: Minister of Supply & Services.

Goodwin, S. (1992). Nurses and purchasing. *Senior Nurse, 12*(6), 7–11.

Gottlieb, L. (1992). Nurses not heard in the health promotion movement. *Canadian Journal of Nursing Research, 24*(4), 1–2.

Guldan, G.S. (1996). Obstacles to community health promotion. *Social Science & Medicine, 43*(5), 689–695.

Jewkes, R., & Murcott, A. (1996). Meanings of community. *Social Science & Medicine, 43*(4), 555–563.

Labonte, R. (1993a). *Health promotion and empowerment: Practice frameworks.* Toronto: Centre for Health Promotion.

Labonte, R. (1993b). *Health promotion—Knowledge development.* Paper presented at the Health Promotion Knowledge Development Meeting, January 27–28, 1993, Toronto.

Lalonde, M. (1974). *A new perspective on the health of Canadians.* Ottawa: Information Canada.

Mahler, H. (1985, June). Nurses lead the way. *Who Features,* No. 67.

McMillan, B., Florin, P., Stevenson, J., Kerman, B., & Mitchell, R.E. (1995). Empowerment praxis in community coalitions. *American Journal of Community Psychology, 23*(5), 699–727.

Minister of Supply & Services Canada. (1994). *Strategies for population health: Investing in the health of Canadians.* Ottawa: Author.

Mitchell, A. (1994, November 30). Native tuberculosis rate "unbelievable." *Globe and Mail,* p. A5.

O'Neill, M. (1997). Health promotion: Issues for the year 2000. *Canadian Journal of Nursing Research, 29*(1), 71–77.

Pan American Health Organization. (1996). *Health promotion: An anthology.* Washington, DC: Author.

Pederson, A., O'Neill, M., & Rootman, I. (Eds.). (1994). *Health promotion in Canada: Provincial, national and international perspectives.* Toronto: W.B. Saunders.

Raeburn, J., & Rootman, I. (1998). *People-centered health promotion.* Chichester, UK: John Wiley & Sons.

Reilly, S.M. (1998, revised). *The Community Health Promotion Practice model.* Copyright by the author.

Rissel, C. (1994). Empowerment: The holy grail of health promotion. *Health Promotion International, 9*(1), 39–47.

Smith, G. (1996). *Community and communitarianism: Concepts and contexts.* (Online: http://www.btwebworld.com/communities/greg/gsum.html)

Sohng, S.S.L. (1996). Participatory research and community organizing. *Journal of Sociology and Social Welfare, 23*(4), 77–95.

Stacy, S., Down, E., & Donaghue, S. (1987). Primary Health Care: A new focus and challenge for nursing. *Australian Nurses Journal, 16,* 44–45.

Sutherland, R.W. (1996). *Will nurses call the shots? A look at the delivery of health care twenty years from now.* Ottawa: Canadian Nurses Association.

University of British Columbia Institute of Health Promotion Research. (1995). *Study of participatory research in health promotion: Review and recommendations for the development of participatory research in health promotion in Canada.* Ottawa: Royal Society of Canada.

Wilkinson, M. (1997). Health promotion planning: A liberal communitarian perspective. In J.S. Bright (Ed.), *Health promotion in clinical practice.* London: Bailliere Tindall.

Williams, D.M. (1989). Political theory and individualistic health promotion. *Advances in Nursing Science, 12*(1), 14–25.

World Health Organization (WHO). (1978). *Primary Health Care: Report of the International Conference on Primary Health Care, Alma Ata, USSR.* Geneva: Author.

World Health Organization (WHO). (1988). *The Adelaide recommendations: Healthy public policy.* Copenhagen: Author.

World Health Organization (WHO). (1991). *To create supportive environments for health. The Sundsvall handbook.* Geneva: Author.

World Health Organization (WHO). (1997). *New players for a new era: Leading health promotion into the 21st century.* Geneva: WHO & Ministry of Health, Republic of Indonesia.

World Health Organization (WHO), Health & Welfare Canada (HWC), & Canadian Public Health Association (CPHA). (1986). *Ottawa charter for health promotion.* Ottawa: Canadian Public Health Association.

CHAPTER 21

Community development

John C.B. English

Participating in community development is part of a newly expanded role for most community health nurses. This chapter explores community development as a mechanism for public participation in community health. This approach represents a change from the traditional model that advocated "caring for" to one that advocates "caring with" clients. In community health, the change came about, in part, because of the Ottawa Charter for Health Promotion and the Healthy Cities initiative. A case study exemplifying community development in the prairie city of Brandon, Manitoba, concludes the chapter.

LEARNING OBJECTIVES

In this chapter, you will learn:

- to differentiate community development activities from those traditionally associated with community health nursing
- to understand how the process of change fits the various models of community development
- how to cultivate community development in the context of everyday nursing practice
- how the Healthy Communities movement relates to the concept of community development

Introduction

Community health teaching preceded the idea of health promotion in Canada (English, 1994; Raeburn & Rootman, 1998). In community health teaching, a health educator would identify a health problem within a community, for example, by reviewing health statistics for that community. After validating the problem with individual community members, a teaching plan would be developed and delivered to a target group.

This approach was effective when the problem was attitudinal or was due to lack of knowledge and/or skills. However, it has not been effective in addressing environmental and community-wide problems that have an impact on health. Problems such as substandard housing, pollution, or unequal access to health services require community-wide action.

Given such broad health-related problems, community health nurses need to be familiar with the principles of community development to be effective agents for change. In this chapter, various approaches to community development are described, leading to a framework that can assist community health nurses to promote public participation in health and health care. Rather than simply "caring for" clients, community health nurses must work with clients in a "caring with" model. A brief overview of two of the factors that led to the introduction of community development as an approach to community health are described, namely, the *Ottawa Charter for Health Promotion* (World Health Organization [WHO], Health & Welfare Canada [HWC], & Canadian Public Health Association [CPHA], 1986), the Healthy Cities initiative (WHO, 1988a–e), and the *Jakarta Declaration on Leading Health Promotion into the 21st Century* (WHO, 1998). A community development project in Brandon, Manitoba, is described to illustrate the principles of community development in action.

What is community development?

The United Nations (1955), Dunham (1970), and Hoffman and Dupont (1992) have all defined community development. Their varied definitions share common themes: goals for improvement of the community, organized change processes, and empowerment of people. For community development to be successful, health workers must facilitate and encourage community members in the work necessary to bring about change.

Health promotion practitioners see community development as a philosophy, a process, or a project, or as all three at once (Feather, 1994). As a philosophy, community development entails the fundamental democratic belief that people can identify and solve their own problems; as a process, it supports groups as they find their own power to effect change; and as a project, it entails work with community representatives to bring about specific change in their community. Both of the following definitions of community development incorporate these three viewpoints:

Community development is people taking charge of their own futures. It is people identifying commonly-felt problems and needs and taking steps to resolve the problems and meet the needs. It is people struggling to make their community a better place to live out their lives than it ever was before. (Four Worlds Development Project, 1984, p. 7)

Community development is a process through which all members of the community gain an increase of the control over their lives, as well as the life of the community, by attaining equal access to participate in determining, and making decisions about their needs, and in the development and implementation of strategies which utilize their collective power to meet those needs. (City of Toronto Department of Public Health, 1991, p. 2)

The first definition recognizes the process of identification of community needs or problems by community members, who own responsibility to solve the problems or meet the needs. The word "struggle" captures the toil inherent in effective community development work. The second definition seems to express frustration with the control (power) that bureaucracies and government sometimes exercise over the lives of people and the communities in which they live. The democratic requirement for equality, control, and collective power is reflected in this definition. Both definitions suggest disadvantaged or oppressed people working together to change their relationship with their oppressors and to improve their economic and/or social conditions. There is striking congruence between these two definitions and the ideology expressed within the widely accepted definition of health promotion adopted by the World Health Organization in 1984: "Health promotion is the process of enabling individuals and communities to increase control over the determinants of health and thereby improve their health." (See also deLeeuw, 1989; Hancock, 1986; Kickbusch, 1981, 1986a, 1986b; Milio, 1986a, 1986b, 1987; WHO 1988a–e, 1998.)

It is intrinsic to community development that community representatives participate in identifying broad issues or problems, plan remedial actions, and act on these plans. "Participation is essential to sustain efforts. People have to be at the centre of health promotion action and decision-making processes for them to be effective" (WHO, 1998). A community health nurse can participate as team member, consultant, or facilitator when invited by the community. Clearly, this is different from a program planned by health professionals, who have their own agenda for solving a health problem and who recruit the support of the community in implementing it. Put into action, all these ideas and approaches to community development culminate in community and social change.

Models of community and social change

Various models of social change have emerged in the literature over the years, of which community development is one. Warren (1977) describes two types of change that affect communities: deliberative or purposive change and crescive change. Crescive change refers to change in communities that continually occurs outside a community group's planned change. For example, one community group's plan to provide "Wheels to Meals" (rides to a community kitchen) for the elderly will be crescive change; another community group may provide "Meals on Wheels" (meals delivered to homes) for the same target group.

Warren (1977) also delineated social change, describing the objective (behavioural, relational, or ideal change), the target system, resistance, and stabilization of change.

Objective of change

The greater the care taken in thinking through the change, the more likely the community will be able to identify its consequences before the change takes place. Strategies for change can then be more carefully chosen. Behaviour, relationships, and ideas are the three foci for community change objectives. *Behaviour* is the target of all purposive change. Changing individual behaviour can eventually bring about social change, such as change in discriminatory practices, attitudes toward physical exercise, or smoking. (Consider changes wrought in the workplace because of actions directed toward sexual harassment or discriminatory hiring practices.) *Relationships* are part of individual behaviour and are reflected in the way community groups and formal organizations are developed and how they function. Community groups and formal organizations can also be targets of change, as well as intra- or inter-organizational and interpersonal networks. *Ideas* refers to a focus on people's attitudes, values, and beliefs. An example of community and social change in this area is the environmental movement, which has influenced the way people think and feel about ecology, resource development, and conservation.

Target system

Identification of the target system puts attention at the level of the system that will be the focus of the change from individual to international relations. Designating the target system level will influence the choice of strategies. The change-inducing system alludes to the organization of people who work to cause the desired change. For example, the community health nurse who assesses the need for creating a new drop-in centre for single parents will need a steering committee responsible for planning, a fund-raising committee, a committee on building design, a program design committee, and so on. The strategies for change available to a community health nurse within a change-inducing system fall into two distinct categories: those within the target system and those outside the system.

Strategy for change

Cooperative strategies are used when there is significant agreement on the objective. Coalition building (where small groups of like-minded individuals join to exert their influence) and collaboration are examples of cooperative strategies. *Campaign strategies* are used when there is no consensus on the need for change, but it is believed that agreement can be achieved by using persuasive tactics. Coalition building and use of the media are examples of campaign strategies. *Contest strategies* refer to power struggles that result when there is no agreement about a change objective. Use of the media, coalition building, negotiation, and confrontations such as demonstrations and strikes exemplify these strategies.

Resistance is a natural phenomenon, in itself neither good nor bad. Resistance can prevent the change-inducing system from causing changes that could be catastrophic. Several sources of resistance have been identified, such as habit, vested interests, ideology, psychopathology, and rational conviction (Paul & Miller, 1955; Watson, 1967).

Stabilization of change needs to occur if the change is to be lasting, to assure supporters within the target system of the continuation of the change, and to buffer against external forces that may try to eliminate it.

Models of community development

Cox and Erlich (1974) described three models of community intervention: locality development, social action, and social planning. The community development models most pertinent to community health nurses are locality development and social action.

Practitioners of *locality development* assume that change is accomplished by the involvement of a broad spectrum of people in the process of change. It is best applied within a confined geographic location and is frequently concerned with issues in the local community. Initial approaches used to create change will likely be collaboration and campaign strategies.

The *social action* model is concerned with social justice and democracy and organizes disadvantaged groups to make demands on the larger community. This approach seeks to redistribute power, resources, or decision making in the community and to change basic policies of formal organizations. Conflict strategies are typically used. The women's movement, gay liberation, and insurgent labour unions typify this approach. The community health nurse would apply the principles of community development in the local community to implement social action changes affecting the determinants of health.

The *social planning* model of community intervention advocates a rational, deliberately planned and controlled approach to community problem solving by expert agents for change. The level of community involvement may vary depending on the nature of the community problem. Building community capacity or fostering radical social change does not play a central part

(Warren, 1977). An example of such social planning change in Canada was the planned elimination of the Imperial system of weights and measures in favour of the SI metric system.

Labonte (1992) has identified five essential principles of community development: empowering services (direct care is applied with dignity and cultural sensitivity), connective processes (bringing people together into a sympathetic group working with common purpose), organizational actions (groups organize to act as agents for change within community structures), collaborative strategies (individuals, groups, and organizations work together), and advocacy that challenges control. Conflict is seen as a healthy part of community development, just as it can be of human relations.

While community development seeks empowerment for all, it also struggles with an empowerment in which the powers that some gain are balanced by the powers that some lose or give up (Labonte, 1992, p. v). The changes sought by a community group can meet with resistance from stakeholders with vested interests. The challenge is to keep conflict at a level that is healthy for all parties affected by the process of change.

Community development is a fundamental approach in health promotion. The strategy benefits those groups that are at greatest risk for poor health and often the most difficult to reach through traditional approaches.

Community development and community health nursing

Making the paradigm shift from the expert caregiver to the agent for community development and change has been difficult for some community health nurses. (See also Chapters 16 and 18.) Jackson, Mitchell, and Wright (1989) relate three ways in which nurses in community health centres initially reacted to the notion of community development: ignoring community development, hiring special workers to "do" community development, and allocating some portion of time a day, or half a day per week, for community development (Jackson et al., 1989).

Although they need to adjust to new role expectations, most community health nurses can subscribe to the philosophy of community development. Community development is grounded in a set of values that fit well with existential nursing philosophies such as those espoused by Parse (1981) and Watson (1985), and with nursing theories based on systems theory. For example, the Neuman (Campbell & Keller, 1989) and King (1981) systems' conceptual frameworks encompass an approach that recognizes that the physical, psychological, social, and spiritual parts of an individual's world are intimately and reciprocally related.

Jackson et al. (1989) generated a model to illustrate the fit of community development to the range of practice in community health centres. Each of the identified actions (explained in the list below) facilitates the assumption of power. Although the model was originally presented as a continuum, it more accurately represents the forms that community development can assume in community health nursing practice.

- *Developmental casework.* This conventional approach tended to foster dependency on the community health practitioner and concentrated on developing the client's capacity to make informed decisions. Community development occurs when the client can stop relying on the health practitioner and start sustaining others in like circumstances.
- *Mutual support.* The goal here is to strengthen natural relationships with family, friends, and neighbours or, if necessary, to form new support groups. Mutual support can develop community members' networks of support, which enable them to deal confidently with broader community health issues.
- *Issue identification and campaigns.* This form of development brings community networks and/or individuals together around a common social, political, or health issue to plan deliberate, joint action. This point marks the transition from participation for survival to participation to achieve change (Jackson et al., 1989, p. 104).
- *Participation and control of services.* The community sets up boards of directors (such as regional boards, in some provinces) or advisory committees of established organizations or founds new organizations. Community health nurses must be open to community members participating in the control of their own organization. Clients must feel comfortable expressing their views of community health nursing services and proffering suggestions for improvement.
- *Social movements.* This pervasive form of community development leads to a fundamental change in decisions and in the decision-making process. The target system has the power to exercise control over peoples' lives. Community organization, discussions, presentation of briefs, use of the media, and public protests are some strategies that can be used by the community health nurse to bring about needed change.

Hoffman and Dupont (1992) compare community development in health to community economic development. They point out that the experience and capacity that a community gains through solving problems in one area may be valuable in another (p. 24). For example, a community group that organized a cooperative soup kitchen will have cultivated a network of people and organizational skills that could be applied to another issue.

In health, community development typically starts with a community's examination of the physical and psychosocial risk factors in the process of identifying its own health problems. It is the process of enabling communities to make decisions necessary to plan and carry out strategies to achieve better health (Labonte, 1990, p. 104). Community-managed strategies for change are usually broad and socially and politically based. The roles of health professionals shift to consultation and support. To be effective in community development, community health nurses need to be competent in coalition building, networking, advocacy, mutual support group facilitation, facilitation of empowerment, and use of the media (English & Hicks, 1992, p. 64).

Healthy Communities and community development

The Healthy Cities initiative was started first in the European Division of the World Health Organization (WHO) and has burgeoned into a worldwide movement (WHO, 1988a–e). A healthy city is a community that is active in working out its own fate. It does not lie passively waiting for politicians to apply solutions to problems; it develops its own community (Sherman, 1988, p. 22). This perspective is remarkably similar to the definition of community development by Labonte (1990).

Canada's Healthy Communities project was initiated in 1988. Sponsored by the Canadian Public Health Association, Canadian Association of Municipalities, and City Planners Association, this two-year project established Healthy Communities across the country. Community health nurses often found themselves educationally unprepared for engagement in new activities related to issues of community concern. In addition, this new responsibility sometimes resulted in internal role conflict or conflict of loyalties for community health nurses employed by governments.

The development of an understanding of the community and the change processes operating within it requires a conceptual framework to organize pertinent concepts. A framework can enhance nurses' understanding of community dynamics and facilitate the development of an action plan. A systems-in-transition paradigm developed by English and Hicks (1992) provides one framework for community development. Briefly, this framework organizes the community into five mutually and inextricably linked subsystems: production–distribution, socialization, mutual support, social control, and social participation. The transition processes include the system's development and change over time and the internal adjustment to social stresses (which can involve system conflict). Using the language of this framework, the authors proffered a definition of a healthy community:

A healthy community is a system which promotes its own growth, development and health by managing community conflict through effective communication between its subsystems and with other systems, has people who strive for physical, mental and spiritual health for all, and who recognize the impact of community decision-making on the health of the inhabitants and the habitat. (English & Hicks, 1992, p. 63)

This definition assumes that the fundamental principles of community development will apply to the development of a healthy community. The following case study illustrates a community development project that emerged because of Brandon's Healthy Communities philosophy.

Case study

This is the story of an organization of citizens in southwestern Manitoba ("Westman") called the Westman Association for Terminal Care in Hospice (WATCH). This organization was formed when the only palliative care facility in Westman was closed. WATCH is in the process of becoming fully established. Even at this stage, however, it provided a good illustration of community development.

Brandon, a city of approximately 40 000 and the second largest city in Manitoba, is in the southwest corner of the province. Principal employers are manufacturers of agricultural chemicals, a general hospital, the university, and a technical college. It is the cultural heart of the region, and the retail centre for the surrounding agricultural communities.

Like hospitals all over Canada in the early 1990s, Brandon General Hospital's administration was forced to make difficult choices because of a drastically reduced budget and health system reform. The hospital's palliative care program was an early casualty. Its team was disbanded, and the six remaining beds of the 22-bed unit were dispersed throughout the hospital.

The palliative care unit was a source of pride to the community, especially to its volunteers, who had devoted time, effort, and money to its development and maintenance. News of its demise spread quickly, and letters decrying the closure of the unit came pouring in to the editor of the local newspaper, The Brandon Sun. *Surviving family members liberally praised the staff who had selflessly provided comfort and solace on the last journeys of so many community residents.*

Coalition building

News of another cut of $1.3 million made it clear that the palliative care unit was eliminated at Brandon General Hospital. As a nurse concerned with the health of the community, the author wrote a letter to the *Sun* suggesting the possibility of establishing a hospice for Brandon and invited readers to a meeting to hear the administrator of Jocelyn House, a free-standing hospice in Winnipeg, explain what a hospice was and how it operated. Following the presentation, the 43 citizens present formed a small group to study the feasibility of establishing a hospice in Brandon.

The feasibility study group included members from diverse sectors of the community and comprised various disciplines. Members included clergy, a nursing professor, a biology professor, AIDS support group members, Alzheimer Society members, physicians, palliative care nurses and volunteers, a community health educator, and a parent of a deceased child. An informal survey of the community sought information from neighbours, friends, family members, physicians (especially those treating people with terminal illness), volunteer agencies, ministerial associations, social workers and nurses in community health, and palliative care nurses.

The respondents were informed about the purpose and goals of a hospice and asked their opinion about the necessity of a hospice for Brandon and whether they thought that a program entailing volunteer service would be sustainable. It was their unanimous opinion that not only was a hospice needed for Brandon, but for the entire region of Westman. This need was further supported by statistics on usage of the former palliative care unit. One disease-specific voluntary organization, however, expressed the opinion that there may not be sufficient volunteers in the community to support a new organization.

The change-inducing system

After such emphatic validation of the need, the hospice feasibility study group assumed the responsibility for forming the Westman Association for Terminal Care in Hospice (WATCH). After the constitution had been written, a board of directors was elected at the first annual meeting. Many members of the original feasibility study group were elected, including the community health educator, who was a nurse. A bishop, a former palliative care nurse, and a nun from a local religious order were added to the board.

Developing objectives

The purpose of WATCH, clearly identified in its constitution, was

. . . to sustain dying persons and their families by providing a caring community in which patients may live life to the full, and to support families into the future. This mission will be carried out through offering residential Hospice services to selected terminally ill patients and their families, and by providing home care service which eases dying at home. (WATCH, 1992, p. 1)

Six goals (grouped according to Warren's framework for social change) were articulated to support the mission statement:

Changing ideas, beliefs, and attitudes

1. to increase public awareness of the need for hospice and home care for the terminally ill in Western Manitoba
2. to provide opportunities for the training of volunteer hospice workers in Western Manitoba

Organizational relationships

3. to establish free-standing hospices in the Western region of Manitoba
4. to establish and maintain contacts with those groups concerned with the provision of terminal care

Behavioural changes

5. to provide support for the terminally ill and their families within the home environment
6. to raise the necessary funds for the establishment and maintenance of facilities and programs for the terminally ill in the Westman region

To ensure that all the directors shared the same vision of WATCH, a statement of philosophy (see Table 21.1) was developed. These beliefs were drawn from the precepts of the American Palliative Care Association, with clauses added concerning non-discrimination on the basis of race, colour, age, gender, marital status, religion, sexual orientation, and diagnosis. Some clauses particularly pertinent to principles of public participation include beliefs that

* self-esteem can be maintained and/or promoted in the dying person and his or her family by fully involving them in decisions affecting their care
* the living will or similar document representing the dying person's intentions will be respected as one of the determinants in the total pattern of care
* opportunities should be provided for experiencing the final moments of life in a way that is meaningful to the dying person
* dying persons and their families should have the opportunity to discuss dying, death, and related emotional needs with representatives of WATCH
* a mutual support network should exist among the members of WATCH, encompassing both the socio-emotional and technical dimensions of working with dying people and their families.

The range of services focussed on provision of support to families and/or friends to maintain dying persons at home ("outreach") and to provide a residential service ("hospice") for those for whom dying at home was not possible.

Table 21.1
Philosophy of WATCH

We, the board of WATCH, believe that:

- self-esteem can be maintained and/or promoted in the dying and his or her family by fully involving them in decisions affecting their care,

- remission of symptoms and pain control are treatment goals for people in the terminal stages of illness,

- the living will or similar document representing the dying person's intentions will be respected as one of the determinants in the total pattern of care,

- dying persons should have a sense of basic security and protection in their environment,

- opportunities should be provided for leave-taking with the people most important to the dying person,

- opportunities should be provided for experiencing the final moments in a way that is meaningful to the dying person,

- dying persons and their families should have the opportunity to discuss dying, death, and related emotional needs with representatives of WATCH,

- families should have the opportunity for privacy with the dying person both while living and newly dead,

- care-giving members of WATCH should have adequate time to form and maintain personal relationships with the dying and his or her family,

- a mutual support network should exist among the members of WATCH, encompassing both the socio-emotional and technical dimensions of working with dying people and their families,

- the hospice services provided by WATCH should encompass a program of palliative and supportive services which provide physical, psychological, social and spiritual care for dying persons and their families,

- we should offer services by professional and lay volunteers and staff in the person's home or in a free-standing hospice setting,

- home care should be provided on a part-time intermittent, regularly scheduled, round-the-clock basis, and bereavement services should be available to the family,

- admission to hospice program services should be on the basis of patient and family need, and

- there should be no discrimination on the basis of diagnosis, race, colour, creed, marital status, age, or sexual orientation.

WATCH (1992). Used with permission.

The members of WATCH were recruited to serve on six standing committees of the board in charge of fund raising and public relations, developing relationships with professional groups, organizing the outreach program, organizing the in-house program, training and nurturing volunteers, and acquiring and maintaining property. The sixth task was completed quickly. An unused but well-equipped and well-maintained 12-bed personal care home in the local convent became available for lease. The facility needed fire safety upgrading, but included beds and nursing equipment.

The target system
The community of Brandon and surrounding municipalities (Westman) formed the primary target system. During planning and implementation other target systems emerged, primarily Manitoba Health and the Brandon General Hospital. Cooperative relationships with all systems needed to be forged, and support for the venture elicited.

Strategies for change
Community organization of WATCH was the initial strategy. Public meetings, the local press, radio, and television ensured that the Westman community was kept informed. Raising sufficient funds ($125 000) to open the Westman Hospice necessitated the presentation of briefs to foundations, Manitoba Health Services Development Fund (lotteries money), and service clubs. The fledgling organization was daunted by the magnitude of the task of finding so much money. Hence, they retained the services of an administrator who agreed to raise the necessary funds, including his own salary. The initial strategy was to campaign for funds from government coffers.

Foundations rarely fund an organization if it is not established and functioning. Consequently, fund raising for seed money at first focussed on the acquisition of a grant from the provincial lotteries fund. The Minister of Health resisted all petitions for funding, despite rational arguments that referred to the health system reform principles of Manitoba Health and the fiscal benefits of the project.

Resistance encountered
Because of this strong resistance, the board first planned contest strategies. Arguments put to the power elite were to be printed in the media, and public protests through letter-writing campaigns were to be launched. The inequity of the palliative care services available in Winnipeg and in Western Manitoba was to be again drawn to the attention of the public.

Sober reflection led the board to abandon these plans in favour of reviewing alternatives and becoming more creative. The administrator was charged with developing a new tactical plan. Meanwhile, efforts were renewed to raise the profile of WATCH in the community through the media. Stories of the people affected by the WATCH outreach program were shared, and efforts were revitalized to acquire funds.

Early forms of resistance came from a few hospital nurses who feared that their jobs would be jeopardized. These sources of resistance diminished as understanding of the role of WATCH evolved and cooperative relationships with other volunteer organizations developed. Judging from comments and the increase in membership, the community came to support the new organization. The active supportive membership grew to more than 200 citizens and now includes hospital and community health nurses and home care personnel. A cooperative linkage with the hospital's palliative care committee was forged.

Despite fiscal limitations, a volunteer education program was launched, and the outreach team became operational. The volunteer services offered by the team were in such demand that a Coordinator of Volunteers, a social worker, was hired to keep the service organized. WATCH was poised to open a free-standing hospice when sufficient funding was available. As this book goes to press, funding for a free-standing hospice is not yet available. However, WATCH is collaborating with government and non-governmental agencies in the community to develop a proposal for an integrated and comprehensive palliative care service for those living with terminal illness in the health region. This approach is consistent with the Jakarta declaration, which advocates strengthening existing partnerships:

Partnerships offer mutual benefit for health through the sharing of expertise, skills and resources. Each partnership must be transparent and accountable and be based on agreed ethical principles, mutual understanding and respect. (WHO, 1998)

Conclusion

The emerging mission of community health calls for intersectoral and interdisciplinary participation in community development to influence the determinants of health. This mission arises from social change related to health promotion and health system reform across Canada and is consistent with the future direction of health promotion (WHO, 1998).

Various theories of community and social change enable community health nurses' participation in community development. Community health nurses' use of cooperative, campaign, and contest strategies will ensure the increasing implementation of community development in health promotion.

The case study presented in this chapter represents a classic example of coalition building and illustrates the process of locality development. It also demonstrates the extensive planning needed to launch a new community organization. The key is to keep the community members motivated and to have a plan to deal with the inevitable opposition. Most of all, this case exemplifies the need for sheer determination and confidence to overcome setbacks and appreciate progress.

Nursing research has identified that knowledge and skills in community development will be necessary for community health nurses of the future (Bramadat, Chalmers, & Andrusysyzyn, 1996). Community development is usually learned gradually by both the community health nurse and the community because it is best learned by practice. The heart of community development practice is the authentic commitment to hearing the experiences of people's lives, to understanding these experiences in the words people use to express them, and to negotiating mutual actions to improve those situations people would like to alter (Labonte, 1992, cited in Hoffman & Dupont, 1992, p. 40). The learning process should include reviewing the literature about the principles of community development, practising in partnership with the community, and evaluating interventions to discover what was done well and what could be improved for the future. A mentor can act as a guide to those new to this novel and rewarding domain of community nursing practice.

QUESTIONS

1. What are some of the basic differences between a community development approach in community health nursing and the traditional approach?
2. What roles should community health nurses fill in development in your community?
3. What examples of community development can you identify in your region?
   a. How was the group facilitating the change created?
   b. What was the goal of the proposed change?
   c. What part of the community was targeted for change?
   d. What strategies were used?

REFERENCES

Bramadat, I., Chalmers, K., & Andrusyszyn, M.A. (1996). Knowledge, skills and experiences for community health nursing practice: The perceptions of community nurses, administrators and educators. *Journal of Advanced Nursing, 24*, 1224–1233.

Campbell, V., & Keller, M.B. (1989). The Betty Neuman health care systems model: An analysis. In J.P. Riehl-Siska (Ed.), *Conceptual models for nursing practice* (3rd ed.). Norwalk, CT: Appleton-Century-Crofts.

City of Toronto Department of Public Health. (1991). *Policy on community development.* Toronto: Author.

Cox, F.M., & Erlich, J.L. (1974). *Community action, planning, development.* Itsaca, IL: F.E. Peacock.

deLeeuw, E.J. (1989). *The sane revolution—health promotion: Background, scope, prospects.* Assen, Maastricht: Van Gorcum.

Dunham, A. (1970). *The new community organization.* New York: Crowel.

English, J. (1994). Health promotion in Manitoba. In A.M. Pederson, M. O'Neill, & I. Rootman (Eds.), *Health promotion in Canada: Provincial, national and international perspectives.* Toronto: W.B. Saunders.

English, J., & Hicks, B.C. (1992). A systems-in-transition paradigm for healthy communities. *Canadian Journal of Public Health, 83*(1), 61–65.

Feather, J. (1994). *Reflections on health promotion practice* (Occasional paper no. 2). Saskatoon: Prairie Region Health Promotion Research Centre, University of Saskatchewan.

Four Worlds Development Project. (1984). *Community development* (Discussion paper no. 8 in Adult Education Series). Lethbridge, AB: University of Lethbridge.

Hancock, T. (1986). Lalonde and beyond: Looking back at *A new perspective on the health of Canadians. Health Promotion: An International Journal, 1*(1), 93–100.

Hoffman, K., & Dupont, J.M. (1992). *Community health centres and community development.* Ottawa: Health Services & Promotion Branch, Health & Welfare Canada, Ministry of Supply & Services.

Jackson, T., Mitchell, S., & Wright, M. (1989). The community development continuum. *Community Health Studies, 13*(1), 68–71.

Kickbusch, I. (1981). Involvement in health: A social concept in health education. *International Journal of Health Education, 24* (Suppl.), 3–15.

Kickbusch, I. (1986a). Life-styles and health. *Social Science & Medicine, 22*(2), 117–124.

Kickbusch, I. (1986b). Health promotion: A global perspective. *Canadian Journal of Public Health, 77,* 321–326.

King, I.M. (1981). *A theory for nursing.* New York: Wiley.

Labonte, R. (1990). *Scientific basis for the community development approach* (Paper prepared for the Heart Health Inequalities Program). Ottawa: Health & Welfare Canada, Ministry of Supply & Services.

Labonte, R. (1992). Foreword. In K. Hoffman & J.M. Dupont (Eds.), *Community health centres and community development.* Ottawa: Health Services & Promotion Branch, Health & Welfare Canada, Ministry of Supply & Services.

Milio, N. (1986a). Multi-sectoral policy and health promotion: Where to begin? *Health Promotion: An International Journal, 1*(2), 129–132.

Milio, N. (1986b). *Promoting health through public policy.* Ottawa: Canadian Public Health Association.

Milio, N. (1987). Making healthy public policy: Developing the science of learning the art: An ecological framework for policy studies. *Health Promotion: An International Journal, 2*(3), 263–274.

Parse, R.R. (1981). *Man living health: A theory of nursing.* New York: Wiley.

Paul, B.D., & Miller, W.B. (1955). *Health, culture and community.* New York: Russell Sage Foundation.

Raeburn, J. & Rootman, I. (1998). *People-centred health promotion.* Toronto: John Wiley & Sons.

Sherman, B. (1988). *Cities fit to live in: Themes and variations A to Z*. Whitley, UK: Channel 4 Television. [Book].

United Nations. (1955). *Social progress through community development*. New York: Author.

Warren, R.L. (1977). *Social change and human purpose: Toward understanding and action*. Chicago: Rand McNally.

Watson, G. (1967). Resistance to change. In G. Watson (Ed.), *Concepts of social change*. Washington, DC: National Training Laboratories.

Watson, J. (1985). *Nursing: Human science and human care*. Norwalk, CT: Appleton-Century-Crofts.

Westman Association for Terminal Care in Hospice (WATCH). (1992). *Constitution*. Brandon, MB: Author.

World Health Organization. (1988a). *The health promotion program*. Copenhagen: Author. [Brochure].

World Health Organization. (1988b). *Promoting health in the urban environment* (WHO Healthy Cities Papers no. 1). Copenhagen: FADL.

World Health Organization. (1988c). *Five-year planning framework* (WHO Healthy Cities Papers no. 2). Copenhagen: FADL.

World Health Organization. (1988d). *A guide to assessing healthy cities* (WHO Healthy Cities Papers no. 3). Copenhagen: FADL.

World Health Organization. (1988e). *The new public health in an urban context: Paradoxes and solutions* (WHO Healthy Cities Papers no. 4). Copenhagen: FADL.

World Health Organization. (1998). *The Jakarta declaration on leading health promotion into the 21st century*. (Online: http://www.int/hpr/hep/documents/jakarta/english)

World Health Organization (WHO), Health & Welfare Canada (HWC), & Canadian Public Health Association (CPHA). (1986). *Ottawa charter for health promotion*. Ottawa: Canadian Public Health Association.

C H A P T E R   2 2

Community needs and capacity assessment: Critical component of program planning

Nancy C. Edwards and Alwyn Moyer

Community needs assessment and program planning are vital to the implementation of effective Primary Health Care interventions. In this chapter, the program planning cycle is introduced. Qualitative and quantitative approaches to assess community needs are reviewed, and processes to guide the selection of effective interventions are presented.

LEARNING OBJECTIVES

In this chapter, you will learn:

- an appropriate framework to guide a community needs assessment
- a plan for conducting an assessment of community needs and capacity
- qualitative and quantitative techniques and data sources for community needs assessment
- the rationale for using a participatory approach in community needs assessment
- criteria and processes for setting priorities in planning intervention strategies
- the components of a comprehensive program plan

Introduction

Assessing community needs is a important aspect of community health nurses' role (CPHA, 1990) and one that they are well placed to fulfil. Given their large numbers, their dispersion, and the trust they have gained within communities, community nurses are a valuable resource for building capacity for health promotion and disease prevention (Kang, 1995). Not only are they well positioned to gain a broad perspective of community needs, strengths, and resources, they also have contact with marginalized and disadvantaged groups, whose voices are not always heard. This places the community nurse in a unique position to foster community involvement in the assessment process and to advocate for full documentation of health needs. A survey of public health nurses in Ontario revealed that most nurses were conducting community needs assessments and expected it would form an increasing part of future practice (Chambers et al., 1994). Paradoxically, few felt well prepared for this important role. A range of knowledge and skills are required to identify and define needs for programs and policy. This chapter provides an introduction to a systematic and comprehensive approach for assessing community needs and capacity and for planning relevant interventions and programs.

Rationale for conducting a community needs assessment

Community assessment is a necessary first step in the process of developing health programs and services. It presents an entry point for citizen involvement in identifying and describing community health issues, and weighing their relative importance in setting priorities for program planning (Haglund, Weisbrod, & Bracht, 1990). Assessment data can also be used in other ways: to justify the need for health programs, to determine how resources should be allocated, and to serve as a benchmark against which to evaluate change. In reality, needs identification is an iterative process embedded within a cycle of assessment, planning, implementation, and evaluation (Tugwell, Bennett, Sackett, & Haynes, 1985). The process, which can be initiated at many different levels—organizational, community, regional, and national—has many forms:

[In some cases] the focus of the assessment is narrow, concentrating on one issue, or one segment of the population (for example, access to medical care, use of tobacco and alcohol by Latin youth, or motor vehicle injuries). In others, the focus is broader, encompassing a wide range of factors that determine the health of a geo-political population as well as the resources that a community can muster to respond to health needs. (Lasker & The Committee on Medicine & Public Health, 1997, p. 107)

While each level of the system has interests and responsibilities with regard to developing health programs, the assessment of community needs, together with the capacity to meet them, forms an essential component of health planning.

Foundations for community
needs assessment

The way in which community is defined underpins the process of community needs assessment (see Chapter 5). Although definitions of community may vary widely, they usually encompass both a geographical and social dimension. For example, a community is seen as a group of people with social, cultural, or economic ties within a specified location (Israel, Checkoway, Schulz, & Zimmerman, 1994). Hence, information about geographical boundaries, social institutions, patterns of social interaction, and control are important elements of community assessment (Haglund et al., 1990).

In practical terms, the community of interest to a community health nurse is likely an urban or rural locality that forms the catchment area for the provision of health and social services to the population as a whole or certain aggregates. Aggregates may be defined using a variety of criteria, such as socio-demographic group (low-income mothers), behavioural risk status (current smoker), or health problem (diabetes). (See Chapter 19.) Sometimes, community is defined by social settings such as schools or workplaces, which house certain populations and have their own distinctive subcultures.

Models and assumptions about community health frame the community needs assessment. Ecological frameworks of health, which organize a range of concepts about determinants of health and health behaviour, provide a useful perspective (Eng, Salmon, & Mullan, 1992; Hancock, 1993). According to such frameworks, the relationships between people and their environment are central to understanding health needs and resources. Social and personal resources, as well as physical capacities, are important determinants of health. Ecological frameworks incorporate the broader definition of health as a resource for everyday life, not simply the objective of living (WHO, HWC, & CPHA, 1986). To reach states of positive health and well-being, communities must be able to identify and realize aspirations, to satisfy needs, and to change or cope with the environment (Israel et al., 1994; Sheilds & Lindsey, 1998). Prerequisites such as social justice, peace, and a stable ecosystem are fundamental if communities are to take control over and improve their health (Eade, 1997).

The broader conceptualization of community health dictates a more sophisticated process of assessment (Stoner, Magilvy, & Schultz, 1992). Health is no longer seen primarily as an attribute of the individual but as an attribute of the community. A comprehensive community needs assessment must consider people within their social and environmental context (Frankish & Green, 1994; Green & Kreuter, 1991; Hawtin, Hughes, & Percy-Smith, 1994). New types of data are needed to provide a profile of a community and its resources and baseline information about health needs and health behaviours.

Fostering community participation in the identification of needs is in keeping with the empowering orientation of health promotion. With widespread involvement in the assessment of need, a broader range of stakeholders can voice their concerns and the community can document health issues. Furthermore, by initiating a problem-solving process, communities have the opportunity to develop knowledge and skills, transform the environment, and build community capacity (McKnight & Kretzmann, 1990; Srinivasan, 1990). Community participation in needs assessment lays the groundwork for involving community members in activities that can have a positive impact on their health.

A community needs assessment is no longer viewed as an expert-driven compilation of disease prevalence and an inventory of health and social services (Boston et al., 1997; Gaventa, 1993; Hagey, 1997). With the growing recognition that many health problems are rooted in community life, medical, health planning, and community development approaches to conducting a needs assessment have been integrated (Haglund et al., 1990). Programs must build on the values, strengths, and resources of the community and address multidimensional risk factors (Butterfoss, Goodman, & Wandersman, 1993; Francisco, Paine, & Fawcett, 1993; Ostrom, Lerner, & Freel, 1995). Indeed, McKnight (1985) argues that the main aim of a community needs assessment should be to gain an understanding of community values and to map the resources that are currently or potentially available to bring about change. The two goals can be melded into a unified approach that fosters public participation and builds the problem-solving capacity of a community to address local needs and concerns.

Conducting a community needs assessment

Ultimately, a needs assessment is undertaken to identify priorities for intervention and to guide the development of programs that are tailored to the needs and characteristics of a community. When operating from an ecological framework, three principles guide the community needs assessment. First, data collection should identify the community's needs and health-related problems as well as its strengths and resources. Second, the application of participatory approaches in a community assessment helps to build consensus toward the identification of priorities for action. (See Chapter 28.) Third, it is essential to use a systematic approach and scientifically sound techniques for collecting, analyzing, and interpreting data.

Often, community assessment involves a two-stage process. The initial stage is directed at the larger community and is intended to identify priorities for program development and implementation. Both priority target groups and priority health problems will be identified. This data collection and priority setting is often part of a strategic planning process of a region or an organization. As such, it will reflect the current mandates, policy documents, organizational climate, and uniqueness of the community. The second stage shifts to a data collection process that supports the design and implementation of an evidence-based program to address priority health issues.

Stage 1: Identifying priorities for program development and implementation

A variety of approaches can be used to conduct a needs assessment. Examples include reviewing health and social indicators, gathering health service utilization data, undertaking community surveys, holding a community forum, or conducting key informant interviews with service providers and community leaders (Aboud, 1997; Illinois Department of Health, 1996; Morris & Almagor, 1993). The approaches can vary on several dimensions: the data gathered (qualitative or quantitative); the need considered (health or illness); the representativeness of the target population (convenience or random sample); and the perspective of need (population, service user, or service provider). Each approach has advantages and disadvantages. An ecological approach suggests that data from various sources should be accessed to provide a comprehensive overview of community health issues and challenges (Schultz & Magilvy, 1988). Involvement of the community has the potential to provide a more valid portrayal of community need (Morris & Almagor, 1993). The community health nurse can facilitate the assessment process by being familiar with approaches to identifying needs and by helping community groups gain access to data sources and data interpretation.

Socio-demographic and health indicators. Community health nurses should be familiar with epidemiological techniques used to group and display data using standard rates and measures (Beaglehole, Bonita, & Kjellstrom, 1993; Kelsey, Whittemore, Evans, & Thompson, 1996; Streiner & Norman, 1996). (See Chapter 29.) Epidemiological methods enable comparisons within and between communities or in relation to norms. Table 22.1 summarizes some commonly measured socio-demographic and health indicators, along with examples of data sources. It is time-consuming and expensive to collect new data, so it is important for the community health nurse to be knowledgeable about existing data sources and their strengths and limitations.

Many health status reports generated by various planning groups across the country provide a detailed overview of the health problems and needs within a community as well as existing resources. These reports have been produced in recent years to inform the process of health system reform (Table 22.1).

Table 22.1
Summary of health indicators, data sources, and health status reports for community needs assessment

Socio-demographic and Health Indicators	Data Sources	Health Status Reports
Demographic and Socioeconomic • Age distribution • Population growth rate • Immigration rates • Mobility rates • Population density • Labour force participation rates • Education, marital, and income status • Family type and household composition • Percentage of population living below poverty line • Unemployment rates	• Census data base • Immigration reports • Demographic and income statistics for postal areas • Social survey data • Taxation statistics • Population profile report of Correctional Services • Labour force surveys	Canadian Public Health Association, 1997 Dumas, 1993 Immigration Canada, 1994 *Small Area Data Guide*, 1991 Statistics Canada, 1995a Statistics Canada, 1995b

(continued)

Table 22.1 (*continued*)

Socio-demographic and Health Indicators	Data Sources	Health Status Reports
Mortality and Morbidity • Crude mortality rate • Age- and sex-specific mortality rates • Cause-specific mortality rates • Incidence and prevalence rates • Quality-adjusted life years • Life expectancy at birth • Quality of life	• Canadian mortality data base • Homicide statistics reports • Provincial vital statistics • Canadian cancer statistics (http://www.cancer.ca/stats) • Birth defects registries • Notifiable communicable disease reports • Provincial and national health surveys • Injury data base (e.g., CHIRPP, Workers' Compensation) • Statistics Canada life tables • Quality-of-life indicators	Cochrane, Goering, & Rogers, 1997 Federal, Provincial, & Territorial Advisory Committee on Population Health, 1996 Hill, Forbes, Lindsay, & McDowell, 1997 Joseph & Kramer, 1997 Lipman, Offord, & Boyle, 1997 Makomaskilling & Kaiserman, 1995 Raphael, Renwick, Brown, & Rootman, 1996 Rosenberg & Moore, 1997 Statistics Canada, 1994 Statistics Canada, 1995c Wade & Cairney, 1997
Lifestyle • Knowledge • Attitudes • Behaviour patterns	• Regional, provincial, and federal population health surveys • Statistics Canada	Bondy & Ialomiteanu, 1997 Canadian Fitness & Lifestyle Research Institute, 1995 EKOS Research Associates Inc., 1995 Kerdall, Kipskie, & MacEachern, 1997 Single, McLennan, & McNeil, 1994 Statistics Canada, 1995a–c

(*continued*)

Table 22.1 *(continued)*

Socio-demographic and Health Indicators	Data Sources	Health Status Reports
Environmental		Ashley, Bull, & Pederson, 1995
Physical environment	• Canada Mortgage and Housing Corporation	Burnett, Brook, Yung, Dales, & Krewski, 1997
• Building hazards	• National Air Pollution Surveillance monthly summaries	deGuia et al., 1998
• Accessibility of buildings		Health Canada, 1995
• Industrial hazards		Health Canada, 1998
• Pollution levels		National Clearinghouse on Tobacco & Health, 1995
Social environment	• Regional, provincial, and federal population health surveys	Stephens & Mitchell, 1996
• Social norms		Stieb et al., 1995
• Levels of social support		
• Neighbourhood cohesion		
Policy and regulatory environment	• Regional, provincial, and federal surveys	
• Existence of legislation, by-laws and organizational policy	• Government documents	
• Levels of support for policy change		
• Regulation enforcement		
Health Services	• Provincial health insurance data	Choi, Robson, & Single, 1997
• Hospital admission rates	• Hospital separation data	Goel et al., 1996
• Health care utilization rates	• Health provider manpower data	Health Canada, 1996
• Health provider:population ratios	• Drug utilization data	Hogan & Ebly, 1995
• Regional variations in medical procedure rates	• Hospital morbidity and mortality reports	Kestin, Rebuck, & Chapman, 1993
• Direct and indirect costs of health care		Snider et al., 1996
		Sutcliffe, Deber, & Pasut, 1997
		Wen, Liu, & Fowler, 1998
		Williams & Young, 1996

Community profile. The community profile complements and expands the health status report. Whereas the health status report describes the burden of illness and identifies affected segments of the population, the community profile provides information about community characteristics, resources, and perceptions of its health and its ability to solve community problems (Nova Scotia Department of Health, 1997a).

In addition to providing factual information on which to plan programs, compiling the community profile enables cooperation among decision makers, concerned groups, and individuals and creates awareness of community needs and resources. It is important to be clear about the dimensions of community, the scope of the assessment, and how the public will be involved in designing and implementing programs.

Several techniques can be used to assemble a community profile (Table 22.2). Drawing mainly on qualitative approaches, they provide a more immediate picture of the community. For example, interviews with community residents and service providers can raise awareness about subtle changes, emerging needs, and political forces. The broad contextual information provided by qualitative approaches also helps in understanding and interpreting survey data. It is important for the community nurse to be familiar with qualitative approaches, such as conducting focus groups and key informant interviews, to gain a representative picture of the community.

Priority setting. Once quantitative and qualitative data are assembled, a systematic process can be used to determine which health issues should be a priority for resource allocation (Hadorn, 1991; Nova Scotia Department of Health, 1997b). Commonly, setting priorities involves the application of explicit criteria in rank ordering the identified health problems. Both objective and subjective criteria can be used. Examples of objective criteria include magnitude of the problem, availability of effective interventions to prevent or treat the problem, and costs of alternative interventions. Examples of subjective criteria include leverage (i.e., to what extent does implementing this intervention increase the likelihood of additional resources for priority problems); acceptability of interventions to community leaders, target groups, or service providers; interventions' congruence with the mandate of the organization; and potential for the program to strengthen networks or partnerships (Kennedy, Sheeska, & Edwards, 1993; Shuster & Goeppinger, 1996).

Stage 2: Planning intervention strategies

In the second stage of a needs assessment, the focus shifts from identifying priority health problems and target populations to planning intervention strategies. The scope and orientation of this assessment will be determined by the nature of the health problems, the target group(s), and the community. An appropriate program planning framework is essential. At a minimum, the framework should be ecologically sound, systems-based, and informed

Table 22.2
Qualitative approaches for community needs assessment

Qualitative Approaches	Description of Approaches and Examples	References
Ethnographic (observations and description of community characteristics)	"Windshield" survey; walking the community; observing how people interact; talking informally to community residents to identify potential issues; participant observation	Aboud, 1997 Babbie, 1989 Bogdewic, 1992 Jordan & Yeomans, 1995
Document analysis	Examination of community plans, reports, and maps to understand community history and future plans	Srinivasan, 1990
Community forum	Open meetings to elicit community perspective on social needs, strengths, and resources	Hawtin, Hughes, & Percy-Smith, 1994 Scrimshaw, Carballo, Ramos, & Blair, 1991

(continued)

Table 22.2 (*continued*)

Qualitative Approaches	Description of Approaches and Examples	References
Key informant interviews	Semi-structured or unstructured interviews with community leaders, health and social service providers, and members of the community provide an opportunity to gather a wide range of views from different vantage points to	Boyce et al., 1997 Gilchrist, 1992 Morris & Almagor, 1993
	• identify health problems	Schultz & Magilvy, 1988
	• identify community leaders	Barker et al., 1994
	• document how community gives and receives help (using interviews with municipal government, media, educational and religious institutions, local groups and organizations)	Eng, Salmon, & Mullan, 1992
	• elicit opinions on community competence, democratic participation style, crime, resource adequacy and use, and decision-making interactions (using a telephone survey of community members)	Goeppinger & Baglioni, 1985

(continued)

Table 22.2 (continued)

Qualitative Approaches	Description of Approaches and Examples	References
Focus groups	Semi-structured group discussions to elicit information about issue of interest, led by a moderator posing open-ended questions; encourage expression of diverse opinions and perceptions	Basch, 1992 Morgan, 1993 Weinriech, 1996
Social network mapping	Mapping of social networks and relationships within and between communities identifies social supports, key resources and resource control, communication channels, tensions, and boundaries within community	Weller-Molongua & Knapp, 1995

by theory (Richard, Potvin, Kishchuk, Prlic, & Green, 1996). An example of such a framework is the Ottawa–Carleton Framework for Health Department Programs (Edwards, Murphy, Moyer, & Wright, 1995) (see Figure 22.1). Based on an ecological understanding of health and grounded in experience, this framework describes three types of intervention—building self-care capacity and action; strengthening collective-care capacity and action; and creating supportive environments—which work in synergy to form a healthy community. Interventions identified in this framework aim to increase healthy lifestyle practices, strengthen community partnerships, and foster environments for healthy choices. Such changes are linked to improvements in health status and community capacity. The framework can be used to guide a participatory assessment of community needs, strengths, and resources.

The second stage involves three steps: (a) prepare a "web of causation" to examine the problem and its causes, (b) use components of the framework (i.e., self-care capacity and action, collective-care capacity and action, and supportive environments) to identify potential interventions and facilitators or barriers, and (c) determine the optimal sequence and combination of intervention components. The steps involved in a second-stage assessment are described next, using smoking during pregnancy and postpartum as an illustration.

Web of causation. A web of causation is a technique for examining the relationships and interconnections among various determinants of health problems. One asks the questions "What factors are contributing to the problem?" and "What issues does each problem cause?" Problems and issues may be based on actual data from your community or on evidence from other sources (e.g., research and technical reports, provincial or national studies). Anticipated links among these problems may be based on expert opinion, research findings, and theory. An example is presented in Figure 22.2. All important factors related to the health issue should be included in a fully developed web.

The web of causation looks like a hierarchy. The uppermost problems reflect the longer-term goals of community health interventions. For example, a program targeting smoking during pregnancy and postpartum aims to reduce the health effects of smoking (e.g., incidence of low birth-weight babies, prevalence of chronic ear infections among young children). Problems at the next level reflect shorter-term objectives (e.g., reduce the percentage of women who relapse during the postpartum period, decrease the proportion of infants exposed to second-hand smoke). The middle and lower segments of the web suggest intervention strategies (e.g., increase smoking cessation and smoking relapse prevention counselling for pregnant women; include partners in relapse prevention counselling; work with pregnant women who quit smoking to build skills that help them resist high-risk

Figure 22.1
Framework for public health programs

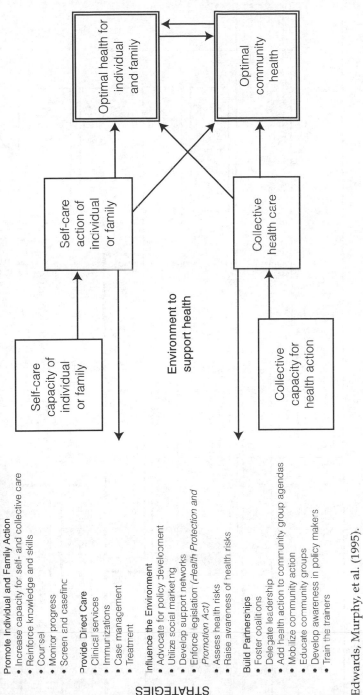

Promote Individual and Family Action
- Increase capacity for self- and collective care
- Reinforce knowledge and skills
- Counsel
- Monitor progress
- Screen and casefind

Provide Direct Care
- Clinical services
- Immunizations
- Case management
- Treatment

Influence the Environment
- Advocate for policy development
- Utilize social marketing
- Develop support networks
- Enforce legislation (*Health Protection and Promotion Act*)
- Assess health risks
- Raise awareness of health risks

Build Partnerships
- Foster coalitions
- Delegate leadership
- Add health action to community group agendas
- Mobilize community action
- Educate community groups
- Develop awareness in policy makers
- Train the trainers

STRATEGIES

Edwards, Murphy, et al. (1995).

Figure 22.2
Partial web of causation

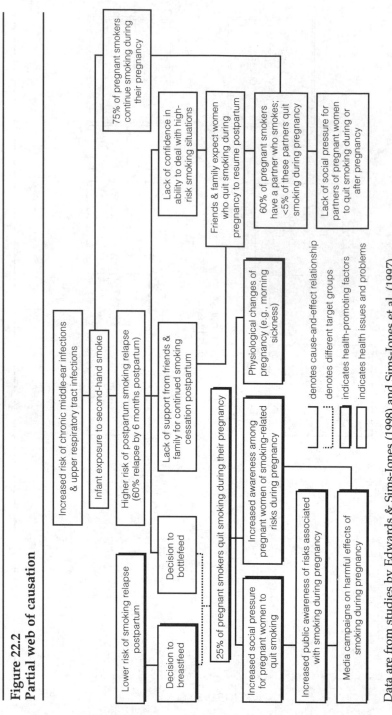

Data are from studies by Edwards & Sims-Jones (1998) and Sims-Jones et al. (1997).

smoking situations in the postpartum period; and use social marketing techniques to shift norms) (Edwards & Sims-Jones, 1998; Sims-Jones et al., 1997).

Finally, in developing a web of causation, it is important to consider the domains of issues in the guiding framework. The domain of self-care capacity and action focusses attention on the population directly affected by the health problem(s) (in this example, pregnant women, fetuses, and young children). Examining elements of the supportive environment will help to identify additional target groups for intervention (in this example, social supports for a woman to stop smoking during pregnancy and to maintain cessation afterward, include partners, family, friends, co-workers, and the larger community, as reflected in social norms). The dimensions of collective capacity and action are useful in mobilizing broader societal support and action for change.

Intervention strategies. The next step involves identifying intervention strategies within each domain of the framework. The experience of the community, other health providers, and a knowledge base informed by theory and research can generate a comprehensive list of potential interventions. For example, the web of causation (Figure 22.2), indicates that several groups are at risk for postpartum smoking relapse: women whose partners smoke; women who plan to bottlefeed their babies; and women with low self-efficacy for dealing with high-risk smoking situations. Within the domain of self-care capacity and action, interventions might include face-to-face and telephone counselling, provision of health education materials, and group meetings. These strategies could be used in settings such as prenatal classes, ultrasound and antenatal clinics, hospital maternity wards, and breastfeeding or well-baby clinics. Many smoking mothers could be reached by mobilizing the large array of health providers who are in contact with ante- and postpartum women in these settings (e.g., hospital staff nurses, public health nurses, prenatal class teachers, midwives, physicians, nutritionists, lactation consultants).

For each potential intervention, factors that would support or jeopardize its implementation in the community of interest need to be considered (Kretzman & McKnight, 1993). For example, barriers to having prenatal class teachers offer smoking cessation counselling might include lack of familiarity with smoking cessation counselling techniques and inadequate continuing education resources for skills training. Facilitators might include the large proportion of primiparous women who access prenatal classes early in the pregnancy and attendance of partners at prenatal classes.

Sequence and combination of interventions. Priority setting aims to determine the optimal mix and sequence of interventions. Promising interventions are compared. The criteria previously outlined in the needs assessment process may be useful. Two other priority-setting criteria should also be considered. First, in reviewing each intervention, community health nurses should identify prerequisites for implementation. For example, home visit counselling cannot be undertaken successfully unless community health nurses know how to use a smoking cessation intervention with pregnant women. Similarly, physicians are not going to refer clients at risk for postpartum smoking relapse unless they are aware of the program and believe it can make a difference. Second, it is important to consider the potential for synergies among intervention strategies (Schooler, Flora, & Farquhar, 1993; Simons-Morton, Simons-Morton, Parcel, & Bunker, 1988). Although on its own an intervention may have limited impact, it may increase the effectiveness of another intervention strategy. For example, the effect of smoking cessation counselling by public health nurses may be enhanced if a mass media campaign on the risks of smoking during pregnancy is also launched.

Through this second stage, a comprehensive program plan can be prepared. It should include program goals and objectives that address priority community needs; effective strategies that build on the strengths and resources within the community; timelines and estimates of resource requirements for program implementation; and indicators to monitor and evaluate program activities.

Conclusion

A community needs assessment is a two-stage process that draws on a variety of quantitative and qualitative data sources. Considerable resources are required of health care agencies, health providers, and the community to conduct a community needs assessment. However, a systematic assessment constitutes an essential step in the program planning cycle, guiding the identification of priority problems and target groups, the determination of goals and objectives, and the selection and implementation of intervention activities. Community health nurses play a critical role in all steps of the program planning cycle and are key to the full engagement of community members and other partner agencies in this process.

QUESTIONS

1. How would you engage community members in the process of needs assessment in your catchment area?
2. What epidemiological methods and qualitative approaches would you use in conducting a needs assessment?
3. What criteria for priority setting would you use for a health issue or target group of interest in your community?

4.   Identify the barriers and facilitators for implementing interventions for a selected target group in your community.
5.   Prepare a web of causation, and use this to identify program objectives for a health problem in your region.

REFERENCES

Aboud, F. (1997). Methods from social sciences: Overview of qualitative and quantitative methods. In J. Pickering (Ed.), *Health research for development: A manual*. Canadian University Consortium for Health in Development (pp. 101–131). Montréal: McGill Printing Services.

Ashley, M.J., Bull, S.B., & Pederson, L.L. (1995). Support among smokers and non-smokers for restrictions on smoking. *American Journal of Preventive Medicine, 11*, 283–287.

Babbie, E. (1989). *The practice of social research*. Belmont, CA: Wadsworth.

Barker, J.B., Bayne, T., Higgs, Z.R., Jenkin, S.A., Murphy, D., & Synoground, G. (1994). Community analysis: A collaborative community practice project. *Public Health Nursing, 11*(2), 113–118.

Basch, C.E. (1992). Focus group interviews: An underutilized research technique for improving theory and practice in health education. *Health Education Quarterly, 19*(1), 411–448.

Beaglehole, R., Bonita, R., & Kjellstrom, T. (1993). *Basic epidemiology*. Geneva: World Health Organization.

Bogdewic, S.P. (1992). Participant observation. In B.F. Crabtree & W.L. Miller (Eds.), *Doing qualitative research: Multiple strategies* (pp. 45–69). Newbury Park, CA: Sage.

Bondy, S.J., & Ialomiteanu, A.R. (1997). Smoking in Ontario 1991 to 1996. *Canadian Journal of Public Health, 88*(4), 225–229.

Boston, P., Jordan, S., MacNamara, E., Kozolanka, K., Bobbish-Rondeau, E., Iserhoff, H., Mianscum, S., Mianscum-Trapper, R., Mistacheesick, I., Petawabano, B., Sheshamush-Masty, M., Wapachee, R., Weapenicappo, J. (1997). Using participatory action research to understand the meanings Aboriginal Canadians attribute to the rising incidence of diabetes. *Chronic Diseases in Canada, 18*(1), 5–12.

Boyce, W., Khanlou, N., Lysack, C., Mulay, S., & Zakus, D. (1997). Evaluating community participation. In J.L. Pickering (Ed.), *Health research for development: A manual*. Canadian University Consortium for Health in Development (pp. 132–162). Montréal: McGill Printing Services.

Burnett, R.T., Brook, J.R., Yung, W.T., Dales, R.E., & Krewski, D. (1997). Association between ozone and hospitalization for respiratory diseases in 16 Canadian cities. *Environmental Research, 72*, 24–31.

Butterfoss, F.D., Goodman, R.M., & Wandersman, A. (1993). Community coalitions for prevention and health promotion. *Health Education Research, 8*(3), 315–330.

Canadian Fitness & Lifestyle Research Institute. (1995). *1995 Physical activity monitor. Progress in prevention* (Bull. No. 3). Ottawa: Author.

Canadian Public Health Association (CPHA). (1990). *Community health–public health nursing in Canada: Preparation and practice*. Ottawa: Author.

Canadian Public Health Association (CPHA). (1997). *Health impacts of social and economic conditions: Implications for public policy.* Board of Directors Discussion Paper. Ottawa: Author.

Chambers, L.W., Underwood, J., Halbert, T., Woodward, J., Heale, J., & Isaacs, S. (1994). 1992 Ontario survey of public health nurses: Perceptions of roles and activities. *Canadian Journal of Public Health, 85*(3), 175–179.

Choi, B.C.K., Robson, L., & Single, E. (1997). Estimating the abuse of tobacco, alcohol and illicit drugs: A review of methodologies and Canadian data sources. *Chronic Diseases in Canada, 18*(4), 149–165.

Cochrane, J.J., Goering, P.N., & Rogers, J.M. (1997). The mental health of informal caregivers in Ontario: An epidemiological survey. *American Journal of Public Health, 87*(12), 2002–2007.

de Guia, N.A., Cohen, J.E., Ashley, M.F., Ferrence, R., Northrup, D.A., & Pollard, J.S. (1998). How provincial and territorial legislators view tobacco and tobacco control: Findings from a Canadian study. *Chronic Diseases in Canada, 19*(2), 57–61. (Online: http://www.isr.yorku/ISR)

Dumas, J. (Ed.). (1993). *Population aging and the elderly: Current demographic analysis.* Ottawa: Statistics Canada. (Cat. No. 91-533E)

Eade, D. (1997). *Capacity-building: An approach to people-centred development.* Oxford: Oxfam.

Edwards, N., Murphy, M., Moyer, A., & Wright, A. (1995). *Building and sustaining collective health action: A framework for community health practitioners.* Ottawa: Community Health Research Unit. (Pub. No. DP95-1)

Edwards, N., & Sims-Jones, N. (1998). Smoking and smoking relapse during pregnancy and postpartum: Results of a qualitative study. *Birth, 25*(2), 95–101.

EKOS Research Associates Inc. (1995). *An assessment of knowledge, attitudes and practices concerning environmental tobacco smoke.* [Report prepared for Health Canada]. Ottawa: EKOS.

Eng, E., Salmon, M.E., & Mullan, F. (1992). Community empowerment: The critical base for primary health care. *Family and Community Health, 15*(1), 1–12.

Federal, Provincial, & Territorial Advisory Committee on Population Health. (1996). *Report on the Health of Canadians. Technical appendix.* Ottawa: Health Canada Communications. (Cat. No. H39-385/1-1996E)

Francisco, V.T., Paine, A.L., & Fawcett, S.B. (1993). A methodology for monitoring and evaluating community health coalitions. *Health Education Research: Theory and Practice, 8*(3), 403–416.

Frankish, C.J., & Green, L.W. (1994). Organizational and community change as the social scientific basis for disease prevention and health promotion policy. *Advances in Medical Sociology, 4,* 209–233.

Gaventa, J. (1993). The powerful, the powerless and the experts: Knowledge struggles in an information age. In P. Park, M. Brydon-Miller, B. Hall, & T. Jackson (Eds.), *Voices of change: Participatory research in the United States and Canada.* Toronto: Ontario Institute for Studies in Education.

Gilchrist, V.J. (1992). Key informant interviews. In B.F. Crabtree & W.L. Miller (Eds.), *Doing qualitative research: Multiple strategies* (pp. 70–89). Newbury Park, CA: Sage.

Goel, V., Williams, J.I., Anderson, G.M., Blackstein-Hirsch, P., Fooks, C., & Naylor, C.D. (1996). *Patterns of health care in Ontario. The ICES practice atlas* (2nd ed.). Toronto: Institute for Clinical Evaluative Sciences in Ontario.

Goeppinger, J., & Baglioni, A.J. (1985). Community competence: A positive approach to needs assessment. *American Journal of Community Psychology, 13*(5), 507–523.

Green, L.W., & Kreuter, M.W. (1991). *Health promotion planning: An educational and environmental approach.* Mountain View, CA: Mayfield.

Hadorn, D.C. (1991). Setting health care priorities in Oregon. *Journal of the American Medical Association, 265*(17), 2218–2225.

Hagey, R.S. (1997). The use and abuse of participatory action research. *Chronic Diseases in Canada, 18*(1), 1–4.

Haglund, B., Weisbrod, R.R., & Bracht, N. (1990). Assessing the community: Its services, needs, leadership and readiness. In N. Bracht (Ed.), *Health promotion at the community level* (pp. 91–108). Sage Sourcebooks for the Human Services, Series 15. Newbury Park, CA: Sage.

Hancock, T. (1993). Health, human development and the community ecosystem: Three ecological models. *Health Promotion International, 8*(1), 41–47.

Hawtin, M., Hughes, G., & Percy-Smith, J. (1994). *Community profiling: Auditing social needs.* Philadelphia: Open University Press.

Health Canada. (1995). *Smoking by-laws in Canada 1995.* Ottawa: Health Canada.

Health Canada. (1996). *National health expenditures in Canada, 1975–1994. Summary report.* Ottawa: Minister of Supply & Services Canada. (Cat. No. H21-99/1994-2)

Health Canada. (1998). *Health and environment. Partners for life.* Ottawa: Minister of Supply & Services Canada.

Hill, G.B., Forbes, W.F., Lindsay, J., & McDowell, I. (1997). Life expectancy and dementia in Canada: The Canadian study of health and aging. *Chronic Diseases in Canada, 18*(4), 166–167.

Hogan, D.B., & Ebly, E.M. (1995). Regional variations in use of potentially inappropriate medications by Canadian seniors participating in the Canadian Study of Health and Aging. *Canadian Journal of Clinical Pharmacology, 2*(4), 167–174.

Illinois Department of Health. (1996). *Illinois Project for Local Assessment of Needs (IPLAN). Unit I and II training manuals and overview.* (Online: http://www.idph.state.il.us)

Immigration Canada. (1994). *Immigration plan 1994: Annual report to Parliament.* Ottawa: Author. (Cat. No. IM-094-01-94)

Israel, B.A., Checkoway, B., Schulz, A., & Zimmerman, M. (1994). Health education and community empowerment: Conceptualizing and measuring perceptions of individual, organizational and community control. *Health Education Quarterly, 21*(2), 149–170.

Jordan, S., & Yeomans, D. (1995). Critical ethnography: Problems in contemporary theory and practice. *British Journal of Sociology Education, 16*(3), 389–408.

Joseph, K.S., & Kramer, M.S. (1997). Recent trends in infant mortality rates and proportions of low-birth-weight live births in Canada. *Canadian Medical Association Journal, 157*(5), 535–542.

Kang, R. (1995). Building community capacity for health promotion: A challenge for public health nurses. *Public Health Nursing, 12*(5), 312–318.

Kelsey, J.L., Whittemore, A.S., Evans, A.S., & Thompson, W.D. (1996). *Methods in observational epidemiology* (2nd ed.). New York: Oxford University Press.

Kennedy, A., Sheeshka, J., & Edwards, N. (1993). Directing our future: Objective-oriented program planning by public health nutritionists. *Canadian Journal of Public Health, 84*(6), 408–409.

Kerdall, O., Kipskie, T., & MacEachern, S. (1997). Canadian health surveys, 1950–1997. *Chronic Diseases in Canada, 18*(2), 70–90.

Kestin, S., Rebuck, A.S., & Chapman, K.R. (1993). Trends in asthma and chronic obstructive pulmonary disease therapy in Canada, 1985 to 1990. *Journal of Allergy and Clinical Immunology, 92*(4), 499–506.

Kretzmann, J.P., & McKnight, J.L. (1993). *Building communities from the inside out: A path toward finding and mobilizing a community's assets.* Chicago: ACTA Publications.

Lasker, R.D., & The Committee on Medicine & Public Health. (1997). *Medicine and public health: The power of collaboration.* New York: New York Academy of Medicine. (Online: http://www.nyam.org/pubhlth)

Lipman, E.L., Offord, D.R., & Boyle, M.H. (1997). Single mothers in Ontario: Sociodemographic, physical and mental health characteristics. *Canadian Medical Association Journal, 156*(5), 639–645.

Makomaskilling, E.M., & Kaiserman, M.J. (1995). Mortality attributable to tobacco use in Canada and its regions, 1991. *Canadian Journal of Public Health, 86*(4), 257–265.

McKnight, J. (1985). Looking at capacity, not deficiency. In M. Lipsitz (Ed.), *Revitalizing our cities.* Chicago: The Fund for an American Renaissance and the National Center for Neighborhood Enterprise.

McKnight, J.L., & Kretzmann, J.P. (1990). *Mapping community capacity.* Evanston, IL: Centre for Urban Affairs & Policy Research, Northwestern University.

Morgan, D.L. (Ed.). (1993). *Successful focus groups. Advancing the state of the art.* Newbury Park, CA: Sage.

Morris, B., & Almagor, G. (1993). Identifying and responding to community need. In M. Bass, E.V. Dunn, P.G. Norton, M. Stewart, & F. Tudiver (Eds.), *Conducting research in the practice setting. Research methods for primary care.* Newbury Park, CA: Sage.

National Clearinghouse on Tobacco & Health. (1995). *Federal and provincial legislation in Canada: An overview.* Ottawa: Author.

Nova Scotia Department of Health. (1997a). *Developing a community health profile.* Community Health Planning Guidebook Series: 2.1. Halifax: Author.

Nova Scotia Department of Health. (1997b). *Which issues are more important?* Community Health Planning Guidebook Series: 3.2. Halifax: Author.

Ostrom, C.W., Lerner, R.M., & Freel, M.A. (1995). Building a capacity of youth and families through university–community collaborations: The development-in-context evaluation (DICE) model. *Journal of Adolescent Research, 10*(4), 427–448.

Raphael, D., Renwick, R., Brown, I., & Rootman, I. (1996). Quality of life indicators and health: Current status and emerging conceptions. *Social Indicators Research, 39,* 65–88.

Richard, L., Potvin, L., Kishchuk, N., Prlic, H., & Green, L.W. (1996). Assessment of the integration of the ecological approach in health promotion programs. *American Journal of Health Promotion, 10*(4), 318–328.

Rosenberg, M.W., & Moore, E.G. (1997). The health of Canada's elderly population: Current status and future implications. *Canadian Medical Association Journal, 157*(8), 1025–1032.

Schooler, C., Flora, J.A., & Farquhar, J.W. (1993). Moving toward synergy: Media supplementation in the Stanford Five-City Project. *Community Research, 20*(4), 587–610.

Schultz, P.R., & Magilvy, J.K. (1988). Assessing community health needs of elderly populations: Comparison of three strategies. *Journal of Advanced Nursing, 13*, 193–202.

Scrimshaw, S.C.M., Carballo, M., Ramos, L., & Blair, B.A. (1991). The AIDS rapid anthropological assessment procedures: A tool for health education planning and evaluation. *Health Education Quarterly, 18*, 111–123.

Sheilds, L.E., & Lindsey, A.E. (1998). Community health promotion nursing practice. *Advances in Nursing Science, 20*(4), 23–36.

Shuster, G.F., & Goeppinger, J. (1996). Community as client: Using the nursing process to promote health. In M. Stanhope & J. Lancaster (Eds.), *Community health nursing: Process and practice for promoting health* (4th ed.) (pp. 289–314). St. Louis: Mosby.

Simons-Morton, D.G., Simons-Morton, B.G., Parcel, G.S., & Bunker, J.F. (1988). Influencing personal and environmental conditions for community health: A multilevel intervention model. *Family and Community Health, 11*, 25–35.

Sims-Jones, N., Chamberlain, M., MacLean, L., Edwards, N., Hotte, A., Hotz, S., & Cushman, R. (1997). *Smoking behaviour during pregnancy and postpartum: Living with tobacco use in childbearing families.* Ottawa: Community Health Research Unit. (Pub. No. M97-7)

Single, E., McLennan, A., & MacNeil, P. (1994). *Horizons 1994: Alcohol and drug use in Canada.* Ottawa: Health Canada, Health Promotions Directorate Studies Unit & the Canadian Centre on Substance Abuse.

Small area data guide: A list of sources. (1991). Toronto: ICURR Press.

Snider, J., Beauvais, J., Levy, I., Villeneuve, P., & Pennock, J. (1996). Trends in mammography and Pap smear utilization in Canada. *Chronic Diseases in Canada, 17*, 108–117.

Srinivasan, L. (1990). *Tools for community participation: A manual for training trainers in participatory techniques.* New York: PROWWESS/UNDP–World Bank Water & Sanitation Program.

Statistics Canada. (1994). *Health status of Canadians. Report of the 1991 General Social Survey.* Ottawa: Industry, Science, & Technology Canada. (Cat. No. 11-6122E)

Statistics Canada. (1995a). *Life tables, Canada and the provinces, 1990–1992.* Ottawa: Industry, Science, & Technology Canada. (Cat. No. 84-537)

Statistics Canada. (1995b). *Profile of census tracts in Ottawa Hull—Part A. 1991 Census of Canada.* Ottawa: Industry, Science & Technology Canada. (Cat. No. 95-350)

Statistics Canada (Health Statistics Division). (1995c). *National Population Health Survey 1994–95. Public use microdata file documentation and users guide.* Ottawa: Industry, Science, & Technology Canada.

Stephens, T., & Mitchell, B. (1996). *Reducing ETS exposure in public places frequented by children.* Toronto: Ontario Tobacco Research Unit.

Stieb, D.M., Pengelly, L.D., Arron, N., Taylor, S.M., & Raizenne, M.E. (1995). Health effects of air pollution in Canada: Expert panel findings for the Canadian Smog Advisory Program. *Canadian Respiratory Journal, 2*(3), 155–160.

Stoner, M.H., Magilvy, J.K., & Schultz, P.R. (1992). Community analysis in community health nursing practice: The GENESIS model. *Public Health Nursing, 9*(4), 223–227.

Streiner, D., & Norman, G. (1996). *PDQ epidemiology* (2nd ed.). St. Louis: Mosby.

Sutcliffe, P.A., Deber, R.B., & Pasut, G. (1997). Public health in Canada: A comparative study of six provinces. *Canadian Journal of Public Health, 88*(4), 246–249.

Tugwell, P., Bennett, K.J., Sackett, D.C., & Haynes, R.B. (1985). The measurement iterative loop: A framework for the critical appraisal of need, benefits and costs of health interventions. *Journal of Chronic Disease, 38,* 338–351.

Wade, T.J., & Cairney, J. (1997). Age and depression in a nationally representative sample of Canadians: A preliminary look at the National Population Health Survey. *Canadian Journal of Public Health, 88*(5), 297–302.

Weinreich, N.K. (1996). *Research in the social marketing process.* The Social Marketing Place, Weinreich Communications. (Online: http://users.aol.com/weinreich/)

Weller-Molongua, C., & Knapp, J. (1995). Social network mapping. In R. Slocum, L. Wichhart, D. Rocheleau, & B. Thomas-Slayter (Eds.), *Power, process, and participation—Tools for change.* London: Intermediate Technology.

Wen, S.W., Liu, S., & Fowler, D. (1998). Trends and variations in neonatal length of in-hospital stay in Canada. *Canadian Journal of Public Health, 89*(2), 115–119.

Williams, J.I., & Young, W. (1996). *Inventory of studies on the accuracy of Canadian health administrative databases.* Toronto: Institute for Clinical Evaluative Sciences in Ontario. (Pub. No. 96-03-TR)

World Health Organization (WHO), Health & Welfare Canada (HWC), & Canadian Public Health Association (CPHA). (1986). Ottawa charter for health promotion. *Canadian Journal of Public Health, 77*(6), 425–427.

C H A P T E R   2 3

Nursing practice in outreach clinics for the homeless in Montréal

Marie-France Thibaudeau and Hélène Denoncourt

The homeless have been identified as one of the most vulnerable groups in society. This chapter presents the results of an exploratory study examining the practice of one nurse working in outreach clinics located in shelters and day centres in down-town Montréal. The characteristics and needs of the homeless, the nurse's interventions and discussions with them, her perceptions of the paradigm guiding her work, and those of her co-workers concerning her role are described. The limits of commu-nity health nursing practice for this serious social problem are presented.

LEARNING OBJECTIVES

In this chapter, you will learn:

- factors that contribute to the development of homelessness
- barriers that prevent the homeless from using the health care system appropriately
- the role of community health nurses in working with the homeless and with the community resources that serve them
- the basic components of community nursing care for the homeless
- strategies in the organization of health care services to the homeless to prevent their ghettoization

Introduction

Vulnerable populations are at risk for poor physical, psychological, and social health (Aday, 1997). Vulnerability is characterized by personal factors that interact with the environment to influence health. Thus, if vulnerable individuals are exposed to hazards within a non-supportive environment, they are likely to develop health and social problems. Homeless persons are vulnerable because their social condition, lifestyle, and environment dimin-ish their ability to stay healthy or to take the necessary steps to seek health care. Homeless persons live on the streets, in day centres, in night shelters, and in boarding houses. They seldom use health and welfare services; they do so only when their health has deteriorated. They distrust health services for being too bureaucratic and normative, especially as homeless people frequently lose their identification or health cards. In Montréal, a special committee, set up in 1987, defined a homeless person as an individual who does not have an address or a decent and safe home for the next 60 days, who has little or no revenue and no social network, and is therefore isolated and excluded (Comité des sans-abri de la Ville de Montréal, 1987).

In the province of Québec, the local community service centre (CLSC) is a Primary Health Care service with responsibilities for illness prevention, health promotion, and home care within a district. The CLSC des Faubourgs is responsible for the health of an estimated 8000 homeless persons in central Montréal. In 1988, the CLSC set up a Team for the Homeless composed of one part-time general practitioner, one part-time psychiatrist, two full-time nurses, one part-time and two full-time social workers, and other support personnel.

When interviewed, a nurse and a social worker from the Team for the Homeless saw the homeless as vulnerable. They believed that these individuals feared health and social services, that their health condition was poor, and that they had few social networks. In other words, the homeless showed personal factors that, in interaction with a non-friendly environment, put them at risk for being wounded or experiencing deterioration of their health. In 1991, the nurse and the social worker set up outreach clinics in shelters and day centres in the district of the CLSC to offer care to homeless persons. At a set hours four days a week, the community health nurse sees individuals who need her attention. She works closely with the community workers in these centres, with other members of the Team who act as consultants, and with key professionals in the community and in the local hospitals. The social worker who accompanies her intervenes only when asked to do so, unless the homeless individual seeks him out first because he already knows him. The nurse's long-term aim is to develop self-care abilities in the homeless and to help them to utilize appropriate health services.

The main aim of this exploratory study was to analyze the practice of the nurse in outreach clinics for homeless individuals who used hostels and day centres in downtown Montréal and to describe the context of this community health nursing practice. The specific objectives were: (a) to identify the demands and needs that the homeless presented to the outreach nurse, (b) to identify the main characteristics of these homeless individuals, (c) to describe the settings in which community nursing care was given, (d) to describe the nursing interventions, (e) to describe the nurse's participation in the multidisciplinary team, (f) to describe the perceptions of other team members and community workers concerning the nurse's role, and (g) to describe factors that facilitated or hindered the nurse's practice.

Literature review

Health problems of the homeless

Until 1985, there were few studies of the physical health problems of the homeless. Researchers and services had concentrated on psychiatric problems and drug and alcohol abuse (Wright & Weber, 1987). Since then, U.S. studies have shown a high rate of physical and mental illness in all groups of homeless persons in 16 cities (Committee on Health Care for Homeless People, 1988). The physical problems noted most often are acute illnesses and trauma (about 25 percent of the homeless population), infectious diseases, upper respiratory tract infections, digestive problems, food poisoning, and skin problems. Moreover, an exarcerbation of chronic illnesses is observed. Psychiatric problems (25 to 50 percent of homeless persons) are often associated with alcohol and drug abuse. The Institute of Medicine reports a prevalence of 15 to 60 percent of alcohol abuse in this population. The Street Health Project in Toronto revealed that 40 percent of their clientele had been beaten in the last year; 20 percent of women had been raped (Crowe & Hardill, 1993). In 1991, a study of 124 clients of hostels in Vancouver showed that 52.4 percent presented a health problem, 58 percent complained of dental problems, and 40 percent complained of mental health problems (Acorn, 1993). In Montréal, Fournier (1991) observed that 40 to 50 percent of 299 subjects who used shelters and missions suffered from mental illness. Raynault, Battista, Joseph, and Fournier (1994) compared hospitalization records of the homeless (n=245) with the records of the 3553 residents of the same area admitted to the same hospital in Montréal over a period of one year. The results show that mental diagnoses were more frequent (homeless, 62.9 percent; residents, 12.9 percent), while cardiovascular diagnoses were rarer (homeless, 3.7 percent; residents, 10.8 percent). The number of visits to the emergency room by these homeless individuals varied from one to 19 (mean = 4.6) during the year.

Services for the homeless

Missions, shelters, day centres, and soup kitchens are places where the homeless can find temporary shelter, food, clothes, and hygiene facilities. Cohen and Isemberis (1991) mention that homeless persons suffering from mental illness utilize emergency services; this is mostly true for vulnerable persons suffering from alcohol and drug abuse and chronic illnesses. In an extensive review, Fournier and Mercier (1996) present a wide array of barriers that the homeless face in accessing regular psychiatric and general health services. These barriers, related to personal factors of the homeless as well as to the functioning of the services, include lack of a health card, inability of the homeless to follow the rules of health services (e.g., making an appointment and turning up on time), waiting in an emergency clinic, filling in forms that have little relevance to the homeless' problems, or following medical recommendations (e.g., the diabetic who lacks a permanent home and cooking facilities) (Carter, Green, Green, & Dufour, 1994; Crowe & Hardill, 1993).

Nursing services for the homeless

Nurse-managed free clinics in one Georgia city are an effective means of serving the needs of the homeless and indigent population (Carter, Green, Green, & Dufour, 1994). Primary Health Care programs staffed by nurse practitioners include the Cross-Over Health Clinic for homeless persons (Richmond, Virginia), which uses the services of other health or welfare professionals when needed (Bowdler, 1989). The extraordinary work of Lenehan and her colleagues at Pine Street Inn, Boston (Lenehan, McInnis, O'Donnell, & Hennessey, 1985), is another example of nursing services adapted to the needs of the homeless population. In Toronto, the Street Health Project (Crowe & Hardill, 1993) is a community-based nursing organization that operates clinics for women and men who are homeless or underhoused. Four nurses operate nursing stations in various drop-in centres and shelters.

Although most studies do not describe the work of the nurses, they do identify attitudes to adopt and appropriate interventions. These centre on the development of a trusting relationship; giving first aid, support, counselling, and clear and precise information; adopting the initial interview to the situation; and offering realistic treatments (Bowdler, 1989; Jackson & McSwane, 1992; Sebastian, 1992). Crowe and Hardill (1993) recommend sensitizing emergency room staff to the needs of homeless persons. Most authors suggest case management and advocacy. Although the literature describing the health needs of the homeless and the nursing street clinics that strive to meet these needs is voluminous, few nursing models have been developed or adapted from known models to guide care. Berne, Dato, Mason, and Rafferty (1990) proposed effective interventions for homeless families using Pesznecker's model of poverty. According to this model, people develop health-promoting or health-damaging responses to the stress of poverty, which are shaped by interactions between the individual/group and the environment. This comprehensive model provides direction for interventions with the homeless that address individuals, families, the environment, and society. The more explicit grounded theory of Jezewski (1995) explored the ways in which nurses in nurse-managed shelter clinics cared for homeless persons and facilitated the delivery of health care. This study influenced the authors' data collection method.

Method

The design consisted of an exploratory study that collected data on the practice of a nurse who held drop-in clinics in six shelters and day centres.

Interviews were conducted with workers in these shelters, as well as with members of the Team for the Homeless housed in the CLSC.

Sample and settings

The researcher studied nursing situations (i.e., encounters between the nurse and the homeless individual and the context of these situations). A situation lasted from 10 to 30 minutes. The nurse saw an average of 30 to 50 individuals a week. An individual could be seen many times during the course of the study. The researcher also carried out interviews with two members of the Team for the Homeless (physician and social worker) and key workers in eight shelters.

The shelters and centres provide services to the destitute and homeless over 18 years of age. Day centres offer a meal (either breakfast or lunch), clothes, and facilities to wash clothes. Night shelters provide a bed, shower facilities, clothing, and two meals (breakfast and supper). Three shelters cater to a female population, three to men; two have a mixed clientele, but few women go to the mixed centres. One centre for men has a mandate of education and services for alcoholics and drug addicts. Others administer welfare cheques and offer counselling for work placement. Most centres for women offer help with social rehabilitation and legal assistance. The nurse provided health care in all milieux that she visited once a week for a period of two to three hours.

Data collection and analysis

Four research instruments were used:

- One form requested information on the client's characteristics in terms of age, residence, needs, and demands; the nursing interventions; and topics discussed with the client. Checklists were developed, composed of 37 categories of nursing actions and 22 topics discussed with clients and tested during nursing situations.
- Notes were taken by an observer and completed by the nurse on other nursing actions for the client (not in the client's presence), including group activities, such as teaching prevention and care of upper respiratory tract infections.
- The interview guide for the nurse consisted mainly of open-ended questions focussed on values, attitudes, and behaviours related to the four concepts of the nursing paradigm: person, health, environment, and nursing care. It also raised questions concerning the factors that facilitated or hindered the nurse's work with the homeless.
- The interview guide for Team members and for workers in shelters consisted of open-ended questions centred on perceptions of the nurse's role with the homeless and their collaboration with her. All interviews were recorded.

The researcher or the research assistant accompanied the nurse to the shelters for 10 visits. The researcher observed the nurse giving care to the clients during 15 situations. The nurse completed the forms for 199 situations. Both recorded comments about the homeless person's situation and the nurse's work. Considering the aim of the study, it is not so much the number of nursing interventions that is important as the spectrum of these interventions or the variety of themes covered. Data were collected over a period of three months.

Frequency tables were created for nursing activities *with* and *for* clients. The recordings of the taped interviews were transcribed and subjected to content analysis. Similar themes were grouped. The activities observed and the respondents' comments related to these activities were integrated.

For ethical reasons, no homeless person was interviewed. Since it is well known that the homeless distrust intrusion into their lives and considering the aim of the study, the researcher did not solicit their opinions concerning the nurse's work in order to protect her relationship with her clients. Shelters are not identified by name in order to protect the identity of the workers.

Results

The population

During the collection of data, the nurse saw 132 individuals, and 199 situations were coded (i.e., some individuals were seen more than once). There were 110 men; 105 spoke French, 16 English. Seventy persons were already known to the nurse, and 40 were seen for the first time (no information is available on the other 22). The ages ranged from 22 to 75 years (mean age = 40). Most (n=41) were on welfare, and four had no revenue. Twenty-four lived in shelters, 23 had a room in a boarding house, and 46 had no address. Fifty-one individuals were known to have health problems, 15 had a psychiatric diagnosis, and 36 had varied conditions. The high rate of information not recorded arises from the fact that the homeless go to the nurse not to fill in complex questionnaires, but to obtain relief from pain and answers to their health-related questions. The homeless person volunteers information and controls the visit.

Initial demands and needs of the homeless

The first 11 categories shown in Table 23.1 account for 93 percent of individuals' demands. Except for 14 requests (mostly dealing with housing and money), all demands and needs are closely related to health matters.

Themes discussed by the nurse with the homeless

In contrast to Table 23.1, Table 23.2 shows a large number of themes that do not centre directly on health, such as activities of daily living, housing, and plans for the future. Psychological conditions are the focus of interaction in

Table 23.1
Initial demands of homeless persons to the nurse in the outreach clinic (N=132)

Demands (Health)	N	%	Demands (Non-health)	N	%
Physical and mental health care	167	76%	12. Wants help with housing	6	
1. Follow-up: dressings, tests, wounds, cuts, abscesses	58		13. Wants help managing welfare cheque	4	
2. Care of feet	34		14. Needs money for rent	3	
3. Wants medication, ointment, etc.	25		15. Wants to be removed from blacklist in shelters	1	
4. Various infections	23				
5. Requests information	11				
6. Wants to talk, seeks comfort	11				
7. Wants help to manage medication	5				
Utilization of health services	37	17%			
8. Wants reference for test, MD, etc.	19				
9. Follow-up with nurse	11				
10. Wants help with hospital appointment	5				
11. Wants detoxification program	2				
Total	204	93%		14	7%

30 percent of situations. If the themes are grouped into two categories, those directly related to health and the utilization of health and welfare services and those related to other aspects of life, the latter accounts for 44 percent of all themes. Although the authors noted initial demands of the clients, it is evident that the homeless raised further issues, many related to subjects other than health, with which they required assistance.

Interventions with homeless persons

As shown in Table 23.3, one-third (32 percent) of the nursing interventions consisted of exploring the individual's need for help, listening, and asking the individual's opinion. The category "offers disapproval/negative feelings" was related to the inappropriate behaviour of an individual, such as putting his hand on the nurse's thigh or requesting money from the nursing clinic when it was prohibited by court order.

In a typical interaction with an individual, the nurse centres attention first on what the person requests. She does not conduct a systematic inquiry related to the person's health or life; rather, she deals with the immediate need. The nurse does not make any moral judgements. If a dressing is required, the nurse shows the person how to do it. She gives the person the necessary supplies and may invite him or her to come back, either to the CLSC or to the shelter clinic. The person typically raises another issue, such as the loss of a health card or of pills. The following case study exemplifies this process.

Robert comes to the clinic with a blister on one foot. The nurse deals with the problem (care, shoe, prevention, etc.). Robert tells the nurse that he misses his "peanuts" (illegal drugs). The conversation centres on his psychiatric problem (he is a chronic schizophrenic). Since he abuses alcohol, the nurse asks if he has considered a detoxification cure (which he has mentioned to her in the past). She gives information and offers suggestions; he gives his opinion. Robert requests an appointment with the psychiatrist at the CLSC, and the nurse arranges this. Before he leaves, Robert sees the social worker, who helps him to obtain a new health card.

Interventions for homeless persons

Observations of the nurse in the outreach clinics and in the CLSC show five groups of activities: (a) those with shelter workers (information sessions for the homeless are also attended by shelter and clinic workers), (b) those with the Team for the Homeless, (c) clerical work (e.g., statistics, individuals' files, orders for medical and nursing material), (d) indirect clinical duties (e.g., taking blood tests to the lab; preparing weekly medications for patients) and public health activities (e.g., organizing clinics for hepatitis B or flu vaccination, TB testing; participating in surveys by the public health unit), (e) meetings or telephone conversations with the family of the homeless person.

Table 23.2
Themes discussed by the nurse with the homeless (N=132) during 199 situations

Related to Health		Not Directly Related to Health	
General condition	84	Activities of daily living	71
Psychological condition	58	Housing	65
Wounds of all types	51	Plans for the future	63
Nutrition and sleep	44	Social and family relations	24
Medications and treatments	49	Welfare problems	23
Behaviour	24	Appointment with social services	21
Compliance with regimen	13	Transportation	15
Detoxification cure	9	Budget planning	14
Utilization of health services	51	Clothes	2
Total	383 (56%)	Total	298 (44%)

Table 23.3
Nursing interventions during 199 nursing situations with the homeless (N=132)

	N	%
Identification of needs	490	32%
Explores, clarifies person's request	258	
Listens (96), observes person's condition (68)	164	
Asks person's opinion	68	
Physical exam and objects given	130	9%
Gives physical exam, care	99	
Gives object (booklet, medication, socks, cards, etc.)	31	
Psychosocial care	708	47%
Offers encouragement, positive feelings, support, approval, reassurance, praise	179	
Gives responsibility to person, requests participation	149	
Gives information, explanation, demonstration	131	
Gives suggestion, advice	103	
Offers opinion	81	
Offers disapproval, negative feelings, refusal	30	
Negotiates contract	20	
Jokes	15	
Utilization of services	190	12%
Arranges appointment, follow-up	75	
Makes referral(s)	74	
Introduces person to another Team member	37	
Accompanies person	4	
Total	1518	100%

The nurse's perception of her practice

The nursing paradigm

To understand the nurse's practice, the authors felt it was necessary to know her values and views on various aspects of the nursing paradigm. During an interview, the nurse responded to a series of questions about health, individuals, environment, and nursing interventions. The nurse's view of her care is described here.

Health is a state of equilibrium among various dimensions: physical, psychological, and environmental. To be healthy is to have quality of life. However, a healthy environment will help the individual to maintain or achieve that state. All individuals want to develop their potential to the maximum; they want to live an active life, and they want to be healthy. The *environment* includes the physical setting in which a person lives, together with its material resources; social class, with its norms and conventions; and relationships with people

Nursing care is helping people to take care of themselves. The community health nurse recognized that two nurse theorists have influenced her most. Nightingale's vision of health and of the community helped her to realize that basic hygiene, food, and a clean physical environment are central to health. Virginia Henderson viewed the client as an individual with basic needs, an insight that is particularly relevant in dealing with the homeless.

According to this nurse, short-term goals in working with the homeless include improving their overall quality of life, their physical health, and their social interactions. If nurses succeed in improving the health of the homeless, in giving them needed medication, in making sure they eat good meals and have a place to stay, then we have given some comfort and taken the first steps to improve their difficult situation. Quality of life is thus enhanced. The long-term goal is to bring the homeless into the mainstream of society, to help them utilize appropriate health and welfare services, and to lead them on the road to empowerment.

Knowledge, attitudes, and skills needed to work with the homeless

Primary Health Care *knowledge* is basic to nursing the homeless. It means knowing techniques to care for various kinds of wounds, infections, and other ills with little means and resources. It requires diversified experience as well as techniques in screening. Knowledge includes an understanding of epidemiology, as well as an awareness of communities, community resources and mutual aid, and public health problems—how they develop and how they are solved. It also entails an ability to work with groups and to enlist collaboration.

Three basic *attitudes* are required of the nurse working with the homeless. First, the nurse has to abandon preconceived ideas concerning the homeless. Prejudices often arise from exaggerated media coverage and social misrepresentations. Second, the nurse must be patient. Nurses working in highly technical milieux and in acute care hospitals are used to working fast and expecting patients to comply with the medical regimen and with health care regulations. Since the hospital stay must be as short as possible, nurses expect patients to cooperate fully in order to learn self-care quickly. By contrast, when working with the homeless, the nurse allows the individual to set the pace: the individual's speed is the nurse's speed. This is the *sine qua non* condition of care. The third attitude is flexibility—with the homeless themselves and with the network of community and health care resources. Changes in the lives of the homeless can be drastic and sudden. Since they depend on an unreliable environment, they often find themselves without resources to cope with new and unexpected situations. Therefore, the nurse must accept noncompliance, forgetfulness, and deviations from good intentions and promises.

The nurse working with the homeless needs various *skills:* skills in treatments and in screening an individual quickly to determine if the condition is serious. Nurses must make clear decisions and give clear explanations, as homeless individuals can be anxious and confused (especially if using illegal drugs or alcohol). The nurse must also be very resourceful, as illustrated in the following case study.

Marie, a homeless woman over 50, had been brought to a night shelter after many months of outreach interventions from the nurse. Marie never spoke; she was believed to be schizophrenic. She had developed an enormous abscess on the back of her neck which caused her excruciating pain. The night worker informed the nurse, who arranged to go regularly to the park next to the shelter to give Marie antibiotic medication and to change her dressings until she was well again. Thus, the nurse adjusted her behaviour to the circumstances and adapted her treatments to the milieu.

The nurse's perception of the homeless

The nurse perceives homeless persons as having many physical and social needs basic to survival: problems with their feet and skin, pulmonary infections, and other ailments, including chronic and severe psychiatric conditions. All have problems with medication (prescriptions not filled, or lost). Their daily activities are focussed on survival. They want to be healthy to cope with their hard lives.

According to the nurse, being homeless involves losing one's pride and identity. Hence, homeless persons have low self-esteem; many are ashamed of themselves. They feel awful ("ils se sentent mal dans leur peau"), and that feeling prevents them from making friends. Lack of significant relationships, together with poor self-discipline, lack of competence due to poor schooling, lack of a home, and financial and psychological problems, are the main factors that keep the homeless from entering mainstream society.

The nurse's first priority is to deal with physical ailments and medicines. Other problems are more difficult to handle, including psychiatric conditions, drug and alcohol abuse, and poor budget administration. Further, some homeless have been barred from all shelters because of their disruptive behaviour, mostly associated with drug and alcohol abuse. They may ask the nurse to intervene for them to regain acceptance at a particular centre. Few homeless have contact with their families; therefore, the most meaningful persons for them are the workers in the shelters.

Often, homeless individuals do not feel responsible for what is happening to them. Some become aggressive as a way of denying or coping with a painful situation. However, "after they get to know me, they see me for all kinds of reasons, from therapy to housing, from welfare cards to health information." Willingness to go to the CLSC clinic for tests, results, or referrals, or to discuss problems and possible solutions, is an indication that the homeless individual is establishing trust in the nurse. This trust is later transferred to other professionals.

Nursing the homeless

The nurse identified two steps: (a) respond to the homeless person's request (relief of aches and pains) and (b) later, investigate other needs. The five nursing interventions seen to be most helpful are: (a) giving physical care, (b) giving badly needed resources such as food, socks, pills, bus tickets, etc., (c) giving attention and listening, (d) referring the client to the social worker, who will deal immediately with welfare cheques, the court, housing problems, etc., and (e) arranging follow-up with various professionals.

The whole array of interventions is adapted to the need for help and to the homeless person's understanding and willingness to participate. The nurse invites the homeless individual to participate through demonstrations; she teaches and gives the necessary materials. She helps the individual to take immediate steps to solve problems, even if the steps are small (e.g., a telephone call to the appropriate professional). She establishes a partnership with the individual, or she proposes a partnership with a worker in the shelter. Contracts are negotiated, but the responsibility resides with the individual. This nurse believes that once homeless persons have felt the "goodness of comfort and the pleasure of possessing money," they will want to experience this feeling again. She encourages them to avoid problems by recalling difficult situations (e.g., going to jail), to be compliant with medication (already packaged in dosages), and to work closely with the workers in the shelters. In other words, she teaches homeless individuals to win over their environment. She gives visible signs of her involvement, such as making an appointment or supplying a card with names and telephone numbers. The nurse adds that at times she will accompany a homeless individual to a health or social service agency or to a community organization.

The nurse and Team members aim to help the homeless get back into society, not to establish a parallel system of care or to keep them in a ghetto.

Working with the shelters

The nurse deplores the lack of centres that develop rehabilitation programs for the homeless, such as supervised settings where the homeless can have non-intrusive and humane monitoring, an adequate support system, therapy, and work training. Unfortunately, because of small budgets, many shelters cannot afford experienced and stable staff. They therefore have a high turnover of personnel, with no continuity in care plans for the sickest patients. The nurse has observed that some shelter workers have difficulty putting limits on inappropriate behaviours of some homeless persons. The shelters would benefit from more support and outreach work by the Team in order to prevent the deterioration of timid and withdrawn individuals. The nurse sometimes goes to the shelter outside of her regular visiting hours if an urgent situation arises.

Factors that facilitate the nurse's work

Working in a multidisciplinary team where members can help one another is necessary. No one professional possesses the ability to cope alone with such an overwhelming task nor has the resources to address the whole range of needs of the homeless. The team approach lessens communication problems among providers and addresses homeless individuals' problems through comprehensive care. Members complement one another and think they make better joint decisions, especially with drug abusers who have a tendency to manipulate care providers. Another factor that facilitates nursing practice is the establishment of partnerships with shelter workers, which help to promote continuity and coordination of care.

Within the Team, the nurse has a clearly defined role; she is the first person to whom the homeless go. She plans, organizes, and gives the care. She has privileged communications with doctors, psychiatrists, and coordinators in the hospitals. *She opens the door to the health care system.*

Factors that hinder nursing practice

Bureaucracy in hospitals, welfare agencies, and governmental offices, as well as restrictive mental health laws, places constraints on the work of the nurse.

The shortage of staff also limits rehabilitation work with the homeless and systematic evaluation of activities. Since the Team knows the needs of the homeless and often plays an advocacy role, members believe it should undertake a more active political role in order to bring about change in social housing policies and in the deinstitutionalization process.

Team members' and shelter workers' perceptions of the nurse

Team members perceive that the nurse, with her Primary Health Care skills, is the pivot of the Team. The social worker states:

The trust the homeless establish in her [as their initial contact] is transferred to me, and I can start helping them with other needs such as money, housing, court orders, etc. . . . We share the burden of the work. The homeless present all types of problems; often, we can better understand their situation if there are two of us. After many years of working together, we know exactly who should handle what problem. . . . We complement each other. There has never been a power game between us. Our population is composed mainly of men. Many have had difficult relations with women before. They are now helped by a professional woman who is firm and non-judgemental. It is difficult for them to deal with that. It was not easy for the nurse at the beginning to cope with these situations. She now knows what reactions to expect; she is firm but she never withdraws her help.

According to the physician, the nurse has an important role, as she is the first contact with the homeless:

I seldom go to the shelters. The nurse and the social worker reach out to the homeless and bring them to me in the CLSC. We do not want to create a parallel system of care. My role is secondary to the nurse's. She gives basic care, takes blood pressures and temperatures, dresses sores, wounds, and blisters, treats headaches, etc. When she deals with those aches and pains that have priority for the homeless, she becomes their gateway to the health care system. For example, many patients are HIV positive. The nurse may take care of what seemed like a simple "sore," then bring the individual in to the CLSC. . . . She is the link between the homeless, the CLSC, the physician, and the psychiatrist. . . . Four elements characterize the nurse: her technical competence and professional judgement; her ability to establish trust; her clearly defined role; and her respect for, and solidarity with, Team members.

Shelter workers said: "Because [the nurse] solves the homeless' problems, their behaviour improves." "The homeless have better follow-up, especially the mentally ill." "[The nurse] answers the needs of the homeless; their health improves. They trust her and they come to the shelter on the days that she visits." The workers appreciate the nurse's presence as it brings them closer to health and social services.

Discussion

The population seen by this community health nurse is similar in terms of sex, age, and housing to the ones surveyed in previous studies in Canada (Crowe & Hardill, 1993; Fournier, 1991; McCormack & Gooding, 1993; Raynault, Battista, Joseph, & Fournier, 1994). Women are less numerous because there are fewer homeless women than men and because the nurse visits more shelters for men than for women. The lack of information on the characteristics of the homeless demonstrates the nurse's awareness that some homeless persons do not want to give information about themselves. They prefer to be anonymous until they trust the professional.

As noted, the nurse deals first with the specific physical problem that the person presents; typically, these are related to health matters. Wiedenbach (1964) called this demand a "need for help," defined as any measure or action required and desired by the individual that has potential for restoring or extending his or her ability to cope with the demands implicit in the situation. The fact that one-third of the nursing interventions are focussed on exploring the client's need for help (see Table 23.3, p. 452) reflects Orlando's (1961) deliberative process. The nurse collects data reflectively rather than systematically. As the interaction progresses, the nurse continually clarifies with the homeless client other needs for help. The client trusts her enough to bring up more needs and demands, and will accept more help from her.

Although health is related to all aspects of human life, it is not usual for health professionals to deal with housing and transportation issues. The fact that 44 percent of all the themes discussed with the homeless (Table 23.2, p. 451) consisted of subjects other than health matters indicates the broad spectrum of the nurse's interventions.

Although she cannot solve all homeless persons' problems, the nurse ensures that others on the Team continue the care. This behaviour is consistent with the nurse's belief that human beings "want to be independent and responsible for self-care but, at the same time, also want to be taken care of by somebody"; "Beliefs are the bedrock of our behaviour and the essence of our affect. . . . We *are* our beliefs" (Wright, Watson, & Bell, 1996, pp. 19, 25). The nurse's perceptions of the life of the homeless are similar to those of many nursing authors (Acorn, 1993; Jackson & McSwan, 1992; Lenehan et al., 1985; Sebastian, 1992), although her comprehension of their suffering and loneliness seems deeper. She has observed, analyzed, and thought through the phenomenon of homelessness and raised questions about the meaning of life, freedom, solitude, and social justice.

The great emphasis that the nurse puts on the support of the interdisciplinary Team shows how coordination of all services is crucial in order to have some positive impact on the self-care behaviours of the homeless. Equally important are the relationships with the shelters and day centres where the nurse holds outreach clinics. The workers in these centres are often the only social network of the homeless; they contribute to the homeless' quality of life.

In essence, the nurse's practice with the homeless follows the phases of nursing as described by Wiedenbach: (a) identification of clients' need for help; (b) delivery of the help that is needed, with an emphasis on Primary Health Care and on the relief of pain as measures to establish trust; (c) validation that the help provided was useful; and (d) coordination of the resources and of the help provided.

Conclusion

Homelessness in Canada is a social problem that has roots in the individual as well as in major changes that have occurred in our economy and in our value system. This study has examined the practice of one nurse working in outreach clinics with homeless persons. This practice was developed to serve the specific needs of this vulnerable population and illustrates the wide spectrum of physical, psychological, and social actions that can be performed in the context of community health practice.

Acknowledgement
This project was supported by the Fondation de recherche en sciences infirmières du Québec.

QUESTIONS

1. What factors contribute to homelessness that are outside the control of the individual?
2. How do people in your area describe the homeless? What values are reflected in their choice of words? Do you share these values? Explain.
3. Describe at least three links that the community health nurse must establish to facilitate care for the homeless.
4. What actions can a community health care team take to improve the living conditions of the homeless?
5. Can you think of another vulnerable group that could benefit from this type of community health nursing practice? Explain.

REFERENCES

Acorn, S. (1993). Mental and physical health of homeless persons who use emergency shelters in Vancouver. *Hospital and Community Psychiatry, 44*(9), 854–857.

Aday, L.A. (1997). Vulnerable populations: A community-oriented perspective. *Family and Community Health, 19*(4), 1–18.

Berne, A.S., Data, C., Mason, D.J., & Rafferty, M. (1990). A nursing model for addressing the health needs of homeless families. *Image: Journal of Nursing Scholarship, 22*(1), 8–13.

Bowdler, J.E. (1989). Health problems of the homeless in America. *Nurse Practitioner, 14*(7), 44–51.

Carter, F.K., Green, L., Green, R.D., & Dufour, T.L. (1994). Health needs of homeless clients accessing nursing care at a free clinic. *Journal of Community Health Nursing, 11*(3), 139–147.

Cohen, N.L., & Tsemberis, S. (1991). Emergency psychiatric intervention on the street. *New Directions for Mental Health Services, 52*, 3–16.

Comité des sans-abri de la Ville de Montréal. (1987). *Vers une politique municipale pour les sans-abri.* Montréal: Ville de Montréal.

Committee on Health Care for Homeless People. (1988). *Homelessness, health and human needs.* Washington, DC: Institute of Medicine, National Academy Press.

Crowe, C., & Hardill, K. (1993). The Street Health Report. *Canadian Nurse, 89*(1), 21–24.

Fournier, L. (1991). *Itinérance et santé mentale à Montréal.* Verdun: Hôpital Douglas, Unité de recherche psychosociale.

Fournier, L., & Mercier, C. (Eds.). (1996). *Sans domicile fixe—au delà du stéréotype.* Montréal: Éditions du Méridien.

Jackson, M.P., & McSwane, D.Z. (1992). Homelessness as a determinant of health. *Public Health Nursing, 9*(3), 185–192.

Jezewski, M.A. (1995). Staying connected: The core of facilitating health care for homeless persons. *Public Health Journal, 12*(3), 203–210.

Lenehan, G.P., McInnis, B.N., O'Donnell, D., & Hennessey, M. (1985). A nurse's clinic for the homeless in America. *American Journal of Nursing, 85*(11), 1237–1240.

McCormack, D., & Gooding, S.B. (1993). Homeless persons communicate their meaning of health. *Canadian Journal of Nursing Research, 25*(1), 33–50.

Orlando, I.J. (1961). *The dynamic nurse–patient relationship.* New York: G.P. Putnam's Sons.

Raynault, M.F., Battista, R.N., Joseph, L., & Fournier, L. (1994). Motifs d'hospitalisation et durée de séjour d'une population d'itinérants de Montréal. *Revue canadienne de santé publique, 85*(4), 274–277.

Sebastian, J.G. (1992). Vulnerable populations in the community. In M. Stanhope & J. Lancaster (Eds.), *Community health nursing* (pp. 374–379). St. Louis: Mosby.

Wiedenbach, E. (1964). *Clinical nursing: A helping art.* New York: Springer.

Wright, J.D., & Weber, E. (1987). *Homelessness and health.* Washington, DC: McGraw-Hill.

Wright, L.M., Watson, W.L., & Bell, J.M. (1996). *Beliefs: The heart of healing in families and illness.* New York: Basic Books.

C H A P T E R   2 4

Effects of health system reform on helping relationships

Jean R. Hughes

This chapter discusses implications of health system reform for the helping relationship between the client and the community health nurse. The impact of Primary Health Care on the choice of theoretical framework and the principles guiding the helping relationship are examined. Critical premises include client centredness, client determination, health orientation, and client–nurse partnership. Specific examples illustrate issues and demonstrate nursing approaches to the helping relationship.

LEARNING OBJECTIVES

In this chapter, you will learn:

- how Primary Health Care, as a driving force of health system reform, influences the helping relationship between community health nurse and client
- the relevance and capacity of interaction theories in nursing for guiding practice in a reformed health system
- how the nursing role may be strengthened to enhance the helping relationship in keeping with principles of reform

Introduction

Throughout the 1990s, the Canadian health system has undergone sweeping reform. There is general agreement that a system focussing more on services than on needs, more on curing illness than on promoting health, and more on unidimensional views than on comprehensive perspectives cannot enhance the capacity of individuals, families, and communities to function optimally or to improve their social and physical environments (Health & Welfare Canada, 1987, 1988; Marmor, Barer, & Evans, 1994; National Forum on Health, 1997). As a result, every province and territory throughout the country has embarked on a major effort to restructure its health system. Unfortunately, most of this change has attended more to economic restructuring than to true system reform. Until the principles and mechanisms underlying the health system are transformed, Canadians are unlikely to see significant improvement in their health status (Angus, 1991; Marmor et al., 1994; National Forum on Health, 1997; Rachlis & Kushner, 1994).

What would real reform look like? How would the principles, philosophical framework, and mechanisms underlying the health system have to change? What effect would fundamental reform have on the ways in which community health nurses think about clients as people, about our relationships with clients, about the helping processes we use to assist them, and about the ways in which we think about health and illness?

Underlying principles and mechanisms

Until recently, principles underlying the medical model governed the Canadian health system and, in turn, community health nursing. The professional is considered the authority who is in sole possession of the expert knowledge necessary for resolving professional-identified client problems. The client, who seeks prescriptive guidance from the professional, is considered deficient. Reform principles advocate an alternative model to guide the professional–client relationship. Under the partnership model, professionals and clients hold shared values of responsiveness, interaction, reciprocity, and public participation. This means professionals work in ways that share control and promote empowerment (Fawcett et al., 1995).

The partnership model is not fully supported by all professionals. Rather than viewing it as a more effective way of working with clients, some nurses consider the model a threat to their professional role and integrity (e.g., Glenister, 1994; Sully, 1996). These nurses feel powerless in their relationships with clients when they lack sole control of the knowledge base. Other nurses, who have been rendered powerless by their workplace, view sharing control with the client as a further undermining of their professional integrity (Chalmers & Bramadat, 1996). Some professionals argue that clients prefer a role of dependence and consider notions of client participation as an abdication of professional responsibility (Waterworth & Luker, 1990).

There is no common view of the partnership model among its supporters. Regardless of the definition, however, the partnership model means more than merely having a voice (Sullivan & Scattolon, 1995). Some professionals (Deber, 1995) argue that a true partnership model involves equal but different role responsibilities. Using this approach, the professional provides clinical knowledge (health-related facts) and proceeds with problem solving, while the client provides experiential knowledge (personal information and cultural values/traditions) and proceeds with decision making (choosing among alternatives, for which the ability to weigh risks and benefits according to individual values is important). Other authorities (Donovan & Blake, 1992) maintain that the partnership model involves professionals and clients working collaboratively to solve problems related to health matters. Still others (Dunst, Trivette, & Deal, 1988) hold that the most effective partnership model is one in which the professional provides clinical knowledge and skills to facilitate the relationship, while the client identifies the need, provides experiential knowledge, and makes the final decisions.

Client

The medical model has permeated our understanding of the client. This model focusses on client deficits (problems) and reinforces social structures that create and maintain unequal power relationships (Cowger, 1994). Its influence on practice is quite dramatic, yet the messages are simple and clear—for example, "clients *lack* competence," "clients need the professional to do for them, or to tell them what to do," "professional help is the only legitimate expertise." Such models victimize clients, render them dependent, and undermine their personal and social power.

In contrast, a reform model establishes a fundamentally different view of the client (Dunst, Trivette, & Deal, 1988). First, it takes a proactive stance by assuming that people who seek help from professionals are competent or have the capacity to become competent. Second, the reform model creates opportunities for "enabling" experiences that promote proficient individuals who are able to mobilize their social networks to get needs met and attain desired goals (Dunst, Trivette, & Deal, 1988, pp. 88–89). The reform model assumes that failure to display competence is due not to deficits within the client, but rather to the failure of social systems to create opportunities for developing or exercising competencies. For example, when clients do not follow prescribed treatment regimes (e.g., they fail to give up smoking despite a respiratory condition), it is not because they lack motivation or interest in their health; rather, it is due to inadequate contextually relevant (i.e., meaningful and acceptable) supports in the environment.

Third, the reform model holds an empowered view by assuming that clients change behaviour *only* when they believe they play a role in making the change. Nursing interventions help clients gain a sense of control over their lives as a result of their own efforts to meet their needs.

Helping processes

Under the reform model, the power balance in the helping relationship is shifted from paternalistic control to collaborative partnership. Rather than focussing on problem solving, the nurse concentrates more on the *processes* involved with enabling and empowering help-seekers (Dunst, Trivette, & Deal, 1994). The professional role shifts access to and control over needed resources to the client. Nurses help clients gain decision-making skills and problem-solving abilities (Dunst & Trivette, 1986). Major attention is placed on strengthening the client's personal social network, which influences coping strategies (Stewart, 1989) and alleviates social isolation (Fisher, Goff, Nadler, & Chinsky, 1988). The professional neither usurps decision making nor supplants the client's support networks with professional services (Dunst, Trivette, & Deal, 1994).

In other words, under the reform model, the community health nurse focusses on assisting clients to develop knowledge and skills that solve client-identified needs using their own resources. The nurse suspends the impulse to "take over" or "rescue" the client. Thus, the mark of a successful relationship is a shift from a focus on solving a *problem* to one of *enhancing* capacity.

Health and illness

A reformed philosophical framework also requires nurses to adopt new ways of thinking about, working with, and evaluating health and illness (Trainor, Pomeroy, & Pape, 1993). A true understanding of health and illness is formed from more than one domain of knowledge. Two critical sources of information, in addition to conventional clinical knowledge, include the client's thoughts/ideas (experiential knowledge) and the client's customs/mores learned from families, friends, and community (customary/traditional knowledge) (Cravener, 1992; PEI Health & Community Services Agency, 1996; Trainor et al., 1993). Such information helps to discern individual values and attitudes as well as cultural practices that influence health and illness patterns. Unfortunately, most professionals either ignore or pay mere lip service to this crucial source of information when working with clients. This omission can have disastrous effects on the helping relationship. Professionals fail to focus on what the client perceives to be the real problem, and clients refuse to follow what they perceive to be an unjustified treatment regime. In such cases, professionals often label clients as resistant, non-compliant, or manipulative (Heszen-Klemens, 1987; Trilling & Jaber, 1993). Under a reform model, the client is less likely to be misunderstood as relationships are more likely to be built around a full appreciation of the client's world.

These changes in philosophical framework are basic to Primary Health Care reform (see also Chapters 2 and 3). For these to take hold, nurses and clients will have to change the ways in which they work together. When the professional–client power relationship is balanced, interactions will be based on client need; decisions will become client-determined; and client understanding, skill, and motivation regarding health will be improved (e.g., Donovan & Blake, 1992; Gyulay, Mound, & Flanagan, 1994; Hughes & Carver, 1990; Smith, 1992). The helping relationship promotes client autonomy—the capacity to self-determine and initiate action (Deci & Ryan, 1991). There is mounting evidence that autonomy (personal control) plays a significant role in healthy functioning (e.g., Bertrand, 1996; Carroll, Davey Smith, Sheffield, Shipley, & Marmot, 1997; Doherty, 1997; Hemingway, Nicholson, Stafford, Roberts, & Marmot, 1997; Marmot, Bosma, Hemingway, Brunner, & Stansfeld, 1997a; Stansfeld, Head, & Marmot, 1998). Autonomy enables clients to take action to meet their health needs in productive and satisfying ways and acts as a buffer against disease (Marmot et al., 1997b).

Given that the helping relationship forms the working mechanism for nursing practice (e.g., Arnold & Boggs, 1989; Brammer & MacDonald, 1996; Hughes & Carver, 1990; Smith, 1992; Varcarolis, 1990), it is important to understand how this essential tool is affected by health system reform. Under these conditions, the historical power differential between nurses and clients is removed to equalize roles and responsibilities (Shoultz, Hatcher, & Hurrell, 1992). Professionals who equalize the power balance in the helping relationship are more likely to promote empowerment (e.g., McWilliam et al., 1997; Trivette, Dunst, & Hamby, 1996) and healthy outcomes in clients (e.g., Williams, 1997). It has also been connected with clients' enhanced sense of personal control over supports and resources (Dunst & Trivette, 1996). A power balance can be found in practices that hold a family-/client-centred or caring (Williams, 1997) orientation.

Under reform conditions, nurses become facilitators who work *with* clients as consumers or citizens. Both clients and nurses share common rights (e.g., choice of actions) and responsibilities (e.g., accountability for these choices). As client capacity for taking appropriate action is assumed, the nurse relinquishes ownership of the decision-making process.

Health outcomes are measured in terms of client ability to function in everyday life. Therefore, nurses focus on building client strengths rather than eliminating deficiencies. One of the more innovative approaches to health system reform adopted by nursing is the "strengths perspective." This model comes from the mental health field and is gradually being tested in other fields of practice, including community health nursing, with promising results (Saleebey, 1996). The strengths perspective builds on existing abilities and promotes optimal capacity in the client (Pray, 1992). It has obvious connections with health reform concepts such as resilience, wellness, natural resources, and holism. Nurses who incorporate the strengths perspective work with opportunities, in contrast to their counterparts using traditional illness models, who work with risks.

Fit between nursing theory and Primary Health Care reform

Given the impact of health system reform on the nurse–client relationship, consider how well nursing's theoretical models support the underlying principles of Primary Health Care. Frameworks oriented toward illness and problems reinforce a deficit orientation and, consequently, a power differential between nurses and clients. Such frameworks are incongruent with conditions for Primary Health Care reform. Most nursing theories that focus on helping relationships fail in this regard (Meleis, 1991). Although several theories acknowledge the importance of the client perspective (e.g., King, 1981; Peplau, 1992; Wiedenbach, 1964), many fail to promote client self-determination (autonomy) (e.g., Orlando, 1961; Wiedenbach, 1964). Those few models that increase client control (e.g., Peplau, 1992) make the transition only gradually as the nurse–client relationship progresses, and the relationship is regulated by the nurse.

In contrast, frameworks that promote client-centred relationships and interactions (client-initiated encounters to address client-identified health needs) support Primary Health Care reform. For example, King's Goal Attainment Theory (1981) encourages nurses and clients to use their unique knowledge to find mutually agreeable ways of reaching client-identified goals. Clients are considered responsible and capable and, therefore, have the ultimate power to accept or reject nursing care. According to this theory, nurses provide clients with accurate and meaningful (i.e., contextually relevant) information to facilitate *client* problem solving. When nurses work with clients in mutual ways, they develop more intense relationships than when they use other approaches (Ramos, 1992). These nurses are able to balance the engagement and detachment processes in their relationships with clients in ways that *affect* outcomes without *controlling* outcomes (Carmack, 1997).

The McGill Model of Nursing (Gottlieb & Rowat, 1987) also supports principles of reform. Its philosophical foundation is client centred and health oriented. The model assumes that individuals, families, and communities are motivated toward and have the potential for health. It also assumes that clients learn best through active participation. Using this model, nurses work in collaboration with clients and assist them to function at client-identified maximum capacity.

In contrast to other nursing theories that reward clients for their submissive, unchallenging behaviour, King's theory and the McGill Model view client decisions (including rejection of care) as a positive step toward building client autonomy. Community health nurses who use these frameworks to guide their practice move in the direction of health system reform based on the Primary Health Care principle of public participation.

The fit between health system reform and client–nursing interactions

A system that relies on active client participation and accountability demands a purposeful and sensitive alliance between clients and nurses. Such an alliance is enhanced by the nurse's use of facilitative affiliation (Rogers, 1996), presence (Osterman & Schwartz-Barcott, 1996), and knowing (Jenny & Logan, 1992). These skills enable the nurse to perceive, feel, and sense the client. Empathy is well recognized as the most critical sensory element for achieving a client-centred helping relationship (Egan, 1994; Gazda, Childers, & Brooks, 1987; Pike, 1990). Empathy is both an attitude (Rogers, 1975) and a skill (Carver & Hughes, 1990; Gazda & Evans, 1990) and has long been considered a fundamental component of nursing (Sutherland, 1995).

Empathy validates and affirms the client (Gazda & Evans, 1990). It plays a significant role in influencing health and well-being (Lancee, Gallop, McCay, & Toner, 1995; Olson, 1995; Olson & Hanchett, 1997; Reid-Ponte, 1992; Wheeler, 1990). Empathy humanizes the health system by creating a caring environment (Holden, 1990; Wheeler & Barrett, 1994). It helps ensure that clients are viewed as unique and are respected for their ability to take primary responsibility for bringing about change in their health. Nurses who use the skill of empathy practise in ways that are consistent with reform. They tend to be facilitative rather than controlling in their relationships and work with clients rather than doing things "to" or "for" them (Carver & Hughes, 1990).

Nurses consider themselves empathic in *attitude* (Coffey & Swirsky, 1988; Rogers, 1986). Community health nurses report significantly higher empathic attitudes than hospital nurses (Coffey & Swirsky, 1988). However, nurses' empathic skills fall far short of their perception (Brunt, 1985; MacKay, Carver, & Hughes, 1990). Indeed, one case study analysis found that nurses used little validation or affirmation in their interactions and attended to their own needs, rather than those identified by the client (Hughes & Carver, 1990). They assumed primary control of the interactions and limited the discussion to physical care issues, while avoiding emotional matters.

Nurses need to enhance their empathic skills to work in a reformed Primary Health Care system. Without empathy, nurses fail to understand the client's perspective, fail to work with client-identified needs, and therefore, it is argued, fail to promote health.

Reformed approach to the helping relationship: Case study

Primary Health Care reform is client-centred and emphasizes a health orientation, a strengths perspective, and public participation. To illustrate how reform principles apply to the practice of community health nursing, the following case study depicts the developmental processes of a helping relationship. The case involves a family learning to live with chronic illness. Helping clients who have chronic health problems manage major emotional adjustments, lifestyle alterations, and treatment requires an empathic, egalitarian relationship (Thorne, 1990).

John MacDonald is a 56-year-old labourer at the shipyards in Halifax, Nova Scotia. He has had 37 years of good marriage to his wife, Susan. Together they have raised three children, who now live in neighbouring communities no more than a day's drive from the MacDonald home. Six months ago, Mr. MacDonald was diagnosed with diabetes following several months of fatigue, thirst, and urinary frequency. Up to that time, he had been a strong, healthy man who prided himself on missing fewer days from work than any of his co-workers.

Mrs. MacDonald called the community health nurse (CHN) because her husband had not been following his diet or regulating his insulin intake carefully for the past two months. Mrs. MacDonald was worried about her husband's health and asked for assistance.

Primary Health Care principles direct the CHN to work with the client-identified need. As Mrs. MacDonald initiated the contact, the CHN will begin her relationship with her rather than her husband. The nurse will begin by establishing the client's perspective of the situation. The following illustrates how the interaction might proceed and explains how the approaches fit the Primary Health Care reform model, in contrast to a more traditional nursing approach.

CHN: I understand you're worried about your husband and his diabetes?

Mrs. M.: Yes. At first my husband did everything he was supposed to do. Neither one of us ever had to deal with anything like this before and so we were both pretty careful. It wasn't easy but the diabetes finally started to make some sense to us. Well, nurse, we were just beginning to get his treatments straight and all that, when he started fooling around with them. He said he didn't need all that stuff.

CHN: It must have been pretty frustrating to have worked so hard together to learn how to manage diabetes and then, just when you started to feel comfortable, your husband decided to change the rules.

If the CHN had used a more traditional response, she might have provided Mrs. M. with the information that her husband's behaviour is consistent with the coping behaviour of other people during the initial stages of chronic illness. However, the CHN who bases her practice on Primary Health Care principles concentrates instead, at this point, on empathy to validate Mrs. M.'s perspective of the situation and refrains from teaching about, or passing judgement on, Mr. M.'s actions. The nurse is careful to focus on the couple and to build on strengths by pointing out their ability to persevere and overcome a health challenge.

Mrs. M.: That's right, nurse. You don't know how scared I am. I keep telling him he's playing Russian roulette. I just can't understand him.

CHN: You thought you both had agreed that John would follow his diabetic regime carefully. I can see why you'd be confused when he started changing his routine. I can also imagine that it is quite frightening for you, and perhaps for your children too, to watch your husband's actions. I think most people get pretty scared when they observe someone they love put themselves at risk. You want to help, yet feel so helpless about which way to turn.

Using a traditional approach, the CHN might try to reassure Mrs. M. that her husband is grieving about the loss of his independence and that he needs to know he still has control in his life. Such an approach minimizes the wife's need to tell her story and predetermines what information the family wants. In contrast, an approach based on Primary Health Care reform strives to increase the CHN's understanding of how Mr. M.'s actions affect his wife and other family members. The nurse continues to work with family strengths by acknowledging the members' love and commitment to help one another. The CHN also normalizes the family's worry by letting Mrs. M. know that most people in her circumstances would share her worry.

Mrs. M.: This is a serious disease! I thought John understood all that stuff. Maybe I was wrong. . . . We've always managed on our own in the past, but now I'm at my wit's end. The kids have been great in listening to my rantings about their father—they're worried, too. Lord knows they've tried to talk to him, but he won't listen. Nurse, that's why I called you. I didn't know what else to do.

CHN: You're afraid that unless John changes his ways something tragic is going to happen and you might lose him. That's a heavy burden to carry on your own. You're most fortunate to be able to share your fears with your children and have their support. Of course, that may be little consolation for you at the moment. But considering that your family has been successful in managing problems in the past, you're in a good position to find ways to solve this situation, too. When you called me, I guess you had an idea of how I might be part of that solution.

A traditional approach might have the CHN take charge of the situation based on the fact that the family has requested the nurse's help and that it is the nurse's responsibility to respond. In contrast, a reform approach, based on Primary Health Care principles, assumes that families have the necessary capacity and motivation to solve problems on their own. Therefore, the CHN confirms that Mrs. M. fears her husband is going to die unless he changes his behaviour. She then points out more of Mrs. M.'s strengths—family support and competencies (e.g., past success with problem solving and ability to seek out resources). In this way, the CHN maintains a facilitator role that creates opportunities for empowerment. The CHN affirms Mrs. M.'s ability to take control using informal supports, rather than formal support from the system. Thus, the CHN begins to work in partnership with Mrs. M. in a way that fits with the MacDonald family values.

Mrs. M. (starts to cry): Oh, what am I going to do? I love him so. We've been through too much together over the last 37 years. Too much to let this problem end it all. I just can't figure him out. It's as if he doesn't care.

CHN: It hurts, and it's disturbing to watch someone you know as a fighter seem to give up all of a sudden . . . makes you wonder whether there is another explanation for his behaviour.

A more traditional approach might take Mrs. M.'s repeated question ("what am I going to do?") as an indication of the client's inability to determine a solution. The CHN might take control by reassuring Mrs. M. that her husband really does care about his family. In contrast, the CHN who practises according to Primary Health Care principles comments on Mr. M.'s success in managing problems in the past. She also reinforces Mrs. M.'s competence by encouraging her to use her own problem-solving skills and reframe the situation by thinking of other explanations for her husband's behaviour.

Mrs. M.: I think of all the troubles we've been through together, like trying to do right by the kids when money was tight, or helping out my brother's family when he got laid off. Things haven't been easy for us but somehow we've always managed. John's always been there for everyone. . . . I guess, now that I think of it, this is the first time he's been the one needing help. He's probably wondering what would happen if he wasn't here. I guess he's scared too. I never thought about him as ever being scared.

CHN: You know him so well. . . . With so many people counting on him, he can't imagine not living up to his responsibilities. However, he may think that keeping his commitment to his family means ignoring his treatment and pretending he doesn't have diabetes. Given your knowledge of the disease, his actions terrify you. You think that he is going to collapse, perhaps even die!

A CHN using a traditional approach might have explained Mr. M.'s fear and, in doing so, would have usurped the opportunity for Mrs. M. to reason things through on her own. In contrast, a CHN who practises according to Primary Health Care principles uses her professional knowledge about the coping patterns of people who have been diagnosed with a chronic illness to guide Mrs. M. through a process of active personal discovery about her husband's behaviour. Moreover, she compliments Mrs. M. on her understanding of the situation ("You know him so well"). In this way, the nurse reinforces the client's capacity for developing insight in her own way, at her own pace, and from her own unique perspective.

At this point Mr. MacDonald comes home from work, sees the CHN, and immediately becomes suspicious: his wife has "brought in the troops" to ensure that he changes his behaviour! Mrs. MacDonald introduces the CHN and explains why she was called.

CHN: Mr. MacDonald, I can imagine you might be surprised, even angry, to come home and find me here today.

Mr. M.: You're right about that! Susan has become a real worry wart lately.

Mrs. M.: It's just that I got so afraid about you not paying enough attention to your diabetes. John, I didn't know what else to do; I don't want to lose you.

Mr. M.: You see, nurse. There she goes again. Susan, I'm not going anywhere. This stuff about my diet and those needles is exaggerated . . . I know I had a spell there a ways back, but you and I figured it out. You took great care of me. (To the nurse) She worries too much, but she means well. She nursed me right back to health. I'm fine now; I just needed a break.

CHN: So you're hoping that you're cured now because you're feeling so much better? I can understand that you might be confused, then, why the doctor wants you to keep up the diabetic routine.

A CHN using a traditional approach might explain that Mrs. M. is justified in worrying and might reinforce information about the realities of this chronic illness. In contrast, a CHN using a Primary Health Care approach maintains a family focus, listens to Mr. M.'s perspective of the situation, and carefully investigates the rationale underlying his actions. Furthermore, she is careful not to pass judgement.

Mr. M.: Dr. Stillman is a good man, but he's young . . . worries too much . . . just like Susan. He doesn't know anything about what a guy like me does all day. I've been working hard labour nearly 40 years and I'm not about to let anything get in my way now. I've got responsibilities, a pension to think about. And I never could stand anyone who used sick leave as a way out of an honest day's work.

CHN: So you're afraid that if you follow the diabetic routine you might have to take more time off or even stop working. In your mind, that would be a lazy man's way out . . . I can see that work and caring for your family are very important to you.

A CHN using a traditional approach might attempt to reassure Mr. M. that his doctor means well and that with proper care he can continue a normal life. In contrast, a CHN using a reformed approach works to gain a fuller understanding of the concerns from Mr. M.'s perspective and makes no attempt to judge his views about treatment and work. Instead, she acknowledges the strong values (hard work and caring for family) that drive Mr. M.'s actions. This approach establishes a critical foundation for future discussions around goal setting.

Mr. M.: I've been the provider since the beginning, and that's the way it's going to stay.

CHN: You are quite a remarkable man. Your concern for your family's welfare has been so important to you that you figured the only way to provide for them was by keeping up with your old work habits. You believed that following the diabetic routine would slow you down somehow—so ignoring parts of the treatment would make your life seem normal again and help you provide for your family just as you always have.

A CHN using a traditional approach might point out to Mr. M. the "flaws" in his thinking. She would try to convince him that his family loves and needs him, in an effort to motivate him to change his ways. This approach uses emotional blackmail and does little to promote meaningful understanding or lasting change. In contrast, a CHN practising according to Primary Health Care principles searches for the motivator of Mr. M.'s behaviour. She learns that, rather than shirking his duties, Mr. M. is willing to sacrifice his health to meet his responsibilities. This "reframing technique" is driven by the assumption that people have the desire to move toward health when it is framed in contextually relevant terms. A strengths perspective allows the client to build on existing family capacity and directs the discussion away from a problem orientation.

Mr. M.: Look, I told you I'm feeling fine. Besides, I'm no sissy; I've always been strong as a horse.

CHN: Because you're a hard worker and have always felt fine, it's difficult to imagine how your health could change if you keep living your life in the same way. I can imagine how angry you must have been when you were told that you had acquired a chronic disease through no fault of your own and, in order to keep feeling as strong as a horse, you would require treatment for the rest of your life.

A traditional approach might simply point out to Mr. M. that he will become seriously ill if he does not adhere to his diabetic regime. In contrast, a CHN using Primary Health Care principles uses the client's perspective of the situation and builds on existing strength. The nurse links Mr. M.'s long-standing belief in hard work and pride in his health with her knowledge about diabetes to help him understand the specific effects of the diagnosis on his life.

Mr. M.: You're right. I was mad as hell! I never did anything to deserve this. The guys at work, my family, everyone . . . they all see me as a real work horse. Everyone counts on me. I go to work no matter what.

CHN: You certainly have a heavy burden to carry. I can see why you've been hoping that if you ignored your diabetes, it might just go away. Given your long history of good health, it seemed reasonable to believe that you could keep going and nothing would happen . . . and you can, to a point. It's true, your type of diabetes cannot be cured and requires some permanent changes in lifestyle to keep you doing what you want. However, your history of good health can make a real difference in how strong you can be and in the control you can have over your illness.

A traditional CHN might reinforce the realities of the management strategies and long-term effects of diabetes in an effort to break through Mr. M.'s "denial." In contrast, in a Primary Health Care role, the CHN discusses diabetes from a positive perspective to promote a new way of viewing his situation that fits Mr. M's value of good health. In this way, the nurse avoids long lectures and, instead, provides information only when the client gives readiness cues. The CHN also acknowledges the heavy burden that Mr. M. carries and, in doing so, affirms Mrs. M.'s earlier insight about the motivation behind her husband's actions.

Mr. M.: My family was real shook up when they heard about my diabetes, so I tried to downplay the whole thing.

Mrs. M.: Oh John, I can see now that you tried so hard to protect us, and we only made things worse for you by badgering you about your health. . . . But when you started ignoring parts of your treatment, we got frightened and thought you didn't care any more.

Mr. M.: I didn't realize that you and the kids were also carrying a heavy load. But I guess, deep down, I knew that you were nagging because you cared. . . . (To the nurse)

Well, if what you say is true and this healthy feeling can only last with treatment, I have no choice but to pay closer attention to it if I want to keep working. Providing for my family means everything to me.

CHN: *Mrs. MacDonald, you called me because you were worried about your husband's health and asked for assistance. I wonder how you see the situation now?. . . Mr. MacDonald, I wonder how you see things?*

A traditional approach might rely on a nursing assessment to evaluate the nursing care plan. It is not uncommon for this procedure to lack client input. In contrast, a CHN using a Primary Health Care approach measures the success of the interaction according to strengthened capacity to achieve client-identified outcomes. For Mrs. M., success is measured in terms of physical health indicators. For Mr. M., success is measured in terms of his ability to provide for his family.

Mrs. M.: Things look a lot different. I'm not so panicky now that I understand what's really been going on. I think our family can get through this, just like we have in the past.

Mr. M.: I agree. Knowing that I can keep on working just as hard for my family, even though I have diabetes, is a big relief to me.

The foregoing example illustrates how the helping relationship proceeds in a reformed Primary Health Care system. The client and nurse engaged in unique roles and developed a collaborative relationship. The nurse refrained from doing "for" or "to" the client and, instead, "worked with" the MacDonalds. She facilitated client decision making. Mr. and Mrs. MacDonald developed a new understanding of their situation that fit their family values. This empathic approach to interaction is critical for the next stage of the helping relationship, problem solving.

Problem solving in a reformed Primary Health Care system

Clients can begin to find appropriate solutions only when they have determined their needs and goals. Unlike a more traditional approach in which the nurse might suggest solutions, the CHN in a Primary Health Care role supports the development of competencies and provides a *framework* to facilitate client problem solving. The nurse refrains from telling clients what to do. Instead, she works in partnership with clients, providing requested information and supporting them in using their skills, capacities, and resources to develop solutions that fit their values. Clients are encouraged to create their own unique ways of managing health-related problems using trusted resources. Therefore, informal resources (e.g., family, friends, support groups) are recognized as primary supports, and formal resources (i.e., professionals) are viewed as complementary supports (Dunst, Trivette, & Deal, 1994).

The CHN might use a problem-solving framework adapted from client-centred principles (e.g., Clunn & Payne, 1982; Egan 1994). Table 24.1 suggests basic questions (left column) that nurses may use as a framework to help clients reach a solution to a problem.

Under these conditions, the nurse uses client knowledge gained earlier in the interaction to facilitate, but not direct, client thinking in a systematic and purposeful way. For example, the nurse might ask Mr. M., "You told me that your biggest concern is being able to continue providing for your family. Tell me, what does that means to you?" This question ensures that both the nurse and client have the same understanding of the client's goal. From Mr. M.'s perspective, being able to support his family could mean that he maintains his job (a likely perception), or it could mean that another source of income is found to meet the family's needs (an unlikely perception). By clarifying the client's perception, the CHN is careful to work toward the client's goal, rather than her own.

The CHN might also ask Mr. M., "What would have to change in order for you to be able to continue working?" This question challenges the client to think realistically about the adjustments needed in his life to make his goal a reality. The nurse refrains from telling Mr. M. that he will have to follow his diabetic regime and from teaching him about specific protocols. She remembers that he is familiar with that information. Indeed, she recalls that Mr. M.'s behavioural change (cutting back on his diabetic routine) occurred after he understood the dynamics of his illness. Indeed, the shift away from treatment was a conscious decision that resulted from a perceived value conflict (dealing with his illness versus providing for family), not a learning problem.

The CHN who practises according to the principles of Primary Health Care proceeds through the problem-solving framework (Table 24.1) by working with client knowledge, enhancing client capacity/competencies, and encouraging informed client decision making. In the case of the MacDonald family, success does not hinge on Mr. MacDonald's knowledge about diabetes or on his compliance with treatment. While such behaviours might meet the nurse's expectations about health, they are not consistent with the client's views and, therefore, are not in keeping with the client-centred principle of Primary Health Care reform. Instead, the test of success is contingent on whether the family can find solutions that enable Mr. MacDonald to continue working and providing for his family's financial needs.

Fit of reform in crisis situations

If the CHN accepts the philosophical underpinnings of reform based on Primary Health Care principles, then these values must guide her practice regardless of the situation. Nurses should assume that clients want and are

Table 24.1
A framework of questions to assist in problem solving

Question	Explanation
If things were different, how would you like them to be? What would that change (or your goal) look like?	The *client-identified goal* becomes the standard against which the success of a solution can be measured. If the client is a couple, family, or group, the CHN asks them to find a common and manageable goal.
What would you have to change in order to achieve this goal?	This question determines the client's priority, which may not be the same as the nurse's. The nurse can help clients to examine their ideas more fully to ensure that the ramifications of their decisions are understood. However, the CHN refrains from casting judgement. The CHN is challenged to provide information to promote *client insight* rather than compliance.
Can you think of some ways that you could achieve these changes?	This identifies the necessary *work for goal attainment*. It is a good idea to have the client identify several possible solutions. In this way, clients can choose from among alternatives and have a back-up solution should one fail.
Tell me about some of the advantages and disadvantages of each of these alternatives. (Ask in a questioning tone.)	This encourages the client to identify the *implications* and potential consequences of each choice. Clients can be asked to think of long-term implications as well as short-term implications to ensure that the selected alternative will bring few undesirable surprises.

(continued)

Table 24.1 (*continued*)

Question	Explanation
Which alternative seems best for *you*?	This question promotes a sense of *client self-determination*. Clients are asked to make a free choice (rather than a forced choice out of fear or guilt) that is consistent with their values (rather than those of an external source, e.g., the nurse).
Is this alternative something you *could* do?	This establishes *client capacities* and potential learning needs.
Is this something you *would* do?	This establishes *client motivation* and helps clients to think realistically.
Are there other people who could help you? Do you need assistance from other sources?	This promotes *partnerships* within the client's natural network and the formal health system. It provides opportunity for discussing skills needed to access resources.
Can you think about how you might carry our your chosen solut on?	This provides the opportunity to talk through, or role play, the logistics of the client's plan. It promotes a sense of reality and identifies potential problems. It also creates an opportunity for the CHN to support and encourage client capacities and competence.

capable of achieving health, even in crisis situations. The CHN acts as the facilitator.

This shift in thinking does not fit with the more traditional perspectives on crises that continue even today (e.g., Aguilera, 1998). The traditional approach views crisis as a transitional period (either maturational or situational) in which resolution cannot be achieved through usual problem-solving methods (Caplan, 1964, 1989). It has a sudden onset, takes the client by surprise, and taxes familiar resources to their capacity. According to this perspective, individuals are rendered incapable of recognizing their feelings or dealing with the problems. Therefore, people in crisis need protection and guidance (Aguilera, 1998). Using this traditional approach, the CHN would define the problem, suggest possible solutions, and give specific directives to clients until the nurse determined that clients were capable of managing on their own.

The theoretical notions contained in crisis theory are derived mainly from psychoanalytic theory and based on research focussed on major life stressors (Caplan, 1964; Erickson, 1963; Lindemann, 1944). This paternalistic medical model, which emphasizes deficits and problem alleviation, remains unaltered in nursing (e.g., Aguilera, 1998; Varcarolis, 1990; Woolley, 1990). In contrast, others have argued that people in crisis do not lose their capacity to help themselves (Hoff, 1995), to make decisions on their own (Hoff, 1995), or to work in partnership with professionals (Hoff, 1995; Phelan, 1979). These critics believe that clients in crisis can make appropriate decisions when given sufficient information and support (Chandler, 1993; Hoff, 1995). They reason that clients in crisis appear incapacitated because the environment lacks supports (Dunst, Trivette, & Deal, 1994). Rather than providing directives, interventions focus on creating more helpful surrounding conditions.

To gain a more complete understanding of how a reformed helping relationship might proceed in a crisis, let us consider a situation in which the CHN is faced with reporting a mother to child protection services for child maltreatment. Using a traditional approach, the nurse might simply tell the family, after the fact, that it was necessary to report the mother's behaviour. Under these conditions, the CHN assumes that the mother lacks the capacity to do anything positive, given her harmful parenting actions.

In contrast, a CHN using a Primary Health Care approach would discuss her observations with the mother and invite her to share her perspective on the situation. The nurse would then explain why a report was necessary and ask the mother how she wanted to participate in the process. For example, the CHN might say:

CHN: We've both noticed that your parenting behaviour is not helping your child grow in a happy and healthy way. Indeed, your parenting practices are causing your child harm. I can appreciate that you want the best for your child and that it took great courage for you to be honest about your parenting. It was very painful and may well have been the toughest thing you ever did. I think you know I have to discuss this situation with the child protection agency. I wonder if you want to participate in that discussion in some way. For instance, you might want to make the first contact with the agency to explain the situation in your own words. If you choose this action, I would be interested in knowing how I can assist you in making the call.

This approach emphasizes the positive features of the mother's actions, and creates an opportunity for her to take some control of an extremely stressful situation in her own way. The nurse establishes her legal responsibilities in a straightforward manner, but expresses her belief that the mother did not intend harm. The nurse also demonstrates her belief in the mother's ability to take appropriate action. The mother retains a measure of control, is presumed to have the capacity to make decisions, and works in a complementary partnership with the nurse in which both have rights and responsibilities (Hoff, 1995).

Consider another crisis situation:

The CHN makes a routine home visit to the Bonner family, who are caring for Mr. Campbell, the wife's elderly father, who has Alzheimer's disease. Although the family made a deliberate decision to care for the grandfather, they underestimated the caregiving expectations superimposed on the demands of a growing family with three preschool children. The nurse finds the grandfather tied in a chair in the family room. He is yelling obscenities at his daughter. Whenever she replies that she will tend to him soon, he repeats his demands to be freed. Mrs. Bonner is struggling to bathe two crying children, while her husband is feeding the third child. The atmosphere is strained, and the parents are visibly exhausted.

Using a traditional approach, the CHN might explain that it is harmful to restrain Mr. Campbell and suggest that the family consider applying for respite care or placing him in a nursing home. However, this approach would only confirm the family's feelings of inadequacy and irresponsibility. In contrast, using a Primary Health Care approach, the CHN would compliment the Bonners' intentions to meet their children's needs and keep their father safe. She might comment, "It's exhausting when everyone needs you at the same time. I can see that you are really trying to tend to everyone." The nurse might also reinforce client control by asking the Bonners, "As it's impossible to be everywhere at once, how can I help right now?" In this way, she encourages the family to use their capacity to make decisions about priorities.

When the immediate chaos subsided, the CHN would comment on Mr. Campbell's restraint to the Bonners: "You want your father to feel that he is still part of the family, yet figuring out ways to keep him safe when you're busy is not easy." In this way, the CHN acknowledges the family goals along with the challenge of making these goals a reality. The nurse would include the grandfather in the discussion, even if he did not appear to comprehend, to ensure that all perspectives are invited and valued. The nurse might then say, "I can see that you, Mr. and Mrs. Bonner, worry about your dad's safety when you are busy and can't be with him. At the same time, the restraint makes you, Mr. Campbell, panicky." Using this approach, the nurse assumes that the family does not intend harm and incorporates both the family's experiential knowledge (i.e., what it is like trying to care for small children and a frail, elderly person who wanders) and her own clinical knowledge (i.e., family development, cognitive disease processes) to gain a full understanding of the situation. The nurse focusses on the two issues (safety and fear) that keep the family from meeting their identified goal: ensuring that the grandfather feels part of the family. Thus, the CHN reframes the discussion on the assumption that the family has the capacity to find appropriate solutions that fit with their values.

Conclusion

Principles of Primary Health Care reform challenge nurses to work with clients in different ways. Community health nurses must work as partners on client-identified needs and in ways that build on client strengths and capacities to achieve client-determined health outcomes.

QUESTIONS

1. What do you consider to be the strengths and limitations of the Primary Health Care approach to the helping relationship?
2. Think about a nurse–client relationship in which you have attempted to use principles of Primary Health Care. Did you work as partners? What kind of partnership evolved? Was the client a full participant? Who identified the need? Who made decisions? What client capacity did you attempt to strengthen? What was the easiest and what was the most difficult principle to apply?
3. Compare the Primary Health Care interaction identified in question 2 with a situation in which you played a more traditional nursing role. What were the differences between the interactions? Compare the outcomes for both the client and yourself. What were your personal thoughts and reactions to each role?
4. Invite a client to discuss your working relationship.
   a. How does the client feel about the Primary Health Care approach? How has it affected his or her ability to resolve health needs?

b.   How might this approach affect the client's relationship with other nurses or with the health system in the future?

REFERENCES

Aguilera, D.C. (1998). *Crisis intervention: Theory and methodology* (8th ed.). St. Louis: Mosby.

Angus, D. (1991). *Review of significant health care commissions and forces in Canada since 1983–1984*. Ottawa: Canadian Medical Association/Canadian Nurses Association/Canadian Hospital Association.

Arnold, E., & Boggs, K. (1989). *Interpersonal relationships: Professional communication skills for nurses*. Philadelphia: W.B. Saunders.

Bertrand, J.E. (1996). *Summary of enriching experiences of children*. Paper commissioned by the National Forum on Health, Ottawa.

Bosma, H., Marmot, M.G., Hemingway, H., Nicholson, A.C., Brunner, E., & Stansfeld, S.A. (1997). Low job control and risk of coronary heart disease in Whitehall II (prospective control) study. *British Medical Journal, 314*(7080), 558–565.

Brammer, L.M., & MacDonald, G. (1996). *The helping relationship: Processes and skills* (6th ed.). Boston: Allyn & Bacon.

Brunt, J.H. (1985). An exploration of the relationship between nurses' empathy and technology. *Nursing Administration Quarterly, 9*, 69–78.

Caplan, G. (1964). A conceptual model for primary prevention. In G. Caplan, *Principles of preventive psychiatry* (pp. 26–55). New York: Basic Books.

Caplan, G. (1989). Recent developments in crisis intervention and the promotion of support service. *Journal of Primary Prevention, 10*(1), 3–25.

Carmack, B.J. (1997). Balancing engagement and detachment. *Image: Journal of Nursing Scholarship, 29*(2), 139–144.

Carroll, D., Davey Smith, G., Sheffield, D., Shipley, M.J., Marmot, M.G. (1997). The relationship between socioeconomic status, hostility, and blood pressure reactions to mental stress in men: Data from the Whitehall II study. *Health Psychology, 16*(2), 131–136.

Carver, E.J., & Hughes, J.R. (1990). The significance of empathy. In R.C. MacKay, J.R. Hughes, & E.J. Carver (Eds.), *Empathy in the helping relationship* (pp. 13–27). New York: Springer.

Chalmers, K.I., & Bramadat, I.J. (1996). Community development: Theoretical and practical issues for community health. *Journal of Advanced Nursing, 24*(4), 719–726.

Chandler, S.C. (1993). Crisis theory and intervention. In B.S. Johnson (Ed.), *Adaptation and growth: Psychiatric–mental health nursing* (3rd ed.) (pp. 661–674). Philadelphia: J.B. Lippincott.

Clunn, P.A., & Payne, D.B. (1982). *Psychiatric–mental health nursing* (3rd ed.). New Hyde Park, NY: Medical Examination Publishing.

Coffey, K., & Swirsky, J. (1988). Comparison of empathy levels between hospital and visiting homes. *Caring, 7*, 10–12.

Cowger, C.D. (1994). Assessing client strengths: Clinical assessment for client empowerment. *Social Work, 39*(3), 262–268.

Cravener, P. (1992). Establishing therapeutic alliance across cultural barriers. *Journal of Psychosocial Nursing, 30*(12), 10–14.

Deber, R. (1997, June). Transferring research information to patients. In National Forum on Health, *Summary report: Changing the health care system—a consumer perspective*. Ottawa: Minister of Public Works & Government Services.

Deci, E.L., & Ryan, R.M. (1991). A motivation approach to the self: Integration in personality. In R. Dienstbier (Ed.), *Nebraska symposium on motivation 1990: Perspectives on motivation* (pp. 238–288). Lincoln, NB: University of Nebraska Press.

Doherty, G. (1997). *Zero to six: The basis for school readiness*. Ottawa: Applied Research Branch, Strategic Policy, Human Resources Development Canada. (Cat. No. R-97-8E)

Donovan, J.L., & Blake, D.R. (1992). Patient non-compliance: Deviance or reasoned decision-making? *Social Science & Medicine, 34*, 507–513.

Dunst, C.J., & Trivette, C.M. (1996). Empowerment, effective helpgiving practices and family-centered care. *Pediatric Nursing, 22*(4), 334–337, 343.

Dunst, C.J., Trivette, C.M., & Deal, A. (1988). *Enabling and empowering families: Principles and practices*. Cambridge, MA: Brookline Books.

Dunst, C.J., Trivette, C.M., & Deal, A. (1994). *Supporting and strengthening families* (Vol. 1). Cambridge, MA: Brookline Books.

Egan, G. (1994). *The skilled helper: A problem solving approach to helping* (5th ed.). Pacific Grove, CA: Brooks/Cole.

Erickson, E.H. (1963). *Childhood and society* (2nd ed.). New York: W.W. Norton.

Fawcett, S.B., Paine, A.A., Francisco, V.T., Schultz, J.A., Richter, K.P., Lewis, R.K., Williams, E.L., Harris, K.J., Berkley, J.Y., Fisher, J.L., et al. (1995). Using empowerment theory in collaborative partnerships for community health and development. *American Journal of Community Psychology, 23*(5), 677–697.

Fisher, J.D., Goff, B.A., Nadler, A., & Chinsky, J.M. (1988). Social psychological influences on help seeking and support from peers. In B.H. Gottlieb (Ed.), *Marshalling social support* (pp. 267–304). Newbury Park, CA: Sage.

Gazda, G.M., Childers, W.C., & Brooks, D.K. (1987). *Foundations of counselling and human science*. New York: McGraw-Hill.

Gazda, G., & Evans, T. (1990). Empathy as a skill. In R.C. MacKay, J.R. Hughes, & E.J. Carver (Eds.), *Empathy in the helping relationship* (pp. 65–77). New York: Springer.

Glenister, D. (1994). Patient participation in psychiatric services: A literature review and proposal for a research strategy. *Journal of Advanced Nursing, 19*(4), 802–811.

Gottlieb, L., & Rowat, K. (1987). McGill Model of Nursing: A practice-derived model. *Advances in Nursing Science, 9*, 51–61.

Gyulay, R., Mound, B., & Flanagan, E. (1994). Mental health consumers as public educators: A qualitative study. *Canadian Journal of Nursing Research, 26*, 29–42.

Health & Welfare Canada. (1987). *The active report: Perspectives on Canada's health promotion survey 1985*. Ottawa: Author.

Health & Welfare Canada. (1988). *Coordinating healthy public policy: An analytic literature review and bibliography* (Health Services & Promotion Branch Working Paper prepared by A. Pederson, R. Edwards, M. Kelner, V. Marshall, & K. Allison, Department of Behavioural Science, University of Toronto). Ottawa: Author.

Heszen-Klemens, I. (1987). Patients' noncompliance and how doctors manage this. *Social Science & Medicine, 24*(5), 409–416.

Hemingway, H., Nicholson, A., Stafford, M., Roberts, R., & Marmot, M. (1997). The impact of socioeconomic status on health functioning as assessed by the SF-36 questionnaire: The Whitehall II study. *American Journal of Public Health, 87*(9), 1484–1490.

Hoff, L.A. (1995). Helping people in crisis. In L.A. Hoff, *People in crisis: Understanding and helping* (4th ed.) (pp. 112–141). Menlo Park, CA: Addison-Wesley.

Holden, R.J. (1990). Empathy: The art of emotional knowing in holistic care. *Holistic Nursing Practice, 5,* 70–79.

Hughes, J.R., & Carver, E.J. (1990). The effects of empathy on the dynamics of professional–patient interaction. In R.C. MacKay, J.R. Hughes, & E.J. Carver (Eds.), *Empathy in the helping relationship* (pp. 133–149). New York: Springer.

Jenny, J., & Logan, J. (1992). Knowing the patient: One aspect of clinical knowledge. *Image: Journal of Nursing Scholarship, 24*(4), 254–258.

King, I.M. (1981). *A theory for nursing: Systems, concepts, process.* New York: Wiley.

Lancee, W.J., Gallop, R., McCay, E., & Toner, B. (1995). The relationship between nurses' limit-setting styles and anger in psychiatric inpatients. *Psychiatric Services, 46*(6), 609–603.

Lindemann, E. (1944). Symptomology and management of acute grief. *American Journal of Psychiatry, 101,* 141–148.

MacKay, R., Carver, E.J., & Hughes, J.R. (1990). The professionals' use of empathy and client care outcomes. In R.C. MacKay, J.R. Hughes, & E.J. Carver (Eds.), *Empathy in the helping relationship* (pp. 120–131). New York: Springer.

MacKay, R.C., Hughes, J.R., & Carver, E.J. (Eds.). (1990). *Empathy in the helping relationship.* New York: Springer.

Marmor, T.R., Barer, M.L., & Evans, R.G. (1994). The determinants of population's health: What can be done to improve a democratic nation's health status? In R.G. Evans, M.L. Barer, & T.R. Marmor (Eds.), *Why are some people healthy and others are not? The determinants of health of populations* (pp. 217–230). New York: Aldine De Gruyter.

Marmot, M.G., Bosma, H., Hemingway, H., Brunner, E., & Stansfeld, S. (1997a). Contribution of job control and other risk factors to social variations in coronary heart disease incidence. *Lancet, 350*(9073), 235–239.

Marmot, M.G., Bosma, H., Hemingway, H., Brunner, E., & Stansfeld, S. (1997b). Contribution of job control and other factors to social variations in coronary heart disease incidence. *Lancet, 350*(9073), 253–259.

McWilliam, C.L., Stewart, M.J., Brown, J.B., McNair, S., Desai, K., Patterson, M.L., Del Maestro, R.L., & Pittman, B.J. (1997). Creating empowering meaning: An interactive process of promoting health with chronically ill older Canadians. *Health Promotion International, 12*(2), 111–123.

Meleis, A.I. (1991). Nursing theory: An elusive mirage or a mirror of reality. In A.I. Meleis (Ed.), *Theoretical nursing: Development and progress* (2nd ed.) (pp. 247–268). New York: J.B. Lippincott.

National Forum on Health. (1997). *Canada health action: Building on the legacy synthesis reports and issues reports.* Ottawa: Minister of Public Works & Government Services.

Olson, J.K. (1995). Relationships between nurse-expressed empathy, patient-perceived empathy and patient distress. *Image: Journal of Nursing Scholarship, 27*(4), 317–322.

Olson, J., & Hanchett, E. (1997). Nurse-expressed empathy, patient outcomes, and development of a middle-range theory. *Image: Journal of Nursing Scholarship, 29*(1), 71–76.

Orlando, I. (1961). *The dynamic nurse–patient relationship: Function, process and principle.* New York: G.P. Putnam's Sons.

Osterman, P., & Schwartz-Barcott, D. (1996). Presence: Four ways of being there. *Nursing Forum, 31*(2), 23–30.

PEI Health & Community Services Agency. (1996). *Circle of health: Prince Edward Island's health promotion framework.* Charlottetown: Author.

Peplau, H.E. (1992). Interpersonal relations: A theoretical framework for application in nursing practice. *Nursing Science Quarterly, 5,* 13–18.

Phelan, L.A. (1979). Crisis intervention: Partnership in problem-solving. *Journal of Psychiatric Nursing & Mental Health Services, 17,* 22–27.

Pike, A.W. (1990). On the nature and place of empathy in clinical nursing practice. *Journal of Professional Nursing, 6,* 236–240.

Pray, J.E. (1992). Maximizing the patient's uniqueness and strengths: A challenge for home health care. *Social Work in Health Care, 17*(3), 71–79.

Rachlis, M., & Kushner, C. (1989). *Strong medicine: How to save Canada's health care system.* Toronto: HarperCollins.

Ramos, M.C. (1992). The nurse–patient relationship: Theme and variations. *Journal of Advanced Nursing, 17*(4), 496–506.

Reid-Pointe, P. (1992). Distress in cancer patients and primary nurses' empathy skills. *Cancer Nursing, 15*(4), 283–292.

Rogers, C.R. (1975). Empathic: An unappreciated way of being. *Counselling Psychologist, 5,* 2–9.

Rogers, I.A. (1986). The effects of undergraduate nursing education on empathy. *Western Journal of Nursing Research, 8,* 329–342.

Rogers, S. (1996). Facilitative affiliation: Nurse–client interactions that enhance healing. *Issues in Mental Health Nursing, 17*(3), 171–184.

Saleebey, D. (1996). The strengths perspective in social work practice: Extensions and cautions. *Social Work, 41*(3), 296–305.

Shoultz, J., Hatcher, P.A., & Hurrell, M. (1992). Growing edges of a new paradigm: The future of nursing in the health of a nation. *Nursing Outlook, 40,* 57–61.

Smith, S. (1992). *Communications in nursing* (2nd ed.). St. Louis: Mosby Year Book.

Stansfeld, S.A., Head, J., & Marmot, M.G. (1998). Explaining social class differences in depression and well-being. *Social Psychiatry & Psychiatric Epidemiology, 33*(1), 1–9.

Stewart, M.J. (1989). Nurses' preparedness for health promotion through linkage with mutual aid self-help groups. *Canadian Journal of Public Health, 80*(20), 110–114.

Sully, P. (1996). The impact of power in therapeutic relationships. *Nursing Times, 92*(41), 40–41.

Sullivan, M.J.L., & Scattolon, Y. (1995). Health policy planning: A look at consumer involvement in Nova Scotia. *Canadian Journal of Public Health, 86,* 317–320.

Sutherland, J.A. (1995). Historical concept analysis of empathy. *Issues in Mental Health Nursing, 16*(6), 555–566.

Thorne, S.E. (1990). Constructive non-compliance in chronic illness. *Holistic Nursing Practice, 5,* 62–69.

Trainor, J., Pomeroy, E., & Pape, B. (1993). *A new framework for support: For people with serious mental health problems.* Toronto: Canadian Mental Health Association.

Trilling, J.S., & Jaber, R. (1993). Formulation of the physician/patient impasse. *Family Systems Medicine, 11*(3), 281–286.

Trivette, C.M., Dunst, C.J., & Hamby, D. (1996). Characteristics and consequences of help-giving practices in contrasting human services programs. *American Journal of Community Psychiatry, 24*(2), 272–293.

Varcarolis, E.M. (1990). *Foundations of psychiatric mental health nursing.* W.B. Saunders.

Waterworth, S., & Luker, K. (1990). Reluctant collaborators: Do patients want to be involved in decisions concerning care? *Journal of Advanced Nursing, 15,* 971–976.

Wheeler, K. (1990). Perception of empathy inventory. In O. Strickland & C. Waltz (Eds.), *Measurement of nursing outcomes: Measuring client self-care and coping skills as nursing outcomes* (Vol. 4) (pp. 81–198). New York: Springer.

Wheeler, K., & Barrett, E.A.M. (1994). Review and synthesis of selected nursing studies on teaching empathy and implications for nursing research and education. *Nursing Outlook, 42,* 230–236.

Wiedenbach, E. (1964). *Clinical nursing: A helping art.* New York: Springer-Verlag.

Williams, S.A. (1997). Caring in patient-focused care: The relationship of patients' perceptions of holistic nurse caring to their levels of anxiety. *Holistic Nursing Practice, 11*(3), 61–68.

Woolley, N. (1990). Crisis theory: A paradigm of effective intervention with families of critically ill people. *Journal of Advanced Nursing, 15,* 1402–1408.

Part 5
Community Health Nursing Research

The development of the knowledge base that guides community health nursing practice is derived in part from theoretical foundations (see Part 2) and in part from research. Therefore, in this section, one chapter (Chapter 25) peruses the links between practice and research, one chapter (26) scrutinizes the status and contributions of community health nursing research in Canada, and three chapters (27, 28, and 29) portray pertinent methodologies and approaches.

In Chapter 25, Clarke clearly elucidates the research–practice gap and the importance of research–practice links. She examines the need for research-based practice and interprets pertinent issues such as infrastructure and change.

For Chapter 26, Chalmers and Gregory conducted a comprehensive review of the literature to identify published research. They analyze funding sources and barriers; describe types of studies, methodologies, and theoretical frameworks; and examine practical barriers to research. This chapter offers an excellent overview of current contributions of community health nursing research and researchers. It reveals research focussed on health promotion, illness prevention, families, aggregates, needs assessment, and evaluation; however, it also uncovers the neglect of cost analysis, theory testing, health determinants, and communities.

Gottlieb and Feeley (Chapter 27) also focus on change and on practice-relevant research—specifically, intervention studies; these authors deliberate on complex methodological challenges and offer astute guidelines for the design of intervention projects and for evaluation of outcomes of interventions. In Chapter 28, Dickson reflects on the suitability of participatory designs for community health nursing research and its appropriateness in terms of Primary Health Care principles—in particular, public participation and reduction of inequities. Finally, Brunt (Chapter 29) delineates the salience of epidemiology to community health nursing research. This methodology is appropriate for the study of health promotion (another Primary

Health Care principle), population health, and determinants of health of individuals, families, groups, and communities. The authors of these three coherent and comprehensive methodological chapters illustrate their points with superb examples from their own research.

Clearly, community health nursing research will need to bridge the gaps identified in Chapter 25. As well, investigators will need to inform and expand research-based practice and apply appropriate methodologies in their Primary Health Care research.

C H A P T E R   2 5

Research-based practice in community health nursing

Heather F. Clarke

This chapter discusses important issues related to the promotion and implementation of research-based practice in community health nursing. Health care systems issues—cost–benefit and infrastructures—are discussed. Issues related to the professional practice of community health nurses—partnerships and innovation adoption behaviour—are explored and utilization frameworks are presented. Research-based community health nursing practice, grounded in the principles of Primary Health Care, is also explored. To stimulate readers' critical examination of community health nursing practice and work environments and to facilitate fruitful discussion with colleagues, questions related to these issues are posed.

LEARNING OBJECTIVES

In this chapter, you will learn:

- what factors influence promotion and implementation of research as a basis for community health nursing practice
- the benefits of basing community health nursing practice on research
- why research utilization is relevant to community health nursing in a Primary Health Care context

Introduction

With the evolving reform of the health care system in Canada, delivery of public or community health services is changing. The role of the community health nurse (CHN) is also evolving, albeit more slowly (Mills, 1994). Restricted and reallocated health care funds, refined or reformed program delivery systems, and decentralized and regionalized decision making require CHNs to be more accountable for their practice. CHNs need to evaluate what they do, determine the difference it makes, and modify their practice accordingly. A less frequently articulated requirement of these changes is that practice, programs, and policy must be based more on research-generated knowledge.

Not only are CHNs being called upon by health care reform to reorient their practice consistent with Primary Health Care principles; they also are required to participate in program and policy development and evaluation and to articulate their practice and its effectiveness within a multidisciplinary context (Hayward, Ciliska, Mitchell, et al., 1993a, 1993b). Although CHNs predict that these roles will change further in the future, they also note that nurses are inadequately prepared to meet many challenges (Chambers et al., 1994; Clarke, Beddome, & Whyte, 1993). CHNs write comparatively little about their practice (Mills, 1994) and conduct a meagre amount of research (Hayward, Ciliska, Mitchell, et al, 1993a, 1993b). A recent review of effectiveness research in nursing revealed that therapeutic and rehabilitation nursing were most often studied, especially in practice involving adult hospitalized patients. Children and elderly people were seldom studied, and economic evaluation was lacking. No reference was made to community contexts (Pirjo & Perala, 1998). In addition, few, if any, data captured and stored in health information data bases reflect the contributions of nursing care. Health care and nursing systems cannot continue with untested, unsubstantiated, traditional practices. Clearly, there is a need to move to and to evaluate research-based practice. Where evidence is weak or non-existent, research must be undertaken, and interventions, programs, and policies must be evaluated. CHNs need to participate in the development of health information systems to provide data for evidence-based decision making in clinical practice, administration, education, and research.

Promoting and implementing research-based practice is not a simple task, nor is it solely reliant upon CHNs in the field. Forces affecting the advancement of research-based practice operate within both the health system and community health nursing. Within the public health system, there are costs and requirements for supportive infrastructures. Within the profession, perceived barriers hinder development of collaborative partnerships within and among agencies and limit integration of innovations in clinical practice.

This chapter discusses issues related to the promotion of research-based community health nursing practice through the utilization of research. Research utilization is "use of research as a means of verifying or as a basis for changing nursing practice . . . [and] the purpose of such . . . is to substantiate or improve the quality of nursing practice" (Horsley, 1985, p. 135). Research utilization is a planned, logical process of implementing research findings in practice. Although not addressed in this chapter, research-based administration should also be valued and implemented. This chapter does consider issues of costs–benefits and infrastructures in the health care system, and suggestions are given for strategy development. Issues specifically related to the professional practice of CHNs are also explored, and utilization frameworks are presented as a strategy to promote research-based practice grounded in the principles of Primary Health Care.

Assumptions

The following assumptions are identified because they affect thinking about research-based practice in community health nursing:

- Standards for nursing practice require nurses to participate in the research process, basing their practice on knowledge derived from research and other relevant evidence.
- There are codes of ethics for practice and research that nurses must reflect in their practice.
- The research process is iterative (i.e., we ask questions, conduct research, apply research, disseminate findings, and ask further questions).
- Community health nurses practise in multidisciplinary contexts that require collaboration and empowerment in the research process.
- Shared community health information systems and data bases require CHNs to articulate the uniqueness of their practice and also to contribute to the broader context.
- Health care reform includes moves to regionalization and amalgamation; development of new ministries and program structures; and involvement of different team members.

Public health system issues

The predominant themes in contemporary health systems include cost containment, cost effectiveness, and quality improvement, with emphasis on the use of evaluation methods to measure outcomes of practice and document the effectiveness of care. More than ever, there is need for nursing to use in practice the findings and methods of research in order to show that interventions improve client outcomes and are cost effective. Research utilization is a professional responsibility and is increasingly included in practice standards set for the profession (Crane, 1995; RNABC, 1998).

Costs and benefits

It has been difficult to sway decision makers about investing in nurses and nursing research because of the overriding emphasis on worth or "pay-off" inherent in cost–benefit analysis rather than in cost-effectiveness analysis.

Focussing solely on monetary aspects neglects the essential human and social costs and benefits.

Cost–benefit analysis weighs the inherent worth or consequences of a program or intervention expressed in numerical terms, almost always dollars (Fordyce, Mooney, & Russell, 1982). The focus is on the "whether" of decision making: whether costs are justified by benefits. Cost-effectiveness analysis focusses on the "how" of decision making. It weighs the relative merit of one program against another, based on clearly identified objectives and outcomes. Monetary and non-monetary outcomes, such as preventing death, reducing disability, and improving client activity levels, are considered (Fordyce et al., 1982).

In promoting research-based community health nursing practice, it is imperative that the cost effectiveness of a program be considered, rather than merely its costs–benefits. Recent attention to outcomes research, in both nursing and health care in general, supports a cost-effectiveness perspective. This perspective includes measures of effectiveness (degree to which an action can accomplish a purpose or help to bring about an expected outcome) and of efficiency (ability to accomplish a task with a minimum expenditure of time and effort).

In the past, community health nursing has experienced limitations in determining its cost effectiveness. Not only is there a paucity of research evaluating effectiveness of nursing interventions (Hayward, Ciliska, Mitchell, et al., 1993a), there is also confusion over the terms "nursing outcome" and "nursing-sensitive outcome" (Shamian, 1993). Any single discipline's approach is too narrow and limited to address the wide variety of structures and interventions that influence outcomes (Marek & Lang, 1993; Shamian, 1993). Given the complex context of community health nursing, it is essential that CHNs actively participate in multidisciplinary efforts to determine which outcomes are salient to clients (individuals and aggregates) and which outcomes are particularly sensitive to community health nursing interventions.

However, before CHNs can participate as equal partners in this effort, it is necessary to name and categorize health status, intervention, and outcome variables from a nursing perspective. Following publication of the papers of the Nursing Minimum Data Set Conference (CNA, 1993), a national working group, supported by the Canadian Nurses Association, is developing consensus on essential nursing care data elements to be included in health information systems and defining those elements for consistent application. In addition, through the Partnership Program of the Canadian Institute for Health Information, CNA is participating in working groups to ensure attention to nursing's requirements and health promotion and population health concepts. Meanwhile, community-based information systems are being developed at provincial, territorial, regional, and local levels, with or without nursing input.

Despite these limitations, nursing research has demonstrated the effectiveness of nursing care in terms of improved client care and client satisfaction. It has also demonstrated that high-quality, research-based care can be delivered at reduced cost to an agency, even though an explicit cost–benefit analysis was not done. Three major categories of effectiveness outcome indicators have been used in nursing research (Marek & Lang, 1993; Shamian, 1993):

- client-related indicators—physiological, psychosocial, and functional measures (e.g., behaviour, knowledge, symptom control, quality of life)
- environment-related indicators—resolution of nursing diagnoses or problems, family and caregiver strain, home functioning, goal attainment
- organization-related indicators—utilization of service, safety.

Examples of cost-effectiveness research
A landmark study by Brooten and her colleagues (1986) demonstrated that, with care provided by a nurse specialist, very low birth-weight infants could be discharged safely an average of 11 days earlier, at a cost savings to the health care system of $18 560 (U.S.) for each infant. Although studies of this magnitude are rare in community health nursing, success stories include mothers recovering from postpartum physical and emotional illness; women leaving abusive relationships, finding safe housing, or no longer using chemicals; and youth using birth control, finishing school, and being employed (Zerwekh, 1991). Clarke and colleagues (Clarke, Joseph, et al., 1998; Hislop et al., 1996) have developed culture-specific interventions to promote early and regular Pap smear testing to reduce the discrepancy of cervical cancer mortality rates between First Nations women and other women. If these successes were translated into cost-effectiveness frameworks, think of the potential for decision making in policy and program development—even though it is difficult to attribute health outcomes unequivocally to a community health nursing intervention.

Costs of research-based community health nursing practice
There are both hidden and visible costs associated with research-based nursing practice. Agency resources must be allocated to the research process. Visible costs may include a position for a nurse with research expertise, library services, computers and relevant software, computer time and assistance, and consultation fees. Hidden costs are associated with time and resources needed to review, summarize, and synthesize the literature; develop and implement a research utilization framework; develop or revise practice or program protocols; and monitor and evaluate change. Such activities may require nurses with research and clinical expertise, staff nurses, and secretarial support staff. As well, there are hidden costs of professional

development and impact of change on other disciplines and departments (RNABC, 1991). An evaluation of the Research Consultation Services of the Registered Nurses Association of British Columbia (1990) indicated that nurses were unable to carry out their research-related activities within their working day, but did so in off-hours. Thus, the total costs of research-based nursing practice may be invisible to nurse administrators and not included in agency budgets.

As agency support of research-based nursing practice improves nurses' work satisfaction (Kenneth & Stiesmeyer, 1991), such support can be viewed as an investment. In a research-friendly environment, staff begin to question their practice and systematically document problems. This fosters a sense of accountability and professionalism, which leads to increased job satisfaction and lower staff turnover (Smeltzer & Hinshaw, 1988).

Fagin's (1982) review of the economic value of nursing research demonstrated the cost effectiveness of primary nursing, innovative staffing plans, research-based patient teaching plans, and nurse-delivered primary care to both home care clients and public school client populations. Fagin concluded that nursing research and its utilization are severely underfunded and that investment leads to "a terrific economic payoff" (p. 1849). Nearly two decades later, the same conclusions are apparent in the current emphasis on quality improvement programs and outcome-focussed accreditation standards (CCHFA, 1993). Crane (1995) states: "[t]he ultimate goal is not the use of research, it is to deliver high quality, cost-effective care and to achieve desirable patient outcomes; and to deliver care from a professional practice model" (p. 575).

Research-based nursing practice ensures that quality and cost effectiveness of nursing care will be the best that they can be. However, evaluation of community health nursing interventions presents unique problems for research methodology. In particular, the health outcomes that CHNs consider to be valid indicators of effectiveness are often measured clinically by small changes over long periods of time. In addition, the contexts of multidisciplinary practice and client participation in care complicate the ability to determine clear cause–effect relationships attributable to CHN practice. Kitson (1998) suggests that successful utilization is a function of the relationship between the nature of the evidence, the context in which the proposed change is to be implemented, and the mechanisms by which the change is facilitated. Thus, instead of a hierarchy of cause and effect, each of these dimensions should be considered simultaneously.

Infrastructures

When respondents of the RNABC (1990) evaluation study were asked what resources would facilitate their research efforts, they indicated that consultants (statisticians and nurse consultants), libraries, release time, administrative support, collegial support, and seed money were essential but often missing. Other authors add that access to research reports, time to read and critique them, start-up and maintenance funding, academic preparation or relevant in-service education, and autonomy to implement research findings in practice also require resources (Champion & Leach, 1989; Funk, Champagne, Wiese, & Tornquist, 1991; Lynn & Moore, 1998; Moore & Lynn, 1998; Sayner, 1984). It is clear that research-based community health nursing practice requires a supportive infrastructure. Infrastructure can be defined as structures, policies, and facilities in an agency that support specific activities, such as the research process and use of findings in practice. Infrastructure elements include a nursing committee with responsibility for research-based practice, key positions that have responsibility for research leadership, services, time, communication, and consultation.

Nursing committees. Nursing research committees serve as a powerful and visible means of facilitating the use of nursing research (Stetler, 1983). Generally, their functions include promotion of interest and participation in research-based nursing practice and coordination of policies and procedures for qualified nurse researchers to access agency resources and clients (Kenneth & Stiesmeyer, 1991). Committee activities may include presenting research findings, publishing a research newsletter, consulting on proposal writing, promoting or providing research-related education, and liaising between nursing staff and research programs (Edwards-Beckett, 1990; Kenneth & Stiesmeyer, 1991; RNABC, 1993a, 1993b; Thurston, Tenhove, & Church, 1990).

In the early 1990s, agency-based nursing research committees began to emphasize promotion of the use of research. This shift in focus from the conduct and support of research reflects changes in nursing practice and agency accreditation standards (which require evidence of research-based nursing practice) and pressures from the health care system for cost-effective care with demonstrable outcomes. In 1994, one newly formed committee in a metropolitan public health department made research use its primary goal. To achieve this goal, they undertook four major initiatives: (a) revised a research utilization framework (Clarke, 1995) to fit the department's structure and the staff's resources, (b) pilot-tested the framework in both prevention and home care programs, (c) wrote a user-friendly manual, and (d) disseminated their work internally and externally. Subsequently, the health department adopted the framework and made research-based community health nursing practice the foundation of their programs.

By the mid-1990s many nursing research committees were integrated with multidisciplinary research committees, nursing practice committees, or quality improvement committees. The terms of reference for such committees tend to include responsibility for evidence-based practice and use of research as the preferred evidence.

Clinical nurse researchers. Clinical nurse researchers (CNRs), along with senior nurse administrators and managers, are responsible for creating an organizational environment that supports the conduct and use of nursing research. The CNR is a doctorally prepared nurse with research skills, an astute understanding of nursing practice, and leadership abilities, who fosters and coordinates nursing research (Crane, 1995; Knafl, Bevis, & Kirchhoff, 1987; Shamian, Nagle, Duffey-Rosenstein, Evans, & Strada, 1998). The CNR's responsibilities may include (a) education of staff, educators, and management nurses; (b) leadership of the nursing research committee; (c) consultation on the development and conduct of research; (d) liaison with appropriate groups to discuss current nursing issues and to develop potential research questions (Eagle, Fortnum, Price, & Scruton, 1990); (e) implementing a research utilization framework throughout the nursing department; (f) critiquing, translating, and disseminating research results for use in practice; and (g) evaluating outcomes of research utilization. Although this role is not yet prevalent in community health nursing, nursing research and practice have been brought into closer alignment.

Services and time. A third infrastructure element, services, provides CHNs with space and resources for participating in the research process (e.g., computers, libraries, secretarial services). A fourth, and related, element is provision of adequate release time. Even motivated CHNs have difficulty engaging in research activities during their regular work hours. Lack of motivation has been cited as a barrier to using nursing research (e.g., Funk et al., 1991; Varricchio & Mikos, 1987). However, recent surveys have found that lack of time, recognition, and meaningful rewards are equally, if not more, important (Davies & Eng, 1991; Nagy, Lumby, McKinely, & Macfarlane, 1998; RNABC, 1993a, 1993b). In addition, nurses need access to the research literature and integrative research reviews that may be published electronically (e.g., Sigma Theta Tau International's *Online Journal of Knowledge Synthesis for Nursing*) and in journals (e.g., *Evidence-based Nursing*).

Communication. Several authors cite poor communication as a major barrier to research utilization (Bock, 1990; Chambers, 1989; King, Barnard, & Hoehn, 1981; Repko, 1990). CHNs have difficulty finding relevant studies (Hayward et al., 1993a); those that are relevant may be presented in an inaccessible or unreadable form (Pank, Rostron, & Stenhouse, 1984). Or, nurses may lack preparation to analyze research critically (Wells & Baggs, 1994). Researchers often present findings in tentative terms in response to hypothetical inquiries and discuss results as they relate to theory and the need for further inquiry. This style of communication provides little foundation on which nurse clinicians can base their care (King et al., 1981). Furthermore, Canadian CHNs lack a national journal or special editions of generalist journals that focus on community health nursing and rarely have CHN-specific national conferences. Finally, CHNs tend not to use electronic communication systems beyond their agencies. In fact, Hayward, Ciliska, Underwood, and Dobbins (1998) found that the preferred medium for receiving systematic reviews was hard copy of the full paper rather than the summary, abstract, or disk copy. The latter options are generally more accessible and easier to read and use in decision making.

Consultation. The fifth infrastructure element is consultation. Access to both nurse and non-nurse consultants (e.g., statistician, computer expert) is desirable. A recent survey of all clinical agencies (hospitals and community health) in British Columbia found that few of these infrastructure elements were in place, particularly in public health units and home care departments (RNABC, 1993b). Little recognition had been given to the responsibilities for research-based nursing practice in community health nursing job descriptions. This suggests that even though nurses might be involved in research activities and changes in practice based on research findings, it is unlikely that they will receive agency support or recognition in their performance appraisal. Despite this lack of support, the majority of public health agencies expected their staff nurses to question their practice and to use research findings.

Approaches to infrastructure development

Two approaches have been suggested for establishing an infrastructure for research-based nursing practice—decentralized and centralized (Crane, 1995; MacKay, Grantham, & Ross, 1984). A third approach should also be considered—one that is integrated into an existing structure with responsibility for "best" practice. Linking research activities with a mandated process for accreditation and professional practice increases their viability. The integrated approach also increases the probability that research will be related to client care and that successful quality improvement approaches will be shared with others inside and outside the agency. Given the multidisciplinary context in which CHNs practise and the multidimensional aspects of community health care, a multidisciplinary approach to infrastructure development is important. This is most advanced in teaching units where there is a research mandate and involvement of academic researchers. A multidisciplinary, agency-based research committee has responsibilities similar to the nursing research committee. Although this model has many advantages, especially for obtaining essential infrastructure supports, CHNs must ensure that they are part of the research committee and decision-making process.

Relevant British Columbia survey results

Little attention has been paid, on a national level, to assessing infrastructure for research-based practice in workplaces of CHNs. In British Columbia, a survey of 174 health care agencies in the province, including 28 community health departments, was undertaken to assess agency-based nursing research development (RNABC, 1993b). Results indicated that only 13.3 percent of the health units had a mission statement that included research or had a nursing philosophy that explicitly referred to nursing research. No nursing departments had a definition of nursing research to guide the development of research programs or research-based practice, nor were there any nursing research committees.

The 1997 Member Survey of the Registered Nurses Association of British Columbia (1997) revealed that, for nurses practising in community-based agencies, open communication within all levels of their organization and an agency culture that encouraged change based on evidence were present less than 50 percent of the time. These findings indicate that urgent attention should be paid to the establishment and maintenance of supportive infrastructures if research-based community health nursing practice is to become a reality. Wells and Baggs (1994) concluded that "[a] supportive organization, which provides tangible resources and rewards for research activity, has been identified as an important factor for using and conducting research" (p. 146).

Professional practice issues in community health nursing

In addition to the barriers within the health system, professional barriers plague the development of research-based practice in community health nursing. The lack of collaborative partnerships within and among agencies is a critical issue. A second, and equally important, issue concerns the integration of research findings and innovations into clinical practice, a process that needs to be better understood in community health nursing.

Partnerships for research in community health nursing practice

The research process does not end when the study is completed, nor does it end with the dissemination of results. It also involves assessment of the findings for clinical application, use of the findings to improve community health nursing care, and evaluation of the clinical outcomes of research-based practice. Who is responsible for this complex set of activities? Nurses in administration, education, and clinical practice must develop collaborative partnerships with researchers. Although interdisciplinary collaboration is often desirable in community health research, developing harmonious partnerships within nursing is the crucial first step.

Administrative partnerships. Administrative partnerships should include intradisciplinary collaboration. At the senior management level, nurse administrators implement a philosophy that places value on research-based practice in three ways: (a) setting nursing policies and procedures that are based on research findings; (b) developing job descriptions for supervisors, program managers, clinical nurse specialists, and staff nurses that include research responsibilities; and (c) making infrastructure support available within and beyond the agency. At the operational level, supervisors or program managers are responsible for establishing a climate that encourages identification of clinical problems; organizing release time for staff nurses to read, critique, and synthesize research; and assisting with the application and evaluation of appropriate findings. In addition, they can make available access to data bases (e.g., Cochrane Library).

Senior nurse administrators' and managers' collaborative efforts can ensure that

- CHNs feel free to question practice
- consultation is available to support their efforts
- time is provided for research activities and professional development
- agency resources are allocated to research-based nursing practice
- opportunities are provided to incorporate research findings into practice and to evaluate clinical outcomes
- staff who participate in research activities receive due recognition.

Nurse educators. A second partnership in research-based nursing practice involves nurse educators (both academic and clinical educators). It has been observed that developments in nursing practice have been hampered by the formal separation of teachers, researchers, and practitioners (Wilson-Barnett, Corner, & DeCarle, 1990). Some educators, who undertake research as part of their required scholarly activities, may choose to conduct non-clinical research to avoid an uncomfortable atmosphere in the agency (Wilson-Barnett, Corner, & DeCarle, 1990). Other studies found that agency staff do not perceive faculty who are in their agency for education or research purposes as potential consultants (RNABC, 1993b) and believe that university faculty do not appreciate the potential contribution of staff nurses to research projects (Alcock, Carroll, & Goodman, 1990). Faculty–clinician collaboration can be facilitated by joint appointments between schools of nursing and health units/boards and by having a faculty member on the agency's nursing research committee or its equivalent.

Agency clinical instructors and educators face the challenge of encouraging staff nurses to incorporate nursing research into their practice. Many CHNs either do not understand the relevance of findings, or they are unable to apply them to nursing decisions or nursing actions (Chambers et al., 1994; Hunt, 1981; Kramer, Albrecht, & Miller, 1985). Clinical educators have a significant role in in-service programs aimed at enhancing knowledge and skills in using nursing research.

Clinical nurse specialists. Clinical nurse specialists (CNSs) should be part-ners and leaders in the research utilization process. They assume the roles of consultant and agent for change (Hamilton et al., 1990). The CNS is respon-sible for five essential steps in research utilization: (a) assessment of system readiness for research utilization; (b) design of the research utilization plan; (c) implementation of a research utilization process; (d) evaluation of the innovation, with revisions as necessary; and (e) report of findings, for repli-cation and further research, to clinical nurses and nurse researchers (Hickey, 1990). One approach to carrying out these responsibilities involves the estab-lishment of an agency-based nursing research interest group (Pearlman, Laitinen, Rebelo, Trieu, & Williams, 1998). Organizational support for the research responsibilities of the clinical nurse specialist and for research part-nerships forged with staff nurses and managers is important. Although it is not yet a common occurrence, CNSs are being employed with increasing fre-quency by community health agencies.

Staff nurses. Key players in partnerships are staff nurses. Survey findings indicate that staff nurses value research in nursing (Alcock et al., 1990; RNABC, 1993a, 1993b; Wells & Baggs, 1994). Wells and Baggs (1994) found that nurses who value research highly were five times more likely to use it, and that those who had taken a greater number of statistics courses were 1.6 times more likely to use research. This ought to bode well for CHNs who report greater interest in research and more experience and education in this area (RNABC, 1993b). Staff nurses are also in an excellent position to collab-orate with other clinicians, educators, administrators, and researchers and to implement clinical practice changes that will have a positive impact on the quality, efficacy, and cost of health care (Alcock et al., 1990).

It is partnerships, rather than any one person or factor, that influence the degree to which research use occurs in community health nursing practice. Successful partnerships require mutual respect and commitment to research-based practice that leads to meaningful, demonstrable client out-comes (Clarke & Mass, 1998).

Research adoption

The use of research findings in nursing practice requires adoption of an inno-vation—a new idea, a different way of thinking about an issue, or a change in behaviour. Like other nurses, CHNs tend to be perfectionists, looking for absolute proof of all facts before a piece of research is considered usable (Wood, 1992). Adopting an innovation is a complex process and involves several stages.

Process. Although several models of innovation adoption exist, Rogers's Diffusion Innovation Theory (1997) is particularly useful. Diffusion and adoption of innovations are conceptualized as occurring in stages through which all individuals, including CHNs, must pass. The first stage, the *knowledge stage,* occurs as CHNs become aware of the innovation. Next, in the *persuasion stage,* they form a favourable or unfavourable attitude toward the innovation. Third, they take action to adopt or reject the innovation on a trial basis—the *decision stage.* Finally, in the *implementation stage,* CHNs use the innovation on a regular basis. If a new practice is mandated without practitioners moving through these appropriate stages, it is unlikely that the innovation will be implemented consistently or as intended.

Several factors can affect the research adoption process. The source of new knowledge influences the rate at which individuals pass through the first stage. Influential sources for adopting innovations are professional nursing literature (especially the journal *Nursing Research*), research-oriented conferences and in-service programs, and role models (Brett, 1987; Coyle & Sokop, 1990). Factors influencing nurses in the persuasion stage are perceived agency policy, procedure manuals, and the opinions of other professionals (Brett, 1987). In the last two stages, the most common barriers identified by clinicians were organizational. Nurses' perceptions that they lack authority and do not have the support of administration to change nursing practice inhibit adoption of innovation.

The following issues related to innovation adoption need to be addressed:

- *Availability of research-based knowledge:* Is it available in clinically focussed journals, conferences, or electronic communication systems?
- *Acceptability and readability of that knowledge:* Is it worded in jargon that only a researcher can understand?
- *Credibility of the study:* Do CHNs believe the findings, given their understanding of the research methods?
- *Relevancy of the findings:* How relevant are the findings to clinical practice, the sociocultural context of practice and clients, and organizational structures?
- *Support and reinforcement to adopt and maintain the innovation:* Are supportive persons and materials available to assist CHNs to adopt and practise the innovation?

Research utilization framework. A research utilization framework can facilitate the research adoption process and resolve some of these issues. A framework provides a structure that guides the process of making research the foundation for nursing practice. The four best-known decision-driven frameworks are (a) the Western Interstate Commission for Higher Education in Nursing, also called WICHEN (Krueger, Nelson, & Wolanin, 1978), (b) the Conduct and Utilization of Research in Nursing, or CURN (Horsley, Crane, & Bingle, 1978), (c) NCAST (King et al., 1981), and (d) Stetler/Marram (Stetler, 1994). The WICHEN and CURN frameworks are both based on the concepts of diffusion of innovation and planned change; NCAST focusses solely on diffusion of innovations; and the refined Stetler/Marram framework is an interactive, staged model.

Based on the work of Stetler (1983) and the expressed needs of nurses and health agencies in British Columbia, a decision-driven model for utilization of research findings in practice was developed, tested, and published (Clarke, 1995). Application of this framework requires partnerships among nurses with clinical expertise, research experience, and administrative responsibilities. Each of the four phases requires particular nurses to be involved, decisions to be made, and resources to be accessed. Consistent with decision-driven models, the framework's basic assumption is that knowledge is used when it is implemented as part of a new practice protocol or intervention (Cronenwett, 1995). The framework can be modified by individual agencies, thus making it relevant to staff needs, organizational structure, and integration of evidence-based clinical tools (Clarke, 1996).

How well a given framework will serve a situation or agency depends on the framework's efficacy, the type of problem, and the congruence of the framework's theoretical base with nurses' decision making (Stetler, 1985). As well, the framework must fit with the organization's structure, philosophy of nursing practice, and available resources. Using a framework fosters an inquiring attitude, resulting in problem identification and resolution and in adoption of innovations in practice.

Behavioural change strategies. Changing behaviour is complex and involves many systems. Behavioural change strategies need to be considered for their evidence of providing effective outcomes. A taxonomy of interventions to improve practice has been developed by the Cochrane Collaboration on Effective Professional Practice (Thompson, 1998). Consistently effective strategies include education outreach visits, reminders, multifaceted interventions, and interactive educational meetings. Those with mixed effects include audit and feedback, local opinion leaders, local consensus process, and client-mediated interventions. Sadly, those strategies having little or no effect are the ones most frequently used—distribution of educational materials and didactic educational meetings. In preparing to introduce new research findings, nurses need to pay attention to preparing the context and selecting the most appropriate intervention strategies.

Research utilization and Primary Health Care principles

CHNs facilitating research utilization in practice will encounter challenges. The first is to demonstrate the cost effectiveness of research-based nursing practice and to justify the allocation of resources and personnel. The second challenge is to reduce the time gap between when knowledge is developed and when it is used. The third is to create agency infrastructures. Using research in community health nursing practice within a Primary Health Care context poses additional challenges. These can be readily identified when consideration is given to the seven elements contained in the World Health Organization definition of Primary Health Care (WHO, 1978).

Essential health care

Primary Health Care is essential health care. The challenges here are to explicate the research basis of community health nursing practice, to identify and measure outcomes that are sensitive to nursing interventions, and to use these practice-based research findings in health promotion and illness prevention. To meet these challenges, CHNs require knowledge of different types of research approaches, both quantitative (e.g., epidemiology) and qualitative (e.g., ethnography). Related challenges include access to health information data bases and research reports; ability to read, understand, and critique research; and integration of findings into practice.

Universal accessibility

Services should be made universally accessible. Relevant questions to be answered include: What human resources are needed? How many nurses should be prepared, and at what levels? What advanced preparation do CHNs require to gain competencies in promoting and evaluating research-based nursing practice and its accessibility? To what extent do CHNs have the knowledge, skills, and experience to engage in comprehensive assessments of community assets and deficits? Tenn and Niskala's (1994) survey of Canadian university schools of nursing revealed that approximately 60 percent of schools report only a "reasonable" degree of integration of Primary Health Care into their curricula.

Acceptable care

Care should be acceptable to those receiving it. Increasingly, Canada is made up of many different cultural groups coming from all over the world. As well, the health of First Nations people is of particular concern. The challenge for CHNs is to be knowledgeable about the cultures of these different groups (Krebs, 1983). What are their customs, values, beliefs, and taboos? How do they perceive the promotion and maintenance of health—of individuals, of families, and of communities? New and culturally relevant approaches to research-based nursing practice and evaluation are needed, including application of critical ethnography and participatory action research (Clarke, 1997; Hayward, Ciliska, Mitchell, et al., 1993b; Thomas, 1993).

Public participation

The hallmark of Primary Health Care is health care "by the people"; the public should participate fully. The related challenges for basing practice in research include involving clients as partners in the research process; empowering them with research-based knowledge to advocate and lobby for change; using community development strategies in research; and applying, in a critical way, research findings from other disciplines. Joint evaluation with clients of the effect of Primary Health Care interventions on the health of individuals, groups, and communities will be needed (Clarke & Mass, 1998).

Affordability

Care should be given at a cost that the community and country can afford. The challenges, again, are many. Are CHNs ready to examine critically what they are doing and how they are doing it (Krebs, 1983)? How will CHNs react if some of their present activities are carried out by others, including, eventually, members of the family? Is there a "dose–response" effect of community health nursing interventions? What are the implications of an "overdose" or "underdose"? Estimating the costs of the services of CHNs is an enormous challenge, given that outcomes are most likely to be influenced by any number of factors clearly beyond that of a particular CHN intervention. What difference does having a CHN make on the health team? How can this be demonstrated?

Determinants of health

Primary Health Care forms an integral part of the overall social and economic development of the community. Research-based community health nursing practice involves understanding the health of communities in the context of economic and social development, as well as health development. According to Chambers and colleagues (1994), CHNs do not have extensive or explicit roles in policy formulation, research and evaluation of resource management, planning, and coordination. Although CHNs report that they are not well prepared for these roles, they expect them to increase in significance for developing community health programs in the future (Chambers et al., 1994; Clarke, Beddome et al., 1993; Hayward, Ciliska, Mitchell, et al., 1993b).

Conclusion

Primary Health Care is the nucleus of the country's health system. In essence, this could mean that CHNs are at the nucleus—not at the periphery. CHNs practise where people live, work, and play and where services are being reoriented in health system reform. Research-based practice to support this shift challenges CHNs to participate in policy formulation and program development within a multidisciplinary context. Current and future community health initiatives that include CHNs must be evaluated with criteria that are sensitive to community health nursing practice. The challenge is to develop collaborative relationships that respect, value, and integrate the research-based knowledge and experience brought by each discipline.

The everyday decisions that CHNs make are complex and require accurate, reliable information upon which to predict individual, family, community, and health system outcomes of nursing interventions and programs. Research is the means by which this vital nursing knowledge is generated and validated. The research process must not stop with the conduct of research; it must also include dissemination, use, and evaluation of findings.

Acknowledgements

The author wishes to acknowledge the contributions of Ann Syme, Research Assistant, during the early conceptualization of RNABC's promotion of research-based nursing practice and of Nora Whyte, former New Directions Coordinator of RNABC, for her thoughtful critique, especially with respect to its relevancy to Primary Health Care.

QUESTIONS

1. What value does your clinical agency/school place on research and research-based nursing practice? How is this demonstrated? What steps can be taken to reinforce the value placed on research and research-based nursing practice?
2. How are the nursing components of health information data bases being developed in your clinical area? What is the role of the CHN in this development?
3. Does your school/clinical agency have supportive infrastructures for research-based nursing practice? If so, what are they? How might they be strengthened? If not, what would you suggest?
4. What resources are needed for creating or maintaining a nursing research committee in a community health nursing agency? What barriers and supports can you identify for having a nursing research committee in a community health nursing agency? What alternative structures are available?
5. What policies need to be in place to promote a collaborative approach to the use of research and research-based nursing practice in a CHN agency? How should CHNs' job descriptions be worded to involve them more directly in research utilization and research-based nursing practice?

6.   What are the advantages and disadvantages of using a framework to promote research-based community health nursing practice?

REFERENCES

Alcock, D., Carroll, G., & Goodman, M. (1990). Staff nurses' perceptions of factors influencing their role in research. *Canadian Journal of Nursing Research, 22*(4), 7–18.

Bock, L. (1990). From research to utilization: Bridging the gap. *Nursing Management, 21*(3), 50–51.

Brett, J.L.L. (1987). Use of nursing practice research findings. *Nursing Research, 36*(6), 344–349.

Brooten, D., Kumar, S., Brown, I.., Butts, P., Finkler, S., Bakewell-Sachs, S., Gibbons, A., & Delivoria-Papadopoulos, M. (1986). A randomized clinical trial and home follow-up of very-low-birth-weight infants. *New England Journal of Medicine, 315*(15), 934–939.

Canadian Council on Health Facilities Accreditation (CCHFA). (1993). *Community health services standards* [1994 draft]. Ottawa: Author.

Canadian Nurses Association (CNA). (1993). *Papers from the Nursing Minimum Data Set Conference*. Ottawa: Author.

Chambers, C. (1989). Barriers to the dissemination and use of research in nursing practice. *NRIG Newsletter, 8*(2), 2–3.

Chambers, L.W., Underwood, J., Halbert, T., Woodward, C.A., Heale, J., & Isaacs, S. (1994). 1992 Ontario survey of public health nurses: Perceptions of roles and activities. *Canadian Journal of Public Health, 85*(3), 175–179.

Champion, V., & Leach, A. (1989). Variables related to research utilization in nursing: An empirical investigation. *Journal of Advanced Nursing, 14*, 705–710.

Clarke, H.F. (1995). Using research to improve the quality of nursing care. *Nursing BC, 27*(5), 19–22.

Clarke, H.F. (1996). Integrating evidence-based clinical tools with practice. *Nursing BC, 28*(5), 19–22.

Clarke, H.F. (1997). Research in nursing and cultural diversity: Working with First Nations people. *Canadian Journal of Nursing Research, 29*(2), 11–25.

Clarke, H.F., Beddome, G., & Whyte, N. (1993). Public health nurses' vision of their future reflects changing paradigms. *Image: Journal of Nursing Scholarship, 25*(4), 305–310.

Clarke, H.F., Joseph, R., Hislop, T.G., Deschamps, M., Band, P., & Atleo, R. (1998). Reducing cervical cancer among First Nations women. *Canadian Nurse, 94*(3), 36–41.

Clarke, H.F., & Mass, H. (1998). Comox Valley Nursing Centre: From collaboration to empowerment. *Public Health Nursing, 15*(3), 216–224.

Coyle, L.A., & Sokop, A.G. (1990). Innovation adoption behavior among nurses. *Nursing Research, 39*(3), 176–180.

Crane, J. (1995). The future of research utilization. *Nursing Clinics of North America, 30*(3), 565–577.

Cronenwett, L.R. (1995). Effective methods for disseminating research findings to nurses in practice. *Nursing Clinics of North America, 30*(3), 429–438.

Davies, B., & Eng, B. (1991). *Final report: Survey of nursing research programs in children's hospitals*. Vancouver: British Columbia Children's Hospital.

Eagle, J., Fortnum, D., Price, P., & Scruton, J. (1990). Developing a rationale and recruitment plan for a nurse researcher. *Canadian Journal of Nursing Administration, 3*, 5–10.

Edwards-Beckett, J. (1990). Nursing research utilization techniques. *Journal of Nursing Administration, 20*(11), 25–30.

Fagin, C. (1982). The economic value of nursing research. *American Journal of Nursing, 12*, 1844–1849.

Fordyce, J.D., Mooney, G.H., & Russell, E.M. (1982). Economic analysis in health care. *Health Bulletin, 39*(10), 21–38.

Funk, S.G., Champagne, M.T., Wiese, R.A., & Tornquist, E.M. (1991). Barriers: The barriers to research utilization scales. *Applied Nursing Research, 4*(1), 39–45.

Hamilton, L., Vincent, L., Goode, R., Moorhouse, A., Hawker Worden, R., Jones, H., Close, M., & DuFour, S. (1990). Organizational support of the clinical nurse specialist role: A nursing research and professional development directorate. *Canadian Journal of Nursing Administration, 3*(3), 9–13.

Hayward, S., Ciliska, D., Mitchell, A., Thomas, H., Underwood, J., & Rafael, A. (1993a). *Evaluation research in public health nursing (Paper 93-3)*. Hamilton, ON: Quality of Nursing Worklife Research Unit.

Hayward, S., Ciliska, D., Mitchell, A., Thomas, H., Underwood, J., & Rafael, A. (1993b). *Public health nursing and health promotion (Paper 93-2)*. Hamilton, ON: Quality of Nursing Worklife Research Unit.

Hayward, S., Ciliska, D., Underwood, J., & Dobbins, M. (1998). Transferring public health nursing research to health system planning: Assessing the relevance and accessibility of systematic reviews. *Research utilization: Preparing for the new millennium*. Proceedings of the First International Research Utilization Conference, Toronto, April 24–25.

Hickey, M. (1990). The role of the clinical nurse specialist in the research utilization process. *Clinical Nurse Specialist, 4*(2), 93–96.

Hislop, T.G., Clarke, H.F., Joseph, R., Deschamps, M., Band, P.R., Smith, J., Le, N., & Atleo, R. (1996). Cervical cytology screening in British Columbia First Nations women living in a large urban setting. *Canadian Family Physician, 42*, 1701–1708.

Horsley, J. (1985). Using research to practice: The current context. *Western Journal of Nursing Research, 1*, 135–139.

Horsley, J., Crane, J., & Bingle, J. (1978). Research utilization as an organization process. *Journal of Nursing Administration, 8*, 4–6.

Hunt, J. (1981). Indicators for nursing practice: The use of research findings. *Journal of Advanced Nursing, 6*, 189–194.

Kenneth, H., & Stiesmeyer, J. (1991). Strategies for involving staff in nursing research. *Applied Nursing Research, 10*(2), 103–107.

King, D., Barnard, K., & Hoehn, R. (1981). Disseminating the results of nursing research. *Nursing Outlook, 3*, 164–169.

Kitson, A. (1998). Major issues related to research utilization. *Research utilization: Preparing for the new millennium*. Proceedings of the First International Research Utilization Conference, Toronto, April 24–25.

Knafl, K., Bevis, M., & Kirchhoff, K. (1987). Research activities of clinical nurse researchers. *Nursing Research, 36*(4), 249–252.

Kramer, M., Albrecht, S., & Miller, R. (1985). A team approach to nursing research. *Nursing Forum, 22*(1), 19–21.

Krebs, D. (1983). Nursing in Primary Health Care. *International Nursing Review, 30*(5), 141–145.

Krueger, J., Nelson, A., & Wolanin, M. (1978). *Nursing research: Development, collaboration, and utilization.* Germantown, MD: Aspen.

Lynn, M.R., & Moore, K.A. (1998). Barriers to research utilization for staff nurses. *Research utilization: Preparing for the new millennium.* Proceedings of the First International Research Utilization Conference, Toronto, April 24–25.

MacKay, R.C., Grantham, M.A., & Ross, E.M. (1984). Building a hospital nursing research department. *Journal of Nursing Administration, 6*(4), 23–27.

Marek, K.D., & Lang, N.M. (1993). Nursing sensitive outcomes. *Papers from the Nursing Minimum Data Set Conference,* Edmonton, October 27–29, 1992 (pp. 100–120). Ottawa: Canadian Nurses Association.

Mills, K. (1994). The changing practice of public health nurses. *Canadian Journal of Public Health, 85*(3), 153–154.

Moore, K.A., & Lynn, M.R. (1998). Barriers to research utilization for nurse managers. *Research utilization: Preparing for the new millennium.* Proceedings of the First International Research Utilization Conference, Toronto, April 24–25.

Nagy, S., Lumby, J., McKinely, S., & Macfarlane, C. (1998). Solving problems in research utilization: An organization-based approach. *Research utilization: Preparing for the new millennium.* Proceedings of the First International Nursing Research Utilization Conference, Toronto, April 24–25.

Pank, P., Rostron, W., & Stenhouse, M. (1984). Using research in nursing. *Nursing Times, 80*(11), 44–45.

Pearlman, L., Laitinen, A., Rebelo, J., Trieu, T., & Williams, A. (1998). A program-based nursing research interest group: A strategy for research utilization. *Research Utilization: Preparing for the new millennium.* Proceedings of the First International Research Utilization Conference, Toronto, April 24–25.

Pirjo, P., & Perala, M.L. (1998). Towards evidence-based practice: A systematic literature review of effectiveness research. *Research utilization: Preparing for the new millennium.* Proceedings of the First International Research Utilization Conference, Toronto, April 24–25.

Registered Nurses Association of British Columbia (RNABC). (1990). *Report on the evaluation of member services of the Research Consultation Services.* Vancouver: Author.

Registered Nurses Association of British Columbia (RNABC). (1991). *Making a difference: From ritual to research-based nursing practice.* A discussion paper. Vancouver: Author.

Registered Nurses Association of British Columbia (RNABC). (1993a). *Nursing and research in undergraduate education programs: A B.C. survey.* Vancouver: Author.

Registered Nurses Association of British Columbia (RNABC). (1993b). *Nursing and research in clinical agencies: A B.C. survey.* Vancouver: Author.

Registered Nurses Association of British Columbia (RNABC). (1997). *1997 membership survey.* Vancouver: Author.

Registered Nurses Association of British Columbia (RNABC). (1998). *Standards for nursing practice in British Columbia.* Vancouver: Author.

Repko, L. (1990). Turn research reports into an assessment challenge. *RN, 53*(8), 56–61.

Rogers, E.M. (1997). *Diffusion of innovations* (4th ed.). Toronto: Collier MacMillan.

Sayner, N. (1984). Research in the clinical setting: Potential barriers to implementation. *Journal of Neurosurgical Nursing, 16*(5), 279–281.

Shamian, J. (1993). Response to K.D. Marek's and N.M. Lang's paper on nursing sensitive outcomes. *Papers from the Nursing Minimum Data Set Conference,* Edmonton, October 27–29, 1992 (pp. 121–126). Ottawa: Canadian Nurses Association.

Shamian, J., Nagle, L., Duffey-Rosenstein, B., Evans, S., & Strada, ME. (1998). Creating an environment of knowledge-based nursing practice and management. *Research utilization: Preparing for the new millennium.* Proceedings of the First International Research Utilization Conference, Toronto, April 24–25.

Smeltzer, C., & Hinshaw, A. (1988). Research: Clinical integration for excellent patient care. *Nursing Management, 19*(1), 38–44.

Stetler, C. (1983). Nurses and research: Responsibility and involvement. *National Intravenous Therapy Association, 6*(3), 207–212.

Stetler, C. (1985). Research utilization: Defining the concept. *Image: Journal of Nursing Scholarship, 17*(2), 40–44.

Stetler, C. (1994). Refinement of the Stetler/Marram Model for application of research findings to practice. *Nursing Outlook, 42*(1), 15–25.

Tenn, L., & Niskala, H. (1994). *Primary Health Care in the curricula of Canadian university schools of nursing* (Final report to the Canadian Nurses Foundation). Vancouver: University of British Columbia School of Nursing.

Thomas, J. (1993). *Doing critical ethnography.* Newbury Park, CA: Sage.

Thompson, M.A. (1998). Closing the gap between nursing research and practice. *Evidence-based Nursing, 1*(1), 7–8.

Thurston, N., Tenhove, S., & Church, J. (1990). Hospital nursing is alive and flourishing. *Nursing Management, 21*(5), 50–54.

Varricchio, C., & Mikos, K. (1987). Research: Determining feasibility in a clinical setting. *Oncology Nursing Forum, 14*(1), 89–90.

Wells, N., & Baggs, J.G. (1994). A survey of practicing nurses' research interests and activities. *Clinical Nurse Specialist, 8*(3), 145–151.

Wilson-Barnett, J., Corner, J., & DeCarle, B. (1990). Integrating nursing research and practice—the role of the researcher as teacher. *Journal of Advanced Nursing, 15,* 621–625.

Wood, M. (1992). Shaping practice through research. *Clinical Nursing Research, 1*(2), 123–126.

World Health Organization (WHO). (1978). *Primary Health Care: Report of the International Conference on Primary Health Care.* Geneva: Author.

Zerwekh, J.V. (1991). At the expense of their souls. *Nursing Outlook, 39*(2), 58–61.

C H A P T E R   2 6

Community health nursing research: Looking toward the future

Karen I. Chalmers and David M. Gregory

The purpose of this chapter is to analyze research conducted in the area of community health nursing and to provide an overview of the major strengths, limitations, and opportunities for research development. Theoretical, methodological, practical, and future challenges facing community health nurse researchers are discussed.

LEARNING OBJECTIVES

In this chapter, you will learn:

- the theory that guides community health nursing research
- the diversity of methodological issues and challenges inherent in community health nursing research
- the practical challenges encountered when conducting community health nursing research
- some future initiatives that will foster the development of research and the use or "uptake" of research findings

Introduction

A major goal in nursing today is the systematic development of a body of knowledge, through research, to guide nursing practice. The need for research in community health nursing is well documented (Association of Community Health Nursing Educators [ACHNE], 1992; Canadian Public Health Association [CPHA], 1990). The context of community health nursing practice, however, presents unique challenges to the conduct of research. Although standard steps in the research process are described in nursing texts, issues related to community health nursing research are seldom discussed.

Community health nursing differs from other types of nursing practice in many ways. It is generally considered to represent the synthesis of both public health and nursing sciences (ACHNE, 1993; CPHA, 1990). As a result, the focus of practice encompasses a range of clients, including individuals, aggregates, groups, and the community as a whole. Interventions may be directed at one or more of these client levels and each may have physical, emotional, psychological, and social health needs. The knowledge needed to offer care along this client continuum is extensive.

Community health nursing recognizes the need to act on the determinants of health, and not just the health-related outcomes of these influencing forces. For example, community health nurses attempt to "work upstream" on health problems to prevent or minimize negative health outcomes (Butterfield, 1990). This involves focussing on the underlying determinants of poor health, such as poverty, education, gender, inadequate social support, and marginalization. Actions to address these underlying determinants may entail not only direct intervention with the individual client (e.g., immunizations), but also intervention with the family and the community (e.g., community development initiatives to prevent child abuse). The goal of community health nursing is enhancement of the health of the community, an emphasis that is congruent with the tenets of Primary Health Care.

The purpose of this chapter is to analyze research conducted in the area of community health nursing and to identify the major strengths and limitations of and opportunities for research development. The authors define community health nursing research as the systematic study of the interrelationships between the community and its components (i.e., individuals, families, groups, and aggregates). Ideally, this research should contribute to the enhancement of the community's health in theory or in practical ways.

To support our discussion of the theoretical, methodological, practical, and future challenges of community health nursing research, we examined the abstracts of published research (listed in the CINAHL and Medline data bases during the years from 1992 to the early part of 1998). The review was not intended to be an exhaustive critique of all research relevant to community health nursing. The literature was searched using the keywords "community health nursing," "research," and "study"; and "public health nursing," "research," and "study." Subsequently, in an attempt to identify additional articles, searches using the keywords "health policy," "community assessment," and "community development" were conducted.

Abstracts provided information about nurse researchers, their institutional affiliations, and the location of the study. The articles included in the review met the following criteria: at least one author was a nurse affiliated with a Canadian agency or educational institution; the articles were written in English; and they were empirically based. Doctoral dissertations were excluded because of cost and accessibility issues. In keeping with the definition of community health nursing research, the authors did not include studies of patients receiving care in the community (e.g., palliative care patients) or their caregivers (e.g., home care nurses). In total, 43 published studies were included.

Content analysis of the 43 studies examined the focus of each study, the research design, method of sampling, client level, and use of a conceptual framework. These studies serve to supplement the following discussion of theoretical and practical challenges in community health nursing research.

Theoretical challenges

The theoretical challenges facing community health nursing research are discussed under two headings. The first relates to a need to develop a sound theoretical base for research and practice. The second concerns the foci that have occupied community health nurse researchers in recent years.

Need to develop a theoretical base
for research and practice

Generation of nursing knowledge is based on the interplay among theory, research, and practice. A fundamental issue related to nursing knowledge development is the beginning level of theory-based research. Community health nursing research, in particular, is in the early stages of establishing and advancing relationships among these three elements. Conducting research without a theoretical framework limits the value of research and hinders advancement of theory and practice.

Approximately 50 percent of the Canadian studies reviewed incorporated either nursing or non-nursing theoretical frameworks or key concepts. Primary Health Care was the most commonly cited perspective (Beddome, Clarke, & Whyte, 1993; Chalmers, Bramadat, & Sloan, 1997; Clarke, Beddome, & Whyte, 1993; Kulig, 1994; Tenn, 1995). Although this represents only 12 percent of the studies, this is an increase from the previous review (Chalmers & Gregory, 1995), in which only two studies applied a Primary Health Care framework to guide community health nursing research. These studies addressed the following topics: public health nurses' vision of the premises of their future practice; the development of the Primary Health Care Questionnaire (PHCQ); and community health needs assessment based on intersectoral collaboration (Chalmers, Bramadat, et al., 1997).

Non-nursing theoretical perspectives were evident. For example, Duncan (1992) examined ethical concepts in community health nursing, while an ecological framework directed an intervention study focussed on tertiary prevention of child abuse (MacMillan & Thomas, 1993).

Several published reports were identified that made use of qualitative methods, including grounded theory (Chalmers, 1992a, 1992b, 1993). There was evidence of critical–theoretical frameworks associated with feminist research (Stewart et al., 1996) or action research (Battle Haugh & Spence Laschinger, 1996; Russell, Gregory, Wotton, Mordoch, & Counts, 1996). These studies reported programs developed to address the needs of people, a goal common to community health nurses (Allen, 1987).

Given the centrality of collaborative partnerships in community health nursing, there were relatively few studies completed within a participatory action research (PAR) framework. This process entails active involvement of participants from conceptualization to completion of the project (see also Chapter 28). From a theoretical perspective, this approach to research is in keeping with the basic premises of Primary Health Care and community health nursing, ideologies rooted in participatory principles.

Only one study was identified in which nursing theory was used. Peplau's conceptual framework for psychodynamic nursing served as the theoretical guide to examine the orientation phase of the nurse–client relationship (Forchuk, 1992). Nursing theories have been criticized for their limited relevance to community health nursing (Hanchett & Clarke, 1989), as they tend to be individualistic and non-participatory and neglect social and economic environments. Given this limited relevance, researchers may avoid the use of nursing theory in their studies, thereby reinforcing the schism between nursing theory and research conducted in community health nursing.

Many contend that theories specific to community health nursing should be developed (Hamilton, 1991). This may entail developing new theory and/or adapting existing theories from other disciplines such as psychology, sociology, anthropology, and economics. The principles of Primary Health Care may also serve as a framework for research.

Focus of community health nursing research

The research conducted by Canadian nurses revealed the scope inherent in community health nursing. Studies focussed on many areas, such as practice, nursing education, characteristics and perceptions of community health nurses, the delivery of community health nursing services, and many target groups and populations, such as high-risk aggregates and the well elderly. Poulin, Gyorkos, MacPhee, Cann, and Bickerton (1992) developed and evaluated an interview technique for contact tracing of rural community populations at risk for hepatitis B. Their successful approach may provide a useful strategy for other rural communities. Ploeg and colleagues (1994) evaluated public health nursing home visits that promoted either safety behaviours or influenza immunization in a group of community-based elderly clients. They found that the two client groups (who received information about safety or immunization) made approximately equal changes in their behaviour after the intervention. In another study, Ciliska et al. (1996a), using a trisectoral collaborative approach (hospital, health department, university school of nursing), evaluated the efficacy and efficiency of referral decisions by hospital staff nurses and public health liaison nurses. With additional education, maternity staff nurses more effectively identified mothers needing follow-up in the home by public health nurses. As well, this study demonstrated cost savings to the health system.

In addition to studies of community health nursing practice with specific aggregates, projects also investigated issues related to the delivery of community health nursing services. These studies are particularly helpful in documenting the unique components of community health nursing practice. For example, Duncan (1992) explored ethical challenges in community health nursing. Public health nurses reported that situations involving high-risk parenting presented the most serious ethical challenges to them. Beddome and colleagues (1993) used a delphi approach to identify issues and directions for future public health nursing practice in British Columbia. This study revealed that nurses believed their future practice would be based on Primary Health Care and community development models. The results of one study (Mitchell et al., 1993) were ultimately used to change policy concerning discharge planning for postpartum women. Referrals to public health nurses are now made by hospital nurses on maternity wards, with public health liaison nurses available as consultants. A study of British community health nurses, conducted by a Canadian nurse, examined the processes involved in identifying health needs in the community. Nurses and clients both controlled the interactions by selectively giving and receiving information (Chalmers, 1992b, 1993).

Historical methods, although used infrequently, help to illuminate the origins of practice issues. Stuart's (1992) historical study analyzed public health nurses' practice in the early 20th century. Similarly, Zilm and Warbinek (1995) investigated early tuberculosis nursing in British Columbia. Such studies situate today's practice problems within the broader issues of power, control of women, surveillance, and the nursing profession's response to societal needs.

Program evaluation research is an important domain within community health nursing. Existing programs need to be evaluated to ensure that they are meeting the needs of groups in the community. This is particularly important during periods when resources are limited and programs must demonstrate their value. Davies, Matte-Lewis, O'Connor, Dulberg, and Drake (1992) conducted an evaluation study of the "Time to Quit" Self-Help Smoking Cessation Program.

One area that has received limited research attention is the organization and administration of community health. With respect to public health nursing work environments, Battle Haugh and Spence Laschinger (1996) documented that nurse managers are in a pivotal position to enhance job effectiveness and quality nursing care. Nurses' workload has traditionally been organized within geographically defined districts in the community.

More recently, there is a move to have nurses work with specific target populations such as postpartum women, the elderly, or at-risk families.

Most community health nursing studies focussed on individuals and aggregates. Few studies focussed on the community level of practice. With the exception of studies incorporating community health assessments (Kulig & Wilde, 1996; Russell et al., 1996) and community development approaches (Edwards, Ciliska, Halbert, & Pond, 1992), no other study addressed community mobilization, community development, or community-wide health promotion.

Methodological challenges

One of the unique dimensions of community health nursing is the context of nursing practice. Community nurses engage in fieldwork that occurs in naturalistic settings such as homes, worksites, community clinics, and schools. There is a good fit between qualitative or naturalistic methods and community health nursing practice. A range of qualitative methods, evident in the studies reviewed, included grounded theory (e.g., Chalmers, 1992a, 1992b, 1993), ethnography (e.g., Kulig, 1994; Purkis, 1997), phenomenology (e.g., Leipert, 1996), and historical research (e.g., Stuart, 1992; Zilm & Warbinek, 1995).

The world of community health nursing can be known through a variety of research lenses. Survey designs are commonly used by researchers in the area of community health (Beddome, Clarke, & Whyte, 1993; Spence Laschinger, Goldenberg, & Dal Bello, 1995). Surveys are convenient, administered with relative ease, fairly cost effective, useful, and important.

PAR engenders a collaborative approach between participants and researchers in which both define the problem needing study and participate in the research process (Aryanwu, 1988; Dickson & Tutty, 1996; Holter & Schwartz-Barcott, 1993; Kirkpatrick, 1990). Participatory action approaches have been used to study the educational preparation of students for community health practice and to assess community needs (e.g., Bramadat, Chalmers, & Andrusyszyn, 1996; Russell et al., 1996).

Intervention studies enable community health nurses to test new strategies and to evaluate the outcomes of their practice. These studies usually require large numbers of participants who can be randomized into control and experimental groups. For example, Edwards and Sims-Jones (1997) conducted a three-group randomized control trial (RCT) to determine the effectiveness of a postpartum telephone visit by a public health nurse on infant care behaviours of new mothers. Gagnon et al. (1997) also conducted an RCT to study the impact of an early postpartum program on health outcomes of newborns and the competence of mothers. These studies are important because the rigorous design, including random sampling and large sample size, permits testing of the effectiveness of the intervention.

Replication studies are not common in nursing research and are rare in community health nursing. They increase confidence in research findings and have implications for policy changes related to service delivery as well as health promotion (e.g., increasing resources for workplace smoking cessation programs). Policy and programs are more likely to be changed when replication studies across different sites lend support.

In summary, the research reviewed for this chapter addressed many target groups found in the community setting. A number of research designs were used by researchers from both the qualitative and quantitative perspectives. Areas for future methodological development in community health nursing research include expanding the repertoire of methods to include more feminist research, critical theory, and action research. Additional research is also needed on issues relevant to Primary Health Care, community mobilization, community development, policy evaluation, and community as client.

Practical challenges

Many challenges face the researcher attempting to study community health nursing practice. These affect the questions that can be addressed through research, the methods of study, and the outcomes of projects. Three areas are particularly challenging: funding, infrastructure, and implementing research designs.

Funding for research projects

Access to adequate funding is a prerequisite for nursing research today. Most research money in the health sciences is directed toward the study of biological processes. Within the applied or health disciplines, fundable proposals usually require a focus on specific high-risk populations, such as people exposed to HIV or low birth-weight infants. Few resources are available to explore other health promotion issues or the holistic approach used by community health nurses with a range of client groups, health problems, and client levels.

Little money is available to carry out early, descriptive assessment research prior to intervention studies. Pilot work and feasibility studies are useful approaches to test research protocols prior to designing intervention studies. For example, MacMillan and Thomas (1993) conducted a pilot study to assess the feasibility of designing an intervention for high-risk families with histories of abuse. Through this work, they were able to describe and refine the specific intervention used by public health nurses on their visits to the families prior to mounting a larger study.

Intervention studies are expensive to mount because of the costs of recruiting and following large numbers of subjects over time. Gagnon et al. (1997) recruited 360 postpartum women from three sites to evaluate the effectiveness of the delivery of two interventions (telephone versus home visits). Insufficient funding limits the size of samples that can be recruited into projects and hence decreases confidence in the findings. Health promotion interventions may require long-term monitoring in order to detect any impact on the health status of the participants. Additionally, funding for some applied research, such as action research or qualitative research, may be difficult to secure because these approaches are unknown to and/or discredited by some reviewers.

Studies conducted in the community have many additional costs. Data collection is expensive when costs for recruitment, travel to participants' homes, telephone charges, and other expenses are considered. Some innovative approaches to intervention studies have been conducted while containing costs. Davies et al. (1992) used senior baccalaureate nursing students to deliver the research intervention in the "Time to Quit" Self-Help Smoking Cessation Program. By having each participating student recruit two subjects, a sufficiently large sample size (N=312) was secured to carry out the quasi-experimental study. Approaches to curtailing costs while maintaining research standards include the use of naturally occurring focus groups, town hall meetings, and telephone surveys.

There is evidence of increasing funding opportunities for nurses. Thibaudeau (1995) surveyed community health nursing/public health nursing research between 1990 and 1993. One-third of the projects received funding from national research agencies such as Health Canada (e.g., the National Health Research & Development Program [NHRDP]) and national foundations. Approximately 40 percent of the projects were funded by provincial agencies (e.g., Manitoba Health Research Council). The remaining studies were funded by nursing foundations and associations and by universities.

Given the continual preparation of nurses with research training at the doctoral level, nurse researchers will be better situated to compete for research grants. A nurse with a doctoral degree was the principal investigator or co-investigator in most (80 percent) of the studies published in the past four years reviewed for this chapter. In the earlier review (Chalmers & Gregory, 1995), fewer than half of the researchers were prepared at the doctoral level. This finding reflects a maturation of researchers in community health nursing.

Agency infrastructure for research

Community health nursing services are delivered through numerous agencies and organizations, such as provincial and municipal departments of health and non-governmental organizations. Because of the numbers of agencies and their relatively small size (compared with hospitals and universities), many settings do not have the resources to support nursing research initiatives (e.g., a nursing research centre) evident in tertiary institutions. Such centres develop procedures for access within the institution, link researchers with clinicians, and assist with other aspects of the research process. As well, such centres provide visibility for nursing research efforts within the organization.

More recently, community health agencies have begun to develop the infrastructure needed to support research efforts. For example, the Hamilton–Wentworth Health Department has an active teaching unit linking university and public health agency staff for educational, research, and practice development initiatives. An infrastructure that supports research and links university nursing researchers with community health agencies would facilitate community health nursing research. This linkage can promote the conduct of research and also aid the diffusion and implementation of research findings.

As the infrastructure supports for research in community health agencies increase, opportunities for developing collaborative multi-site research projects nationally and internationally will expand. This is particularly important when large sample sizes are needed for specific research designs or when phenomena occur less frequently in populations. Larger multi-site projects can avoid "overloading" participants in follow-up studies in single-site locations. As with any multiple-site research, however, agency and ethical approval procedures can be complex.

Implementing research designs

Implementing research designs may present challenges in community settings. Identifying populations for sampling may be difficult because people are often not recruited through health care facilities. For example, specific populations at risk for breast cancer because of family history cannot be accessed readily through hospital or community clinics, since few services exist. This may result in expenditures of considerable time and budget in the recruitment phase of projects. As well, recruitment through public mechanisms, such as newspaper advertisements, newsletters, and community organizations, may limit sampling to specific segments of the population. People with decreased resources (time, finances, or energy) may not be represented using these approaches.

Sample accrual may be time consuming when many agencies need to be accessed concurrently to secure participants. Because of the decentralized service delivery in community health agencies, recruitment may involve numerous sites that yield relatively few participants. This increases researcher time and study costs. With the move toward regionalization of health care in many provinces, a researcher carrying out a study throughout the province would be required to obtain permission from all the Regional Health Authorities (RHAs). In Manitoba, for example, this means working with 11 RHAs.

Since many people in the community are mobile, securing a sample may not necessarily guarantee that participants will be available for the duration of a study. This may be a particular problem in longitudinal studies of high-risk populations.

Ethical review committees familiar with traditional research designs may find the more interactive methodologies, such as participatory action research, problematic. Time may need to be devoted to convincing committees of the authenticity of the research design prior to attending to ethical issues.

Experimental and quasi-experimental studies are difficult to conduct in community settings. Random assignment to intervention and control groups may be possible, but controlling for contamination of the intervention from the intervention group or exposure in the general population may be difficult. Designs that allow for more control, and hence more confidence in the findings, may need to be forfeited in consideration of participants' needs. For example, Edwards, Ciliska, et al. (1992) in their study of health promotion with immigrants—some of whom had experienced torture and political oppression—opted to forgo a matched post-test so that participants could be offered complete anonymity.

In summary, there are numerous practical challenges to be addressed when conducting community-based research. These challenges are present at all stages of the research process and include securing adequate funds and designing and implementing studies in the field. As the number of well-prepared nurse researchers grows and the structures to support community health research develop, many of these barriers to research will decrease. Continuing challenges for community health nurse researchers include taking advantage of funding opportunities at the local, regional, and national levels and promoting agency infrastructure for research.

Future challenges

Future community health nursing research will be fostered through the following initiatives and efforts:

- systematic knowledge development, whereby research priorities at the local, provincial, and national levels are defined
- programmatic research initiatives that address knowledge deficits
- interdisciplinary research that capitalizes on the strengths of other disciplines, such as community medicine, epidemiology, and social work

- policies and structures to ensure appropriate dissemination of findings to governmental departments, health agencies, and educational centres
- purposeful uptake of new community health nursing knowledge by program planners and relevant policy decision makers.

Limitations of the review

Not all studies found in the search results included an abstract. Therefore, some excellent studies may not have been included in this overview. Also, occupational health or home nursing studies were not reviewed. Although care was taken to search the CINAHL and Medline data bases thoroughly, it is possible that Canadian articles published in non-indexed journals may have been overlooked. Researchers may also contribute to the invisibility of community health nursing research by not indexing their work with descriptors or keywords such as those used to review the data bases for this chapter. For example, a study of Indian health transfer policy (Gregory, Russell, Hurd, Tyance, & Sloan, 1992), despite its relevance for this review, was not retrieved through multiple searches. Similarly, Kulig's (1995) work among Cambodian refugee women was not accessed through the search process. As well, completed research that has not yet been published was not included in the review, as there is a time lag between the completion of research projects and publication.

Conclusion

This discussion of theoretical, methodological, practical, and future challenges has highlighted many positive developments in community health nursing research. Of particular note are the breadth in focus of the studies, the emphasis on many aspects of nursing practice (e.g., evaluation of outcomes), and the attention to several high-risk target groups in the community. Many gaps and challenges will need attention by community health nursing researchers in the future. Individuals (including members of selected high-risk groups) and aggregates are emphasized, whereas families, the community as client, macro-level structures and processes, policy, and community development are neglected. There is also little evidence of programmatic research; single, unrelated projects appear to be the norm. The scope of the field of community health nursing may influence nurse researchers to mount many lines of inquiry and thus may deter a focus on knowledge development. However, despite these limitations, community health nursing research shows promise of developing the knowledge needed to enhance and develop practice.

QUESTIONS

1. To what extent does nursing theory guide community health nursing research? Justify your answer.
2. Identify research methods that are congruent with the philosophy of community health nursing practice.
3. Community health nursing research has traditionally focussed on individuals, particularly those who are members of high-risk groups. Which clients have been overlooked?
4. What are the priority areas for future community health nursing research?

REFERENCES

Allen, D.G. (1987). Critical social theory as a model for analyzing ethical issues in family and community health. *Family and Community Health, 10*(1), 63–72.

Aryanwu, C.V. (1988). The technique of participatory research in community development. *Community Development Journal, 23*(10), 11–15.

Association of Community Health Nursing Educators (ACHNE). (1992). *Research priorities for community health nursing.* Lexington, KY: Author.

Association of Community Health Nursing Educators (ACHNE). (1993). *Differentiated nursing practice in community health.* Lexington, KY: Author.

Battle Haugh, E., & Spence Laschinger, H. (1996). Power and opportunity in public health nursing work environments. *Public Health Nursing, 13*(1), 42–49.

Beddome, G., Clarke, H.F., & Whyte, N.B. (1993). Vision for the future of public health nursing: A case for primary health care. *Public Health Nursing, 10*(1), 13–18.

Bramadat, I.J., Chalmers, K., & Andrusyszyn, M.A. (1996). Knowledge, skills and experience for community health nursing practice: The perceptions of community nurses, administrators and educators. *Journal of Advanced Nursing, 24*(6), 1224–1233.

Butterfield, P. (1990). Thinking upstream: Nurturing a conceptual understanding of the societal context of health behaviour. *Advances in Nursing Science, 12*(2), 1–8.

Canadian Public Health Association (CPHA). (1990). *Community health/public health nursing in Canada: Preparation and practice.* Ottawa: Author.

Chalmers, K. (1992a). Working with men: An analysis of health visiting practice in families with young children. *International Journal of Nursing Studies, 29*(1), 3–16.

Chalmers, K.I. (1992b). Giving and receiving: An empirically derived theory on health visiting practice. *Journal of Advanced Nursing, 17,* 1317–1325.

Chalmers, K.I. (1993). Searching for health needs: The work of health visiting. *Journal of Advanced Nursing, 18,* 900–911.

Chalmers, K.I., Bramadat, I.J., & Sloan, J. (1997). Development and testing of the Primary Health Care Questionnaire (PHCQ): Results with students and faculty in diploma and degree programs. *Canadian Journal of Nursing Research, 29*(1), 79–96.

Chalmers, K.I., & Gregory, D.M. (1995). Community health nursing research: Theoretical and practical challenges. In M.J. Stewart (Ed.)., *Community Nursing: Promoting Canadians' health* (pp. 600–617). Toronto: W.B. Saunders.

Ciliska, D., Mitchell, A., Baumann, A., Sheppard, K., Van Berkel, C., Adam, V., Underwood, J., & Southwell, D. (1996). Changing nursing practice—trisectoral collaboration in decision making. *Canadian Journal of Nursing Administration, 9*(2), 60–73.

Clarke, H., Beddome, G., & Whyte, N. (1993). Public health nurses' vision of their future reflects changing paradigms. *Image: Journal of Nursing Scholarship, 25*(4), 305–310.

Davies, B.L., Matte-Lewis, L., O'Connor, A.M., Dulberg, C.S., & Drake, E.R. (1992). Evaluation of the "Time to Quit" self-help smoking cessation program. *Canadian Journal of Public Health, 83*, 19–23.

Dickson, F., & Tutty, L.M. (1996). The role of public health nurses in responding to abused women. *Public Health Nursing, 13*(4), 263–268.

Duncan, S.M. (1992). Ethical challenge in community health nursing. *Journal of Advanced Nursing, 17*, 1035–1041.

Edwards, N., Ciliska, D., Halbert, T., & Pond, M. (1992). Health promotion and health advocacy for and by immigrants enrolled in English as a second language classes. *Canadian Journal of Public Health, 83*(2), 159–161.

Edwards, N.C., & Sims-Jones, N. (1997). A randomized controlled trial of alternative approaches to community follow-up for postpartum women. *Canadian Journal of Public Health, 88*(2), 123–128.

Forchuk, C. (1992). The orientation phase of the nurse–client relationship: How long does it take? *Perspectives in Psychiatric Care, 28*(4), 7–10.

Gagnon, A.J., Edgar, L., Kramer, M.S. Papageorgiou, A., Waghorn, K., & Klein, M.C. (1997). A randomized trial of a program of early postpartum discharge with nurse visitation. *American Journal of Obstetrics & Gynecology, 176*(1), 205–211.

Gregory, D., Russell, C., Hurd, J., Tyance, J., & Sloan, J. (1992). Canada's Indian health transfer policy: The Gull Bay Band experience. *Human Organization, 51*(3), 214–222.

Hamilton, P. (1991). Theoretical and methodological considerations for research in community health nursing. In B.M. Chambers (Ed.)., *State of the art in community health nursing education, research and practice* (pp. 42–51). Louisville, KY: ACHNE.

Hanchett, E., & Clarke, P. (1989). Nursing theory and public health science: Is synthesis possible? *Public Health Nursing, 5*(1), 2–6.

Holter, I., & Schwartz-Barcott, D. (1993). Action research: What is it? How has it been used and how can it be used in nursing? *Journal of Advanced Nursing, 18*, 298–304.

Kirkpatrick, S.M. (1990). Participatory nursing research: A promising methodology in third world countries. *Western Journal of Nursing Research, 12*(3), 282.

Kulig, J.C. (1994)."Those with unheard voices": The plight of a Cambodian refugee woman. *Journal of Community Health Nursing, 11*(2), 99–107.

Kulig, J.C. (1995). Cambodian refugees' family planning knowledge. *Journal of Advanced Nursing, 22*, 150–157.

Kulig, J.C., & Wilde, I. (1996). Collaboration between communities and universities: Completion of a community needs assessment. *Public Health Nursing, 13*(2), 112–119.

Leipert, B.D. (1996). The value of community health nursing: A phenomenological study of the perceptions of community health nurses. *Public Health Nursing, 13*(1), 50–57.

MacMillan, H., & Thomas, H. (1993). Public health nurse home visitation for the tertiary prevention of child maltreatment: Results of a pilot study. *Canadian Journal of Psychiatry, 38*, 436–442.

Mason, R.A., & Boutilier, M.A. (1995). Unemployment as an issue for public health: Preliminary findings from North York. *Canadian Journal of Public Health, 86*(3), 152–153.

Mitchell, A., Van Berkel, C., Adam, V., Ciliska, D., Sheppard, K., Baumann, A., Underwood, J., Walter, S., Gafni, A., Edwards, N., & Southwell, D. (1993). Comparison of liaison and staff nurses in discharge referrals of postpartum patients for public health nursing follow-up. *Nursing Research, 42*(4), 245–249.

Ploeg, J., Black, M.E., Hutchison, B.G., Walter, S.D., Scott, E.A.F., & Chambers, L.W. (1994). Personal, home and community safety promotion with community-dwelling elderly persons: Responses to a public health nurse intervention. *Canadian Journal of Public Health, 85*(3), 188–191.

Poulin, C., Gyorkos, T., MacPhee, J., Cann, B., & Bickerton, J. (1992). Contact-tracing among injection drug users in a rural area. *Canadian Journal of Public Health, 83*(2), 106–108.

Purkis, M.E. (1997). The "social determinants" of practice? A critical analysis of the discourse of health promotion. *Canadian Journal of Nursing Research, 29*(1), 47–62.

Russell, C.K., Gregory, D.M., Wotton, D., Mordoch, E., & Counts, M.M. (1996). ACTION: Application and extension of the GENESIS Community Analysis Model. *Public Health Nursing, 13*(3), 187–194.

Spence Laschinger, H.K., Goldenberg, D., & Dal Bello, D. (1995). Community health nurses' HIV care behavior. *Journal of Community Health Nursing, 12*(3), 147–159.

Stewart, M.J., Gillis, A., Brosky, G., Johnston, G., Kirkland, S., Leigh, G., Persaud, V., Rootman, I., Jackson, S., & Pawliw-Fry, B. (1996). Smoking among disadvantaged women: Causes and cessation. *Canadian Journal of Nursing Research, 28*(1), 41–60.

Stuart, M. (1992). "Half a loaf is better than no bread": Public health nurses and physicians in Ontario, 1920–1925. *Nursing Research, 41*(1), 21–27.

Tenn, L. (1995). Primary health care nursing education in Canadian university schools of nursing. *Journal of Nursing Education, 34*(8), 350-357.

Thibaudeau, M.F. (1995). Status of community health nursing research in Canada. In M.J. Stewart (Ed.), *Community nursing: Promoting Canadians' health* (pp. 558–576). Toronto: W.B. Saunders.

Zilm, G., & Warbinek, E. (1995). Early tuberculosis nursing in British Columbia. *Canadian Journal of Nursing Research, 27*(3), 65–81.

C H A P T E R   2 7

Nursing intervention studies: Issues related to change and timing

Laurie N. Gottlieb and Nancy Feeley

A variety of challenges confront clinicians and researchers involved in developing and testing community nursing interventions or programs for children and their families. Many of these challenges relate to the issues of change and timing. This chapter discusses some of the critical questions that must be considered when designing and evaluating interventions with this particular population. The authors propose that careful consideration of these questions will improve the design of intervention studies and the evaluation of their outcomes, as well as contribute to the development of knowledge in this domain.

LEARNING OBJECTIVES

In this chapter, you will learn:

- several key conceptual issues related to change and timing that must be considered when designing intervention studies and the methodological implications that arise from these issues
- the advantages and disadvantages of providing a standardized intervention and alternatives that may be utilized
- three perspectives concerning the conditions that influence change in children and/or families
- two reasons why control or comparative groups should be considered in the design of studies that assess change in children or families

Introduction

The issue of change is at the heart of nursing practice and the conduct of nursing science. Nursing interventions are typically employed to help clients and families bring about a desired change. Evaluation studies seek to examine to what extent an intervention has resulted in the desired change in the target population (those individuals, families, groups or communities to which the intervention is directed). Recent trends in health promotion intervention research indicate a broadening of focus to include not only changes in self (e.g., health behaviours and lifestyles), but also changes in environment (e.g., physical, social, economic). How researchers conceptualize change and change processes will shape the ways they choose to work with individuals and families and the methodologies they select to evaluate effectiveness.

Although change is ubiquitous, it often escapes scrutiny (Mahoney, 1991). Yet, such scrutiny of change in client outcomes is necessary in community nursing practice. Limited financial resources and the demand for evidence of the effectiveness and efficiency of health care services have resulted in the recognition that there is a compelling need for research assessing the impact of community nursing practice on client health outcomes (Barriball & Mackenzie, 1993; Goeppinger, 1988; Kristjanson & Chalmers, 1991).

When designing intervention studies, researchers and clinicians are faced with two major decision-making areas. The first concerns decisions related to change. Such questions need to be considered as: What are we trying to change? Whom are we trying to change? How does change come about? How can we determine that change can be attributed in part to the intervention? The second area concerns decisions related to the timing of the intervention. It is impossible for clinicians and researchers to consider change without confronting issues of timing. Timing is important, as it relates to the design and implementation of the intervention and the measurement of its impact. The types of questions that need to be addressed here are: When should the intervention occur? How long does an intervention have to continue to effect long-lasting change? Another set of questions concerns timing as it relates to the point at which outcome measures should be taken: When can we expect change to occur? How long will the change last?

These were some of the questions that the authors confronted in designing a randomized control trial study to evaluate the effectiveness of a year-long, home-based nursing intervention to enhance the psychosocial adjustment of children with a chronic condition (Pless et al., 1994). The nursing intervention was guided by the McGill Model of Nursing (Gottlieb & Rowat, 1987; Kravitz & Frey, 1989). The major features that characterize this model include a focus on overall health rather than illness and treatment, on all family members rather than the patient alone, on family goals rather than the nurse's, and on family strengths rather than deficits. According to this model, nursing takes place within a collaborative relationship wherein both the nurse and the family jointly assume responsibility. The nurse's role is to structure learning experiences that empower families and enable them to define their issues of concern and arrive at approaches to meet their goals.

The purpose of this chapter is to identify some issues and challenges specifically related to change and timing that need to be considered in intervention research with children and families in the community. The authors will draw on their experience in conducting the above study, as well as other empirical research, to illustrate the conceptual issues and their methodological implications.

Conceptual and methodological issues involving change

Several conceptual and methodological issues relate specifically to the process of change itself, including understanding the phenomenon, deciding who should be the focus of the change intervention, identifying the pathways that can lead to change, and evaluating whether the intervention effected the change. Depending on the kind and quality of change that is desired, the questions involved in understanding the process of change can be complex.

What are we trying to change?
Understanding the phenomenon

The impetus for conducting an intervention study often comes about because clinicians and/or researchers identify an area in need of change and believe they know how to effect change. The first and most fundamental question that they must ask when designing an intervention study is: What is the nature of the phenomenon that is being targeted for change? The answer to this question is premised on theoretical understanding about the phenomenon targeted for change and knowledge about change and change processes. A thorough understanding of the phenomenon and its characteristics is required because certain phenomena are more amenable to change than others, and different methodological implications will arise depending on the nature of the phenomenon.

For example, specific behaviours such as children's temper tantrums might be more readily changed than children's shyness. Temper tantrums are shaped by the type and amount of reinforcement (negative and positive) given by parents and others, whereas shyness is a temperament trait that is genetically influenced.

A subset of questions that need to be addressed to clarify the researcher's understanding of the characteristics of the phenomenon under study include: What purpose does the phenomenon serve to the system's integrity and/or to its maintenance and organization? How does the phenomenon develop over time? How long has it been in place? This knowledge will determine the type of change that can be expected and will help forecast how long the change should take to achieve.

For example, phenomena that involve core processes, such as the con-struction of self (self-esteem, identity), values (valence), reality (order), and power (control), are more difficult to change because they develop slowly, involve deep structural changes within the organism and system, and main-tain the system's integrity (Mahoney, 1991). Thus, an intervention of short duration would be unlikely to alter a child's self-esteem. This implies that intervention studies that target core processes need to be long-term to effect any perceptible, long-lasting changes. We will return to the issue of length and intensity of an intervention later in this chapter.

Another characteristic to consider is the form the phenomenon takes at various phases of development. This is particularly relevant to the study of young children. The issue here is that the phenomenon of interest may exhibit itself differently at different ages, as it evolves and changes.

For example, if the researcher is interested in children's gross motor devel-opment, the researcher would observe turning and crawling in the infant, but with toddlers, walking and running would be more appropriate indicators of gross motor development. Thus, the challenge for the researcher is to deter-mine what constitutes "same" and "analogous" behaviours across ages (Kessen, 1960). Consequently, when repeated assessments of the phenome-non are made over time as children grow and develop, different instruments may be required to measure the same phenomenon at different ages.

In our study, we assessed children's self-esteem with the Perceived Competency Scale for Children (Harter, 1982). Two different versions of this measure were used, one for children under seven years of age, and another for children older than age seven. Harter developed these different versions because as children develop, their notion of self-esteem becomes more com-plex and differentiated. For example, in younger children self-esteem is man-ifested in four areas (maternal acceptance, peer acceptance, and physical and cognitive competence), whereas for older children there are five specific domains of self-esteem (scholastic, athletic, and social competence; physical appearance; and behavioural conduct) and a general domain of global self-esteem.

The wide variability in the expression of the phenomenon of interest within age groups must also be considered. Variability can be affected by a multitude of factors such as genotype, gender, maturity determinants (e.g., taking on age-appropriate roles and responsibilities), cultural factors, co-occurrence of other life course events (e.g., entry to school), and social/contextual factors (e.g., support, poverty, maternal employment) (Aldous, 1990; Walsh, 1983). This underscores the importance of including control or comparison groups in order to attribute change to the intervention and not to the factors listed above. We shall return to this point later.

Yet another question that must be addressed concerns the purpose of the intervention. Does the intervention seek to develop the phenomenon, change it, or maintain it? This is an important distinction both for shaping the intervention and for determining the types of outcomes to measure. If the goal of the intervention is to develop a new set of behaviours, then the intervention should focus on helping parents and children acquire new knowledge and develop new skills. Prenatal classes and parenting programs are examples of interventions by community health nurses aimed at developing new knowledge and skills. When evaluating the effectiveness of the intervention, one would expect to find little evidence of the skill pre-intervention and some evidence of its development post-intervention.

On the other hand, if the goal of the intervention is to change or alter a behaviour, the intervention may focus on extinguishing old behaviours, introducing new ones, and reinforcing them. For example, programs that are designed to alter unhealthy behaviours, such as behavioural training programs for parents who have abused their children (Wolfe & Wekerle, 1993), would fall within this category. The analyses would focus on examining patterns of change and trends across time for the various behaviours.

Finally, if the goal of the intervention is maintenance, the intervention would focus on support and reinforcement. Stability and consistency across time would be used as indices of maintenance.

Whom are we trying to change?
Deciding on the target for change

When working with children and families, it is not always readily apparent who should be the focus of the intervention and subsequently the target of evaluation. In practice, community health nurses work at various levels of the family system and the larger environment to effect change. In designing a nursing intervention study, the researcher may decide to focus on (a) individuals (e.g., mother, child), (b) subsystems (e.g., mother–child relationship), and/or (c) the family as a system, including its relationships with other social systems (e.g., extended family, health care system). Issues such as the knowledge of change and change processes, the potential different rates of change among different family members, and the person(s) who can best evaluate change need to be considered when making this decision.

Knowledge of change and change processes. It is important to understand the conditions that influence change in children and families and the mechanisms by which change takes place. These understandings usually derive from foundational knowledge about change and change processes. Researchers and clinicians need to articulate the theoretical bases of their perspective in planning and measuring change.

For example, if the researcher subscribes to the theoretical position that the child is active and shapes the social environment (Sameroff, 1987), then the intervention would focus on the child only, and measures of change would focus on child outcomes. The child's social environment consists of the patterns of interactions and relationships that transpire between the child and other individuals.

On the other hand, if the researcher subscribes to the belief that the child is a passive agent whose behaviour is shaped by the social environment, then the intervenor would elect to work with the mother alone to change the child's behaviour. Assessment, therefore, would be concerned primarily with child outcomes and secondarily with parent outcomes.

However, if the researcher subscribes to a constructivist view of development (Mahoney, 1991; Scarr, 1992) in which both the child and the environment are active, responsive agents, the nurse would work with both the child and the mother. Changes in both the child and the environment would be the focus of measurement.

In the authors' intervention study with chronically ill children and their families, we were concerned with effecting change in both the child and the family environment. Hence, the nurses worked with the child, siblings, parents individually, and/or various dyads and triads within the family. There is empirical support for the effectiveness of such a multipronged approach to intervention. Reviews of the research on early childhood intervention programs and programs for maltreating parents have concluded that comprehensive interventions aimed at multiple levels of the child and family system are likely to be most effective in bringing about the desired outcomes in child development (Seitz, Rosenbaum, & Apfel, 1985; Wolfe & Wekerle, 1993; Zigler, Taussig, & Black, 1992).

A second theoretical notion underlying our study, as well as many models of family nursing, is that of Family Systems Theory. Family Systems Theory posits that each individual and subsystem within the family operates interdependently, influencing and being influenced by the others (Minuchin, 1985). Change in one part of a family system may affect the total system, as well as its subsystems (Mercer, 1989). Although an intervention may be targeted at one family member, change in other family members and the system as a whole may also occur.

For example, an intervention focussed on the child may result in unexpected changes at other levels of the system (Gray & Wandersman, 1980). To capture these unexpected outcomes, multiple measures should be employed within and across domains of potential health outcomes for different individuals and subsystems.

To continue with the example from our study, the authors used several standardized measures of child, parent, and family outcomes to measure the *a priori* hypothesized mechanisms and outcomes. In addition, we included a qualitative component to capture the unexpected. We interviewed the chronically ill child's primary caregiver (usually the mother) to explore that person's perceptions about what changes had occurred and how these changes had come about (Ezer, Bray, & Gros, 1994). Mothers reported several outcomes that had not been captured with the standardized measures we had chosen. For example, they described the child taking more responsibility for the management of the chronic illness, gaining in self-confidence, and doing better in school.

Different rates of change within families and between families. Traditionally, researchers have been concerned with measuring rates of change among different families. More recently, attention has turned to examining rates of change within families. The impetus for this trend is the growing recognition that children, other family members, subsystems within the family, and the family system as a whole have their own developmental trajectory. When families are being formed, experiencing novel events, or dealing with stressful situations, change will be more rapid because family processes (e.g., communication, decision making) are being reoriented and re-established. This implies that depending on the kind of change desired, the intensity and the duration of nursing involvement required within and across families may vary. When selecting an approach to intervening, the researcher should consider tailoring the intervention to the unique needs of each person and family. We will return to the issue of tailoring interventions later in this chapter.

Who will assess change? An important decision that the researcher faces is who in the family will be asked to assess whether change has occurred. The most obvious choice is the individual targeted for change. However, in research with children and families this choice is not always straightforward, because children are often too young to respond to self-report measures. In the past, research has relied on mothers' reports to assess change in their children, as well as change in the family (Ball, McKenry, & Price-Bonham, 1983), because of their intimate knowledge of family life, the amount of time that mothers spend with their children, and their availability to researchers. Although mothers' responses are important, theirs is just one of many perspectives on children and family life.

It has been commonly assumed that everyone in the family has one shared family environment and experiences that environment in the same way. However, recent empirical studies have pointed out that this is not the case. Each family member has a different experience in the family and creates his or her own subjective meanings (Dunn & Plomin, 1990). For example, first-born children have inexperienced parents, whereas later-born children have experienced parents. Moreover, each child has his or her own personality, which may have a differential effect on how parents respond. These findings have important consequences for designing intervention studies. The implication of this principle is that the respondent must be kept constant across repeated measures.

For example, in our study we were concerned with changes in the child's behaviour prior to and after the intervention. We asked parents to complete a standardized child behavioural checklist prior to the start of the intervention. If the mother completed the report at baseline and the father completed the assessment at the end of the intervention, we excluded these data from the analyses because mothers' perceptions and experiences may differ from those of fathers.

A second implication that arises as a result of the notion of non-shared environments concerns the use of multiple respondents. Traditionally, researchers have used triangulation as a test of the validity of a measure. Triangulation is a term that commonly refers to the use of multiple measures to converge on a construct (Breitmayer, Ayres, & Knafl, 1993). Nonetheless, other purposes for triangulation have also been described (Knafl & Breitmayer, 1989). Multiple respondents have been considered necessary in family research in order to capture the complexity of family systems and obtain a comprehensive view of the family (Moriarty, 1990). However, given the current understanding, different family members' reports of the same phenomenon should be expected to diverge rather than converge.

For example, when trying to assess how well children have done as a result of the intervention, the researcher may want to know whether change is apparent to both parents, as well as to those outside the family. She or he may also want to know whether the child's behaviour is consistent at home or at school. To this end, the researcher may elect to collect information about the child from the child him/herself, the child's siblings, peers, parents, teachers, and anyone else of relevance. However, the researcher should expect moderate correlations among individuals because children's behaviour is fairly consistent, but there is variability within this consistency. Children and adults may respond differently in different situations with different people.

How does change come about?
Pathways toward change
Many evaluations of program effectiveness have failed to recognize that processes of development, individual differences in development, and environmental and contextual factors will lead to some children and families benefiting from an intervention, while others will remain the same, and some may even be harmed by it. Increasingly, researchers are recognizing that the question is not: Does this intervention work? but rather, What intervention works with whom, in what domain of functioning, and under what circumstances (Dunst, Synder, & Mankinen, 1989; Gray & Wandersman, 1980)? Two approaches to data analysis may facilitate an understanding in this area: (a) an examination of overall group differences (between-group differences)

and (b) an examination of within-intervention group differences through case or profile analysis (Bergman, 1992; Gray & Wandersman, 1980). These two approaches to analysis should complement each other.

Careful documentation of the intervention will allow the researcher to track the processes that occur during the intervention and will also yield the data needed for the profile analyses that may provide important insights into why the intervention worked for some children but not for others.

For example, in our study the first set of analyses examined the differences between children who received nursing care and those who did not with respect to child behaviour problems, role skills, and self-worth. To understand why and how some children benefited while others deteriorated over the course of the intervention, we conducted a profile analysis. This was accomplished by compiling a profile of children's scores on many variables collected from many different sources (e.g., parent report on standardized measures, nurses' description of each contact with the families during the course of the intervention, and parent interviews conducted post-intervention) (Gottlieb & Feeley, 1996). Improvement in child psychosocial adjustment was shown to be linked to the ability of the mother and/or child to become engaged in the intervention, the nature of the issues worked on, and the nurse's direct involvement with school-age children and adolescents.

How can we know that the intervention contributed to the observed change?

Although it is difficult to attribute change solely to the intervention, nonetheless there are research procedures that, if followed, allow the researcher to infer that some of the change can be attributed to the intervention. This issue is all the more salient in research with children. Because change occurs at a more rapid pace in children, it is sometimes difficult to determine whether a change is due to another event occurring at the same time as the intervention, to the intervention itself, or to a naturally occurring developmental shift in the child (Rutter, 1983).

To illustrate: After the birth of a second child, mothers commonly report an increase in toileting accidents in their preschool first-borns (Stewart, 1990). However, it is difficult to know if this is due to the preschoolers' way of dealing with the stress accompanying the sibling's birth or whether it is due to a natural lapse that is part of the course of toilet training.

The use of a control or comparative group is the most common strategy to address this issue. Control is particularly important to establish in the study of both children and families to counter the argument that change may have occurred as a result of maturation (Bailey & Simeonsson, 1986). In experiments, control is obtained through comparison of the participants who did and did not receive the intervention (Fugate-Woods, 1988). In addition, random assignment of study participants to either the intervention or the control group (a critical feature of experimental design) reduces the likelihood of systematic bias in the two groups with respect to any variables that might be linked to the outcome of interest (Polit & Hungler, 1989). The groups that are formed following random assignment should be comparable with respect to a variety of background characteristics.

In the event that one cannot use a control group, then comparative groups are a reasonable alternative. When studying naturally occurring events, such as the birth of a sibling, it is impossible to randomly assign first-borns to families having a new baby and those not. Instead, a comparison group can be selected from individuals known to be similar to those who will receive the intervention with respect to several pertinent characteristics that have been found to affect the phenomenon (Friedman, 1987).

We will illustrate this point with an example of children's adjustment to a sibling's birth. In a study undertaken by Gottlieb and Baillies (1995), the phenomenon under study concerned understanding first-borns' reactions during their mother's pregnancy. A group of only children whose mother was not pregnant served as the comparison. The comparison group was matched with the "pregnancy group" children by age, because age had been found to influence first-borns' reactions to a sibling's birth (Gottlieb & Mendelson, 1990).

In summary, before undertaking the design and implementation of an intervention study with children and families in the community, nurse researchers and clinicians need to spend considerable time gaining a thorough understanding about the phenomenon they are trying to change and the processes by which change comes about. Only when one has acquired this understanding is one ready to proceed to decisions related to timing.

Conceptual and methodological issues involving timing

The issue of timing is critical to the design of intervention studies, particularly as it relates to the timing of the intervention and the measurement of outcomes. There are two specific questions that researchers need to examine: when to intervene and how long an intervention should last.

When to intervene?

When designing an intervention the researcher needs to ask the following questions: When should the intervention begin? At what point would the intervention be most effective in bringing about the desired outcomes? Underlying these questions is knowledge of when change is most likely to occur.

Change is more rapid and more readily achievable during a critical period, such as when core processes are being laid down and/or transformed, as in infancy, early childhood, and adolescence. Many early childhood intervention programs are premised on this assumption (Carnegie Corporation of New York, 1994; Hamburg, 1992). Change is also more achievable during periods of transition, critical life events, or stressful experiences. This is not surprising in light of the theoretical understanding of what happens during these periods (Schumacher & Meleis, 1994). These events make new demands, which in turn cause major disruptions to individuals and families. To meet these demands, individuals and families must master new ways of coping, redefine existing relationships, learn new roles, and/or restructure a different sense of self. In attempting to meet these challenges, individuals and families are more vulnerable and consequently more open to change at these times.

Therefore, transitions, critical life events, and stressful experiences are important periods for growth. Nurses have a key role to play in promoting growth and change. If the goal of the intervention is to change core processes and develop new insights, knowledge, and skills, then these periods provide the best opportunity for entrée into the family.

In our study, we decided to include families who had been living with the child's chronic condition for at least a year, and we excluded those whose child had been recently diagnosed. Our choice may have made it more difficult to bring about change in child psychosocial adjustment, because families had been living with the chronic illness for at least one year and as many as 14 years.

There is some empirical evidence to suggest that the timing of an intervention plays a role in the process of change. Larson (1980) found that the timing of a home visitation program for mothers was critical in effecting positive mother–infant outcomes. Mothers who began the intervention during their pregnancy benefited more than mothers who began in the postpartum period. This suggests that interventions aimed at effecting change may be potentially more effective during transitional periods in child and family development, such as the birth of the first child or when a child enters school, or during stressful periods, such as the diagnosis of a chronic illness. Although theoretically this seems to be the case, there have been few systematic studies to support these notions. Kristjanson and Chalmers (1991) observed that there is currently little knowledge in the community health nursing literature concerning the most effective timing of interventions with families.

Even during critical periods, change is a dynamic process punctuated by phases of change intermingled with periods of stability (Mahoney, 1991). In contrast to the view that change and continuity are distinct and independent constructs (Fawcett, 1989; Hall, 1981, 1983), we believe that change and continuity are separate but integrally related, co-dependent constructs (Liddle & Saba, 1983; Mahoney, 1991). Mahoney (1991) argues that stabilizing processes are self-protective inasmuch as they enable the person or family to function in the face of new demands without disintegrating or becoming disorganized. For example, when a new child is born the family roles and relationships will change to incorporate the needs of the new child. But at the same time, the family will adhere to old patterns of functioning (e.g., maintaining usual daily routines).

The co-existence of change and self-stabilizing processes helps to explain why change is difficult to achieve. Despite the need for longitudinal research, granting agencies tend to favour short-term intervention studies. Researchers may be confronted with having to choose between intense interventions with a small number of families and less intense interventions with a greater number of families (Gray & Wandersman, 1980).

The aim of our study was to improve the psychosocial adjustment of children with a chronic illness and to prevent deterioration. We decided on a year-long intervention because we recognized that the study nurses would require time to develop relationships with the families and to help families work on bringing about the change they desired. Furthermore, we were aware that some families would take more time to develop a relationship with the nurse, and some would be resistant to the nurse's efforts to develop a relationship.

Our understanding of the balance between the need to change and the need to stabilize implies that nurses have to be sensitive to people's energy levels and readiness to change. Interventions must be tailored to the needs of families. The McGill Model of Nursing (Gottlieb & Rowat, 1987) recognizes the importance of timing and pacing. Moreover, there is empirical support for this position. Interventions conducted with children and parents in early childhood have been shown to be more effective when the intervention is tailored to the needs, values, interests, and readiness of the participants and/or the community (Dunst et al., 1989).

However, the clinical realities of timing potentially conflict with the imperatives of experimental designs. In spite of this understanding about change and stability, many disciplines, nursing included, still subscribe to the belief that a key to sound design of intervention studies is the standardization of interventions (Edwards, 1993). Standardization means that all participants receive the same intervention and is premised on the assumption that all individuals have the same needs and will respond in the same fashion.

One potential solution to this dilemma is to establish a "minimum" intervention and tailor further intervention to each family's needs. This was the method we employed in our study of families with a child with a chronic illness. The design called for a minimum number of contacts (one per month) that every family would receive regardless of need over the 12-month period (Pless et al., 1994). Additional contacts were scheduled based on families' needs. Each family, in collaboration with the nurse, determined the "dose" of nursing they received and set the agenda for their work together.

To be able to attribute change to the intervention, the nurses documented numerous details for each contact with the families. Therefore, they maintained contact logs, which described who was present, how long the visit lasted, the location, and who initiated the contact. As well, they described the nature of families' concerns, goals, and types of nursing strategies they used. This enabled us to describe the intervention in depth and to examine the effects of the intervention on outcomes (Gottlieb & Feeley, 1996). The advantage was that the researcher could examine what actually happened for each participant. These data were important for the profile analysis described earlier.

Another potential solution is that used by Webster-Stratton (1992) to evaluate the effectiveness of a parenting program for parents of children with conduct disorders (Webster-Stratton, 1984). Groups of parents view a predetermined series of videotaped vignettes of parent–child interactions. Although the overall program format and content are standardized, the actual administration of the program centres on the interests and concerns of the particular group.

When an intervention is standardized, documentation can still be important. It cannot be assumed that the intervention will be the same for all participants, particularly when the intervention takes place in the home or is delivered by several intervenors (Gray & Wandersman, 1980). A number of factors may contribute to variations in the intervention across participants. Thus, the researcher should acknowledge that there will probably be a discrepancy between the planned and actual intervention and document as completely as possible the actual intervention that participants received (Goeppinger, 1988). Mechanisms for documenting the intervention (such as those described in the example from the authors' study) must be developed prior to beginning the intervention. The difficulty the researcher will encounter is that documentation and analysis of these data are time consuming and tedious for both the nurses and the researcher and seldom considered worthwhile by funding sources.

How long should the intervention last?

How long does an intervention have to be to effect long-lasting change? How frequent should it be? These questions underlie decisions about the intensity of the intervention.

Researchers have little empirical data to guide them in answering these questions, as little is known about what "dose" of community nursing intervention is required to bring about change (Kristjanson & Chalmers, 1991). Research is needed to address this issue. However, knowledge of change processes suggests that an intervention needs to be of reasonable duration to bring about change and should include "boosters" of the intervention (Clarke & Clarke, 1989). The effects of short-term early childhood interventions seem to fade, while more successful programs provide intervention over time, supporting the child and the family through various phases of development (Zigler et al., 1992).

There is some evidence that more intense interventions (high contact over a relatively short period of time) may be more effective. As a result, models currently in use in the domain of infant mental health and psychiatry advocate intensive work with the mother and child (Emde, 1988).

When should change be measured?

Another aspect of timing that needs to be considered is when to measure change and then how to determine whether its effects are long lasting. Although we suggested earlier that it may be best to intervene at the time of a transition, critical life event, or stressful experience, this may not be the best time to assess the outcomes of an intervention. Rather, the researcher should assess outcomes once the transition has been completed.

A thorough understanding of the phenomenon of interest will be helpful. Specifically, knowledge of the timetable under which events unfold is needed to decide when to assess change. Good descriptive studies of developmental transitions, life event trajectories, and the development of phenomena of interest to nurses are needed. Although there is great variability among individuals, the outer ranges of behaviour can be determined. For example, women between the ages of 18 and 45 are considered to be best equipped to meet the challenges and demands of motherhood. Currently, there is debate about the desirability and impact of a woman having a baby at 13 or 60.

Intervention studies typically assess change at just one point in time, for example, immediately following the nursing intervention. The problem with this practice is that researchers may fail to observe change that has yet to emerge (Type II error) or may detect change that is only transitory (Type I error). Only repeated observations of sufficient duration after the completion of the intervention and replication studies will answer questions concerning the permanency of change.

Nurse researchers often expect short-term effects from any intervention. However, some have noted that this may be highly unrealistic, especially in infancy and early childhood when the effects of intervention may not be stable (Emde, 1988). The possibility of delayed effects must also be considered in the design of intervention studies with children and families in the community. Developmental psychologists have become increasingly aware of the possibility of sleeper or delayed effects from follow-up studies of early child intervention programs (Emde, 1988). One major problem has been obtaining the funds for follow-up assessments. Furthermore, it may also be difficult to assess how long a follow-up is required (Emde, 1988).

A case to support the need for multiple points of measurement of change is the study by Stein and Jessop (1991). At the end of the intervention, children who received the year-long home-care intervention were better adjusted than children in the control group, who received routine care. In a five-year follow-up study, the investigators found that the psychosocial adjustment of children who received the intervention continued to improve, while children in the control group remained stable. Thus, the gap between the children who received the intervention and those who did not grew over time. Without these repeated measurements, the long-term effects of this intervention would have gone undetected and the impact of the intervention would have been undermined.

Conclusion

The past two decades of research have yielded rich descriptions of many nursing phenomena. As nursing develops, the discipline will continue to require this descriptive work. Nonetheless, in some domains nurses have accumulated sufficient knowledge to guide work with clients and families to bring about desired changes. As Ellis (cited in Pressler & Fitzpatrick, 1988) argued, nursing is a practice discipline and needs to conduct investigations that will improve practice and the knowledge upon which practice is based. Furthermore, as nursing moves forward in this decade of increasing accountability, there will be mounting pressure to demonstrate its outcomes and effectiveness. In response to these forces, nurses are already encountering evidence of a growing number of intervention studies. This avenue of research will yield knowledge about how to work with children and families and the effectiveness of approaches with whom and when.

As more researchers embark on this path, they need to pay heed to some of the fundamental questions that we have raised in this chapter. Although the issues and questions we have raised are particularly salient when conducting research with children and families, many are highly relevant to the study of adults as well.

While we have proposed answers to these questions, it can be anticipated that other nurse researchers' experiences will provide different answers and raise other questions. It is imperative that clinicians and researchers share these questions, insights about change, and approaches to the assessment of change with others. Continued discussion is clearly needed of the conceptual and methodological issues related to conducting intervention studies in the community with children and their families. This discussion should give rise to the development of new methodological knowledge and new approaches to the design and conduct of intervention studies.

Acknowledgements

We are grateful to Sarah Parry, who assisted with the review of the literature for this chapter; to Dr. Kathleen Rowat for her careful reading of this manuscript and helpful suggestions; and to Evelyn Malowany, director of nursing at the Montréal Children's Hospital, for her continued support of our efforts.

QUESTIONS

As a community health nurse, you have been asked to develop a parenting program for families with preschool children.

1. List the factors you would need to consider when planning the program. Provide a rationale explaining why these particular factors are important.
2. What information would you need to gather to plan the program? Where would you get this information?
3. List three different approaches to evaluating the program. Discuss when each approach should be used and its unique features.
4. What outcomes would you select to assess the effectiveness of the parenting program? Provide a rationale for the outcomes selected.
5. When would you assess these outcomes? Why?
6. Who would assess whether these outcomes have been achieved?

REFERENCES

Aldous, J. (1990). Family development and the life course: Two perspectives on family change. *Journal of Marriage and the Family, 52,* 571–583.

Bailey, D.B., & Simeonsson, R.J. (1986). Design issues in family impact evaluation. In L. Bickman & D.L. Weatherford (Eds.), *Evaluating early intervention programs for severely handicapped children and their families* (pp. 209–230). Austin, TX: Pro-ed.

Ball, D., McKenry, P.C., & Price-Bonham, S. (1983). Use of repeated-measures designs in family research. *Journal of Marriage and the Family, 80,* 885–896.

Barriball, K.L., & Mackenzie, A. (1993). Measuring the impact of nursing interventions in the community: A selective review of the literature. *Journal of Advanced Nursing, 18,* 401–407.

Bergman, L.R. (1992). Studying change in variables and profiles: Some methodological considerations. In J.B. Asendorpf & J. Valsiner (Eds.), *Stability and change in development: A study of methodological reasoning* (pp. 143–149). Newbury Park, CA: Sage.

Breitmayer, B., Ayres, L., & Knafl, K. (1993). Triangulation in qualitative research: Evaluation of completeness and confirmation purposes. *Image: Journal of Nursing Scholarship, 25*(3), 237–243.

Carnegie Corporation of New York. (1994). *Starting points: Meeting the needs of our youngest children. The report of the Carnegie Task Force on meeting the needs of our youngest children.* New York: Author.

Clarke, A.M., & Clarke, A.D.B. (1989). The later cognitive effects of early intervention. *Intelligence, 18,* 289–297.

Dunn, J., & Plomin, R. (1990). *Separate lives: Why siblings are so different.* New York: Basic Books.

Dunst, C.J., Synder, S.W., & Mankinen, M. (1989). Efficacy of early intervention. In M.C. Wang, M.C. Reynolds, & H.J. Walberg (Eds.), *Handbook of special education: Research and practice* (pp. 259–293). Oxford: Pergamon Press.

Edwards, N. (1993). Primary care research in the community. In M.J. Bass, E.J. Dunn, P.G. Norton, M. Stewart, & S. Tudiver (Eds.), *Conducting research in the practice setting.* Newbury Park, CA: Sage.

Emde, R.N. (1988). Risk, intervention and meaning. *Psychiatry, 51*(3), 254–259.

Ezer, H., Bray, C., & Gros, C. (1994). Families' description of the nursing intervention in a randomized control trial [Abstract]. In *Third Annual International Family Nursing Conference: Program and abstracts.* Montréal: McGill University School of Nursing.

Fawcett, J. (1989). *Analysis and evaluation of conceptual models of nursing.* Philadelphia: F.A. Davis.

Friedman, G.D. (1987). *Primer of epidemiology.* Montréal: McGraw-Hill.

Fugate-Woods, N. (1988). Selecting a research design. In N. Fugate-Woods & M. Catanzaro (Eds.), *Nursing research: Theory and practice* (pp. 117–132). Toronto: Mosby.

Goeppinger, J. (1988). Challenges in assessing the impact of nursing service: A community perspective. *Public Health Nursing, 5*(4), 241–245.

Gottlieb, L.N., & Baillies, J. (1995). Firstborns' behaviors during a mother's second pregnancy. *Nursing Research, 44*(6), 356–362.

Gottlieb, L.N., & Feeley, N. (1996). The McGill Model of Nursing and children with a chronic condition: Who benefits and why? *Canadian Journal of Nursing Research, 28*(3), 29–48.

Gottlieb, L.N., & Mendelson, M. (1990). Parental support and firstborn girls' adaptation to a new sibling. *Journal of Applied Developmental Psychology, 11,* 29–48.

Gottlieb, L.N., & Rowat, K. (1987). The McGill Model of Nursing: A practice derived model. *Advances in Nursing Science, 9*(4), 51–61.

Gray, S.W., & Wandersman, L.P. (1980). The methodology of home-based intervention studies: Problems and promising strategies. *Child Development, 51,* 993–1009.

Hall, B.A. (1981). The change paradigm in nursing: Growth and persistence. *Advances in Nursing Science, 3,* 1–6.

Hall, B.A. (1983). Toward an understanding of stability. *Advances in Nursing Science, 5,* 15–20.

Hamburg, D.A. (1992). *Today's children.* New York: Times Book.

Harter, S. (1982). The perceived competence scale for children. *Child Development, 53,* 87–97.

Kessen, W. (1960). Research design in the study of developmental problems. In P.H. Mussen (Ed.), *Handbook of research methods in child development* (pp. 36–70). New York: Wiley.

Knafl, K.A., & Breitmayer, B.J. (1989). Triangulation in qualitative research: Issues of conceptual clarity and purpose. In J. Morse (Ed.), *Qualitative nursing research: A contemporary dialogue* (pp. 209–220). Rockville, MD: Aspen.

Kravitz, M., & Frey, M.A. (1989). The Allen nursing model. In J. Fitzpatrick & A.L. Whall (Eds.), *Conceptual models of nursing: Analysis and application* (2nd ed.) (pp. 313–329). Norwalk, CT: Appleton & Lange.

Kristjanson, L.J., & Chalmers, K.I. (1991). Preventive work with families: Issues facing public health nurses. *Journal of Advanced Nursing, 16,* 147–153.

Larson, C.P. (1980). Efficacy of prenatal and postpartum home visits on child health and development. *Pediatrics, 66*(2), 191–197.

Liddle, H.A., & Saba, G.W. (1983). Clinical use of the family life cycle: Some cautionary guidelines. In J.C. Hanson & H.A. Liddle (Eds.), *Clinical implications of the family life cycle* (pp. 161–175). Rockville, MD: Aspen.

Mahoney, M.J. (1991). *Human change processes: The scientific foundations of psychotherapy.* New York: Basic Books.

Mercer, R. (1989). Theoretical perspectives on the family. In C.L. Gilliss, B.L. Highley, B.M. Roberts, & I.M. Martinson (Eds.), *Toward a science of family nursing* (pp. 9–36). Toronto: Addison-Wesley.

Minuchin, P. (1985). Families and individual development: Provocations from the field of family therapy. *Child Development, 56,* 289–302.

Moriarty, H.J. (1990). Key issues in the family research process: Strategies for nurse researchers. *Advances in Nursing Science, 12*(3), 1–14.

Pless, I.B., Feeley, N., Gottlieb, L., Rowat, K., Dougherty, G., & Willard, B. (1994). A randomized control trial of a nursing intervention to promote the adjustment of children with chronic physical disorders. *Pediatrics, 94*(1), 70–75.

Polit, D.F., & Hungler, B.P. (1989). *Essentials of nursing research: Methods, appraisal and utilization.* New York: J.B. Lippincott.

Pressler, J.L., & Fitzpatrick, J.J. (1988). Contributions of Rosemary Ellis to knowledge development for nursing. *Image: Journal of Nursing Scholarship, 20*(1), 28–30.

Rutter, M. (1983). Stress, coping and development: Some issues and some questions. In N. Garmezy & M. Rutter (Eds.), *Stress, coping and development in children.* New York: McGraw-Hill.

Sameroff, A.J. (1987). The social context of development. In N. Eisenberg (Ed.), *Contemporary topics in developmental psychology* (pp. 167–189). New York: Wiley.

Scarr, S. (1992). Developmental theories for the 1990s: Development and individual differences. *Child Development, 63,* 1–19.

Schumacher, K.L., & Meleis, A.I. (1994). Transitions: A central concept in nursing. *Image: Journal of Nursing Scholarship, 26*(2), 119–127.

Seitz, V., Rosenbaum, L.K., & Apfel, N.H. (1985). Effects of family support intervention: A ten-year follow-up. *Child Development, 56,* 376–391.

Stein, R.E.K., & Jessop, D.J. (1991). Long-term mental health effects of a pediatric home care program. *Pediatrics, 88*(3), 490–496.

Stewart, R. (1990). *The second child: Family transitions and adjustments.* Newbury Park, CA: Sage.

Walsh, F. (1983). The timing of symptoms and critical events in the family life cycle. In J.C. Hanson & H.A. Liddle (Eds.), *Clinical implications of the family life cycle* (pp. 120–133). Rockville, MD: Aspen.

Webster-Stratton, C. (1984). A randomized trial of two parent training programs for families with conduct disordered children. *Journal of Consulting & Clinical Psychology, 52,* 666–678.

Webster-Stratton, C. (1992). *Working with parents of conduct-disordered children: A collaborative process.* Unpublished manuscript. University of Washington, Seattle.

Wolfe, D.A., & Wekerle, C. (1993). Treatment strategies for child physical abuse and neglect: A critical progress report. *Child Psychology Review, 13*(6), 473–500.

Zigler, E., Taussig, C., & Black, K. (1992). Early childhood intervention: A promising preventative for juvenile delinquency. *American Psychologist, 47,* 997–1006.

C H A P T E R   2 8

Participatory action research: Theory and practice

Geraldine (Gerri) Dickson

Participatory action research (PAR) is evolving as a new-paradigm approach to research. It fosters Primary Health Care by giving renewed importance to the principles of community participation and control, equity, intersectoral collaboration, and use of indigenous knowledge. Explicitly, PAR challenges power inequities, which result in gaps in social and health status. PAR creates opportunities for oppressed people to analyze and critique their own reality. The purpose of this chapter is to describe PAR's theoretical base, its practical application, and its links with health promotion. The reader is invited to reflect on the application of PAR to community health nursing practice.

LEARNING OBJECTIVES

In this chapter, you will learn:

- how research can play a role in empowerment of communities and community development
- how community health nurses can conduct research with communities
- how to use participatory action research
- how participatory action research was used in one health promotion project

Introduction

Community health nurses working with Aboriginal people, single parents, the physically disabled, and other marginalized groups in Canada will likely have heard the statement, often expressed in anger and frustration, "We've been researched to death and never get anything out of it!" Does research commonly leave subjects, especially minority people, with the sense of being the objects of scrutiny for someone else's benefit? Partially in response to dissatisfaction with traditional methods of research, an alternative approach, called participatory action research (PAR), has evolved over the last several decades.

This chapter introduces participatory action research: its theory, including an overview of methodology, relevance to health promotion, expected benefits, and challenges and limitations. Next, the discussion shifts to a health promotion project in which PAR was used as the methodology to conduct a health needs assessment with older Aboriginal women in an urban setting.

PAR in theory

PAR is an approach to research that blends scientific inquiry with education and political action. It has features complementary to the intent and process of health promotion. PAR stresses a sociopolitical analysis to problems, shifting the interpretation of problems from an individual to a societal context. Described another way, PAR is the inquiry component of community development, wherein those involved decide that research is to be a part of their collective initiative.

Typically, PAR is conducted by a research team composed of both community members and external researchers who together work to understand and resolve community problems. PAR may employ a variety of research methods, including individual, in-depth interviews emphasizing personal experience; surveys; and secondary analysis of public documents. Most commonly, qualitative methods are emphasized. The interview style is usually based on Freire's (1968, 1974) concept of "problem-posing dialogue," in which research participants are encouraged to analyze parts of their lives that they might not ordinarily acknowledge or question (Maguire, 1987). "Dialogue," which means talking as equal partners in an exchange of information, sentiment, and values, is a feature of the methodology that distinguishes PAR from other social and health research (Park, 1993).

Cancian and Armstead (1990) identify five distinguishing qualities of PAR: participation in the research by the people being studied; inclusion of popular knowledge, personal experiences, and other non-scientific ways of knowing; a focus on empowerment and power relations; consciousness raising and education of the participants; and political action.

Maguire (1987) describes a number of underlying assumptions of PAR. For example, it is assumed that the ability to shape both common lay and scientific professional knowledge is a source of power for dominant social groups. Furthermore, it is assumed that ordinary people have indigenous knowledge or experiential knowledge based on first-hand experience (Borkman, 1990) and, when provided with tools and opportunities, are capable of critical reflection and analysis, knowledge creation, and mobilization of human resources to solve social and health problems. Additionally, it is important for community members and external researchers to identify, discuss, and clarify assumptions that each hold about conducting research together, so as to avoid misunderstandings.

It is important to distinguish between PAR and other research that may use some participatory methods. In PAR, control of the research process lies firmly with the community, and the research explicitly aims to empower participants and redress power inequities.

Methodology

There are various ways to describe the stages and steps of PAR. Any attempt to standardize this process is done with caution so as not to predetermine the direction that the research participants decide to take. Ideally, a PAR project is initiated by a group of people who are seeking assistance in understanding and resolving a particular problem, such as a group of citizens concerned about pollution from a nearby factory. In reality, PAR projects more commonly are initiated by a researcher who enters a community with a certain issue in mind and establishes relationships and a working group (Cancian & Armstead, 1990). Typically, there are four general stages of the PAR process (Cancian & Armstead, 1990): orientation to a community, dialogue with groups of people to clarify community problems and to raise consciousness, collective research, and collective action.

Orientation to a community. This stage includes the steps of entering a community, experiencing its reality, getting to know the issues, building relationships, and developing interest regarding collective research (Maguire, 1987).

Dialogue with community groups. The dialogue stage involves both researcher and community participants in identifying specific problems, finding out what they already know, and critically analyzing this knowledge (Cancian & Armstead, 1990; Parker, Schulz, Israel, & Hollis, 1998).

Collective research. The research stage is what distinguishes PAR from community organizing and development. The formal research component in a PAR project may be large, but more typically it is small. The participation of community members in this stage ranges from overall management and operation, to serving on a project advisory committee, to being trained to assist in the data collection and analysis, all the while being in control of the research.

Collective action. The collective action stage involves addressing some of the problems identified through the group dialogue and research (Cancian &

Armstead, 1990). Some projects result in major social changes; others produce small or transient changes.

The internal dynamic of PAR is reflection–action, with participants engaged in three learning cycles:

- *Education and analysis.* Participants ask: What do we want to know? What are the causes, contexts, and consequences of the problem? What could be achieved?
- *Investigation.* Participants ask: What other information is needed? Why? From where? By whom? What is that information?
- *Action.* Participants ask: What can be done about the problem? What are the hurdles and resources? Who will do what? What will we call success? How can this new knowledge be shared with others? (adapted from Smith, Pyrch, & Lizardi, 1993)

Role of PAR in health promotion

The literature on PAR describes a type of research that is consistent with health promotion. Four key concepts associated with both constructs are control, powerlessness, empowerment, and participation.

Much health promotion research employs conventional approaches in which the subjects of research function principally as sources of data. This role does not contribute directly to the subjects' empowerment or encourage action by those experiencing the problems studied. By contrast, the term *participants* or *co-researchers* is used in PAR rather than *subjects* to distinguish the unique partnership in this collective research. Some writers (e.g., Hancock & Draper, 1989) have claimed that PAR is potentially a more appropriate and useful methodology for research in health promotion than traditional methodologies.

It is reasonable to assume that control and health are related and that those with more control over their lives and destinies enjoy a higher status of health. The World Health Organization (1986) definition of health promotion shifted emphasis from individual responsibility to control over determinants of health. This emphasis on determinants speaks to "real control" and refers to "the extent to which individuals are able to make things happen the way they want" (Green, 1991, p. 1). Control is also related to health by its interaction with self-esteem: if you respect and value yourself, you are more likely to look after yourself; and being able to control your life increases your self-esteem. Persons with high self-esteem may demonstrate this self-care in a variety of ways. They may adopt behaviours to prevent disease and promote health; resist social pressures to act in ways risky to good health; cope constructively with stress and other health threats; or avoid dissonance between self-concept and unhealthy behaviours (Green, 1991; Tones, 1991).

PAR emphasizes empowerment of research participants through their participation in the research process, their focus on power relations associated with problems, and their education regarding the problems studied. PAR also emphasizes a sociopolitical analysis of problems, shifting the interpretation of problems from an individual to a societal context.

Health promotion emphasizes empowerment (see also Chapters 12, 14, and 16). The World Health Organization (1986) defines health promotion as the process of enabling people to increase control over the determinants of health and thereby to improve their health. This increased control is synonymous with empowerment. Health promotion recognizes the socio-ecological (defined as the interaction between individuals and their environment) aspects of well-being and challenges the health sector to examine these determinants of health and tackle the multiple causes of disease. It recognizes the influence of social determinants, such as gender and income, on health status. Health promotion encourages action on the part of individuals, communities, and policy makers to improve health (Pederson, O'Neill, & Rootman, 1994; WHO, HWC, & CPHA, 1986).

In a comprehensive article, Wallerstein (1992) reviews the health and social science research "relevant to both the role of powerlessness as a risk factor for disease, and the role of empowerment as a health-enhancing strategy" (p. 197). Powerlessness is defined as "lack of control over destiny" (Wallerstein, 1992, p. 197) or "the expectancy held by the individual that his [or her] own behavior cannot determine the occurrence of the outcomes . . . he [or she] seeks" (Seeman, 1959, p. 784). Powerlessness, as a subjective (perceived) phenomenon, is equated with external locus of control and learned helplessness. As an objective (actual) phenomenon, people in some situations do lack power in political and economic terms. There is a strong relationship between powerlessness and social class; powerlessness is experienced by those who are poor, low in the social hierarchy, and living in chronic hardship. Powerlessness "is itself a broad risk factor that increases susceptibility to higher morbidity and mortality rates" (Wallerstein, 1992, p. 199). The social and health professions often benefit from keeping clients dependent and perpetuate, rather than alleviate, the very conditions of victimization that are to be changed (Lord & McKillop Farlow, 1990).

In contrast to powerlessness, empowerment is "the participation of individuals and communities in a social action process that targets both individual and community change outcomes" (Wallerstein, 1992, p. 202). It is the process of increasing people's ability to choose and capacity to define, analyze, and act upon problems (Kent, 1988). Participation is a cornerstone of Primary Health Care, health promotion, and PAR. The premise is that community members must be active participants in the processes that are intended to improve their lives (Bopp, 1994). This includes initiatives aimed at the individual and the setting upon which health and well-being depend.

Empowerment interventions emerge as a strategy for health promotion programs, directly addressing control over destiny. Services that contribute to empowerment are personalized and interactive and reduce dependency (Lord & McKillop Farlow, 1990).

PAR aims to empower participants through their participation in and control of the research agenda, process, and findings; their critical awareness of the causes of the problems studied; and the establishment of individual and community change as a planned outcome. Insofar as these aims are achieved, PAR can function as an empowerment strategy for health promotion. It can reduce the risk of ill health due to powerlessness and promote health by increasing control of individuals, families, groups, and communities over their lives.

Benefits of PAR

Hancock and Draper (1989) propose that the use of PAR can achieve different health-promoting outcomes. These include

- enriching data through the use of participants' expertise regarding problems studied
- raising in participants' minds questions they might never otherwise ask themselves
- giving the powerless a voice and creating opportunities for that voice to be heard beyond their group
- establishing processes that link people who normally never speak to each other
- moving from "power over" to "power with"
- linking research purposely with community action and change
- establishing ongoing processes of community change that activate, mobilize, and empower individuals and communities
- developing research skills in, and transferring other resources to, community people
- writing research results into different languages for different audiences
- taking information and results back to the community, which assumes ownership.

Challenges and limitations of PAR

For community health nurses and other researchers, there are many challenges to the use of PAR:

- Using PAR means working simultaneously in several different contradictory worlds and in diverse languages (Hancock & Draper, 1989).
- As in Primary Health Care, using PAR requires active intersectoral collaboration.

- Time and commitment needed to pursue this type of research may be seen as impractical, given the demands of the community health nurse's work life.
- Researchers using this methodology will have to struggle both for legitimacy within academic and research circles, because PAR lies outside conventional research paradigms, and for an egalitarian, facilitating role with community groups.
- The health care system is hierarchical, which is inconsistent with an egalitarian research methodology; institutions within the system may have difficulty embracing this approach.
- The community group may find it difficult to work with a nurse researcher without being unduly influenced by the researcher's interests and authority; members may defer to the expertise that they perceive lies with the professional and not develop their own.

There are also limitations associated with the methodology:

- To date, much PAR has been male-centred; little attention has been paid to gender issues, although examples of feminist influence are increasing (Maguire, 1987).
- Because of its emphasis on unequal power relations, PAR is often used with oppressed groups who may not have the capacity to devote time to any endeavour that does not deal with basic survival needs or who may not be represented by an organized body with whom a researcher can work.
- If the analysis of the socioeconomic and political elements of the problem under study shows that they are resistant to change, the research may heighten research participants' frustration and dissatisfaction with the status quo, with little apparent resolution in sight (Conchelos & Kassam, 1981).

PAR in community-based practice

As a community health nurse and academic, I believe PAR is particularly appropriate for community-based practice and research. I used and examined PAR as the subject of my doctoral studies. First, I facilitated a health needs assessment using PAR in a project with older Aboriginal women. Second, based on this experience, I assessed the relationship between PAR and health promotion; the results were positive and impressive. In the remainder of this chapter, I will describe that project as an example of PAR.

The community clinic in my city had been awarded funding from the federal government for a health promotion project with older Aboriginal women. The proposal for this project had arisen out of the clinic's earlier initiative on women's health, which revealed many unmet health needs among older Aboriginal women in the city. The project aimed to conduct a health needs assessment of this population using a participatory approach and to support the older Aboriginal women by offering health promotion programs, facilitating leadership development, and liaising with relevant services.

Using the four stages of PAR described above (see "Methodology"), I will show how the theory underpinning this method can be used in practice.

Stage 1: Orientation to the community

Upon learning that the older Aboriginal women's health project might match my interests, I contacted the project director in November 1992. The two new Aboriginal project staff, the director, and I met to discuss the facilitation of the needs assessment.

In January 1993, I met with the recently formed project advisory committee, composed of Métis and Treaty First Nations women, to seek their approval for my involvement. I wanted them to understand my views on health and research, so that they could make an informed choice about my participation. I introduced myself by showing photos of my family and explaining my personal and professional background. Then, I explained my beliefs about health and well-being by telling a story of a woman in a developing country whose baby has diarrhea and dies. Through a visual approach to building a chain of causes and consequences, we together analyzed what factors determined the state of health of that family and related that situation to one in their community. I next gave a brief introduction to PAR, community development, and needs assessment from my perspective. As the meeting concluded, the advisory committee members all consented to have me work with them in the project. It was satisfying to be invited to join the project and to find this home for my interests in PAR.

Although not the ideal, this situation is more typical because the impetus for research comes from an agency or academic who perceives a need. In this case, the need had been identified in the earlier initiative, and the Community Clinic staff developed a proposal for the follow-up health promotion project, including further needs assessment research. Moreover, as there was no identifiable organization of older Aboriginal women in the city, there was little likelihood that an expressed research question would come from them. Normally, people live their problems in their daily lives and may not identify specific issues that need investigation and are amenable to action. Raising awareness of the existence and nature of these lived problems is part of the PAR process.

The next step for me was to start meeting the project participants, older Aboriginal women, hereafter referred to as "grandmothers." The staff had been contacting local agencies, groups, schools, and other possible sources for potential participants; informing them about the project; and inviting referrals. The initial stages of the project included home visits to grandmothers, a weekly get-together on Tuesday mornings, advocacy, and agency networking. The Tuesday meetings were conceived as health education sessions on common health and disease topics, alternating with healing circles in which the grandmothers would discuss their personal joys and sorrows in a supportive and confidential environment.

Based on the set of assumptions that apply to PAR in general (Maguire, 1987; see "PAR in theory," above), I identified personal assumptions that influenced how I functioned in this specific project. For example, one of my assumptions was that Aboriginal people have the right to control their own health care system, which would emphasize holism and balance social, cultural, spiritual, physical, and emotional health.

Within the scope of the project, I had three groups with whom I related: staff, grandmothers, and advisory committee. With members of all three groups, I strove to develop trust, build relationships, and engender common interest in collective research.

Stage 2: Dialogue with community groups

My most immediate and frequent contacts were with the two project staff (a coordinator and a part-time outreach worker); both were women my age—in their late forties. My relationship with the two staff developed through the planning and carrying out of the Tuesday morning group sessions with the grandmothers. The staff were cautious about how the research and my principal role would be communicated to the grandmothers. More than five months of project activities took place before we broached the idea and language of research with the grandmothers. Initially, I was introduced as a nurse and found an accepted role in the Tuesday morning groups by facilitating educational sessions on such topics as diabetes, nutrition, and menopause. I also helped by picking up the grandmothers who needed rides and preparing the coffee and tea for the group. Gradually, as the staff felt more comfortable talking about the research component of the project, I was identified to the grandmothers as a researcher as well.

The second group with whom I worked were the clients of the project, the grandmothers themselves. Most were contacted about the project by word of mouth through the Aboriginal community. We had about 60 women on our list, ranging in age from 40 to 85 years. Of these, between four and 15 came to the Tuesday morning group, with a core group of eight to 10. Even though the women may have known of one another through common friends or relatives, many had not socialized with each other during their time in the city.

After five months of participation in the Tuesday groups, I knew a few of the grandmothers well enough to start home visiting. Some of the others preferred speaking in their native language or were more comfortable with our Cree-speaking coordinator or the outreach worker.

The third contact group was the project advisory committee, composed of nine Aboriginal women. Initially, I saw this group as my principal collaborators in the research team. Although the advisory committee had monthly, two-hour meetings to give direction to the project, attendance was irregular. Additionally, several days were scheduled for workshops to organize the health needs assessment.

Through working with the project on a regular basis over 2.5 years, I felt well accepted by the grandmothers and staff. We phoned one another at home, dropped in for visits or a more structured interview, and went to cultural and other events together. At times I even drew upon my clinical skills, for example, changing surgical dressings in the home.

In the first year, during a circle discussion of spirituality and health, I told of a moving personal experience in which an Aboriginal elder's story gave me clear guidance on how to relate to the Aboriginal mother of my adopted son with whom he had recently reunited. This vignette showed a side of me other than the white, middle-class academic and paved the way for the staff, grandmothers, and I to communicate more deeply as women and mothers.

Stage 3: Collective research

Research design. The actual research component of our work was planned in workshops with the advisory committee. By the end of the first workshop of 2.5 days, we had covered many topics: PAR and community development; the continuum between conventional research and PAR; terms of agreement for all participants in the research; informed consent; aspects of life in which empowerment may be assessed and the potential impact of change seen; principles to guide the project; assumptions underlying the research questions regarding the health needs of older Aboriginal women; methods to record the research findings; and the timeline for research activities.

Table 28.1 summarizes the research design for this PAR health assessment study and illustrates the kind of information that was needed. The brainstorming work of the advisory committee produced the content that I then clustered into 10 themes. Much of the further information was to come from the grandmothers themselves and would include anecdotes and stories that could later be organized to provide a new knowledge base.

As we ended the second workshop, I suggested to the advisory committee that I could organize the research design into a guide for a "community listening survey." During the summer months, each member could listen for information on the various questions and jot findings in a diary. This community listening survey approach met with limited success, however, and

Table 28.1
Health needs assessment research design

What Do We Want to Know? (from brainstorming and theme clusters)	Why?	What Do We Know Already?	Where to Find Out/Whom to Ask	What Kind of Info Needed?
Specific Information				
• How many grandmothers are there in Saskatoon? • Where did they come from? • If they moved to town, why? • What ages are they? • What is their financial state?	• To understand situation, what resources/services are required, entitlements • Needs vary according to age	• Many on pension and/or Sask. Assistance Plan	• Grandmothers • Medical Services Branch • Provincial Health • Sask. Health Board	• Numbers • Stories
Language and Culture				
• What are the grandmothers' first languages? • What are their values and beliefs related to health? • What knowledge do they have about traditions? • Who practises a traditional way of life? • Who practises traditions in the city? • Who makes decisions about them? • What do they do for fun, recreation?	• Need for interpreters • Differences in cultures/beliefs • Lack of traditional First Nations voice in the city (role confusion) • To identify elders, traditions	• Some ideas • Ask about home practices • Need to document differences/commonalities	• Grandmothers • Elders • Literature	• Stories • Photo essay • Story book • Video presentation
Social Relationships				
• What and how are their relationships in the city with family? • With friends? • With the community at large? • With local and Aboriginal leaders?	• To identify needs of future generations • To interrelate with other generations • To find support systems in the city	• Need to find out and document	• Grandmothers • Family members • Community leaders	• Personal stories • Anecdotes

(continued)

Table 28.1 (continued)

What Do We Want to Know? (from brainstorming and theme clusters)	Why?	What Do We Know Already?	Where to Find Out/Whom to Ask	What Kind of Info Needed?
Concept of Health • What do the grandmothers mean by "health" and "disease"? • What do they believe leads to good health? • What leads to ill health? • What is their sense of power/control over health and health care?	• To understand their thinking and plan action accordingly	—	• Grandmothers	• Personal description
Health Status • How would the grandmothers describe their own health: poor, fair, good, excellent? • What are their health problems? • How many grandmothers are physically handicapped? • What diseases do the grandmothers have?	• To understand the situation • To know types of resources required to meet needs	—	• Grandmothers • Hospitals • Physicians • Clinics	• Personal description • Anecdotes • Medical records
Health Practices • What do the grandmothers do for self-care? • What do they do for their health and well-being that is based on tradition? based on Western learning? • What are their spiritual practices? How do these relate to health?	• To understand the situation • To know types of resources required to meet needs	—	• Grandmothers	• Personal description • Anecdotes • Medical records

(continued)

Table 28.1 (continued)

What Do We Want to Know? (from brainstorming and theme clusters)	Why?	What Do We Know Already?	Where to Find Out/Whom to Ask	What Kind of Info Needed?
Health Services				
• Where do the grandmothers go for services (Western/traditional)? • What kinds of services do they use, and why? • What are Western professionals' attitudes toward healing? • What do the grandmothers know about the various levels and systems (federal, provincial, municipal, self-government)?	• To know existing resources; if any/none used; any bad/good experiences • To understand influence of religion • Are explanations needed for access to benefits • Do current services enable rather than help with problems?	—	• Grandmothers • Western professionals	• Personal stories • Anecdotes
Society in General				
• What are society's attitudes about Aboriginal people? Attitudes in the city? • How do society's "isms" affect the grandmothers (institutionalism, racism, classism, sexism, judgementalism)? • What are the Western systemic rules and regulations about health?	• To look at society's assumptions	• Some ideas; need more	• Grandmothers • General population • Literature	• Personal stories/ description • Research and literature • Health system's operating principles

(continued)

Table 28.1 (*continued*)

What Do We Want to Know? (*from brainstorming and theme clusters*)	Why?	What Do We Know Already?	Where to Find Out/Whom to Ask	What Kind of Info Needed?
Issues				
• What are the grandmothers' greatest worries? • What are their most emotional issues? • Which issues do they most desire to act upon?	• Need to name and understand causes/consequences of problems in order to act on them	—	• Grandmothers	• Personal stories/ description
Strengths				
• What do the grandmothers say are their strengths? What do others see as their strengths? • What contributions have grandmothers made to family and community life?	• To empower by working from positive accomplishments	• Some ideas; need more	• Grandmothers • Family/ community members • Leaders	• Personal stories/ description • Anecdotes • Literature

only three of the expected seven diaries were ever submitted. I later realized that it was a task that made sense to me but had not arisen out of the committee itself and thus was not owned and well understood by the members.

Also at the end of the second workshop, I asked each advisory committee member and staff to participate in an individual, audiotaped interview with me on her own life focussed on the aspects of empowerment that we had discussed in the initial workshop. They all agreed, with the understanding that we would repeat this interview a year later to assess changes following their more intense involvement with the research. This would give us some information regarding the impact of involvement in PAR on their personal level of empowerment. Later, each respondent was given her own copy of the transcribed notes from the initial interview.

The next research planning workshop was booked for two days to do more work on group building, clarification of purpose and values, and research design. During that workshop, I presented the major findings of a 1989 study by a provincial seniors' group on the unmet needs of off-reserve Aboriginal elderly in Saskatchewan (Troyer, 1989). Findings were presented under the following headings: education; language; employment; economy; housing; living conditions; moving history and housing satisfaction; movement from reserve to city; transportation and activity patterns; health profile; and need for assistance and care. Our advisory committee members commented on the validity of each finding for themselves and other grandmothers whom they knew. Generally, the members believed that the findings accurately described their own situation. Indeed, the "bottom-line" comment was, "We know this. We could have told you all this! They didn't need to do research." Near the end of the second day of this workshop, one of the members observed that an advisory committee was the "white way" of structuring a project. Now that the grandmothers of the Tuesday morning group were more organized, one advisory committee member proposed that they should guide the project and research.

This proposal was approved, and the advisory committee disbanded. Because of this change, the composition of our research team shifted from the advisory committee to the Tuesday morning grandmothers, and the empowerment interviews were not repeated the next year.

Earlier that fall, a conference that featured presentations on PAR with northern people reinforced the importance of research training of local people. I thought we were attending to the training aspect of PAR through the continual orientation I provided to staff, the advisory committee, and participant grandmothers about research. In these northern projects, however, local people were hired and trained formally as researchers. Following discussion with the grandmothers and with their input on recruitment, selection, and contract terms, we secured additional funds and hired two Aboriginal trainees as research associates. These women worked with us for several months, reaching out further into the community to more older women and conducting home visits and interviews for the health needs assessment.

In the first year, while discussing the needs assessment with the grandmothers in the Tuesday morning group, one of them said, "We're not just going to talk about *problems*, are we?" That question reinforced to me that a needs assessment should not only identify deficits, but should also be an inventory of strengths, resources, unique qualities, traits, and experiences. We began to call our activity a *health* assessment rather than a needs assessment and shifted to focussing on strengths. Since the grandmothers lived their problems every day, they preferred to concentrate on their strengths as the basis for tackling some of the challenges that they faced.

Data collection and analysis. Based on that challenge to focus on strengths and the previous research design work done by the advisory committee, the research associates, staff, and I developed a series of three interview guides for use with the grandmothers in their homes. Each guide focussed on one of the following: past strengths; present strengths; and issues, problems, and concerns. We reviewed the series with the group of grandmothers, seeking their input and endorsement, then conducted the interviews individually. The responses were recorded by hand because many grandmothers expressed discomfort about audiotaping.

There were three other sources of data used in the health assessment: my recordings of the Tuesday morning discussions; audio- and videotapes of other group activities; and my own personal journal and study field notes. The grandmothers agreed to have me document our group sessions. After their trust in the project and me increased, they even approved of recording the healing circles, as long as individuals were not identified by name. In time, they became comfortable with audio- and videotaping group events as well and enjoyed seeing themselves on television. My journal and field notes were tools used to follow the progress of our work, more specifically for my own studies.

Data analysis in PAR typically is of two types: the study of the data for content findings and the critical reflection on those findings for deeper, political understanding of the participants' reality. The staff, research associates, and I worked with the data from various sources, collating and coding for common themes. On selected Tuesday mornings, we took the clustered data back to the grandmothers for member checking, validation, and elaboration. This data treatment by the grandmothers as a group provoked great interest and discussion among them, and the resulting responses were enriched and collectively verified. I used Freire's problem-posing dialogue: What do you hear in this? What does this mean for you? Is that how it should be?

Following several sessions, I used line-by-line content analysis of the data—doing the coding by hand and the clustering using Microsoft Word software (Morse, 1991). Four major categories or themes emerged: traditions, disruptions, concerns, and hopes, with subcategories under each. Because the circle is the basic symbol of life and meaning for Aboriginal people, and four is the basic number, I organized these categories as points on a circle, starting with the traditions in the east—the beginning position on the circle—moving clockwise to disruptions, then concerns, and finishing with their hopes, teachings, and vision for the future. I displayed this model on coloured circles and presented it to the grandmothers and staff. After some thought and study, the grandmothers agreed in principle, with some changes to the labels, subcategories, and colours.

Over the next months, we studied the model on several occasions. I then drafted a report of the health assessment from it, and one of the grandmothers' daughters converted it into a format for easy reading. I took copies to 11 of the grandmothers individually in their homes, then returned a few weeks later to record their feedback. After revising the report according to these comments, we reviewed the new draft in a Tuesday morning group. When these changes were included, three grandmothers offered to read the next draft. With their comments incorporated, the report was professionally formatted, including photos. Then 10 grandmothers reviewed it individually again. Next we went over it, section by section, in the group and made final changes. Three of the grandmothers who could not attend that meeting telephoned me with their comments. The seven months of study of the report provided a forum for critical analysis of the data. As the grandmothers reviewed the various drafts, they discussed the meaning and impact of their own and each others' stories, experiences, and opinions. This critical reflection heightened individual and group understanding of the forces and events in their lives.

This document, entitled "Sharing our health circle: The grandmothers' health assessment report," was the tangible outcome. The report has been printed twice and circulated widely. The grandmothers are very satisfied with the process and product of this research project that examined their own health.

Notwithstanding, two limitations of PAR (see "Challenges and limitations," above) were evident in our project: (a) an oppressed group's capacity to devote little time to anything beyond basic survival and (b) the grandmothers' lack of representation by an organized body with whom to do research. Continuously, I was reminded of the complex, burdened lives of many of the grandmothers, which limited their ability to be involved in our project. This was seen in many ways: a home interview postponed four times because of economic crises, hospitalization, and family demands; minimal attendance at several Tuesday morning data feedback sessions because of other priorities such as movement back to the reserve, another committee commitment, hospitalization, a dependent family member's medical appointment, or an out-of-town funeral. Therefore, an extended time-frame, understanding, and flexibility are essential characteristics of PAR, because the obstacles and delays experienced in the process are part of the everyday reality of marginalized people.

Stage 4: Collective action

The grandmothers, staff, and I responded in various ways to issues and concerns that arose through our health assessment and other project activities. These responses gave a public voice to the collective expression of the grandmothers and intervened and advocated for individuals.

The community development staff of the newly restructured city health district organized a full day of consultations with Aboriginal people, and our project was invited to participate. Using the responses from our health assessment individual interviews and group validation, we worked together for several weeks to identify what we wanted to contribute to the consultation. Six grandmothers took part that day in late March 1994, and four continued in the follow-up committee that became a Health Board subcommittee for Aboriginal participation in policy making and programming.

The local city council established annual consultations with Aboriginal people, and our grandmothers were invited to participate. In preparation, they talked about the Council's designated priorities for the year, such as policing, leisure, and housing, so that those attending could represent the collective views. At the Council meeting, the grandmothers conveyed their opinions and were listened to by others.

Health-related issues arose during the individual interviews and group discussions. We responded to these quickly (e.g., making mammogram service information accessible; setting up home emergency alarm systems; negotiating special terms on telephone installations for medical reasons; advocacy regarding inappropriate health service billings; and taking a public stand against proposed uranium waste disposal in our province).

Empowering research fosters both self-advocacy and the transformation of individual, invisible experiences into a public issue (Roe, Minkler, & Saunders, 1995).

Academic and methodological challenges

Because of the developmental nature of PAR and its new-paradigm approach to knowledge creation and ownership, the researcher faces unique challenges from academic institutions, funding agencies, and other institutions familiar only with conventional research.

One major academic challenge I faced was securing ethical approval for the type of informed-consent protocol that the project staff and advisory committee insisted was appropriate. In their minds, asking the grandmothers to sign a formal consent form would break the trust of the relationship being developed between them and the rest of the project team. As well, in PAR the respondents are in partnership with other members of the research team, in contrast to other methods involving an outside researcher asking permission to use respondents' data for his or her own purposes. In PAR, the data that each grandmother contributes will be used by the group of grandmothers to describe and assess their own health picture. Therefore, in my application to the university's ethics committee, I attached a memo of several pages to the standard form, explaining the unique cultural and methodological features of this application. I requested a verbal informed consent for the collective, rather than individual, grandmothers. This was granted.

There is a "catch-22" position in the search either for student fellowship or for research project funding. Typically there has to be a clear, credible research plan submitted, but in PAR the design must be developed collaboratively with the community group. In fact, many groups do not even have a research question, and much developmental work must be done before they can describe their reality in these terms. I would argue that developmental funds, like the National Health Research and Development Program's formulation funding, should be accessible to finance early work with a community to (a) develop a trusting relationship, (b) understand "research" in the members' own terms, and (c) pose research questions to which they are committed and that they have the capacity to pursue.

With disadvantaged people, the stigma of research must be overcome, including the perception that external researchers are exploitive and self-serving. Considerable time and sincerity must be committed to develop relationships of trust and a process that is controlled by and beneficial to the community participants. The project staff's caution about research exacerbated my feelings of discomfort and added an element of deception to my relationship with the grandmothers in the early months. I would have preferred to work with the grandmothers in an open-ended community development way and incorporate the research as they identified issues they were interested in examining, rather than having a predetermined obligation to conduct a needs assessment.

Conclusion

PAR involves inquiry by ordinary people acting as researchers to explore questions in their daily lives, to recognize their own resources, and to produce knowledge and take action to overcome inequities. PAR was used as the methodology to conduct this health assessment with urban Aboriginal grandmothers as part of a larger health promotion project. A number of challenges and points of tension were faced, including a negative perception of research within the group; the fact that the decision to conduct research had been made by the project staff rather than the participants themselves; the "needs" focus to the assessment, which did not interest the grandmothers; the lack of an organized group, so that a community of grandmothers had to be built before research could be conducted; and the limited capacity of the grandmothers to devote much energy to the research because of their position of disadvantage.

Despite these and other challenges, we accomplished many things. We conducted research that was well integrated into the other health promotion project activities. Other than initially deciding to do a health assessment, all decisions and activities of the research were carried out in close consultation with the grandmothers and/or the advisory committee. The assessment took a strengths rather than a needs focus that suited the grandmothers better; data about problems were collected indirectly or in a group setting, which was considered more acceptable. We stressed validation of the grandmothers' worth as the principal goal of the assessment, with data collection, analysis, and dissemination secondary. The initiative became an empowering one for all involved. For the assessment, we guided the grandmothers into opportunities (consultations, meetings, lobbying) that drew out their values, opinions, experiences, and counsel on issues related to their health and well-being. The research was done by a team whose members developed mutual acceptance, trust, friendship, and respect. Caring relationships connected us all.

Implications for community health nurses

PAR is an approach to research that is consistent with the intent and principles of Primary Health Care, health promotion, community development, and community health nursing. I continue to believe firmly and passionately in this form of research. I am convinced that communities and external researchers can work as a team, each bringing valued skills to a collective inquiry process that can contribute to redressing "socio-health" inequities. I believe that nursing is a logical home for PAR because our profession shares with it common values and characteristics of health, well-being, and social justice. Nursing's premise that an individual or community that takes an active role in its own health and health care is healthier than one that is taken care of by service providers applies to research, as well.

Using PAR, it is possible for community health nurses to integrate scientific inquiry into their community development work. This integration demonstrates to community members that research is a useful process that they can take on with partners of their choice. The community health nurse can undertake many functions to support the research, such as initiating interest in investigating an issue, assisting in writing funding proposals, providing or securing organizational and technical expertise, and consulting with community members at any phase of the research.

Acknowledgements

The author acknowledges with gratitude the support of National Health Research and Development Program, Social Sciences and Humanities Research Council of Canada, Canadian Nurses Foundation, University of Saskatchewan and its Colleges of Nursing and Medicine's Department of Community Health and Epidemiology, Seniors Independence Program of Health Canada, Saskatchewan Education, and the local community clinic.

QUESTIONS

1. What common problems do community health nurses see in their practice that would be appropriately investigated by affected community members?
2. What resources—skills, interests, commitment, materials—do members of the community bring to a participatory research initiative?
3. What collective initiatives has your community undertaken in the past? Who have been the gatekeepers to organize these initiatives?
4. What are the various roles and functions that a community health nurse can play in a PAR process with the community?
5. What are the contributions and limitations that a community health nurse brings when conducting participatory research with a community?

REFERENCES

Bopp, M. (1994). The illusive essential: Evaluating participation in non-formal education and community development processes. *Convergence, 27*(1), 23–44.

Borkman, T.J. (1990). Experiential, professional, and lay frames of reference. In T.J. Powell et al. (Eds.), *Working with self-help* (pp. 3–30). Silver Springs, MD: National Association of Social Workers.

Cancian, F., & Armstead, C. (1990). *Participatory research: An introduction.* Unpublished paper available from authors through the Department of Sociology, University of California, Irvine, CA 92717.

Conchelos, G., & Kassam, Y. (1981). A brief review of critical opinions and responses on issues facing participatory researchers. *Convergence, 14*(3), 52–63.

Freire, P. (1968). *Pedagogy of the oppressed*. New York: Seabury Press.

Freire, P. (1974). *Education for critical consciousness*. New York: Seabury Press.

Green, K. (1991, June). *Control, empowerment, and health promotion*. Paper presented at the 82nd Annual Conference of Canadian Public Health Association, Regina.

Hancock, T., & Draper, R. (1989). *Participatory research: A key strategy for health promotion*. Unpublished paper available from the author of the chapter through the College of Nursing, University of Saskatchewan, Saskatoon.

Kent, G. (1988). Nutrition education as an instrument of empowerment. *Journal of Nutrition Education, 20*(4), 193–195.

Lord, J., & McKillop Farlow, D. (1990, Fall). A study of personal empowerment. *Health Promotion*, 2–8.

Maguire, P. (1987). *Doing participatory research: A feminist approach*. Amherst, MA: Center for International Education.

Morse, J. (1991). Analyzing unstructured interactive interviews using the Macintosh computer. *Qualitative Health Research, 1*(1), 117–122.

Park, P. (1993). What is participatory research? A theoretical and methodological perspective. In P. Park, M. Brydon-Miller, B. Hall, & T. Jackson (Eds.), *Voices of change: Participatory research in the United States and Canada* (pp. 1–19). Toronto: OISE Press.

Parker, E.A., Schulz, A.J., Israel, B.A., & Hollis, R. (1998). Detroit's East Side Village health worker partnership: Community-based lay health advisor intervention in an urban area. *Health Education & Behavior, 25*(1), 24–45.

Pederson, A., O'Neill, M., & Rootman, I. (1994). *Health promotion in Canada: Provincial, national and international perspectives*. Toronto: W.B. Saunders.

Roe, K.M., Minkler, M., & Saunders, F.F. (1995). Combining research, advocacy, and education: The methods of the grandparent caregiver study. *Health Education Quarterly, 22*(4), 458–475.

Seeman, M. (1959). On the meaning of alienation. *American Sociological Review, 24*, 783–791.

Smith, S.E., Pyrch, T., & Lizardi, A.O. (1993). Participatory action-research for health. *World Health Forum, 14*, 319–324.

Tones, K. (1991). Health promotion, empowerment and the psychology of control. *Journal of International Health Education, 29*(1), 17–26.

Troyer, E. (1989). *A study of the unmet needs of off-reserve Indian and Métis elderly in Saskatchewan*. Regina: Saskatchewan Senior Citizens' Provincial Council.

Wallerstein, N. (1992). Powerlessness, empowerment, and health: Implications for health promotion programs. *American Journal of Health Promotion, 6*(3), 197–205.

World Health Organization (WHO), Health & Welfare Canada (HWC), & Canadian Public Health Association (CPHA). (1986). *Ottawa charter for health promotion*. Ottawa: CPHA.

C H A P T E R   2 9

Epidemiology in community health nursing: Principles and applications for Primary Health Care

J. Howard Brunt and Laurene E. Sheilds

Epidemiology, the study of health events in populations, is a core component of community health nursing. It provides a way for community health nurses to organize and rank the multiple factors that affect the health of individuals, families, groups, and communities. Epidemiology, as a practice-based science, has evolved from simply being a way to discover the causes of disease to an approach that has wide-ranging implications for health promotion. Key concepts underpinning epidemiology and a practical example from community health practice are presented in this chapter.

LEARNING OBJECTIVES

In this chapter, you will learn:

- some basic concepts of epidemiology, including the Host–Agent–Environment Model, webs of causation, and natural history of disease, and various measures of population health
- how epidemiology can be valuable to nurses working in a community setting, particularly when they are engaged in Primary Health Care, prevention, and health promotion practice
- how complex health issues can be examined and analyzed using basic concepts of epidemiology through exploring a case study of hypertension in the Hutterite community

Introduction

This chapter is designed to introduce some of the models and methods used in epidemiology and illustrate how they can be used by community health nurses in their practice. Epidemiology is the study of the distribution and occurrence of health and disease events in populations. It was one of the first methods available to community health nurses and physicians for examining health at a population level. As the Canadian health care system has gradually shifted from a focus on treatment/cure to illness prevention and health promotion, epidemiology has become increasingly important. Far from being a static community health science, it has evolved along with the challenges facing the health of society.

History and traditions of epidemiological research in community health nursing

Epidemiology can be used in community health practice (a) to diagnose the health of a community, (b) to evaluate health services, (c) to examine the impact of diseases in populations over time, (d) to predict future health care needs, (e) to estimate individual risk based on population data, (f) to identify syndromes, (g) to determine causality, and (h) to permit early intervention and prevent further morbidity (Turner & Chavigny, 1988). In recent years, epidemiology has been used to illuminate the social determinants of disease (Evans, Barer, & Marmor, 1994). Further, one field, clinical epidemiology, provides community-based clinicians with tools for meeting public health challenges (Fletcher, Fletcher, & Wagner, 1988). The basic contribution of clinical epidemiology is its emphasis on the need for clinicians to remain current in their understanding of epidemiological research and their application of those results in practice.

Epidemiology has always evolved in response to the health challenges faced by society. It began as a collection of methods for uncovering the causes of infectious diseases and preventing their spread. With the development of better public sanitation methods and the advent of antibiotic therapy, epidemiologists next set their sights on the problems associated with chronic diseases with multifactorial causation, such as heart disease and cancer. Although infectious and chronic diseases continue to receive attention, epidemiologists have more recently turned their attention toward ways to apply epidemiologic methods to clinical practice and health promotion.

Basic methods and models in epidemiology

One of the underlying assumptions of epidemiology is that health and illness are complex phenomena and that any health state is affected by multiple factors, associated with the host, agent, and environment. The Host–Agent–Environment Triad (HAET) model (Figure 29.1) was originally used to understand the causes of infectious disease and continues to be valuable as one way to understand the factors that affect health, not just illness (Valanis, 1992, pp. 20–22).

Figure 29.1
Graphic representation of the Host–Agent–Environment Triad (HAET)

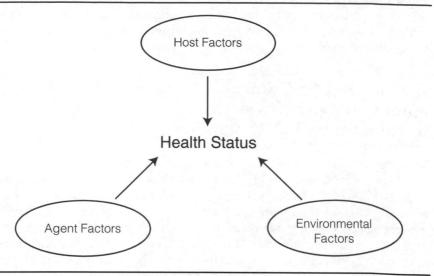

In the HAET model, the "host" refers to those factors intrinsic to the individual or population (e.g., genetic factors, age, sex, ethnicity, physiological state). "Agents" include etiological factors directly associated with the health challenge itself. Such factors may be biological (e.g., bacteria, viruses), chemical (e.g., medications, PCBs), physical (e.g., lifting, exercise), nutritional (e.g., vitamins, calories), or mechanical (e.g., cars, bullets). Finally, "environment" refers to everything external to the host that can influence or mediate the effects of the agent on the health of the host. Examples of environmental factors include such things as socioeconomic variables (e.g., culture, poverty, education), physical surroundings (e.g., temperature, air quality), and biological factors (e.g., immunization rates). As a basic tool of practice, the HAET model may assist a nurse in analyzing community health issues. In the case of teen smoking, host factors may include age and gender; agent factors may include the impact of nicotine on the body; and environmental factors may include advertising or peer group pressure. Within this example, the complexity of causation becomes apparent as agent, host, and environment factors are interrelated.

The creation of a web of causation is an attempt to move beyond the simple classification system of the HAET toward a more complex model that traces the interconnections of the multiple elements affecting health status (Stanhope & Lancaster, 1996, p. 211). Sophisticated statistical modelling

Figure 29.2
Relationship between the three levels of prevention and the natural history of disease

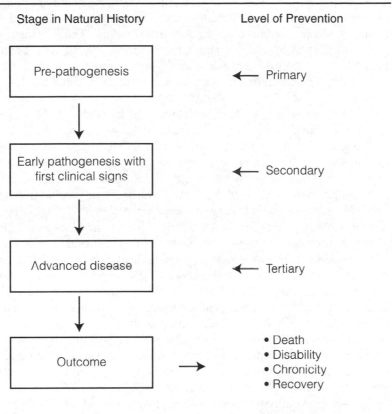

Stage in Natural History   Level of Prevention

Pre-pathogenesis   ← Primary

Early pathogenesis with first clinical signs   ← Secondary

Advanced disease   ← Tertiary

Outcome   →
- Death
- Disability
- Chronicity
- Recovery

techniques have aided epidemiologists in their attempts to understand how multiple factors interact.

An early epidemiologic observation was that challenges to health occur along a continuum; this was first described as the natural history model of disease (Figure 29.2). The natural history concept was first associated with a process of disease progression that ranged from a pre-pathogenesis period through to full-blown disease and ultimate completion of the disease process (Mausner & Kramer, 1985, pp. 6–9). In the pre-pathogenesis stage, the predisposing host–agent–environmental factors are present and begin to interact through a complex web of causation that eventually leads to observable signs of a health disorder. Depending on the disorder in question, a progression of the pathogenesis through various stages of development leads either to its successful treatment, to disability, or to death.

Although a clear description of the progression of a health challenge through its natural history is valuable, understanding how therapeutic interventions can either prevent illness or speed recovery from a disease is of even greater interest to community health practitioners. Thus, epidemiologists have contributed to theories about mechanisms to deal with health challenges through their conceptualization of prevention. Prevention, in community health, has traditionally been conceptualized at three levels: primary, secondary, and tertiary (Valanis, 1992, pp. 25–30).

Primary prevention is aimed at reducing the likelihood that the HAET factors required for developing a challenge to health get an opportunity to interact with one another. Thus, primary prevention activities focus on the pre-pathogenesis stage of the natural history model. Examples of primary prevention include public health measures such as childhood immunization, sex education, and protection from environmental hazards. There continues to be debate over the relationship between primary prevention and health promotion (Stachtchenko & Jenicek, 1990). According to Turner and Chavigny (1988, p. 57), primary prevention strategies are directed toward specific health challenges (e.g., smoking, high-risk groups), whereas health promotion strategies are directed more globally toward maximizing a general state of health and well-being (e.g., meditation). Thus, health promotion can be conceived of as contributing to the prevention of illness as well as to the maximization of health.

Secondary prevention includes those activities that either permit early diagnosis of a health challenge (e.g., Pap smear), permit early treatment that stops or slows the progression of the disorder (e.g., making a dietary change with food allergies), or limit a disability that may result from a health challenge (e.g., preventing foot drop during Guillain-Barré syndrome).

Tertiary prevention strategies are used when rehabilitation is needed to maximize health following a health challenge. For example, cardiac rehabilitation after a myocardial infarction can facilitate an individual's and family's return to maximal functioning.

Figure 29.2 represents the relationship between the three levels of prevention and the natural history of disease. To further understand these concepts, it may be useful to work through a case study using cerebral vascular accident (stroke) as the disease. There has been a deliberate focus on primary prevention through educating the public about the predisposing host–agent–environment factors related to strokes with the goal of reducing the number of strokes that occur. When a person is experiencing signs and symptoms of an impending stroke (e.g., hypertension, dizziness), more focussed secondary prevention activities may be undertaken. Tertiary prevention activities are used with a person who has suffered a stroke to facilitate recovery and prevent further occurrence.

In summary, epidemiologists use four basic tools of analysis: the HAET model, the web of causation, the natural history of disease, and levels of prevention. Additionally, the data that epidemiologists gather are used either to describe the occurrence of or to make inferences about the causes of health conditions in populations.

Epidemiological measures

Epidemiologists use a variety of measures to understand the health and disease of a population. The most notable measures are those that are based on a number of causal factors. Infant mortality, overall mortality rates, and life expectancy are three measures that are used frequently to determine the health of a population. More disease-specific measures, such as morbidity, are used to understand the impact of disease in a population.

Infant mortality rates describe the number of infant deaths in a population, based on the total number of live births in a given year (Stanhope & Lancaster, 1996, p. 216). Infant mortality is a key measure of a population's health because it is influenced by several factors such as poverty, access to health care, and the health of the mother, including physical health factors (e.g., nutrition, age) as well as psychosocial factors (e.g., stress, social support).

$$\text{Infant mortality} = \frac{\text{Number of infant deaths in a given year}}{\text{Number of live births in the same year}}$$

For example, if there were 37 infants (under the age of one year) who died within your region in the past year and there were 4000 live births, the infant mortality rate would be $37 \div 4000 = 0.00925$. This means for every 1000 live births in the past year, nine infants died. This rate can then be compared with other regions in the province, or between provinces and countries. In Canada, the infant mortality rate has decreased dramatically in the past 70 years (from 102 to eight deaths per 1000 live births). However, infant mortality continues to be higher in disadvantaged populations (e.g., Aboriginal communities, those living in poverty) (Angus & Turbayne, 1995).

Similar to the infant mortality measure, *crude mortality rates* are calculated to understand the health of a population. The crude mortality rate represents the proportion of a population who die from any cause during a specific time period (Stanhope & Lancaster, 1996).

$$\text{Crude mortality rate} = \frac{\text{Number of deaths of population in a given year}}{\text{Total population in the same year}}$$

Life expectancy is perhaps the most widely quoted epidemiological measure. Life expectancy answers the question "If an infant was born today, how many years can we expect that infant to live?" Life expectancy data are based upon mortality rates in a population and therefore are affected by the number and causes of death in a population as well as the age at death. For example, in situations where many people die young (in infancy or childhood), overall population life expectancy drops dramatically. Life expectancy differences are evident between men and women and between people with different socioeconomic status (Angus & Turbayne, 1995). In recent years, the United Nations Development Program has used life expectancy to create a "human development index" that includes two other measures (educational attainment and income) to determine the well-being of a population (Ministry of Health & Ministry Responsible for Seniors, 1997).

Epidemiologists use two major methods for determining the occurrence of disease or injury in a population. These measures are prevalence and incidence. *Prevalence* is a statistic that describes the proportion of individuals in a population that have a particular health condition at a particular point in time (Stanhope & Lancaster, 1996, p. 218).

$$\text{Prevalence} = \frac{\text{Number of persons with a given health condition}}{\text{Total number at risk in the population}}$$

Traditionally, prevalence rates have been calculated for disease states. For example, if 200 people in a town of 5000 had a respiratory infection on a given day, the prevalence rate for that day would be $200 \div 5000 = 0.040$. Another way of reporting this finding would be to say that 40 out of every 1000 people had a respiratory infection on the day of the study. With the increased emphasis on factors that promote health, prevalence rates of health factors such as regular exercise and healthy eating habits have been measured (Health & Welfare Canada [HWC], 1988).

Incidence is a measure of the rate of development of a health condition in a population in a given time period (Stanhope & Lancaster, 1996, p. 218).

$$\text{Incidence} = \frac{\text{Number of persons developing a health condition}}{\text{Total number at risk for developing the condition}}$$

For example, if in the same town described above, 75 people developed a respiratory infection during the next week, the incidence rate for the week would be $75 \div 4800 = 0.016$. In other words, for every 1000 residents in the town, 16 persons developed a cold during the week of the study. You will notice that the denominator that was used for computing the incidence rate was 4800, not 5000. That is because the denominator is based on the number of people at risk; 200 people already had the respiratory infection from the previous week, so they are removed from the denominator.

Other descriptive rates and measures used frequently in community health practice include age and cause specific mortality rates, maternal mortality rates, and rates of fertility. For an excellent discussion of these and other descriptive measures, the reader may consult any basic epidemiology text (e.g., Mausner & Lancaster, 1985; Valanis, 1992).

The use of basic descriptive epidemiological measures has become more sophisticated in the past 15 years with the emergence of the field of population health. The intent of population health is, first, to understand what makes and keeps people healthy and, second, to ensure the effectiveness of the health system (HWC, 1994, p. 9). By examining the relationships among such factors as social status, income and education levels, working conditions, and health status, population health experts using epidemiological tools have demonstrated convincingly the impact of social determinants on health.

Canada's Health Promotion Survey (HWC, 1988) used a number of health indicators that went beyond the traditional disease-oriented indicators of the past. For example, the survey gathered prevalence data on attitudes about smoking and drinking, breast self-examination, seat-belt use, home and workplace safety, nutrition, and exercise.

Research designs and determining causality in epidemiology

Descriptive epidemiology is important for understanding and monitoring the health of a community. However, epidemiologists are perhaps better known for their contributions to the understanding of the causes of health challenges. HAET factors that contribute to the development of health problems are called *risk factors*. A number of epidemiological methods and statistical procedures have evolved during the last few decades that have made it possible to tease out risk factors for health conditions from population studies. Three research approaches that are commonly used in epidemiological studies are cross-sectional surveys, retrospective or case-control studies, and prospective or cohort studies (Stanhope & Lancaster, 1996, p. 223).

In cross-sectional surveys, all data about health conditions and risk factors are gathered at a particular point in time. A cross-sectional survey may show that a high proportion of socioeconomically disadvantaged people suffer from poor general health. However, with this design it is not clear whether the poverty preceded poor health or vice versa. Thus, cross-sectional surveys do not provide strong proof of causality. On the other hand, they do generate exciting hypotheses (i.e., predictions) that can be investigated further. The study of hypertension among Hutterites described later in this chapter is an example of a cross-sectional design.

In retrospective, or case-control, epidemiologic studies, individuals with a particular health condition of interest (called "cases") are closely matched with another group of individuals who do not have the condition (called "controls"). The researcher then gathers HAET information from both groups' past (e.g., smoking history) and looks for differences between them. For example, past exposure to second-hand cigarette smoke could be identified via an interview with a group of people with heart disease (cases) and another group without heart disease (controls). Then, the rates of exposure to second-hand smoke for the two groups could be compared. Indeed, research has shown that the odds of being exposed to second-hand smoke are higher in heart disease cases and that exposure to second-hand smoke is a risk factor for heart disease (Dobson, Alexander, Heller, & Lloyd, 1991).

Prospective, or cohort, studies begin with a group of individuals who have been exposed to a possible HAET factor (e.g., regular physical exercise) and another group who have not (e.g., sedentary). Individuals from both groups are then followed for a period of time, and the status of the health condition of interest (e.g., depression) is monitored carefully. The rates of the disorder in the two groups are then compared, and a relative risk for developing the disorder can be determined. Using this method, epidemiologists found that physical exercise provides some protection against depression (Camacho, Roberts, Lazarus, Kaplan, & Cohen, 1991). Because of their ability to monitor and document the development of disease, prospective studies are considered to be the most valid for determining causality, followed closely by well-executed retrospective studies (Lilienfeld & Lilienfeld, 1980, pp. 246–249).

Once a causal link has been established between a risk factor and a health condition, new information is made available to the public and professionals for influencing health choices. This is perhaps best illustrated by the flurry of activity that followed the discovery of the link between smoking and diseases such as cancer and atherosclerosis. Increasingly, epidemiologists are becoming interested in new ways of monitoring the health of populations and understanding the impact of this new information. Despite epidemiology's preoccupation with statistical techniques and quantitative methodologies, many of the more qualitative approaches to population-based research are finding their way into epidemiological research. Classical qualitative techniques such as ethnography and newer methods such as participatory action research show great promise for expanding the horizons, applicability, and meaningfulness of epidemiology (HWC, 1989a).

Relevance and challenges of epidemiology for community health nurses

Community health practice requires that nurses work not only at the individual level, but with families, aggregates, and communities as well. Epidemiology can be applied differently at each of these levels. At the individual and family levels, nurses must recognize the particular factors that may either positively or negatively affect the health of their clients. For example, based on epidemiologic studies, multiple factors, including poverty, strained marital communication, number of children, history of violence, stress, and social isolation, have been identified as risk factors for spousal abuse (Straus, Gelles, & Steinmetz, 1981). If community health nurses are aware of these factors, they may be in a position to intervene.

Recognizing the myriad social, economic, political, and cultural factors that affect the health of the community helps the nurse to plan community-level care. As an example, the close link between AIDS and intravenous substance abuse, which was uncovered by epidemiological methods, has led many community health departments to develop special community-based interventions such as free needle exchange programs (Bardsley, Turvey, & Blatherwick, 1990).

Despite the value of epidemiology for community health nursing, there are some challenges in using it in practice. Gaining access to the epidemiologic data that a nurse may wish to have about the community can prove daunting. There is a wide variation in the quality and accessibility of information across Canada. For example, it is often impossible to find valid, locally relevant information on basic descriptive epidemiology (i.e., prevalence or mortality rates) for health conditions of interest (e.g., malnutrition). This may be caused by a combination of factors, including inadequate reporting mechanisms, lack of funding to support data acquisition and/or dissemination, and competing priorities. Every community health unit should have someone on staff who is aware of available sources of information. Provincial ministries of health and the federal department of health are both excellent sources of information. In many cases, the data are available, but have not been analyzed in a way that makes the information useful. In such cases, it is often possible to have special analyses done.

Another challenge for nurses wishing to use epidemiology in their practice is information overload. By definition, an epidemiologic perspective requires the practitioner to examine multiple factors that may affect health; it is often difficult to set priorities and decide which information is most applicable. Even if a nurse wishes to use current, population-based information in practice, there are often conflicting epidemiological studies on any particular topic (e.g., should you recommend the use of margarine or of butter?). Although there is no simple solution, the community health unit could establish small working groups to sift through information and make consensual decisions about implications for change in practice.

Fortunately, with the advent of more accessible health data bases, community health information systems, and computer-mediated communication systems (i.e., the Internet), the future for relevant data acquisition, storage, retrieval, and analysis should improve over the coming decades.

Application of epidemiological principles to primary prevention and health promotion

Hypertension in the Hutterite community

The remainder of this chapter will demonstrate many epidemiological concepts through an example of a continuing program of community-based research with a unique Canadian cultural group, the Hutterian Brethren.

The Hutterites are an Anabaptist sect related theologically to both Mennonites and the Amish. The Hutterites live on communal agrarian colonies that have between 60 and 140 members. Unlike the Amish, Hutterites do not shun technology; indeed, their farms use the latest equipment, and they make full use of the modern health care system. The 30 000 Hutterites in North America are further subdivided into three endogamous (non-intermarrying) sects, or *leute*. The Hutterite population's genetic isolation and relatively small size have proven to be useful for studying the genetics of chronic disease (Hostetler, 1985).

In 1988, a collaborative program of epidemiological research was launched with the Hutterite communities of Alberta to discover whether they were at increased risk for heart disease (Brunt, 1989). The Hutterites perceived that health problems such as heart disease, stroke, diabetes, and hypertension were too prevalent in some communities. Their part coincided with the first author's interest in population-based studies of cardiovascular disease. In the first study, we found that 60 percent of the males and 29.5 percent of the females, aged 30 to 74 years, had a mean diastolic blood pressure (Dbp) ≥ 90 mm Hg (Brunt & Love, 1992a). The prevalence of elevated Dbp in our sample was between two and four times greater than in the general Canadian population, as reported in the Canadian Blood Pressure Survey (HWC, 1989b). A subsequent study has confirmed our earlier results (Brunt, Reeder, Stephenson, Love, & Chen, 1994).

In an attempt to make sense of this surprising result, the first author used the HAET model to examine factors that might help explain why Hutterites had such a high prevalence of high blood pressure. As a nurse, I was interested particularly in uncovering factors that were amenable to primary prevention interventions.

My first study with the Hutterites was traditional epidemiology, concerning itself primarily with discovering the prevalence of heart health–related problems, including hypertension. As part of that first study, participants were provided with a copy of their individual results, specific recommendations for follow-up, and a pamphlet describing the risk factors for heart disease (Brunt & Love, 1992a). Approximately 1.5 years after the study, participants were contacted and asked to complete a brief questionnaire about lifestyle changes they had made since the intervention. We found that a high proportion of the respondents had made changes such as increasing their surveillance of blood pressure (74 percent), losing weight (36 percent), and reducing their intake of salt (64 percent) and alcohol (48 percent) (Brunt & Love, 1992b).

In an effort to understand the factors that influenced these changes, we undertook further investigations using ethnographic methods. In addition, we began a process of community consultation that fits with the participatory action mode of inquiry and program planning. These epidemiologic findings can be used to support change. First, however, the HAET quantitative and qualitative findings from the research needed further examination.

A number of individual *host factors*, including body mass index (BMI), dietary preference, health-seeking behaviour, heredity, and exercise patterns, have been shown through population-based research to influence blood pressure (Canadian Dietetic Association, 1989; HWC, 1989a, 1989b, 1992). We found that Hutterites had approximately twice the prevalence of an elevated BMI (> 27 kg/m^2) than Canadians in the Canada Health Survey (HWC, 1981). Furthermore, the prevalence of diabetes among Hutterites in our survey was greater than that reported in the Canada Health Survey (HWC, 1981).

Health-seeking behaviour, particularly in relation to preventive health assessments, is essential for early detection of asymptomatic conditions such as hypertension. In our survey, we found that 56 percent of the participants with a Dbp ≥ 90 mm Hg were not aware that their blood pressure was elevated and had not had it checked during the past year by a health professional.

Finally, exercise patterns have been shown to be closely linked to blood pressure, either through direct circulatory effects (Urata et al., 1986) or via their impact on other related mechanisms (e.g., BMI). Moderate to vigorous aerobic physical activity, either on the job or during leisure time, was uncommon in this sample of Hutterites. Increasingly, mechanization has taken over many farm tasks that, in the past, required physical labour. Leisure-time activities tend to be sedentary, and physical activities such as sports are strongly discouraged.

There is considerable evidence supporting a genetic role in familial aggregation of hypertension (Clark, Schrott, Burns, Sing, & Lauer, 1986). Hutterites do not marry outside their own group and, not surprisingly, their coefficient of inbreeding (a measure of how genetically related individuals are) is quite high (Hostetler, 1985). This pooling of genes increases the likelihood of subtle, genetically related expressions of physical signs such as elevated blood pressure. Indeed, in a recent collaboration with geneticists, we have found an angiotensinogen gene associated with blood pressure regulation in the Hutterite population (unpublished data). At a population level, we have determined that blood pressure is significantly different between Hutterite *leute*; this inter-*leute* difference suggests a genetic component to blood pressure (Hegele, Brunt, & Connelly, 1994).

A variety of *agent factors* can affect blood pressure either by their presence or by their absence. Elevated blood pressure among previously diagnosed hypertensives in the Hutterite community was found to be largely uncontrolled and undermedicated (e.g., 76 percent of the Hutterites with a previous diagnosis of hypertension were not controlled). Thus, the absence of adequate pharmacologic treatment in this community plays a significant role in the high prevalence of hypertension in this population.

As discussed above, dietary preferences can expose individuals to particular substances that affect blood pressure. Alcohol consumption, in amounts as little as one or two beverages per day, has been shown to increase blood pressure in some individuals (Weissfeld, Johnson, Brock, & Hawthorne, 1988). Although alcohol abuse is rare in Hutterite society, over half the males and 13 percent of the females drink one or more alcoholic beverages a day. A number of cations (positively charged ions), particularly sodium, potassium, and calcium, have been shown to influence blood pressure in populations (Huttunen, Pietinen, Nissinen, & Puska, 1985). A previous study of the Hutterite diet found a sodium-to-potassium ratio of 4:1, a ratio shown to increase blood pressure (Rokusek-Kennedy, Parry, & Schlenker, 1987). A chronic imbalance in energy requirements and caloric intake can also lead to changes in BMI. Thus, caloric imbalance can be considered an agent that affects blood pressure. In both our study and a study by Schlenker, Parry, and McMillan (1989), excessive dietary intake of calories was identified as contributing to elevated BMI and Dbp in the Hutterite population.

The role of chronic stress in blood pressure elevation remains controversial, although problems with the precision of the instruments used to measure stress may explain why studies report conflicting results (Shoham-Yakubovich, Ragland, Brand, & Syme, 1988). Regardless, based on our survey results, Hutterites appear to have self-reported stress levels similar to those of the general Canadian population.

A number of important *environmental factors* influence the existence of, exposure to, or susceptibility to the agent and host factors described above. One of the most obvious environmental factors in the Hutterite population is their unique cultural milieu and belief systems. For example, Hutterites live their lives based on literal interpretation of the Bible. In a recent ethnographic study (unpublished data), we found that competing biblical interpretations may affect the Hutterites' health-seeking behaviours (e.g., viewing the body as a temple versus a fatalistic acceptance of "God's will"). Although a view of the body as a temple that must be maintained would support health promotion behaviour, a more fatalistic view would suggest that there is little that can be done to prevent premature death. Hutterites have no great fear of death; indeed, they welcome the opportunity to enter heaven. On the other hand, a sudden death is not viewed as a positive event because it prevents important cultural rituals from taking place (Stephenson, 1992).

Sociocultural norms also have a great influence on Hutterian diet and exercise. Many foods commonly consumed are high in saturated fat and sodium content. Although active games and sports are enjoyed by Hutterite children, adults are not permitted to participate, and leisure-time exercise is minimal. Given the high value placed on efficiency, modern equipment has largely displaced the hard physical labour once associated with farm life.

Because the colonies are rural, preventive health services are not as accessible as they would be in urban settings. Indeed, making arrangements for any non-emergency trip to the doctor or the community health clinic is complicated by the isolation of the colonies and the need to coordinate trips to town.

Finally, the physical environment of the colonies, particularly in relation to their water supply, can influence blood pressure. Virtually all colonies in our study rely on well water, much of which is high in sodium. To complicate matters, many colonies also treat their water with water softeners, affecting trace minerals such as calcium and magnesium, which influence blood pressure. Figure 29.3 consolidates many of the factors that affect blood pressure in the Hutterite population into one HAET model.

Figure 29.3
Consolidation of factors that affect blood pressure in the Hutterite population into the HAET model

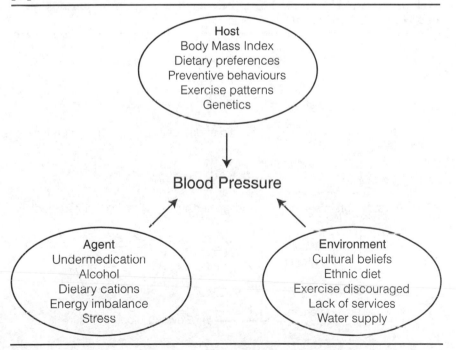

While the HAET model provides an organizing framework for assessing the factors that may affect the blood pressure of Hutterites, it can also be used for identifying and planning prevention and health promotion strategies. In our collaborative research program with the Hutterite community, we linked what we learned from the HAET model with health promotion program planning using a variety of quantitative and qualitative methods.

Having identified individual risk factors, the next step is to examine the interconnections and interactions among them to identify effective ways to reduce the prevalence of hypertension. For example, consideration of the role of sodium in hypertension demonstrated the intricacies of the web of causation (Figure 29.4).

The message from the interconnections among factors is that preventive strategies for reducing hypertension will require multiple culturally relevant approaches. For example, from our continuing research, it would appear that many colonies have made a concerted effort to examine and, in some cases, modify the colony's diet. Salt in the shakers at the table in many colonies has been replaced with a special blend of herbs and spices. Having identified the potential impact of sodium in the Hutterite water supply on blood pressure,

Figure 29.4
Web of causation demonstrating the role of sodium in hypertension in a Hutterite population

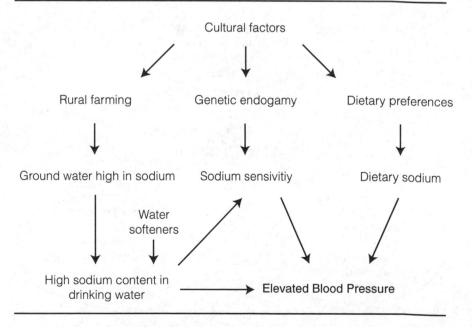

another primary prevention strategy would be to explore ways to increase the hardness of the water. One colony visited recently was examining the feasibility of installing a filtration system that would remove sodium.

From our work with the Hutterites, it became clear that these traditional quantitative approaches (e.g., prevalence) were extremely useful for identifying areas of concern. However, so that we could understand the context of the problem and complete the HAET model in relation to hypertension, other qualitative approaches were necessary.

At the present time, we are analyzing our data from an ethnographic study that examined the meaning of health for Hutterites. From our data, it is clear that belief systems of Hutterites provide many opportunities for developing culturally appropriate health promotion programs. For example, the importance of moderation in all activities and treating the body as a temple appear to predominate over a more fatalistic view of life and death. Health is understood primarily in terms of spiritual health, and taking care of one's physical health is interpreted as a way of living a good life.

To have a richer understanding of what factors affect health promotion decisions, we are conducting another ethnographic study on a group of colonies that have demonstrated either high, low, or intermediate levels of change in response to our previous work. Again, by going beyond the traditional quantitative epidemiological approaches, we believe that we will be in a better position to work collaboratively with the colonies in health promotion program planning. Given the important role played by colony elders, and in particular the minister, manager, and head cook, it is not surprising that colony-wide change appears to be influenced greatly by their beliefs about health promotion.

As helpful as ethnographic methods may prove to be in understanding the context of health promotion within the Hutterite community, it is important that methods drawn from participatory action research be utilized in program planning. A cornerstone of participatory action research is that researchers must give up their need to define health problems and prescribe solutions for communities (Labonte, 1989).

Participatory action research is closely related to the concepts of public participation and empowerment (see also Chapter 28). Public participation involves individual and collective action of people to become involved in and improve their community (Powell, Faghfoury, Hill, & Nyenhuis, 1989, p. 171). In our collaborative work with the Hutterite community, the process of empowerment involves their seeking to (a) identify their problems, (b) assess the social and historical roots of those problems, (c) envision a healthier society, and (d) develop strategies to overcome obstacles in achieving their goals (Wallerstein & Bernstein, 1988). (For a more complete discussion of the cultural aspects of health promotion in the Hutterite community, see Brunt, Lindsey, & Hopkinson, 1997.)

During a recent follow-up visit to 17 colonies identified as having a high prevalence of hypertension, we conducted a community forum in each colony to discuss the colonists' views of their heart health and health behaviour changes that had been or could possibly be made. Although we had anticipated a highly participatory community meeting, we were surprised to find that one or two spokespersons provided the bulk of the information. In retrospect, given the social structure of the colonies with their reliance on elder-based decision making, these group dynamics made perfect sense. Thus, we have found that participatory action for program planning must involve working closely with colony elders. Again, this demonstrates the need for working within the cultural milieu when developing health promotion programs.

Another feature of the Hutterite community is that each colony has its own unique character. Strategies that might work in one colony may have little applicability to any other. Thus, consensus building for action (e.g., health promotion planning) must be done on a colony-by-colony basis. Only in this way can ownership of whatever health promotion program emerges reside with the colony.

In an effort to aid the process of program development, we have also enabled the colonies to locate the internal and external community resources that may prove helpful in the health promotion process. By contacting nurses, dietitians, and physicians in the local community health units, we are compiling a compendium that can be used as a resource by the colonies. This consolidation of diverse resources is an example of the intersectoral and interdisciplinary collaboration that is required for community-based health promotion. In addition, we are gathering information about colony-based resources and documenting their success. For example, in one colony the minister has become proficient in taking blood pressure and regularly offers clinics for colony members. Clearly, if colonies could assume more of the formal responsibility for surveillance and blood pressure monitoring, many problems related to accessibility to health care would be ameliorated.

Conclusion

Traditional epidemiological methods have made an enormous contribution to the understanding of the distribution and causes of many major health challenges facing Canadians. The HAET model is a useful start in taking a holistic view of factors that affect health. However, community health nurses interested in primary prevention and health promotion must draw upon an array of methods to deal with the challenges uncovered by more traditional epidemiologic methods. Ethnography and other qualitative methods are particularly useful for revealing many environmental factors that influence the occurrence of health challenges. The emerging field of participatory action research holds exciting promise for translating the multifactorial determinants of health into positive Primary Health Care and health promotion programs.

QUESTIONS

1. Select a community health issue that you believe is amenable to a primary prevention intervention by nurses, then:
    a. Using the HAET model, outline the multiple factors that influence the health issue.
    b. Draw the interconnections between the various host, agent, and environmental factors (web of causation).
    c. Consider various approaches that could be taken to deal with the health issue, and plot, within the web of causation, where those interventions would have the greatest potential impact.
2. Epidemiology has traditionally focussed on disease, and it is only recently that the notion of "the epidemiology of health" has emerged. Think of an example from your community where epidemiology would be a useful approach to understand factors that enhance health. Based on this example, what would your role as a community health nurse be in promoting health?
3. Based on the community health program of research with the Hutterites described in this chapter, how would you approach assisting this community with its concerns about hypertension? What ethical questions does this type of work raise?

REFERENCES

Angus, D.E., & Turbayne, E. (1995). *Path to the future: A synopsis of health and health care issues*. Ottawa: National Nursing Competency Project.

Bardsley, J., Turvey, J., & Blatherwick, J. (1990). Vancouver's needle exchange program. *Canadian Journal of Public Health, 81*, 39–45.

Brunt, J.H. (1989). *Coronary heart disease among the Dariusleut Hutterites of Alberta*. Unpublished doctoral dissertation, University of Calgary.

Brunt, J.H., Lindsey, A.E., & Hopkinson, J. (1997). Health promotion in the Hutterite community and the ethnocentricity of empowerment. *Canadian Journal of Nursing Research, 29*(1), 17–28.

Brunt, J.H., & Love, E.J. (1992a). Evaluation of hypertension screening in the Hutterite population. *Research in Nursing and Health, 15*, 103–110.

Brunt, J.H., & Love, E.J. (1992b). Hypertension and its correlates in the Hutterite community of Alberta. *Canadian Journal of Public Health, 83*, 362–366.

Brunt, J.H., Reeder, B., Stephenson, P., Love, E.J., & Chen, Y. (1994). A comparison of physical and laboratory measures between two Hutterite leute and the rural Saskatchewan population. *Canadian Journal of Public Health, 85,* 299–302.

Camacho, T.C., Roberts, R.E., Lazarus, N.B., Kaplan, G.A., & Cohen, R.D. (1991). Physical activity and depression: Evidence form the Alameda County Study. *American Journal of Epidemiology, 134,* 220–231.

Canadian Dietetic Association. (1989). The role of diet in the prevention of hypertension: Official position of the CDA. *Journal of the Canadian Dietetic Association, 50,* 12–17.

Clark, W.R., Schrott, H.G., Burns, T.L., Sing, C.F., & Lauer, R.M. (1986). Aggregation of blood pressure in the families of children with labile high systolic blood pressure. *American Journal of Epidemiology, 123,* 67–80.

Dobson, A.J., Alexander, H.M., Heller, R.F., & Lloyd, D.M. (1991). Passive smoking and the risk of heart attack or coronary death. *Medical Journal of Australia, 154,* 793–797.

Evans, R.G., Barer, M.L., & Marmor, T.R. (1994). *Why are some people healthy and others not?* New York: Aldine De Gruyter Press.

Fletcher, R.H., Fletcher, S.W., & Wagner, E.H. (1988). *Clinical epidemiology: The essentials* (2nd ed.). Baltimore: Williams & Wilkens.

Health & Welfare Canada (HWC). (1981). *Canada health survey.* Ottawa: Statistics Canada.

Health & Welfare Canada (HWC). (1988). *Canada's health promotion survey.* Ottawa: Minister of Supply & Services.

Health & Welfare Canada (HWC). (1989a). *Canadian blood pressure survey.* Ottawa: National Health & Welfare.

Health & Welfare Canada (HWC). (1989b). *Knowledge development for health promotion: A call for action.* Ottawa: Ministry of Supply & Services. (Cat. No. H39-147/1989E)

Health & Welfare Canada (HWC). (1992). *Victoria declaration on heart health.* Ottawa: Ministry of Supply & Services.

Health & Welfare Canada (HWC). (1994). *Strategies for population health.* Ottawa: Ministry of Supply & Services.

Hegele, R.A., Brunt, J.H., & Connelly, P.W. (1994). A polymorphism of the angiotensionogen gene associated with variation in blood pressure in a genetic isolate. *Circulation, 90,* 2207–2212.

Hostetler, J.A. (1985). History and relevance of the Hutterite population for genetic studies. *American Journal of Medical Genetics, 22,* 453–462.

Huttunen, J.K., Pietinen, P., Nissinen, A., & Puska, P. (1985). Dietary factors and hypertension. *Acta Medica Scandinavica, 701,* 72–82.

Labonte, R. (1989). Community and professional empowerment. *Canadian Nurse, 85*(3), 21–28.

Lilienfeld, A.M., & Lilienfeld, D.E. (1980). *Foundations of epidemiology* (2nd ed.). New York: Oxford.

Mausner, J.S., & Kramer, S. (1985). *Epidemiology: An introductory text* (2nd ed.). Philadelphia: W.B. Saunders.

Ministry of Health & Ministry Responsible for Seniors. (1997). *A report on the health of British Columbians: Provincial health officer's annual report for 1996.* Victoria: Author.

Powell, M., Faghfoury, N., Hill, K., & Nyenhuis, P. (1989). Fostering public participation. In Health & Welfare Canada, Health Services & Promotion Branch, *Knowledge development for health promotion: A call for action*. Ottawa: Minister of Supply & Services. (Cat. No. H39-147/1989E)

Rokusek-Kennedy, C., Parry, R.R., & Schlenker, E.H. (1987). The nutritional status of Hutterites in South Dakota. *Federation Proceedings, 46*, 1157.

Schlenker, E.H., Parry, R.R., & McMillan, M.J. (1989). Influence of age, sex, and obesity on blood pressure of Hutterites in South Dakota. *Chest, 95*, 1269–1273.

Shoham-Yakubovich, I., Ragland, D.R., Brand, R.J., & Syme, S.L. (1988). Type A behavior pattern and health status after 22 years of follow-up in the Western Collaborative Group Study. *American Journal of Epidemiology, 128*, 579–588.

Stanhope, M., & Lancaster, J. (1996). *Community health nursing: Process and practice for promoting health* (4th ed.). St. Louis: Mosby.

Stachtchenko, S., & Jenicek, M. (1990). Conceptual differences between prevention and health promotion: Research implications for community health programs. *Canadian Journal of Public Health, 81*, 53–59.

Stephenson, P.H. (1992). He died 'too quick': The process of dying in a Hutterian colony. In L.A. Platt & V.R. Persico (Eds.), *Grief in cross-cultural perspective: A casebook* (pp. 293–306). New York: Garland Press.

Straus, M.A., Gelles, R.J., & Steinmetz, S.K. (1981). *Behind closed doors: Violence in the American family*. Garden City, NY: Anchor.

Turner, J.G., & Chavigny, K.H. (1988). *Community health nursing: An epidemiologic perspective through the nursing process*. Philadelphia: J.B. Lippincott.

Urata, H., Tanabe, Y., Kiyonaga, A., Ikeda, M., Tanaka, H., Shindo, M., & Arakawa, K. (1986). Antihypertensive and volume-depleting effects of mild exercise on essential hypertension. *Hypertension, 9*, 245–252.

Valanis, B. (1992). *Epidemiology in nursing and health care* (2nd ed.). Norwalk, CT: Appleton & Lang.

Wallerstein, N., & Bernstein, E. (1988). Empowerment education: Freire's ideas adapted to health education. *Health Education Quarterly, 15*, 379–394.

Weissfeld, J.L., Johnson, E.H., Brock, B.M., & Hawthorne, V.M. (1988). Sex and age interactions in the association between alcohol and blood pressure. *American Journal of Epidemiology, 128*, 559–569.

Part 6
Administration of Community Health Nursing

Community health nurses need to be educationally prepared for Primary Health Care practice and to receive reinforcement and guidance for this type of practice from their administrators. Identification of the unique role of community health nursing administrators is vital to an understanding of the changing practice environment. Recent evidence of the impact of stress on nurses and of their need for occupational support cannot be ignored. Administrators face the challenge of providing a supportive work environment for community health nurses in this era of health system reform.

In Chapter 30, Braunstein, Young, and Beanlands indicate that administration should provide the environment, structure, and leadership for community health nursing services. Recently, decentralization, regionalization, and Primary Health Care principles have been endorsed. Public health nursing programs have become program based. The authors identify issues relevant to public health nursing administration in a reformed health system: paradigm shift, focus on primary prevention, emphasis on populations, provision of universal and targeted services, partnerships and shared decision making, evaluation, and multidisciplinary practice. In this context, administrators must ensure that salient competencies are developed and maintained.

They must also support the changing role of the community health nurse; consider the sociocultural, economic, and environmental determinants of health; and collaborate with communities in developing health public policy. The new competencies include Primary Health Care skills and roles, community development, information technology, policy development, and population-based strategies. Clearly, the community health nursing administrator will require political acumen and knowledge of policy to meet the evolving challenges of health system reform.

C H A P T E R 3 0

Administration in community health nursing

Janet Braunstein, Heather J. Young, and Hope E. Beanlands

The administration of community health nursing within the context of health system reform and renewal is discussed in this chapter. Restructuring, regionalization and decentralization, and evolving administrative structures will continue to have an impact on the administration of public health nursing. These innovations will require the community health nurse administrator to be adaptive, creative, and responsive to the needs of community health nurses and to the political and economic environments in which they work. Seven issues relevant to community health nursing administration are identified. These issues have important implications for administrators, including the need to retool and develop new competencies, assist communities to build capacity for assuming ownership in decisions, and enhance collaborative practice and accountability.

LEARNING OBJECTIVES

In this chapter, you will learn:

- the leadership role of community health nurse administrators in addressing the broad determinants of health as a partner in the health system
- the broad range of competencies required in the administration of community health nursing
- the importance of partnerships and accountability in community health nursing administration

Introduction

The Canadian health system, in general, and community health services, specifically, have undergone major reform and some renewal over the past decade. The Canadian public is demanding an active role in the evolution of a health system that (a) focusses on keeping people well, (b) prevents illness and disability, (c) promotes healthy public policy and reduction of risk, (d) spends treatment dollars wisely on interventions that have a demonstrated result, (e) provides access to treatment services when required, and (f) demonstrates accountability for results.

The administration of community health nursing refers to the process and structure by which a government or an organization uses its resources to deliver community health programs. (Throughout the remainder of this chapter, the term *public health* will also apply to community health.)

The purpose of administration is to provide the structure, leadership, and environment in which public health nursing services are made available to citizens. Administration provides the venue for

- documentation of the mission of public health nursing within an organizational structure
- articulation of goals, objectives, standards, and specific outcomes
- development of public health policies
- development of standards and programs
- implementation of program planning
- development of criteria to achieve quality improvement
- evaluation of the efficacy and efficiency of public health nursing programs
- demonstration of best public health practices
- articulation of accountability and evidence-based decision-making processes.

Leadership in public health nursing administration

The nurse administrator represents the profession, its standards, and the public's health within the public health organization. As a leader, the nurse administrator "creates an empowering environment that fosters creativity, risk taking and growth" (Meilicke, 1990, p. 31).

Public health nurse administrators need an in-depth understanding of the complexity of their role as leaders and an appreciation of the variety of leadership situations. Effective leadership is translated into clear role definitions, balanced work groups, and carefully designed work units (composed of people with complementary knowledge, skill, and style) that implement specific programs or projects (Kernaghan & Siegal, 1991). Administrators must create a work environment that values professionals who embody diversity, critical thought, reflection, commitment to peer and self-evaluation, and dedication to continued learning and skill development.

The values and principles of an organization describe the manner in which work is to be accomplished and the expectations for interactions among team members (Nova Scotia Department of Health, 1997a, pp. 157–160). As an example, the values and principles of the Nova Scotia Department of Health, Public Health Services Division, are shown in Figure 30.1. Organizational support is a key factor in ensuring successful organizational cultural change (Knox & Irving, 1997).

The public health nurse administrator is challenged to provide leadership that facilitates the development and implementation of values and principles for the organization. More importantly, individual team members must be held accountable for reflecting the stated values and principles in their behaviour. It is critical that administrators demonstrate personal commitment to the values and principles of the organization and function as role models in their implementation.

The nurse administrator, using the organization's values and principles, builds diverse work teams and encourages the teams to develop and communicate a clear vision of their work. It is important that the vision for the department or unit be responsive to the ideas generated by team members. This, in turn, will build a strong commitment to the shared vision. There must be trust, respect, and a supportive environment for team members to develop competencies. Administrators who create and sustain this type of work environment can expect team members with high tolerance for ambiguity. There should be an inherent capacity to handle open-ended problems, to analyze situations critically, to establish high standards, to create performance expectations, and to exchange feedback.

Historically, leadership styles have been categorized as autocratic, participatory, and autonomous. Generally, a supportive administration will lead to greater employee commitment and involvement with the work group. Overall, effectiveness is clearly dependent on more than leadership style.

Leadership creates the vision and moves public health nursing toward standards of excellence and achievement of organizational goals. The public health nurse administrator is charged with transforming the vision into reality.

Administrative structures in public health nursing practice

Public health nursing practice in Canada has been administered primarily through provincial government departments, such as departments of health or ministries of health and social services. With regionalization, these structures have been altered significantly, and the public health infrastructure is

Figure 30.1
Example of statement of values and principles

Public Health Services

VALUES

The Public Health Services Division believes that ideals and beliefs are important to people in an organization and are worth striving toward. In this context, values express a vision of how the world should be and they are designed to influence the behaviour of people.

TRUST, HONESTY, INTEGRITY
RESPECT, RECOGNITION
CARING, SUPPORT
JUSTICE, EQUITY,
COMMITMENT/LOYALTY
HEALTHY LIFESTYLE

PRINCIPLES

Principles have also been developed by the Division to serve as a set of guidelines or criteria that support the Division's values. They are also used to determine whether the values are being upheld or violated. They can serve as operating principles and enhance the development of performance assessments. It bears note that the principles are meant to be interpreted collectively and only in concert with the values of the Division.

PRINCIPLE 1
There are generally multiple criteria, which are frequently conflicting, that need to be considered when making and carrying out decisions.

For the Division, major criteria that should always be considered are reflected in the mission statement of the Division:
*The Mission of the Public Health Services Division is **to protect, maintain and contribute to the health of Nova Scotians**.*

PRINCIPLE 2
The Division should have policies and regulations which serve the best interest of the clients.

PRINCIPLE 3
The Division should be sensitive to staff needs and aspirations and be directed to enhance personal growth and development thus enhancing staff's ability to contribute to the goals of the Division.

PRINCIPLE 4
All persons in the Division should know what types of *results* they are responsible for and should agree that they are attainable.

Objectives and evaluation should be focused upon those results which are under the control of the individual.

PRINCIPLE 5
Every individual in the Division should have only one supervisor and know who that individual is.

In general, only the direct supervisor should normally have the authority to set objectives, allocate resources, and direct, veto or evaluate the performance of an individual.

PRINCIPLE 6
Communication should be kept as free and open as possible. Information, assistance, guidance may be obtained from a variety of sources, however in situations involving direction, approval, veto – the lines of authority in the Division must be respected.

PRINCIPLE 7
Authority can be delegated – responsibility cannot.

No one should have the authority to direct or veto any decisions or actions where they are not accountable for the results.

PRINCIPLE 8
Everyone should strive towards promoting and maintaining a strong relationship of mutual trust, confidence and respect among and between all members of the Division.

Everyone has an obligation to actively pursue the foregoing objectives with respect to all individuals in the Division.

PRINCIPLE 9
All individuals in the Division should strive toward absolute integrity in their relationships with all others, both within and outside the Division. Individuals are responsible for their own behaviour and actions and should work to their highest standards.

PRINCIPLE 10
Each individual in the Division should strive to respect and accept individual differences and strive for appreciation of such differences.

PRINCIPLE 11
All individuals in the Division are expected to adhere to their professional and government's code of ethics.

NOVA SCOTIA
Department of Health
April 1993   Printed on paper that contains recycled fibre

Nova Scotia Department of Health, Public Health Services Division (1993). Used with permission.

diverse across Canada (Canadian Public Health Association, 1997). The structure varies depending on the provincial or regional department portfolio (Nova Scotia Department of Health, 1997b). Within the portfolio, public health services are delivered by a multidisciplinary team generally composed of public health nurses, nutritionists, medical officers of health, health inspectors, public health engineers, dentists, dental hygienists, social workers, and educators. Practice is grounded in legislative mandates developed to protect the public's health and safety relative to communicable disease, environmental risks, and lifestyle (e.g., Ontario's *Health Protection and Promotion Act*).

Historically, the system in which public health nurses practised was hierarchical (Smith, 1994; Tappen, 1989). Departments were often headed by a medical health officer and, in more recent years, by administrators who did not have a background in the health professions. Nevertheless, the administrative structure prescribed how public health nurses carried out their activities. During the 1980s, this situation resulted in a controlling system with a vertical approach to decision making. Moreover, public health nurses—and citizens in the community—had almost no say in decision making regarding community health services. This approach fostered overmanagement of the public health nurse and, in turn, stifled nurses' creativity, self-motivation, and citizen participation.

Today, across Canada, fundamental changes are occurring in the health care system. Much of this change has emanated from Royal Commissions and provincial reviews (Rachlis & Kushner, 1994). Across Canada, regionalization and Primary Health Care principles have been endorsed; however, the realization of these principles has been elusive.

Regionalization involves the transfer of power and authority from one group (e.g., government) to a new or pre-existing organization with jurisdiction over smaller specified units or responsibilities (Nova Scotia Minister's Action Committee on Health System Reform, 1994a). Regionalization is based on establishment of regional systems and transfer of power to those systems. In Nova Scotia, the rationale for regionalization and decentralization focussed on

- effective community input into decision making about health care resource allocation
- improved coordination and integration of health services at the community and regional levels
- minimized administrative and overhead costs to allocate more money to services and programs
- reduced disparities among regions in the access, availability, cost, and quality of health care
- funding formula that responds to the health needs of the region

- financial savings through appropriate economies of scale, reduced duplication of services, and competition. (Nova Scotia Minister's Action Committee, 1994b, p. 26)

All provinces have implemented regionalized systems whose approaches vary depending upon operational definition, vision of regionalization, and speed of implementation. Although regionalization may represent decentralization from the provincial government's perspective, it may be a centralizing process from the perspective of local providers and consumers (Blomqvist & Brown, 1994). Regionalization will continue to have major implications for the administration of public health nursing. While nurse administrators can be the catalyst for change, systems and structures are slow in making the necessary organizational changes to move to a Primary Health Care approach.

Some jurisdictions have consolidated Primary Health Care components, resulting in program-based delivery services. Public health nursing programs have been reoriented to become program-based, such as the Early Childhood Initiatives in New Brunswick or the Healthy Baby program in Nova Scotia. Both programs involve interdisciplinary participation. The former position of Director of Public Health Nursing (or equivalent) has been altered; the administrative role is now reflected in such titles as "Manager, Communicable Disease," "Director, Health Promotion," or "Community Care Consultant." These roles represent responsibility for program management and interdisciplinary practice, rather than responsibility for administration of public health nursing solely. However, such changes have made public health nursing less visible and the role of the public health nurse administrator obscure. In future, public health nurse administrators could be eliminated.

The impact of such changes on public health nursing practice has not been fully evaluated. There is a fundamental professional base in public health and public health nursing that needs to be maintained and not marginalized. Program-based practice should ensure high standards.

In summary, Primary Health Care and regionalization have been key themes within the Canadian health care system in the 1990s. These changes have the potential to enhance or diminish public health nursing's contributions and value in the health system.

Administration in public health nursing and healthy public policy

The public health nurse administrator, as a member of the multidisciplinary team, has an important role in facilitating the development of healthy public policy, a mechanism for health promotion. Healthy public policies should reflect the broad determinants of health. The public health nurse administrator is in a position to provide leadership regarding the development of healthy public policy related to health determinants. For example, the public health nursing perspective is critical when governments are creating policies related to nutritional supplements for women on social assistance, introduction of new vaccines, development of day-care programs, or school programs to enhance students' self-esteem and promote responsible health behaviour.

Healthy public policy must be grounded in a philosophy of social justice and consideration of the health-related needs of populations. It can, for example, involve decisions related to gambling. Although gambling establishments may increase revenue and contribute to employment, their negative impact in terms of addictions and community social problems, such as crime and prostitution, is not conducive to overall population health outcomes.

Public health nurse administrators, with their knowledge of population health, expertise in working in partnership with communities, awareness of current research, and membership on multidisciplinary teams, are in a unique position to contribute to the development and implementation of healthy public policy.

Issues related to public health nursing administration in a Primary Health Care system

Public participation is one major element in a Primary Health Care system (Smith, 1994). The realities of transforming all the principles of Primary Health Care into practice are daunting. Issues relevant to public health nursing administration in a reformed health system based on Primary Health Care include (a) paradigm shift in public health administration, (b) focus on primary prevention, (c) focus on populations, (d) provision of universal and targeted services, (e) enhancement of partnerships and shared decision making, (f) accountability and evaluation, and (g) multidisciplinary practice.

Paradigm shift in public health nursing administration

Several administrative changes must occur to accommodate the principles that support Primary Health Care. These changes include shifts from (a) authoritarianism (top-down control) to democratic control (shared responsibility for decision making with nurses and communities), (b) elitism to equality and social justice, (c) uniformity (one way of doing things) to pluralism (different ways of doing things), (d) conformity to self-determination and growth (creative and innovative environment), and (e) stasis to dynamic change (Smith, 1994). The rapid expansion in knowledge and skills required by the public health nurse challenges the administrator to ensure that competencies are maintained. The shift from doing "all things for all people" in a defined geographic area to a programmatic approach now requires the public health nurse to focus on program areas such as sexual health, family health, and child health using principles of Primary Health Care. Community development and health promotion are two key Primary Health Care strategies that must be integrated into practice. Inclusion of citizens is essential, as community action will exert major influence and effect fundamental change over the next decade. The skills required in working with communities are not well developed across the professions. Partnerships with community animators, community developers, and community leaders are required.

Focus on primary prevention

Integration of primary prevention into the Primary Health Care model is essential. Public health nurse administrators must ensure that a focus on primary prevention is maintained. Primary prevention seeks to prevent the initial occurrence of an illness or injury, whereas secondary prevention seeks to arrest or retard existing disease through early detection and appropriate treatment. Tertiary prevention is aimed at avoiding further deterioration of an already existing problem.

Nurses who work in hospitals focus on treatment and varying levels of secondary and tertiary prevention. For instance, nutrition counselling following a myocardial infarction is tertiary prevention. Nutrition counselling for those with risk factors (smoking, high cholesterol levels, sedentary lifestyle) would be secondary prevention. Examples of primary prevention include promoting low-fat diets to young families (a program issue) and working with the agricultural industry and farmers to produce low-fat products (a policy issue).

Evaluation of Primary Health Care activities must ensure that primary prevention interventions, both program and policy, have been implemented. Program planning must include the use of epidemiological data, criteria for primary prevention activities (e.g., those that are acceptable, effective, and targeted), and a policy framework to achieve predetermined outcomes. Public health nurse administrators, as advocates, must lobby for the inclusion of primary prevention in the implementation of Primary Health Care.

Focus on populations

Public health nurse administrators must ensure that programs and policies focus on the health of populations (e.g., youth, children, seniors, immigrants) and the determinants of health (Government of Nova Scotia, 1997/1998). Decisions must be based on epidemiological data and must contribute to improved health status of the population. Measurable targets to achieve population health must be identified. Examples of measurable targets are "By the year 2007, 50 percent of parents and caregivers will demonstrate knowledge, skills, and behaviours appropriate to healthy child growth and development" or "By the year 2007, 80 percent of parents with children aged 18 months to five years will be able to identify the relationship between diet and oral health" (Nova Scotia Department of Health, 1997a).

The usual frame of reference for health professionals is the individual, while policy decisions in public health focus on population groups. The individual frame of reference can be complementary to population-based strategies. One example of a population health intervention is a needle exchange program for intravenous drug users to prevent the spread of HIV. This intervention protects the population at large from the spread of HIV. In contrast, provision of needles to persons with diabetes has an individual frame of reference. The public health nurse administrator must advocate for the integration of the needs of unique populations, such as persons with AIDS, into policy.

Provision of universal and targeted services

Public health nursing practice is the combined art and science of nursing and public health, with Primary Health Care goals of promotion and protection of health and prevention of illness and injury. Universal and targeted services are used to achieve these goals. Universal services include, for example, an immunization program for all children or parenting classes for all parents. Targeted services include parenting classes for socially isolated, financially constrained parents or meningococcal vaccine provided only to at-risk children in a day care. The public health nurse administrator combines universal and targeted services in program and policy decisions.

Targeted services may have a higher cost–benefit ratio and be more desirable than universal services. Finite resources may also dictate the targeting of services. Targeted services challenge the administrator, as every decision to allocate resources to one group is made at the cost of limited or no service to another. Targeted services must be based on principles of social justice. In allocating resources, the public health nurse administrator and others must articulate the ethical principles that underpin targeted or universal services.

Enhancement of partnerships and shared decision making

The implementation of the Primary Health Care principle of public participation in public health nursing practice necessitates shared responsibilities between consumers and professional providers. The use of community development in determining needs and assets, allocation of resources, and delivery of services involves a partnership between communities and public health nurses. Community expertise must be balanced with professional knowledge. This new relationship requires respect, time, and trust.

Public health nurse administrators must support the changing relationship between the public health nurse and the consumer and relevant changes in measures of outcomes. For instance, information systems in public health nursing have historically focussed on quantitative measures (e.g., how many visits, how many students). With the advent of community development, administrators recognize that new methodologies are required to measure outcomes. Communities accept different indicators of success than those traditionally used in health care. For example, a valued community outcome might be the degree to which residents believe that they participate in decision making, not the number of people attending a clinic.

Accountability and evaluation

Public participation demands accountability to the public. Setting clear objectives and measuring results are crucial to accountability. "Accountability is the obligation to answer for a responsibility that has been conferred" (Nova Scotia Department of Health, 1997b, p. 10). Today, because of public accountability, fiscal restraint, and new scientific and sociological information, evaluation has become a crucial component of public health nursing administration. An evaluation plan is an essential part of program planning. The public health nurse administrator must facilitate evaluation and advise on evaluation methodology.

Multidisciplinary practice

The multidisciplinary team in public health recognizes the unique yet complementary skills, competencies, and expertise of all members. Multidisciplinary practice demands mutual respect, trust, and collaborative work toward common goals and outcomes (Nova Scotia Department of Health, 1993). Multidisciplinary practice should be valued and instilled during the educational process—ideally through interdisciplinary courses, field placements, and research (Nova Scotia Task Force on Nursing, 1993).

These seven administration issues, arising from Primary Health Care principles, offer a unique opportunity for leadership and creativity. Public health nurse administrators must facilitate the necessary paradigm shift, advocate for primary prevention, and promote a population-based approach to policy development and program planning. In addition, the public health nurse administrator is expected to facilitate ethical decision making in service delivery, foster partnerships with consumers, and endorse multidisciplinary practice.

Implications for administration in public health nursing

Illness prevention and health promotion are important components of a Primary Health Care system. The rhetoric espousing a shift from a curative, illness-care system to one that values health promotion and illness and injury prevention is becoming reality. Such a shift should position public health nurse administrators to play an important role in population health promotion efforts. Working with clients in a variety of settings, public health nurse administrators contribute to the sociocultural, economic, and environmental determinants of health. These include safe homes and schools, food security, environmental protection, waste management, fiscal accountability, crime prevention, economic development, literacy improvement, and social support (Chambers, 1992). These determinants must be considered in developing healthy public policy. Moreover, public health nursing must work in collaboration with communities in developing such policy. These issues for public health nursing administration necessitate new competencies, capacity for change, and collaborative practice.

New competencies: Retooling for the new millennium

The core competencies required for administrators in public health nursing represent a blend of knowledge, critical thought and decision-making abilities, management expertise, and creative leadership. Core competencies include public health nursing theory and practice, leadership, change theory, financial management, quality assurance, qualitative and quantitative evaluation, information technology, policy development and analysis, evidence-based outcome research, organizational redesign, and political acumen (Beanlands, 1993).

The new competencies required by public health nurses have major implications for the administrator. The competencies required of today's practitioner include knowledge of population-based strategies, the determinants of health, community development, and community activation; partnership and collaborative relationships; and the ability to facilitate the diverse roles of volunteers and informal helpers such as family, friends, and self-help groups (Health & Welfare Canada, 1991). The public health nurse administrator should value these skills and knowledge and allocate professional development time and financial resources to these competencies.

To provide leadership and vision with respect to these new competencies, the public health nurse administrator requires preparation at the graduate level. Graduate educational requirements may be obtained through either an advanced nursing core of knowledge within an administration program or an administrative core of knowledge within a nursing degree program.

The acquisition of new competencies by public health nurses may be threatening to the public health nurse administrator. Acknowledging and celebrating the value of past practice while simultaneously analyzing new best practices are important. Collaboration with educational institutions offers opportunities for the exchange of ideas among faculty, students, administrators, and public health nurses in attaining these new competencies.

Building capacity for change

The capacity to change to a practice founded on Primary Health Care principles is a challenge for public health nurses, administrators, and citizens. Working with targeted populations may increase the intensity and protracted nature of the nurse–client relationship in that solutions may be more difficult to attain and the time to attain goals may be longer. Providers may grieve the loss of the traditional role and may have difficulty abandoning past practices. Citizens may perceive these changes as withdrawal of services. Often, the client has come to depend on the presence of the public health nurse, and the change in practice may highlight the dependent nature of the relationship. Alternatively, the community may facilitate the changing practice by supporting the new provider–client relationship. It is crucial for the public health nurse and administrator to develop partnerships with a broad range of partners: the private sector, community action groups, and all groups that influence the broad determinants of health.

If the public health nurse administrator builds the capacity to change, this enables nurses to practise creatively in a new Primary Health Care system. The administrator can build capacity through mentoring, support, resources, time, commitment to risk taking, and working collaboratively with communities.

Collaborative practice

Collaboration with other health professionals, other sectors related to health determinants, and community members is a challenge for public health nurses and administrators. Multidimensional interventions require multidisciplinary approaches to achieve shared goals. Health practitioners often protect their own practice domain. Although theoretically, public health nurses endorse collaborative practice, the reality can be threatening and time-consuming. Open and honest discussion among providers, clients, and community can delineate roles, functions, accountabilities, and responsibilities. A shared analysis of the organization and its mission, values, programs, and outcomes is important. Mutual respect and trust are critical to collaboration.

Challenges and realities

As efforts to redefine, refocus, and implement a vision for Primary Health Care continue and as health system redesign evolves, the public health nurse administrator must expect change and uncertainty.

The focus on results, outcomes, and evidence-based practice requires sophisticated information systems. This, in turn, requires personnel who possess the ability to use such systems and to analyze data that have an impact on public health interventions. These mechanisms and systems are still being developed in the public health environment. For example, the

Local Public Health Infrastructure Development Demonstration Project, being implemented in the Atlantic Region by Health Canada, will contribute to the development of essential systems and competencies.

In the current atmosphere of restructuring, administrators have had to terminate and then re-hire employees. An aging workforce and an impending nurse shortage will challenge the public health nurse administrator to be proactive and to pursue human resource planning. Relationships with unions have shifted focus from wage issues to job security. Employers are also faced with the challenge of providing continuing education programs to address the changing needs of communities and the health system. These are a few of the challenges and realities facing the public health nurse administrator in the new millennium.

Conclusion

Health system reform will continue to have a significant impact on public health nursing, as well as its administration. In this context, the implementation of Primary Health Care will influence the practice of public health nurses. New and evolving competencies will be required. The public health nurse administrator is in a leadership position to foster these changes. Nurse administrators must ensure that the culture and environment are conducive for the public health nurse to practise Primary Health Care in the newly reformed health system.

QUESTIONS

1. What are the major challenges confronting public health nurse administrators in the move to a Primary Health Care system?
2. What are the administrative implications of the distinctions between individual and population health?
3. What are the advantages and disadvantages of the changing administrative structures in public health nursing practice?
4. What competencies are required by the public health nurse administrator? How can these competencies be developed?

REFERENCES

Beanlands, H.E. (1993). *Competencies and educational requirements of public health nurse managers.* Unpublished report for the Nova Scotia Department of Health, Public Health Services Division.

Blomqvist, A., & Brown, D.M. (1994). *Limits to care*. Toronto: C.D. Howe Institute.

Canadian Public Health Association (CPHA). (1997). *Public health infrastructure in Canada (summary document)*. Ottawa: Author.

Chambers, L.W. (1992). The new public health: Do local public health agencies need a booster (or organizational "fix") to combat the diseases of disarray? *Canadian Journal of Public Health, 83*(5), 326–328.

Government of Nova Scotia. (1997/1998). *Government by design: The tide has turned*. Halifax: Author.

Health Protection and Promotion Act. Revised Statutes of Ontario, 1990, chapter H.7.

Health & Welfare Canada (HWC). (1991). *Report of the working group on the educational requirements of community health nurses*. Ottawa: Author.

Kernaghan, K., & Siegel, D. (1991). *Public administration in Canada*. Toronto: Nelson Canada.

Knox, S., & Irving, A. (1997). Nurse manager perceptions of healthcare executive behaviors during organizational change. *Journal of the Ontario Nurses' Association, 27*(11), 33–38.

Meilicke, C. (1990). Nurses and physicians in the modern hospital: "Watering the garden". *Canadian Journal of Nursing Administration, 3*(4), 19–22.

Nova Scotia Department of Health. (1993). *Values and principles of public health services division*. Unpublished document prepared for the Public Health Services Division.

Nova Scotia Department of Health. (1997a). *Nova Scotia health standards, edition I*. Halifax: Author.

Nova Scotia Department of Health. (1997b). *Accountability in Nova Scotia's health system*. Halifax: Author.

Nova Scotia Minister's Action Committee on Health System Reform (1994a). *Background paper on regionalization*. Halifax: Author.

Nova Scotia Minister's Action Committee on Health System Reform. (1994b). *Nova Scotia's blueprint for health system reform*. Halifax: Author.

Nova Scotia Task Force on Nursing. (1993). *Education subcommittee: Final report*. Halifax: Nova Scotia Department of Health.

Rachlis, M., & Kushner, C. (1994). *Strong medicine: How to save Canada's health care system*. Toronto: HarperCollins.

Smith, D. (1994). *Implementing citizen participation in Primary Health Care: Implications for public health organizations*. Unpublished paper prepared for Faculty of Nursing, Dalhousie University.

Tappen, R. (1989). *Nursing leadership and management: Concepts and practices* (2nd ed.). Philadelphia: F.A. Davis.

Part 7
Vision for the Future

Years ago, in an earlier version of this book (Stewart, 1985), I made seven predictions on the future of community health nursing:

- *There will be an increased proportion of total nursing labour power devoted to community health service delivery.*
- *Health promotion strategies will become the primary focus of community health nursing programs.*
- *Increased efforts of community health nurses will be directed at the community and aggregate levels.*
- *Consumerism will expand as community health nurses emphasize Primary Health Care and self-help.*
- *The community health nurse will provide the leadership for the interdisciplinary community health care team. Concurrently, the increased status of the community health nurse will be demonstrated not only in interdependent but in independent practice.*
- *Community health nurses will eventually be prepared at the master's level for generalist practitioner positions and at the doctoral level for administrative, research, and clinical specialist posts.*
- *Research increasingly will become a respected and mandatory role in community health nursing.*

Regrettably, the first forecast has not transpired. However, in recent years, governments have promised increased commitment to Primary Health Care, health promotion, and community-based care. Thus, this prediction may still come true. Although the sixth prophecy, pertaining to education, has proved premature, the trend continues. The other five predictions are coming to pass, although new challenges continue to arise and tax the ingenuity and dedication of community health nurses as they help to forge a future that promotes Canadians' health.

In this chapter, we review new challenges, many of which are described in more detail in other chapters, and reiterate how the principles of Primary Health Care predominate in discussions of the future context of community health and health care in Canada. Finally, we forecast an agenda for community health nursing in the 21st century.

C H A P T E R   3 1

Community health nursing in the future

Miriam J. Stewart and Beverly Leipert

The changing context of health system reform in Canada poses critical challenges to community health nursing. Regardless of the diversity of settings and roles, Primary Health Care principles should continue to underpin practice. Community theory, family theory, and Primary Health Care theory can contribute core concepts to the creation of community health nursing theory. In the future, funding agencies need to support more community health nursing research. Educational preparation for Primary Health Care roles in the community will expand. Community health nurses should respond to the call for policy development in health and health-related sectors. Clearly, Canadian community health nurses must strive for enhanced status in the 21st century.

LEARNING OBJECTIVES

In this chapter, you will learn:

- the major challenges in the changing societal and health system contexts that will influence the future of community health nursing
- the relevance of Primary Health Care principles to future roles and opportunities in community health nursing practice
- trends in the research, education, and theory domains of community health nursing that will influence knowledge generation over the next decade
- the importance of community health nurses' involvement in health-relevant policy development

Introduction

"Human ventures into outer space; advancements in science and technology; the explosion of information reflected primarily in developments in the areas of computer programming, genetic engineering and international communication; and the exploitation of resources inevitably influence the future health of the community and hence the role of the community health nurse" (Stewart, 1985, p. 738).

Challenges in changing context

As the 21st century approaches, Canada faces critical economic, environmental, technological, and social challenges. These include escalation of total health system costs; the growing population of seniors; new health problems arising from environmental pollutants; re-emergence of communicable diseases; treatment of resistant strains of bacteria and viruses; increases in sexually transmitted illness and HIV infection; continuing costs of cancer, cardiovascular illness, and other chronic conditions; persistent maternal and infant health challenges; and prolongation of physical function by technology. According to Pender, Barkauskas, Hayman, Rice, and Anderson (1992), community health nurses may also face the future challenge of helping communities adapt to life in space and of assessing the effects of weightlessness and altered sensory experiences.

Four trends that threaten the achievement of the World Health Organization's Health for All mandate include managerialism, increasing dominance of market economics and promotion of economic growth at all cost, individualism, and environmental degradation (Baum & Sanders, 1995). Fewer human resources, longer waiting periods, institutional autonomy, and the creation of integrated networks are also critical challenges during health care reform (Nadeau, 1996).

Public health professionals should forge a future that fosters basic requirements for health and protection against illness. Their priorities for the 21st century should focus on equity in the distribution of food, housing, education, employment, income, and health care, and access to better standards of living (McBeath, 1991). Their vision of the future should encompass access to health-promoting measures, such as developing supportive environments, strengthening community action, enhancing people's capacity to cope, building public policy (Kaplun, 1992), and balancing cost containment, quality improvement, and universal access to health care (Chassin, 1997). Health promotion is one of four major thrusts of the World Health Organization, an objective of many international organizations such as UNICEF, and an important goal of numerous developed and developing countries (Rootman, 1995).

In Canada, the National Health Forum focussed on several goals: striking a balance between health care versus illness prevention and health promotion; determinants of health; evidence-based decision making; a universally accessible health system; and public understanding and support of health and health care (National Forum on Health, 1997a&b). The Forum's priorities for action were preserving and protecting medicare; providing a more integrated system (including home care, primary care, etc.); fostering healthy child development; acknowledging employment and economic policies as determinants of health; and promoting community action, Aboriginal health, and a research agenda for health information. (See Chapter 6.)

Similarly, the document "Strategies for Population Health: Investing in the Health of Canadians" proposed three strategic directions for national action: (a) strengthen public understanding about the broad determinants of health and support for actions that improve the health of the overall population, and reduce health disparities experienced by some groups, (b) build understanding about the determinants of health and support for the population health approach among government partners in sectors outside health, and (c) develop comprehensive intersectoral population health initiatives (Federal, Provincial, & Territorial Advisory Committee on Population Health, 1994). Furthermore, the "new public health" recognized the impact of the social services, education, leisure, and justice sectors on health and the importance of public participation (Chambers, 1992). In this context, O'Neill, Rootman, and Pederson (1994) predicted that local communities will become more important in health promotion and that new players will continue to become involved.

Since publication of the Ottawa Charter (WHO, HWC, & CPHA, 1986) and the Epp (1986) framework, health promotion research and health promotion programs have shifted to emphasize socioeconomic, cultural, and environmental determinants of health. Accessibility to these determinants of health is considered as important as accessibility to health care, and supportive environments are highlighted in recent Canadian publications. Indeed, health promotion is viewed as a component of Primary Health Care.

In summary, the five principles of Primary Health Care—accessibility, intersectoral collaboration, public participation, health promotion and illness prevention, and appropriate technology—predominate in these Canadian initiatives. Primary Health Care principles will influence the future context of community health nursing. Certainly, nurses should play a prominent role in the commitment to the goal of Health for All (WHO, 1994) in the new millennium.

Facing challenges in the changing context

As the author predicted in 1985, consumers now play a respected role in health system refo m and renewal in Canada, and interdisciplinary initiatives are more prevalent. The merits of intersectoral collaboration and appropriate technology are espoused in recommendations for reform. Nevertheless, the challenge for community health nurses is to lobby for widespread implementation of Primary Health Care recommendations in all provinces and to push for a major shift of resources from the dominant institutional and illness-oriented sector to health promotion and other community-based programs. Until this reallocation of resources within the health system occurs, and until this is reflected in a concomitant transposition within nursing, resources allocated to community health nursing will be insufficient. Clearly, the proportion of nurses actively engaged in community-based and community-focussed care needs to expand. The World Health Organization (1994) report *Nursing Beyond the Year 2000* recommended a shift in the focus of workforce development in nursing and midwifery to reflect complex health needs. Although the environment is encouraging and the changing context is favourable, community health nurses must demonstrate to other nurses, disciplines, sectors, policy decision makers, and consumers their essential Primary Health Care role in the 21st century.

Challenges in community health nursing practice

Nurses are at the forefront of influencing the health of the community because of their emphasis on community health education, screening, counselling (Brown, Hubbard-Mattson, Newman, & Sirles, 1992), health assessment, health policy development, and assurance of quality health services (Oberle, Baker, & Magenheim, 1994; Salmon, 1993). In Ontario, a study by Chalmers (1994) revealed that although the roles of community developer, policy formulator, researcher/evaluator, and resource manager/coordinator were performed least frequently by community health nurses, they were expected of nurses in the future. Indeed, community health nurses contended that they needed further preparation to perform these roles. According to administrators and educators in Canada, nurses from university programs need a wide variety of knowledge, experience, and skills to begin to practise community health nursing (Bramadat, Chalmers, & Andrusyszyn, 1996).

Decision-making skills of community health nurses in four countries (Canada, Finland, Norway, United States) were influenced by differences in the nature and context of nursing practice (Lauri et al., 1997). Decision making, in turn, influences community nursing assessment (Bryans & McIntosh, 1996).

One recent trend related to practice involves the movement of health care and of acute care nurses into the community (Bryan et al., 1997). Nurses who work in critical care institutions need education to function appropriately and proficiently in community-based settings. Given the increasing demand for home care services (Dittbrenner, 1997), home care nurses also need continuing education as they move into the community (Nemcek & Egan, 1997). (See Chapter 7.) A second trend relates to advanced practice in community health nursing (Abraham & Fallon, 1997; Berger et al., 1996; McDonald, Langford, & Boldero, 1997; Zwanziger et al., 1996). Although advanced practice or clinical nurse specialist roles are emphasized in the international literature, recent discussions indicate that Canadian community health nurses could also consider these roles. The proclaimed value of advanced practitioners is their ability to provide an expanded nursing service for less cost than physicians. How these advanced practice roles would interface with existing community health nursing roles in Canada is unclear.

Community health nurses value their work (Leipert, 1996), but change is needed as health system reform proceeds (Chalmers, 1995; Tappen, Turkel, Hall, Stahura, & Morgan, 1997). Associated challenges for community health nursing practice include the politics of the changing health care system, tensions between physicians and nurses, and legislative acts that allow nurses to provide extended health services such as diagnosis and drug therapy (Kerr & MacPhail, 1996). Strategies proposed by Reutter and Harrison (1996) involve determining essential services and the appropriate use of personnel, removing financial barriers to Primary Health Care, broadening the concept of health, and developing collaborative relationships. The Comox Valley Nursing Centre Project in British Columbia illustrates the potential contributions of Primary Health Care and community-based nursing practice (Mass & Whyte, 1997). Regardless of settings and roles, the five Primary Health Care principles will underpin prospective practice.

Accessibility

Accessibility in the future may be promoted by creating organizational arrangements for group practice that enable movement across practice settings and specialities. Such practice is consistent with predictions by futurists, such as Toffler's (1990) flex firms and Walker's (1994) flexible structures and arrangements.

To be accessible, health promotion and prevention interventions need to address contextual determinants of risk behaviours and changing social influences (Chesney, 1993) and must be tailored to developmental levels and cultural backgrounds. (See Chapters 9, 10, and 23.) Accessibility is an important feature of health promotion initiatives directed at disadvantaged families and aggregates by community health nurses.

Community health nursing practice should empower, rather than pauperize, those who are disadvantaged (Erickson, 1996). Emancipatory community interventions can achieve this aim (Drevdahl, 1995). Class and status differences between nurses and clients, including client communities, should be recognized. The position statement of the Registered Nurses' Association of Nova Scotia regarding third-party payment of RNs and the initiatives of the Alberta Association of Registered Nurses that focussed on increased access to nursing services will influence accessibility. Nevertheless, safety concerns faced by community health nurses in cities and rural neighbour-hoods must be diminished, while striving to enhance accessibility (Gellner, Landers, O'Rourke, & Schlegel, 1994).

Promotion and prevention

Community health nursing is viewed as the way to the future (Hargadon, 1995; Leipert, 1996) because of its cost effectiveness and focus on health promotion and illness prevention. Promotion and prevention activities by community health nurses must expand to varied community settings (Glasgow, McCaul, & Fisher, 1993; Rudd & Walsh, 1993) and to diverse populations and must address the needs of the wider community (Caraher & McNab, 1996).

Clearly, there is a need to move beyond the individual level to the community level (Chesney, 1993). The shift from community health activities for individuals to population-based health promotion demands reorientation of community health nurses. Moreover, nurses require community planning tools for working with the community as client (Oberle, Baker, & Magenheim, 1994). For example, the Planned Approach to Community Health (PATCH) Model, created as a community health promotion and development tool, focusses on mobilizing the community and choosing health priorities and target groups (Oberle et al., 1994). However, such tools must be adapted and tested by community health nurses. Congruent skills for the future include conducting community assessments (Gerberich, Stearns, & Dowd, 1995) and fostering healthy communities (Flynn, 1997; Gebbie, 1997; Porter-O'Grady, 1997).

Intersectoral collaboration

Interdisciplinary practice is integral to health promotion and illness prevention (Pender et al., 1992). As Hudson-Rodd (1994) points out, "No one sphere of knowledge is sufficient and no one group can continue to control and dominate" (p. 124). Collaboration among health professionals can address critical community issues such as violence (Clark, 1997), health of children, and cost containment (Hayes, 1997). Cooperative relationships and transformational leadership styles are needed in the health system of the future (Ferguson-Paré, 1993). Indeed, the future for community nursing lies in collaboration with other providers of community care (Rodrigues, 1992; Trnobranski, 1994).

Browne and colleagues (1995) revealed that 17 percent of community health nursing clients were shared with social services; these clients had more social, emotional, and mental health problems. New collaborative roles for community health nurses involve parish contexts (Rydholm, 1997; Simington, Olson, & Douglass, 1996), work in agromedicine (Malloy, 1994), and delivery of dental care in the community (Armstrong, 1997).

Public participation

Given the growing costs of caregiving assumed by families (Ward & Brown, 1994) and the barriers to family caregivers' use of formal health services, public participation interventions by community health nurses should emphasize social support from family and friends, peer education, self-care, self-help, coping skills, and community development. However, public participation interventions focussed on communities and aggregates have, with few exceptions, been neglected in practice (Courtney, Ballard, Fauver, Fariota, & Holland, 1996). Inadequate support for community participation in health planning may reflect health professionals' reluctance to consult with the public (Hudson-Rodd, 1994). (Chapter 24 offers guidelines for empowering strategies by professionals.)

In a British study, although many people were aware of the health visitor's work in health promotion, very few would contact a health visitor for advice (Kelly, 1996). The invisibility and lack of clarity of community health nurses' work could bring about similar public misunderstanding in Canada. In times of health system restructuring and cost containment, public support and public participation are imperative ingredients in health promotion and illness prevention initiatives by community health nurses.

Appropriate technology

There is recent evidence that telephones and computers can be used to provide support and enhance coping. As noted in Chapter 4, telephone support interventions have been conducted with physically disabled adults; parents of children with chronic conditions; rural persons with AIDS; and low-income, elderly women. Telephone support pairs and groups have been linked with positive health outcomes, such as increased self-care for persons with osteoarthritis (Rene, Weinberger, Mazzuca, Brandt, & Katz, 1992), and with information gain for caregivers of persons with Alzheimer's disease (Goodman & Pynoos, 1988). The advantages of telephone support include anonymity and accessibility.

Computers are another anonymous, community-based medium that can provide access to information and support. They have been employed successfully with individuals who are HIV positive (e.g., Brennan, Ripich, & Moore, 1991), parents of children with cystic fibrosis (Petzel, Ellis, Budd, & Johnson, 1992), physically and emotionally challenged children (e.g., Fallon & Wann, 1994), and family caregivers of persons with Alzheimer's disease (Brennan, Moore, & Smyth, 1991). Computer mutual aid can allow seniors to overcome transportation and functional barriers. Most of the computer links developed across Canada include senior citizens as a special interest group (e.g., Seniors Special Interest Group on the National Capital Freenet, http://cpcug.org/sigs.html). Seniors use this medium regularly for peer interaction and to exchange varied information from health issues to finances. Finally, specialized computer networks for diverse situations and illnesses include Terminal, which links individuals with terminal illness. It is noteworthy that electronic self-help forums (Madara, 1992) are developing at the grass-roots level at a rapid pace.

Regrettably, the potential contributions of these technologies have been overlooked in community health nursing practice, with only a few reported exceptions. For example, community health nurses use a disease management monitoring system in the United States to track clients' health status (Niles, Alemagno, & Stricklin, 1997) and to access the Internet (Webster, 1997). Community health nurses should focus the application of appropriate technology on removing barriers experienced by physically challenged, socially isolated, and disadvantaged populations. Technologies that promote public participation, accessibility, and health should be emphasized.

Facing challenges related to practice

Canadian community health nursing literature reflects increased attention to aggregates and communities, health promotion, consumer participation, and independent and interdependent practice—fulfilling the predictions made by one of the authors in 1985. Nurse practitioner programs in several Canadian universities and community nursing resource centres indicate a shift to independent practice. However, the continuing challenge will be to translate all these trends into the everyday practice of community health nurses in Canada. Community health nurses are challenged to ensure that diverse populations have access to the basic determinants of health as well as to health care. In so doing, community health nurses will need to increase their efforts to collaborate, not only with other health professions, but also with other sectors that influence health (e.g., justice, education, housing, social services, transportation, recreation, religion).

Community health nurses will need to test tools that assess and promote the health of aggregates and communities and new technologies that are appropriate to the needs of the community. The potential of telephones and computers for mobilizing links between and exchanging information with consumers and of computers for generating data bases and interacting with other disciplines and sectors is still largely untapped.

Community health nurses should include consumers and consumer groups as partners in planning, implementing, and evaluating services and programs. The equal importance of consumers' experiential knowledge and community health nurses' professional knowledge in this partnership can be reinforced through community advisory boards, collaboration with self-help mutual aid groups and consumer advocacy groups, consumer satisfaction surveys, and joint consumer–professional applications for program funding. Consequently, consultation and community development roles will undoubtedly predominate in the future practice of community health nurses in Canada.

The impact of health system reform on the practice of community health nurses requires study. Furthermore, interventions and outcomes should be documented and the strengths of community health nursing practice highlighted.

Challenges in theory development

Knowledge development for community health nursing through education, research, and theory faces various challenges. In particular, a relative paucity of theory development persists in community health nursing, and such thinking as exists is at an emergent level (Association of Community Health Nursing Educators [ACHNE], 1995). Community health nursing theory development can be informed by nursing models, family theory, community theory, or Primary Health Care theory.

Nursing models

Which nursing theories can inform community health nursing practice? What are their limitations? Models such as Neuman's Health Care Systems Nursing Model reinforce mutual goal setting with the client and attend to clients' perceptions of their needs, but emphasize stressors rather than supports in the environment. Mutual goal setting is a promising component of King's Open Systems Model and Goal Attainment Theory, yet she limits conceptualization of "interpersonal systems" to individual client–nurse interactions. Although King defines nursing as care of individuals and groups, discussion of nursing in her theory (and other systems theories) is confined to individuals.

Orem's Self-Care Deficit Model, despite intuitive appeal because of its emphasis on self-care, focusses on care of dependent family members and on nurses regulating the capability of "patients" to engage in self-care, rather than on potentiating supportive social networks and lay groups. Conceptualization of groups is restricted to the family and that of environmental change to hospital and home environs. This model (like other developmental models) retains an illness and individualistic orientation and portrays nurses as the final decision makers, rather than reflecting true consumer participation.

In 1995, the Task Force on Community Health Nursing Theory Development of the Association of Community Health Nursing Educators

(ACHNE) reported that the nursing theories most commonly used in community health nursing include Orem's Self-Care Model, Benner's Novice-to-Expert Theory, Pender's Health Promotion Model, and Leininger's Transcultural Nursing (ACHNE, 1995). More recently, Baumann (1997) contrasted the assumptions and concepts of the medical model and Parse's Human Becoming Theory, as applied in community-based nursing practice.

Despite the fact that most conceptual models in nursing refer to person–environment interactions, consideration is typically limited to environmental stressors and to individual nurse–patient interactions, while the social environment is neglected (Stewart, 1990). In contrast, Butterfield's (1990) conceptual interpretation of the societal context of health behaviour indicates that community health nurses should understand social, political, and economic influences on health. Nursing theories are typically limited to individual clients and ignore environmental contexts of health conditions and populations (Hudson-Rodd, 1994). Regrettably, no nursing theories concentrate on groups or the community, and few emphasize the family (Stewart, 1990).

Family theories

The McGill Model of Nursing is the key example of documented nursing theory related to families. It emphasizes family, health, collaboration, and learning. The model conceptualizes *nursing* as complementing the work of other health professionals and *health* as a dynamic, multidimensional construct encompassing coping and development. Health is learned within the family context, and the *person* is an active problem solver and participant in health care (Gottlieb & Rowat, 1987). The model is based on Primary Health Care principles of public participation, health promotion, and intersectoral collaboration.

Future work should be directed toward a clear definition of family, development of germane measures, and creation of middle-range family theory (Stuart, 1991). Nurses could also examine the implications of variations of family structure for health outcomes. To illustrate, there is some evidence that marital ties have an effect on health and that divorce and bereavement can lead to illness. (See Chapter 4.)

Although some family theory developed by other disciplines may be appropriate to community nursing contexts, such as family developmental theory, more research is needed to test these theories in family nursing settings and to isolate important theoretical constructs and propositions that may be unique to family health nursing (Kristjanson & Chalmers, 1991). One germane family theory is the Resiliency Model of Family Stress, Adjustment, and Adaptation (McCubbin & McCubbin, 1993). Families can be considered resilient when they cope with significant stresses and develop collective strength to respond to such challenges. Some of the factors associated with resilient responses by families are stability, cohesiveness, flexibility, ease of communication, adaptability, stress-coping skills, and internal and external supports (Mangham, Reid, & Stewart, 1996; McCubbin, McCubbin, & Thompson, 1992). (See also Chapter 11.) Family theory and community theory are both integral to theory development in community health nursing.

Community theory

The community has been neglected in nursing theories. The theoretical base of community health nursing should be expanded to describe, explain, and predict the health of communities (Hamilton & Bush, 1988).

In the context of health promotion, there is recent speculation that resilience theory could be applied to communities (Manghan, McGrath, Reid, & Stewart, 1994). Indicators of a healthy or well-adjusted (resilient) community might include safety, low pollution levels, green space, public housing (Hayes & Manson-Willms, 1990; Manson-Singer, 1994), self-help and mutual aid organizations, charitable agencies, and community participation. "Community connectedness," as evidenced by community involvement, coping strategies and organizations, and adequate social support, contributes to community resilience. These supportive factors can offset the potentially deleterious effects wrought by economic crises, unemployment, geographic and cultural isolation, and limited educational opportunities (Stewart, Reid, et al., 1996).

Although the Community Change Model and Community Participation Model may be relevant to assessment and intervention at the community level (Chalmers & Kristjanson, 1989), such paradigms must be applied and tested by community health nurses. Community and community development theories can also guide Primary Health Care by community health nurses. (See Chapters 21 and 22.) The relevance of four models of community development—economic development, education, confrontation, and empowerment—to community health nursing practice was analyzed recently by Chalmers and Bramadat et al. (1996). The interactive and organizational model of community as client has been proposed as another relevant conceptual framework for public health nursing (Kuehnert, 1995).

Primary Health Care theories

As public health nurses' visions for the future are congruent with concepts of Primary Health Care, Clarke, Beddome, and Whyte (1993) have proposed some components of a conceptual model pertinent to Primary Health Care. Stewart's (1990) conceptual framework is based on Primary Health Care principles of public participation, intersectoral collaboration, accessibility, and health promotion. The *person* is conceived as an active partner, and the collaborative Primary Health Care roles of the nurse are stressed. There is emphasis on social, physical, psychological, and spiritual health and on the social, economic, political, and physical facets of the environment. This model was tested in the nursing education program at McMaster University (Sword, Noesgaard, & Majumdar, 1994). These Primary Health Care nursing models need further development, integration, and testing.

Other theories

Various other theories and models are being used in community health nursing. Zerwekh's Family Caregiving Model was applied by nursing students in home visits. The Ecologic Health Nursing Model, based on chaos theory, could be another useful model for community health nursing practice (Bellin, Gagnon, Mich, Plemmons, & Watanabe-Hayami, 1997; Vicenzi, 1994). A Partnership Model was examined for its utility in health system reform (Courtney et al., 1996). Kuss and colleagues (1997) proposed a Public Health Nursing Model, encompassing nine concepts, to help define public health nursing roles and practice. The Parish Nursing Model has been proposed as a framework for interpreting community health nurses' contribution to healthy communities (Magilvy & Brown, 1997). (Chapter 16 illustrates the importance of health promotion concepts and principles for community health nursing.)

Facing challenges related to theory

The limitations of traditional nursing theories and inadequate adaptation of interdisciplinary theories to the community health nursing context point to the potential value of generating a unique theory of community health nursing. This theory can be derived in part from family and community theories and in part from embryonic Primary Health Care nursing models. Concepts, assumptions, and relationship statements of this new theory should be congruent with the five Primary Health Care principles. Thus, the *community health nurse* would be conceptualized as a consultant, community developer, collaborator, health promoter, and Primary Health Care provider. The *person* (client) would be conceived as individuals, families, aggregates, and communities, who are equal partners in planning, implementing, and evaluating services and programs and who exchange support and health information. The *environment* would encompass the political, social, economic, cultural, and physical context of communities, aggregates, families, and individuals and the diverse settings in which community health nurses practise. *Health* would be holistic, subsuming the social, psychological, physical, and spiritual well-being of individuals, families, aggregates, and communities. Moreover, the *interactive* element of nursing (Kim, 1994; Meleis, 1991) would need to be integrated into the new theory. Future theory should also be guided by population needs (Meleis, 1992). Canadian community health nursing scholars could lead the way in creating a community health nursing theory that can inform practice and be tested in research.

Challenges in community health nursing research

Community health nursing research faces major challenges in the next decade of knowledge development (Kendall, 1995). Barriers to implementing research in public health nursing practice (Walsh, 1997) include inaccessibility of research reports (Kenrick & Luker, 1996), difficulty implementing random allocation methods, and selection and measurement of appropriate outcomes (Kelsey, 1995). Other challenges relate to funding sources, design issues, and research centres.

Funding sources
By the late 1990s, the priorities of the National Health Research Development Program (NHRDP) focussed on renewal and restructuring of the health system, determinants of population health, health impact of public policies, and transfer and uptake of knowledge. The Medical Research Council (MRC) of Canada now funds health promotion, population health, health services, and psychosocial research. It has taken a lead in establishing a task force to examine a transformative vision of health research. This task force emphasizes evidence-based work and determinants of health. The Social Sciences and Humanities Research Council of Canada's strategic planning emphasizes the importance of health research from a broad, social determinants perspective. Another trend is the link between research and industry represented by the Pharmaceutical Manufacturers Association of Canada and MRC. Major challenges of the future will be to seek industry support for health promotion and illness prevention research and to find a balance among corporate-driven research, curiosity-driven academic research, and policy-driven research. Finally, community health nurses should access new sources, such as the Canadian Foundation for Innovation and the forthcoming Institute of Population/Public Health.

Design issues
In the new millennium, prospective, longitudinal studies are needed to test outcomes of interventions. Public health nurses in the United States ranked foremost research priorities as outcomes in maternal–child and family planning; outcomes in home health services; nurse recruitment, retention, and job

satisfaction; and professional image (Misener, Watkins, et al., 1994). Community health nurses need to develop quality measures and demonstrate outcomes of their interventions (Rodrigues, 1992). For example, a community-based home care program for the management of pre-eclampsia in Winnipeg resulted in a reduction of two days (on average) in the length of hospital stay of 1330 women and cost savings of over $700 000 (Helewa, Heaman, Robinson, & Thompson, 1993). A randomized controlled trial included cost analysis of community health nurses' problem-solving strategies for clients with emotional disorders (Mynors-Wallis, Davies, Gray, Barbour, & Gath, 1997). Although these types of studies can demonstrate the impact of community health nursing interventions and programs, they are rare.

Ciliska and colleagues' (1996) extensive review of research on the effectiveness of home visiting identified such positive outcomes as improvements in children's mental development, mental health, and physical growth and in maternal health, as well as governmental cost savings. Barriers that impede the production and dissemination of outcome research in public health nursing, such as inaccessible graduate education, inadequate research funding, and inappropriate use of intervention studies in public health settings (Hayward et al., 1996), must be overcome.

Process-focussed research is also needed to delineate and document community health nursing interventions and interactions. Qualitative research elucidates process and experiential phenomena, whereas quantitative designs, although capable of testing effects and associations, may not capture the complexity of process. Cowley (1995) used grounded theory methodology to uncover hidden processes and features of health visiting. Issues of validity and reliability associated with qualitative interview data collected in a community setting have been addressed (Appleton, 1995). Nevertheless, debates persist among nurses concerning the rigour of qualitative versus quantitative designs (Morse, 1994). Diverse methodologies have been used in community health nursing research. (See Chapter 25.)

Chesler (1991) contrasts conventional research, in which researchers are detached, objective, and in control, with participatory research, where there is co-control or even participant (subject) control. Participatory action research is consistent with the goals and characteristics of the nursing profession (Rains & Hahn, 1995). Participatory research is one mode of applied research that is particularly relevant to Primary Health Care interventions by community health nurses because of its emphasis on public participation. (See Chapter 28.)

Controlled intervention trials based on theory are needed. Interventions should be evaluated in terms of their positive and negative impact on outcomes, their mixed effects, their side effects, their maintenance over time, and their long-term effects. Furthermore, intervention processes need to be clearly delineated (Gottlieb, in press). Intervention research is needed to inform community health nursing practice, yet gaps in intervention research persist. (Chapter 27 offers excellent guidelines for intervention research in the future.)

Research has implications for practice and programs. (See Chapter 26.) For example, a Canadian project that examined the efficacy and efficiency of referral decisions of hospital nurses and public health liaison nurses later informed planning and program implementation (Ciliska et al., 1996). Practitioners need research tools. The Community Health Intensity Rating Scale is one research tool for measuring the needs of clients and for project-ing required resources (Peters & Hays, 1995). Research also provides evi-dence of practice issues. One study revealed that public health nurses' perceptions of power during program transition were related to access to empowerment structures and to perceptions of their manager's power in the organization (Haugh & Laschinger, 1996). These perceptions could have implications for the success of transformative change during health system restructuring.

Research centres

Creation of new centres for community health research and involvement of existing research centres in more community health projects are challenges for the next decade. Walker (1994) predicted that innovative community nursing centres can raise revenue, measure outcomes related to population needs, develop health policy research, and foster collaboration in research and practice. The Health Promotion Research Centres in Canada continue to play an active role in knowledge development and to build bridges among practitioners, communities, voluntary organizations, the public, govern-ment, and other disciplines and sectors (Stewart, 1997). Although these cen-tres foster interdisciplinary, intersectoral, and participatory research projects and programs relevant to Primary Health Care, they struggle to secure long-term funding. It is noteworthy that nurse researchers played a key role in creating several of these centres and in fostering pertinent partnerships (Stewart, 1997). The Centres of Excellence on Women's Health and on Family Violence have also benefited from nursing leadership.

Facing challenges related to research

As Stewart predicted in 1985, research has become more respected and prevalent in community health nursing. This growth is especially evident in the review in Chapter 26.

Community health nursing research can be expected to expand in scope and extent and to shift from descriptive and exploratory studies to intervention and

theory-testing research during the next decade. Researchers will use both qualitative and quantitative designs to elucidate process and to demonstrate outcomes. Community health nursing scholars will be challenged to conduct their
investigations in collaboration with consumers (i.e., participatory research)
and with other disciplines and sectors (i.e., interdisciplinary research), to
establish pertinent data bases, and to foster population health research. In the
changing context of health systems, they will need to focus their research on
high-risk populations, socioeconomic and cultural determinants of health,
health promotion interventions, technologies appropriate to the community,
and other issues relevant to Primary Health Care. Policy research equips
nurses to enter policy debates with data and to participate as agents of social
change (Rains & Hahn, 1995) and social activism (Rafael, 1997). Recent
trends include a growing expectation that policy and program development
be based on research and that dissemination, transfer, and uptake of research
results occur. Academic researchers, practitioners, policy decision makers,
and consumers should collaborate in setting the research agenda and ensuring that research guides practice and policy.

Funding will increasingly be obtained from national peer-reviewed funding agencies, foundations, and industry. Nursing scholars will require
funded release time to focus on community health and Primary Health Care
research. Pertinent research units, centres, institutes, and programs of
research will continue to be created. If community health nursing research is
to inform practice, programs, and policy, the results of research will need to
be communicated in meaningful ways to diverse audiences: the public, practitioners, other professionals, and policy makers. For example, pamphlets,
fact sheets, newsletters, articles, and television appearances can be used to
communicate research to consumers. All these strategies should make community health nursing research more relevant, timely, and extensive.

Education for community health nursing

Health system reform initiatives indicate that nursing education must prepare nurses for enhanced roles in a community-based, population-focussed
health system. Canadian community health nurses are being challenged to
redefine their roles, and nursing education is a key (Matuk & Horsburgh,
1992).

Preparation for a Primary Health Care role begins at the undergraduate
level and continues into graduate studies. There are emerging examples of
education for Primary Health Care in baccalaureate nursing programs in
Canada. (See Chapter 2.) According to the Canadian Association of University
Schools of Nursing (CAUSN, 1994), future baccalaureate nursing graduates

will have beginning competence in managing a Primary Health Care team. Tenn (1995) found that Canadian university schools of nursing were moving toward integrating Primary Health Care in curricula; approximately 60 percent reported some integration of relevant content.

Education programs prepare baccalaureate nursing students for future practice in community health by emphasizing innovative strategies and models for health system delivery (Williams & Wold, 1996) and by offering experiences that empower students to discover new paradigms of practice in a rapidly changing health care arena (Gauthier & Matteson, 1995), in collaborative community settings (Esheleman & Davidhizar, 1997), and in population-focussed nursing (Duncan, 1996). Neufeld and Harrison (1996) examined educational issues in preparing community health nursing students and practitioners to use nursing diagnoses with populations and groups. (See also Chapter 19.) Nursing education should focus on health in the community, health promotion, healthy environments, and quality of life (Clarke & Cody, 1994) and should value lifelong learning and creative, critical thinking.

In this context, a study of community health nursing students in the United Kingdom revealed that their community experience helped them to think through and develop their own ideas about practice (i.e., reflection in action) (Hallett, 1997). One pilot project tested innovative clinical experiences that promoted understanding of the community health nursing role in health system reform, with emphasis on healthy communities (Jossens & Ferjancski, 1996). Other noteworthy educational strategies involve grant writing to teach community health program planning (Glick & King, 1994), community-based research projects to foster partnership and community empowerment skills (Kelley, 1995), and clinical courses that promote involvement with public policy (Thomas & Shelton, 1994). Additional pertinent undergraduate courses include a community mental health nursing course in Canada (Bunn, 1995) and a Primary Health Care course (Davis & Pearson, 1996).

Appropriate clinical settings are needed to develop skills and knowledge about groups and populations. Excellent sites for students to learn to deliver promotion and prevention strategies include schools, worksites, shelters, ambulatory settings, community meeting places, community agencies, neighbourhood health centres, nurse-managed clinics, homes, outpatient facilities, day cares, rehabilitation centres, student health services, wellness centres (Oermann, 1994; Pruitt & Campbell, 1994; Registered Nurses Association of British Columbia, 1994), local health departments, and community clinics (Pender et al., 1992).

Moreover, clinical experiences in primary care settings help students meet health system reform challenges (McEwen & Kemp, 1994). The use of non-traditional clinical settings, such as McDonald's restaurants and inner-city churches, help students understand Primary Health Care principles and practice (Faller, Dowell, & Jackson, 1995; Sword et al., 1994). These types of community-based experiences should be integrated throughout the undergraduate curriculum.

Graduate nursing programs should emphasize advanced clinical skills in health promotion and disease prevention, as well as expertise in health policy, health research, and surveillance and data systems (Brown et al., 1992; Pender et al., 1992). Doctoral graduates are prepared to develop theories and methodologies relevant to nursing and health promotion (CAUSN, 1994). Some U.S. doctoral programs include community health nursing as a speciality (Clarke et al., 1996). Pertinent graduate education programs in community health reported in the literature include a dual master of nursing and master of public health program (Blaha & Cover, 1994) and a program that prepares nurses for leadership roles and health system reform (Brooking, 1997).

Numerous textbooks suitable for community health nursing education provide important information about educational trends. Furthermore, the International Association of Community Health Nursing Educators (ACHNE) publishes documents that examine community health nursing education issues, trends, and policies.

Educating the nurse of tomorrow requires a community-focussed curriculum. Students need to have a broad perspective on the community's culture, resources, economics, values, and organizations (Oermann, 1994; Pruitt & Campbell, 1994). Nursing students must have early exposure to concepts of health and community; methods of community assessment, community development, and citizen participation and mobilization; politics (McKnight & Van Dover, 1994); and roles of other health disciplines (Koch & Maserang, 1994; Oermann, 1994; Pruitt & Campbell, 1994). More effort should also be expended on education for health promotion (Rootman & O'Neill, 1994; Smillie, 1992). These recommendations reinforce the salience of Primary Health Care principles to curriculum reform.

It is vital that nurse educators be knowledgeable about family and community nursing, public health issues, determinants of and barriers to community health, and interventions that promote the health of aggregates and that they instill positive attitudes toward health promotion in nursing students (Matuk & Horsburgh, 1992). The Registered Nurses Association of British Columbia (1994) recommended that faculty development pertaining to Primary Health Care be a priority. The barriers to widespread implementation of Primary Health Care curricula—similar to those faced in practice (i.e., resources, attitudes, skills, and knowledge)—must be overcome. Clearly, expanded education of nurses to assume Primary Health Care roles will pave the way to an optimistic future for community health nursing.

Facing challenges related to education

There is encouraging evidence that Primary Health Care and community health nursing are encompassed, at least to a certain extent, in the curricula of most Canadian university schools. However, principles of Primary Health Care tend to be confined to a course rather than controlling the direction of the curriculum. To be effective, these principles need to be integrated throughout the curriculum, in both classroom and clinical learning experiences. Students need opportunities to learn to collaborate with consumers, other health professionals, and representatives of non-health sectors in their clinical practice and to assess the appropriateness of technology for the communities in which they work. In nursing educational programs in Canada, theoretical models, assessment tools, and intervention techniques pertinent to aggregates and to communities should co-exist with those relevant to individuals and families.

A variety of traditional and non-traditional community-based settings are needed to introduce students to the diverse roles and sites involved in Primary Health Care nursing and to develop relevant skills in community development and consultation. Input should be solicited from consumers and from practitioners during the development of curricula and selection of learning experiences. Undergraduate students should be socialized to value experiential and professional knowledge equally and to work with clients representing different cultural, educational, and socioeconomic backgrounds. To foster this transition, faculty will need to be reoriented to the principles of Primary Health Care and reaffirmed in their efforts to communicate these principles to students.

Practice specialists with master's preparation are needed to guide and monitor the integration of Primary Health Care principles in community health nursing practice by baccalaureate-prepared nurses. Public health nurses' continuing education needs could be met by both practice and academic communities (Kelly, Cowell, & Stevens, 1997). Innovative education for acute care nurses who make the shift from institutions to community settings is also timely (Gookin, 1996; Meyer, 1997). The issue of specialist versus generalist knowledge pertaining to community health nursing still requires resolution. The gaps in community health nursing theory and research can be bridged by preparing scholars at the doctoral level. Clearly, the challenge to create more community health nurse practitioners and scholars continues.

Challenges related to policy

Community health nurses need to respond to evolving challenges associated with health system reform and health policy development. Nursing centres can capitalize on the opportunities created by the current health policy climate (Barger, 1995). (See Chapter 8.) Coordinated systems of community-based health care delivery (Hayes, 1997) and provider–community partnerships are suitable strategies in the chaotic context of health care reform (Bushy, 1995). Gupton and McKay (1995) examined the Canadian perspective on the influence of health system reform on postpartum home care and on the roles of public health nurses.

Alberta public health nurses expressed concerns that illness prevention and health promotion roles may be curtailed in the future in favour of mandated demands associated with early discharge (Reutter & Ford, 1998). Public health nurses in Vancouver focussed on their ability to provide community services at a cost that was acceptable within a cost-constrained health environment (Leipert, 1996). In a market-oriented and cost-restrictive environment where change is rampant, the marketing of nursing services may be a key to survival during health system reform (Jowett & Vaughan, 1997; Majeski-Felle, 1994; Moore, 1994; Wright, Chamberlain, & Barker, 1996).

Leadership is also important in a climate of health system reform and renewal. Competencies for nursing leadership in public health include political competencies, business acumen, program leadership, and management capabilities (Misener, Alexander, et al., 1997). These can be fostered by paradigms, such as the Manager-as-Developer Model for community-based practice (Brooking, 1997); graduate programs that prepare nurses for leadership roles in health services; and participation in the policy arena (Aroian, Meservey, & Crockett, 1996). (See Chapter 30.)

The World Health Organization has renewed its Health for All policy. This worldwide policy has implications for the directions Canada takes in its development of health and health-related policies and programs. Potential directions in Canadian health system policy also arise from the National Forum on Health and recent provincial health commissions and reports that reinforce Primary Health Care principles (see Chapter 6).

Forging a future for community health nursing

The future of community health nursing can be forecast in part by challenges associated with the changing health system context, intervention initiatives in practice, knowledge development trends, educational experiments, and the influential policy arena. There has never been a more opportune time to shape the destiny of community health nursing in Canada. As governments acknowledge the merits of community-based programs and applaud interdisciplinary and intersectoral collaboration, public participation, cost-effective appropriate technology, and evidence-based decisions, community health nurses can lead the way in the continuing shift to Primary Health Care. Community health nurse practitioners, theorists, researchers, and educators can confront these challenges and create an exciting agenda for the 21st century. This agenda could help to forge a formidable future for community health nursing in Canada.

As we look into our "crystal ball" to predict this agenda, we reaffirm future directions identified in the 1995 edition of this text:

- Community health nursing practitioners will routinely collaborate with consumers, community groups, policy decision makers, other health professionals, and other sectors that influence health.
- Community health nursing practice will focus on health promotion and illness/injury prevention for individuals, families, aggregates, and communities.
- Community health nurses will be partners with the intersectoral health team and with consumers and communities in promoting accessibility to the determinants of health, as well as to health care, for all Canadians regardless of age, education, gender, location, race, religion, sexual orientation, and socioeconomic status.
- Community health nurses will generate and test innovative technologies adapted for use in the community.
- A community health nursing theory, encompassing pertinent concepts from Primary Health Care models and family and community theories, will be created.
- Community health nursing researchers will follow the principles of participatory research, will focus on intervention research and theory-testing research, and will develop programs and centres of research.
- Community health and other Primary Health Care research will be recognized as priorities by interdisciplinary, peer-reviewed funding agencies.
- Community health nursing research will be used to guide health policy.
- Undergraduate nursing programs will emphasize education of students for Primary Health Care roles in the community.
- Graduate programs will focus on preparation of community health nursing scholars for research and theory generation and testing.

The future of community health nursing theory, practice, research, education, and policy must be guided by Primary Health Care principles. We conclude this book as Stewart did the 1985 book, *Community Health Nursing in Canada*: It is imperative that Canadian community health nurses in the realms of service, education, and research take control of their own destiny. It is only by acknowledging our historical and current contributions and deficits that realistic planning can be done for the future. Community health nurses must maintain a visionary stance, as we alone hold the key to our enhanced status in the 21st century (Stewart, 1985, p. 743).

QUESTIONS

1. Which gaps in community health nursing theory need to be bridged in the future?
2. How might community health nursing practice in the 21st century be guided by Primary Health Care principles?
3. What developments in community health nursing research can be expected over the next decade?
4. How can community health nurses influence policy development in a context of health system reform and renewal?

REFERENCES

Abraham, T., & Fallon, P.J. (1997). Clinical exemplar. Caring for the community: Development of the advanced practice nurse role. *Clinical Nurse Specialist, 11*(5), 224–230.

Anderson, K., & Tomlinson, P. (1992). The family health system as an emerging paradigmatic view for nursing. *Image: Journal of Nursing Scholarship, 24*(1), 57–63.

Appleton, J.V. (1995). Analysing qualitative interview data: Addressing issues of validity and reliability. *Journal of Advanced Nursing, 22*(5), 993–997.

Armstrong, M.E. (1997). Expanding the auxiliaries debate. *British Dental Journal, 182*(12), 450–451.

Aroian, J., Meservey, P.M., & Crockett, J.G. (1996). Developing nurse leaders for today and tomorrow: Part 2, Implementing a model of leadership for community-based practice. *Journal of Nursing Administration, 26*(10), 29–34.

Association of Community Health Nursing Educators (ACHNE). (1995). *Task force on community health nursing theory development. Report.* Author.

Barger, S.E. (1995). Establishing a nursing centre: Learning from the literature and the experience of others. *Journal of Professional Nursing, 11*(4), 203–212.

Baum, F., & Sanders, D. (1995). Can health promotion and primary health care achieve health for all without a return to their more radical agenda? *Health Promotion International, 10*(2), 149–160.

Baumann, S.L. (1997). Contrasting two approaches in a community-based nursing practice with older adults: The medical model and Parse's nursing theory. *Nursing Science Quarterly, 10*(3), 124–130.

Bellin, C., Gagnon, M., Mich, M., Plemmons, S., & Watanabe-Hayami, C. (1997). Ecologic health nursing for community health: Applied chaos theory. *Complexity & Chaos in Nursing, 3*, 13–22.

Berger, A.M., Eilers, J.G., Pattrin, L., Rolf-Fixley, M., Pfeifer, B.A., Rogge, J.A.,

Wheeler, L.M., Bergstrom, N.I., & Heck, C.S. (1996). Advanced practice roles for nurses in tomorrow's healthcare systems. *Clinical Nurse Specialist, 10*(5), 250–255.

Blaha, A.J., & Cover, K.M. (1994). Model curriculum for health care reform . . . Dual master of nursing and master of public health degree. *South Carolina Nurse, 1*(3), 8.

Bramadat, I.J., Chalmers, K., & Andrusyszyn, M.A. (1996). Knowledge, skills and experiences for community health nursing practice: The perceptions of community nurses, administrators and educators. *Journal of Advanced Nursing, 24*(6), 1224–1233.

Brennan, P.F., Moore, S.M., & Smyth, K.A. (1991). Alzheimer's disease caregivers' uses of a computer network. *Western Journal of Nursing Research, 14*(5), 662–673.

Brennan, P.F., Ripich, S., & Moore, S.M. (1991). The use of home-based computers to support persons living with AIDS/ARC. *Journal of Community Health Nursing, 8*(1), 3–14.

Brooking, B. (1997). Community systems management: Preparing nurse managers for today and tomorrow. *Seminars for Nurse Managers, 5*(2), 75–78.

Brown, K.C., Hubbard-Mattson, A., Newman, K.D., & Sirles, A.T. (1992). A community health nursing curriculum and Healthy People 2000. *Clinical Nurse Specialist, 6*(4), 203–208.

Browne, G., Roberts, J., Byrne, C., Underwood, J., Jamieson, E., Schuster, M., Cornish, D., Watt, S., & Gafni, A. (1995). Public health nursing clientele shared with social assistance: Proportions, characteristics and policy implications. *Canadian Journal of Public Health, 86*(3), 155–161.

Bryan, Y.E., Bayley, E.W., Grindel, C., Kingston, M.B., Tuck, M.B., & Wood, L.J. (1997). Preparing to change from acute to community-based care. Learning needs of hospital-based nurses. *Journal of Nursing Administration, 27*(5), 35–44.

Bryans, A., & McIntosh, J. (1996). Decision making in community nursing: An analysis of the stages of decision making as they relate to community nursing assessment practice. *Journal of Advanced Nursing, 24*(1), 24–30.

Bunn, H. (1995). Preparing nurses for the challenge of the new focus on community mental health nursing. *Journal of Continuing Education in Nursing, 26*(2), 55–59.

Bushy, A. (1995). Harnessing the chaos in health care reform with provider–community partnerships. *Journal of Nursing Care Quality, 9*(3), 10–19.

Butterfield, P.G. (1990). Thinking upstream: Nurturing a conceptual understanding of the societal context of health behaviour. *Advances in Nursing Science, 12*(2), 1–8.

Canadian Association of University Schools of Nursing (CAUSN). (1994). *CAUSN statement on baccalaureate education.* Ottawa: Author.

Caraher, M., & McNab, M. (1996). The public health nursing roles: An overview of future trends. *Nursing Standard, 10*(51), 44–48.

Chalmers, K. (1994). Difficult work: Health visitors' work with clients in the community. *International Journal of Nursing Studies, 31*(2), 163–182.

Chalmers, K. (1995). Community health nursing in Canada: Practice under transition. *Health & Social Care in the Community, 3*(5), 321–325.

Chalmers, K., & Kristjanson, L. (1989). The theoretical basis for nursing at the community level: A comparison of three models. *Journal of Advanced Nursing, 14,* 569–574.

Chambers, L.W. (1992). The new public health: Do local public health agencies need a booster (or organizational "fix") to combat the diseases of disarray? *Canadian Journal of Public Health, 83*(5), 326–328.

Chassin, M.R. (1997). Public policy. The health care juggling act: Balancing universal access, cost containment, and quality improvement. *Mount Sinai Journal of Medicine, 64*(2), 101–104.

Chesler, M.A. (1991). Participatory action research with self-help groups: An alternative paradigm for inquiry and action. *American Journal of Community Psychology, 19*(5), 757–768.

Chesney, M.A. (1993). Health psychology in the 21st century: Acquired immunodeficiency syndrome as a harbinger of things to come. *Health Psychology, 12*(4), 259–268.

Ciliska, D., Hayward, S., Thomas, H., Mitchell, A., Dobbins, M., Underwood, J., Rafael, A., & Martin, E. (1996). A systematic overview of the effectiveness of home visiting as a delivery strategy for public health nursing interventions. *Canadian Journal of Public Health, 87*(3), 193–198.

Clark, J.F. (1997). Community violence, children and youth: Considerations for programs, policy, and nursing roles. *Pediatric Nursing, 23*(2), 131–137.

Clarke, H.F., Beddome, G., & Whyte, N. (1993). Public health nurses' vision of their future reflects changing paradigms. *International Nursing, 25*(4), 305–310.

Clarke, P.N., & Cody, W.K. (1994). Nursing theory-based practice in the home and community: The crux of professional nursing education. *Advances in Nursing Science, 17*(2), 41–53.

Clarke, P.N., Glick, D.F., Laffrey, S.C., Bender, K., Emerson, S.E., & Stanhope, M. (1996). Doctoral education in community health nursing: A national survey. *Journal of Professional Nursing, 12*(5), 303–310.

Courtney, R., Ballard, E., Fauver, S., Gariota, M., & Holland, L. (1996). The partnership model: Working with individuals, families, and communities toward a new vision of health. *Public Health Nursing, 13*(3), 177–186.

Cowley, S. (1995). Health-as-process: A health visiting perspective. *Journal of Advanced Nursing, 22*(3), 433–441.

Davis, J.H., & Pearson, M.A. (1996). An instructional model for primary health care education. *Public Health Nursing, 13*(1), 31–35.

Dittbrenner, H. (1997). European solutions to home care challenges. *Caring, 16*(4), 24–26, 28, 30.

Drevdahl, D. (1995). Coming to voice: The power of emancipatory community interventions. *Advances in Nursing Science, 18*(2), 13–24.

Duncan, S.M. (1996). Empowerment strategies in nursing education: A foundation for population-focused clinical studies. *Public Health Nursing, 13*(5), 311–317.

Epp, J. (1986) *Achieving health for all: A framework for health promotion.* Ottawa: Health & Welfare Canada.

Erickson, G.P. (1996). To pauperize or empower: Public health nursing at the turn of the 20th and 21st centuries. *Public Health Nursing, 13*(3), 163–169.

Esheleman, J., & Davidhizar, R. (1997). Life in migrant camps for children—a hazard for health. *Journal of Cultural Diversity, 4*(1), 13–17.

Faller, H.S., Dowell, M.A., & Jackson, M.A. (1995). Bridge to the future: Nontraditional clinical settings, concepts and issues. *Journal of Nursing Education, 34*(8), 344–349.

Fallon, M.A., & Wann, J.A. (1994). Incorporating computer technology into activity-based thematic units for young children with disabilities. *Infants & Young Children, 6*(4), 64–69.

Federal, Provincial, & Territorial Advisory Committee on Population Health. (1994). *Strategies for population health: Investing in the health of Canadians.* Meeting of Ministers of Health, Halifax, September 14–15, 1994.

Ferguson-Paré, M. (1993). Women ready to bring excellence to CEO role. *Leadership in Health Services, 2*(3), 12–13.

Flynn, B.C. (1997). Partnerships in healthy cities and communities: A social commitment for advanced practice nurses. *Advanced Practice Nursing Quarterly, 2*(4), 1–6.

Gauthier, M.A., & Matteson, P. (1995). The role of empowerment in neighborhood-based nursing education. *Journal of Nursing Education, 34*(8), 390–395.

Gebbie, K.M. (1997). Using the vision of healthy people to build healthier communities. *Nursing Administration Quarterly, 21*(4), 83–90.

Gellner, P., Landers, S., O'Rourke, D., & Schlegel, M. (1994). Community health nursing in the 1990s—risky business? *Holistic Nursing Practice, 8*(2), 15–21.

Gerberich, S.S., Stearns, S.J., & Dowd, T. (1995). A critical skill for the future: Community assessment. *Journal of Community Health Nursing, 12*(4), 239–250.

Glasgow, R.E., McCaul, K.D., & Fisher, K.J. (1993). Participation in worksite health promotion: A critique of the literature and recommendations for future practice. *Health Education Quarterly, 20*(3), 391–408.

Glick, D.F., & King, M.G. (1994). Grant writing: An innovative project for teaching community health program planning. *Journal of Nursing Education, 33*(5), 238–240.

Goodman, C., & Pynoos, J. (1988) Telephone networks connect caregiving families of Alzheimer's victims. *Gerontologist, 28*, 602–605.

Gookin, L.B. (1996). Partnering for success. *Home Care Provider, 1*(2), 102–104.

Gottlieb, B.H. (in press). Accomplishments and challenges of social support intervention research. In M. Stewart (Ed.), *Chronic conditions and caregiving in Canada: Social support strategies.* Toronto: University of Toronto Press.

Gottlieb, L., & Rowat, K. (1987). The McGill Model of Nursing: A practice-derived model. *Advances in Nursing Science, 9*(4), 51–61.

Gupton, A., & McKay, M. (1995). The Canadian perspective on postpartum home care. *Journal of Obstetric, Gynecologic, & Neonatal Nursing, 24*(2), 173–179.

Hallett, C.E. (1997). Learning through reflection in the community: The relevance of Schon's theories of coaching to nursing education. *International Journal of Nursing Studies, 34*(2), 103–110.

Hamilton, P.A., & Bush, H.A. (1988). Theory development in community health nursing: Issues and recommendations. *Scholarly Inquiry for Nursing Practice: An International Journal, 2*(2), 145–160.

Hargadon, J. (1995). Community nursing is needed more than old buildings. *Community Nurse, 1*(7), 8.

Haugh, E.B., & Laschinger, H.S. (1996). Power and opportunity in public health nursing work environments. *Public Health Nursing, 13*(1), 42–49.

Hayes, J.M. (1997). Coordinated systems of community-based health care delivery: A vehicle for health care reform. *Journal of Pediatric Nursing, 12*(5), 288–291.

Hayes, M., & Manson-Willms, S. (1990). Healthy community indicators: The perils of the search and the paucity of the find. *Health Promotion International, 5*(2), 161–166.

Hayward, S., Ciliska, D., DiCenso, A., Thomas, H., Underwood, E.J., & Rafael, A. (1996). Evaluation research in public health: Barriers to the production and dissemination of outcomes data. *Canadian Journal of Public Health, 87*(6), 413–417.

Helewa, M., Heaman, M., Robinson, M.-A., & Thompson, L. (1993). Community-based home-care program for the management of pre-eclampsia: An alternative. *Canadian Medical Association Journal, 149*(6), 829–834.

Hudson-Rodd, N. (1994). Public health: People participating in the creation of healthy places. *Public Health Nursing, 11*(2), 119–126.

Jossens, M.O., & Ferjancski, P. (1996). Of Lillian Wald, community health nursing education, and health care reform. *Public Health Nursing, 13*(2), 97–103.

Jowett, S., & Vaughan, B. (1997). Making marketing your business. *Nursing Times, 93*(9), 56–58.

Kaplun, A. (1992). A dynamic vision of health. *World Health Organization Regional Publications—European Services, 44*, 415–422.

Kelley, B.R. (1995). Community-based research: A tool for community empowerment and student learning. *Journal of Nursing Education, 34*(8), 384–386.

Kelly, C. (1996). Public perceptions of a health visitor. *International Journal of Nursing Studies, 33*(3), 285–296.

Kelly, C., Cowell, J.M., & Stevens, R. (1997). Surveying public health nurses' continuing education needs: Collaboration of practice and academia. *Journal of Continuing Education in Nursing, 28*(3), 115–123.

Kelsey, A. (1995). Outcome measures: Problems and opportunities for public health nursing. *Journal of Nursing Management, 3*(4), 183–187.

Kendall, S. (1995). Making a difference: Promoting community health nursing research in the 1990s and beyond. *Health & Social Care in the Community, 3*(3), 191–193.

Kenrick, M., & Luker, K.A. (1996). An exploration of the influence of managerial factors on research utilization in district nursing practice. *Journal of Advanced Nursing, 23*(4), 697–704.

Kerr, J.R., & MacPhail, J. (1996). *An introduction to issues in community health nursing.* St. Louis: Mosby.

Kim, H.S. (1994). Practice theories in nursing and a science of nursing practice. *Scholarly Inquiry for Nursing Practice: An International Journal, 8*(2), 145–158.

Koch, C.K., & Maserang, J.W. (1994). Population-oriented nursing: Preparing tomorrow's nurses today. *Journal of Nursing Education, 33*(5), 236–237.

Kristjanson, L.J., & Chalmers, K.I. (1991). Preventive work with families: Issues facing public health nurses. *Journal of Advanced Nursing, 16*, 147–153.

Kuehnert, P.L. (1995). The interactive and organizational model of community as client: A model for public health nursing practice. *Public Health Nursing, 12*(1), 9–17.

Kuss, T., Proulx-Girouard, L., Lovitt, S., Katz, C.B., & Kennelly, P. (1997). A public health nursing model. *Public Health Nursing, 14*(2), 81–91.

Lauri, S., Salantera, S., Bild, H., Chalmers, K., Duffy, M., & Kim, H.S. (1997). Public health nurses' decision making in Canada, Finland, Norway, and the United States . . . including commentary by B. Henry and D.J. Mason with author response. *Western Journal of Nursing Research, 19*(2), 143–165.

Leipert, B.D. (1996). The value of community health nursing: A phenomenological study of the perceptions of community health nurses. *Public Health Nursing, 13*(1), 50–57.

Madara, E.J. (1992). Computerized self-help: The evolving telecommunities. *Social Policy, 23*(2), 32.

Magilvy, J.K., & Brown, N.J. (1997). Parish nursing: Advancing practice nursing. Model for healthier communities. *Advanced Practice Nursing Quarterly*, 2(4), 67–72.

Majeski-Felle, D. (1994). Marketing for community health nurses. *Home Healthcare Nurse*, 12(6), 46–49.

Malloy, C. (1994). Agromedicine: An opportunity for nursing. *Journal of Agromedicine*, 1(1), 85–88.

Mangham, C., McGrath, P., Reid, G., & Stewart, M. (1994). *Resilience: Relevance to health promotion*. Unpublished report to National Health Promotion Directorate, Ottawa.

Mangham, G., Reid, G., & Stewart, M. (1996). Resilience in families. Challenges for health promotion. *Canadian Journal of Public Health*, 87, 373–374.

Manson-Singer, S. (1994). The Canadian Healthy Communities project: Creating a social movement. In A. Pederson, M. O'Neill, & I. Rootman (Eds.), *Health promotion in Canada* (pp. 107–122). Toronto: W.B. Saunders.

Mass, J., & Whyte, N. (1997). Primary health care in action. *Nursing BC*, 29(2), 13–16.

Matuk, L.C.K., & Horsburgh, M.E. (1992). Toward redefining public health nursing in Canada: Challenges for education. *Public Health Nursing*, 9(3), 149–154.

McBeath, W.H. (1991). Health for all: A public health vision. *American Journal of Public Health*, 81(12), 1560–1565.

McCubbin, H.I., McCubbin, M.A., & Thompson, A.I. (1992). Resiliency in families: The role of family schema and appraisal in family adaptation to crises. In T.H. Brubaker (Ed.), *Family relations: Challenges for the future* (pp. 153–177). Newbury Park, CA: Sage.

McCubbin, M.A., & McCubbin, H.I. (1993). Families coping with illness: The resiliency model of family stress, adjustment, and adaptation. In C.B. Danielson, B. Hamel-Bissel, & P. Winstead-Fry (Eds.), *Families, health and illness: Perspectives on coping and intervention* (pp. 21–61). St. Louis: Mosby.

McDonald, A.L., Langford, I.H., & Boldero, N. (1997). The future of community nursing in the United Kingdom: District nursing, health visiting and school nursing. *Journal of Advanced Nursing*, 26(2), 257–265.

McEwen, M., & Kemp, C. (1994). Teaching strategies for operationalizing nursing's agenda for healthcare reform. *Nurse Educator*, 19(1), 10–13.

McKnight, J., & Van Dover, L. (1994). Community as client: A challenge for nursing education. *Public Health Nursing*, 11(1), 12–16.

Medical Research Council of Canada (MRC). (1993). *Interim reports of advisory committees*. Ottawa: Author.

Meleis, A.I. (1991). Nursing theory: An elusive image or a mirror of reality? In A.I. Meleis (Ed.), *Theoretical nursing: Development and progress* (2nd ed.) (pp. 249–267). Philadelphia: J.B. Lippincott.

Meleis, A.I. (1992). Directions for nursing theory development in the 21st century. *Nursing Science Quarterly*, 5(3), 112–117.

Meyer, K.A. (1997). An educational program to prepare acute care nurses for a transition to home health care nursing. *Journal of Continuing Education in Nursing*, 28(3), 124–129.

Misener, T.R., Alexander, J.W., Blaha, A.J., Clarke, P.N., Cover, C.M., Felton, G.M., Fuller, S.G., Herman, J., Rodes, M.M., & Sharp, H.F. (1997). National Delphi study to determine competencies for nursing leadership in public health. *Image: Journal of Nursing Scholarship*, 29(1), 47–51.

Misener, T.R., Watkins, J.G., & Ossege, J. (1994). Public health nursing research priorities: A collaborative Delphi study. *Public Health Nursing*, 11(2), 66–74.

Moore, W. (1994). Taking up the sales challenge. *Health Visitor, 67*(10), 334.

Morse, J.M. (1994). *Critical issues in qualitative research methods.* Thousand Oaks, CA: Sage.

Mynors-Wallis, L., Davies, I., Gray, A., Barbour, F., & Gath, D. (1997). A randomised controlled trial and cost analysis of problem-solving treatment for emotional disorders given by community nurses in primary care. *British Journal of Psychiatry, 170,* 113–119.

Nadeau, J. (1996). Reform of the Quebec health care system. *Leadership in Health Services, 5*(4), 8–10.

National Forum on Health. (1997a). *Canada health action: Building on the legacy (Vol. 1). Determinants of health: Children and youth.* Ottawa: Author.

National Forum on Health. (1997b). *Canada health action: Building on the legacy (Vol. 2). Synthesis reports and issues papers.* Ottawa: Author.

National Health Research & Development Program (NHRDP). (1993). Contributions to health: A profile of the National Health Research & Development Program. *Canadian Journal of Public Health, 84* (Suppl. 2), S2–S40.

Nemcek, M.A., & Egan, P.B. (1997). Specialty nursing improves home care. *Caring, 16*(6), 12–14.

Neufeld, A., & Harrison, M.J. (1996). Educational issues in preparing community health nurses to use nursing diagnosis with population groups. *Nurse Education Today, 16*(3), 221–226.

Niles, S., Alemagno, S., & Stricklin, M.L. (1997). Healthy talk: A telecommunication model for health promotion. *Caring, 16*(7), 46–50.

Oberle, M.W., Baker, E.L., & Magenheim, M.J. (1994). Healthy people 2000 and community health planning. *Annual Review of Public Health, 15,* 259–275.

Oermann, M. (1994). Reforming nursing education for future practice. *Journal of Nursing Education, 33*(5), 215–219.

O'Neill, M., Rootman, I., & Pederson, A. (1994). Beyond Lalonde: Two decades of Canadian health promotion. In A. Pederson, M. O'Neill, & I. Rootman (Eds.), *Health promotion in Canada* (pp. 374–386). Toronto: W.B. Saunders.

Pender, N.J., Barkauskas, V.H., Hayman, L., Rice, V.H., & Anderson, E.T. (1992). Health promotion and disease prevention: Toward excellence in nursing practice and education. *Nursing Outlook, 40*(3), 106–120.

Peters, D.A., & Hays, B.J. (1995). Measuring the essence of nursing: A guide for future practice. *Journal of Professional Nursing, 11*(6), 358–363.

Petzel, S.V., Ellis, L.B.M., Budd, J.R., & Johnson, Y. (1992). Microcomputers for behavioural health education: Developing and evaluating patient education for the chronically ill. *Computers in Human Services, 8,* 3–4.

Porter-O'Grady, T. (1997). Building community health: The real work of advanced practice. *Advanced Practice Nursing Quarterly, 2*(4), 90–91.

Pruitt, R.H., & Campbell, B.F. (1994). Educating for health care reform and the community. *Nursing & Health Care, 15*(6), 308–311.

Rafael, A.R.F. (1997). Advocacy oral history: A research methodology for social activism in nursing. *Advances in Nursing Science, 20*(2), 32–44.

Rains, J.W., & Hahn, E.J. (1995). Policy research: Lessons from the field. *Public Health Nursing, 12*(2), 72–77.

Registered Nurses Association of British Columbia. (1994). *Primary Health Care in nursing education: A survey of British Columbia schools of nursing.* Vancouver: Author.

Rene, J., Weinberger, M., Mazzuca, S.A., Brandt, K.D., & Katz, B.P. (1992). Reduction in joint pain in patients with knee osteoarthritis who have received monthly telephone calls from lay personnel and whose treatment regimes have remained stable. *Arthritis & Rheumatism, 35*(5), 511–515.

Reutter, L.I., & Ford, J.S. (1996). Perceptions of public health nursing: Views from the field. *Journal of Advanced Nursing, 24*(1), 7–15.

Reutter, L.I., & Ford, J.S. (1998). Perceptions of changes in public health nursing practice: A Canadian perspective. *International Journal of Nursing Studies, 35*(1/2), 85–94.

Rodrigues, L. (1992). A bright future for community nursing. *Health Visitor, 65*(10), 363–364.

Rootman, I. (1995). *International developments in health promotion.* Presentation at Dalhousie University, Halifax, March 3, 1995.

Rootman, I., & O'Neill, M. (1994). Developing knowledge for health promotion. In A. Pederson, M. O'Neill, & I. Rootman (Eds.), *Health promotion in Canada* (pp. 139–151). Toronto: W.B. Saunders.

Rudd, R.E., & Walsh, D.C. (1993). Schools as healthful environments: Prerequisite to comprehensive school health? *Preventive Medicine, 22*(4), 499–506.

Rydholm, L. (1997). Patient-focused care in parish nursing. *Holistic Nursing Practice, 11*(3), 47–60.

Salmon, M. (1993). Public health nursing: The opportunity of a century. *American Journal of Public Health, 83*(12), 1674–1675.

Simington, J., Olson, J., & Douglass, L. (1996). Promoting well-being within a parish. *Canadian Nurse, 92*(1), 20–24.

Smillie, C. (1992). Preparing health professionals for a collaborative health promotion role. *Canadian Journal of Public Health, 83*(4), 279–282.

Stewart, M.J. (1985). Planning priorities in service, education and research: Community health nursing in Canada in the year 2000. In M. Stewart, J. Innes, S. Searl, & C. Smillie (Eds.), *Community health nursing in Canada* (pp. 738–744). Toronto: Gage.

Stewart, M.J. (1990). From provider to partner: A conceptual framework for nursing education based on Primary Health Care premises. *Advances in Nursing Science, 12*(2), 9–27.

Stewart, M.J., Ellerton, M.L., Hart, G., Hirth, A., Mann, K., Meagher-Stewart, D., Ritchie, J., & Tomblin-Murphy, G. (1997). Insights from a nursing research program on social support. *Canadian Journal of Nursing Research, 29*(3), 93–110.

Stewart, M., Reid, G., Jackson, S., Buckles, L., Edgar, W., Mangham, C., & Tilley, N. (1996). Community resilience: Strengths and challenges. *Health & Canadian Society, 4*(1), 53–81.

Stuart, M.E. (1991). An analysis of the concept of family. In A. Whall & I. Fawcett (Eds.), *Family theory development in nursing: State of the science and art.* Philadelphia: Davis.

Sword, W., Noesgaard, C., & Majumdar, B. (1994). Examination of student learning about dimensions of health and illness using Stewart's conceptual framework for Primary Health Care. *Nurse Education Today, 14*(5), 354–362.

Tappen, R.M., Turkel, M.C., Hall, R.F., Stahura, P., & Morgan, F. (1997). Nurses in transition: A response to the changing health care system. In *Nursing roles: Evolving or recycled?* (pp. 116–127). Newbury Park, CA: Sage.

Tenn, L. (1995). Primary Health Care nursing education in Canadian university schools of nursing. *Journal of Nursing Education, 34*(8), 350–358.

Thomas, P.A., & Shelton, C.R. (1994). Teaching students to become active in public policy. *Public Health Nursing, 11*(2), 75–79.

Toffler, A. (1990). *Power shift*. New York: Bantam.

Trnobranski, P.H. (1994). Nurse practitioner: Redefining the role of the community nurse? *Journal of Advanced Nursing, 19*(1), 134–139.

Vicenzi, A.E. (1994). Chaos theory and some nursing considerations. *Nursing Science Quarterly, 7*(1), 36–42.

Walker, P.H. (1994). A comprehensive community nursing center model. Maximizing practice income: A challenge to educators. *Journal of Professional Nursing, 10*(3), 131–139.

Walsh, M. (1997). Perceptions of barriers to implementing research. *Nursing Standard, 11*(19), 34–37.

Ward, D., & Brown, M.A. (1994). Labor and cost in AIDS family caregiving. *Western Journal of Nursing Research, 16*(1), 10–25.

Webster, K. (1997). Into the future. A new symptom: Millennium fever . . . telephonic nursing via the Internet. *Telephone Nursing Telezine, 2*(1), 2–5.

Williams, A., & Wold, J.L. (1996). Healthcare for the future: Caring for populations in alternative settings. *Nurse Educator, 21*(2), 23–26.

World Health Organization (WHO). (1994). *Nursing beyond the year 2000*. WHO Technical Report Series 842. Geneva: Author.

World Health Organization (WHO), Health & Welfare Canada (HWC), & Canadian Public Health Association (CPHA). (1986). *Ottawa charter for health promotion*. Ottawa: Canada Public Health Association.

Wright, S., Chamberlain, K., & Barker, P. (1996). Community nurses take on the task of selling themselves. *Nursing Times, 92*(47), 38–40.

Zwanziger, P.J., Peterson, R.M., Lethlean, H.M., Hernke, D.A., Finley, J.L., DeGroot, L.S., & Busman, C.L. (1996). Expanding the CNS role to the community. *Clinical Nurse Specialist, 10*(4), 199–202.

Afterword

Alice J. Baumgart

Primary Health Care took on new life and meaning when it was accepted by the World Health Organization (WHO) and its member nations in 1978 as the cornerstone of a global strategy to achieve Health for All by the Year 2000. As a force for reorienting health systems and health care activities, WHO's model of Primary Health Care put the accent on health promotion and self-reliance of families, groups, and communities in meeting health needs. It also emphasized use of effective and affordable methods and technology and the interplay between health and social-economic development.

Since then, nurses in Canada and throughout the world have been strong advocates for the centrality of Primary Health Care principles to future health policy and sustainable health services. They have also been in the forefront of exploring and testing innovative methods and services consonant with Primary Health Care principles. New scholarship has added to the understandings gained, by drawing out the connections among nursing, women's longstanding responsibility for maintaining family and community health, and the lessons of an earlier era of social reform (Strong-Boag, 1991). A coherent body of theory and practice for implementing, teaching, and researching cost-effective delivery of health services and quality nursing is emerging.

However, the complexity of the goals being pursued should not be underestimated. As a WHO Study Group suggested in *Nursing Beyond the Year 2000* (WHO, 1994), Primary Health Care perspectives often run counter to long-standing attitudes and institutions. As a result, their application requires great change both on the part of individuals, families, and groups who need professional services and on the part of professionals who provide services.

This edition of what has become the definitive reference on community health nursing in Canada provides a timely and important opportunity to take stock of what has been accomplished with regard to Primary Health Care and where new directions still need to be forged. The contributors represent diverse interests in community health nursing theory, practice, administration, education, and research and in health system reform. Their accounts and analyses offer valuable insights into the process of incorporating Primary Health Care perspectives into a broad range of community nursing activity. They also provide a glimpse of the distinctive forces that propel health system reform and health policies in Canada and the dilemmas shaping the shift to community-based care.

During the years since the first book in 1985 and the more recent 1995 edition, significant restructuring of health systems has taken place in every province and territory. Cost pressures of the 1980s, which served as key drivers of reform, have abated, and caps on hospital care and physicians' compensation have been applied. Concurrently, the trend to community-based care and reliance on informal caregivers has accelerated (Angus, Auer, Cloutier, & Albert, 1995). Important initiatives that encourage Aboriginal people to develop their own services are underway and provide an example of community-led and community-managed Primary Health Care. There have also been rapid developments in decentralizing and regionalizing health service decision making across the country, with a view to obtaining greater citizen input and more efficient, locally responsive, and accountable resource use. Beyond these system changes, myriad smaller projects and programs are in place to achieve objectives ranging from cost saving to demonstrating the effectiveness of nurses as a point of entry to the health system.

Nurses have a large stake in these developments. In both the hospital and community sectors, they constitute the largest group of health personnel and one of the main front-line professionals. Their responsibilities are diverse and wide-ranging. Thus, they play fundamental roles in applying health reforms. The necessary commitment to change carries with it transition costs of adjusting to new demands and work arrangements and appraisal of the successes and failures of restructuring. This often requires distinctly political efforts and skilled strategizing, requirements that assume special significance at this critical juncture in the reorientation of health services in Canada.

In speaking of the requisite commitment to change by public health personnel, the eminent public health leader Dr. John Hastings made the cogent observation that changes of this magnitude require "forethought and planning if their impact on the health of the public and morale of those in the system is to be as positive as possible and dislocations kept to a minimum" (Hastings, 1994, p. 8).

A call for political activism should strike a familiar chord. In recent years, nurses worldwide have sought a stronger hand in influencing health policy and programming decisions at all levels of the health system. This growing political consciousness reflects both a frustration with continually having to fight to have their voices heard and the conviction that nurses have a distinctive contribution to make to improving health and shaping health services (ICN, 1985). In the context of community health nursing, Carolyn Williams (1983) identified political activism as a basic responsibility.

To respond to these challenges, nursing associations and unions across Canada have been investing heavily in strengthening nursing's political capacities. This investment has taken many forms, ranging from political education and leadership training for practitioners to enhancing organizational infrastructures to maintain high visibility in the policy arena. Nursing's integration into the policy community in Canada has been aided by its consistent and effective advocacy of Primary Health Care as the route to health system reform. This vision was first set out by the Canadian Nurses Association (1980) in a brief entitled *Putting Health into Health Care.* It continues to be the focal point for nursing perspectives on health system reform across the country.

Nurses must link their policy goals to sound evidence and reasoned analysis. Increasingly, the required currency is information and evidence on health outcomes and on the cost returns of alternative services and interventions. Under the pressure of cost constraints, ethical dilemmas pertaining to how resources can be shared fairly also loom large (Angus et al., 1995). These new dynamics are a helpful reminder that health system reform is an ongoing process, as is political action. While nurses in Canada can be proud of their achievements in advocating and advancing the Primary Health Care approach, there are still many unanswered questions about costs and returns. Much work also remains to be done on how Primary Health Care principles should inform nursing's future goals.

However, there is room for optimism. Predictions of future health care suggest that new demands for services will be heavily dependent on nursing personnel. Similar conclusions can be reached from the results of a major study, released in early 1995, of the cost effectiveness of the Canadian health system (Angus et al., 1995). This study showed that, without sacrificing health outcomes, potential savings of $7 billion could be attained through two measures: an efficient continuing care system in the community and benchmarks to allow comparisons with other provinces and adoption of their best practices. This study also revealed that a relatively small shift in resources from the hospital sector represents a relatively large increase in the budgets of community-based services; for example, transfer of five percent from the institutional sector budgets into home care services translated into an increase of about 120 percent in the estimated global home care budget (Angus et al., 1995, p. 82).

The imperative to get more value for money from the health system is driving reform and renewal. The pathways Canada ultimately chooses to achieve this goal will reflect a distinctive amalgam of social, cultural, economic, and political factors. The choice of one pathway over another emerges out of the struggle over competing conceptions of goals, such as equity, and the ways people exert influence (Stone, 1988). In making choices among available pathways, the perspectives of nursing can enrich the process. This edition of *Community Nursing: Promoting Canadians' Health* makes an important contribution in helping to illuminate the possibilities for Primary Health Care and how nurses can contribute to shaping the shift to the community health services of the future.

REFERENCES

Angus, D.E., Auer, L., Cloutier, E., & Albert T. (1995). *Sustainable health care for Canada: Synthesis report.* Ottawa: Queen's–University of Ottawa Economic Projects.

Canadian Nurses Association. (1980). *Putting health into health care.* Ottawa: Author.

Hastings, J.E.F. (1994). Health reform: Themes, issues and some comments. *CPHA Health Digest, 18,* 8–9.

International Council of Nurses (ICN). (1985). *Guidelines for public policy development related to health.* Geneva: Author.

Stone, D.A. (1988). *Policy paradox and political reason.* New York: HarperCollins.

Strong-Boag, V. (1991). Making a difference: The history of Canada's nurses. *Canadian Bulletin of Medical History, 8,* 231–248.

Williams, C. (1983). Making things happen: Community health nursing and the policy arena. *Nursing Outlook, 31,* 225–228.

World Health Organization (WHO). (1994). *Nursing beyond the year 2000: Report of a WHO study group* (WHO Technical Report Series 842). Geneva: Author.

About the contributors

Margaret May Allemang, BScN, BA (Toronto), MN, PhD (Washington), spent four year as a Nursing Sister with the British Commonwealth Air Training Plan in Canada during World War II, followed by a lifetime career in nursing education. Her teaching responsibilities at the University of Toronto included undergraduate and graduate teaching and research in medical–surgical nursing and in nursing history. Dr. Allemang conducted an oral history project on Canadian Nursing Sisters of World War I; the study now continues with Nursing Sisters of World War II. As co-founder of the Canadian Association for the History of Nursing (CAHN/ACHN) in 1986–87, and as honorary president, she participates in the annual nursing history conference of this organization, which revitalized the discipline of nursing history. The recently incorporated Margaret M. Allemang Centre for the History of Nursing, successor to the Ontario Society for the History of Nursing, also organized in 1986–87, further supports this goal and the eventual establishment of a nursing history archival repository.

Hope E. Beanlands, BN (New Brunswick), MN, MPA (Dalhousie), is Coordinator, Public Health Enhancement, Public Health and Health Promotion, Nova Scotia Department of Health. Her professional career includes working as a public health nurse in New Brunswick and Nova Scotia and in neonatal intensive care, teaching public health nursing, working in nursing research, and home care nursing. She was formerly Assistant Director and Director of Home Care Nursing; Assistant Director, Public Health Nursing; and Coordinator, Communicable Disease Prevention and Control for the Province of Nova Scotia. She was a member of the support team for the Minister's Action Committee on Health System Reform "Blueprint Committee" and a Steering Committee member for the 1995 Nova Scotia Health Survey, and she has presented and written on a variety of nursing and public health issues. She was a founding member of the Community Health Nurses Association of Nova Scotia and has served on the boards of numerous community and professional organizations, including the Registered Nurses Association of Nova Scotia, the Public Health Association of Nova Scotia, the Nova Scotia Commission on Drug Dependency, and Metro United Way.

Janet Braunstein, BSN (Cornell), PNP (Virginia), MPH (Minnesota), holds dual citizenship in the United States and Canada. Ms. Braunstein is currently on secondment to the Government of Nunavut, Canada's newest territory, where she holds the position of Director, Policy and Planning, Nunavut Department of Health and Social Services. Ms. Braunstein has held positions in the Nova Scotia Department of Health as Assistant Director and Director of Public Health Nursing; Administrator of Public Health Services; Senior Director, Planning and Evaluation at the Central Regional Health Board; and Senior Policy Analyst with the Priorities and Planning Secretariat of the Government of Nova Scotia. Ms. Braunstein has been active in the Public Health Association of Nova Scotia and the Canadian Public Health Association. She has published in the areas of health care systems in Canada and the United States.

J. Howard Brunt, BA (Florida), ADN (Vermont), MSN (Yale), PhD (Calgary), is Professor, School of Nursing and Associate Vice President, Research, University of Victoria. Dr. Brunt's clinical practice and research are in the area of population-based cardiovascular health. For the past 10 years, he has engaged in epidemiological research and health promotion planning with the Hutterite communities of Alberta. He is a research grant reviewer for Health Canada (NHRDP), the Medical Research Council (MRC), the B.C. Health Research Foundation, and the Heart and Stroke Foundation of Canada. Dr. Brunt is currently the President of the Canadian Council of Cardiovascular Nurses.

Sharon Ogden Burke, BS (Loma Linda), MN (Washington), MA, PhD (Toronto), is a Professor at Queen's University School of Nursing and a Medical Research Council/National Health Research Development Program Career Investigator. She has cross-appointments to the Department of Paediatrics and the School of Rehabilitation Therapy. In addition, she is Core Researcher and Site Researcher with the Researcher Coordination Unit of Better Beginnings Better Futures, a project funded by the Ontario Ministries of Community and Social Services, Health and Education, and Indian and Northern Affairs. Her research program focusses on disabled and chronically ill children and their families, with particular emphasis on developing and testing clinically feasible approaches to modifying the negative impact on these children. She was co-principal investigator with Dr. Margaret B. Harrison of a clinical trial to test the effects of a preparation program for parents of repeatedly hospitalized children. Dr. Burke's teaching centres on nursing of children and families and on research. Throughout her career, she has published on this topic and has contributed to community and provincial projects that concern children and families. Her newest research is testing an intervention for mothers who use illicit drugs.

Karen I. Chalmers, BScN (McMaster), MSc(A) (McGill), PhD (Manchester), is an Associate Professor, Faculty of Nursing, University of Manitoba, Winnipeg. She conducts research and publishes articles, book chapters, and other reports on community health nursing, health visiting practice, Primary

Health Care, perception of risk of women with primary relatives with breast cancer, and smoking cessation evaluation.

Heather F. Clarke, BNSc (Queen's), MN, PhD (Washington), is currently employed by the Registered Nurses Association of British Columbia as research and policy consultant. Her responsibilities involve the promotion of nursing research and its integration with policy development in nursing and health care. She is also an Adjunct Professor at the School of Nursing and Faculty Associate, Institute for Health Promotion Research, University of British Columbia. Dr. Clarke's nursing career has centred primarily on community and family health nursing as practitioner, educator, manager, and researcher. She has also been in transcultural and international nursing with WHO and ICN. She is currently engaged in research with First Nations and South Asian women regarding their health care practices, including Pap smear screening. She has received funding from national and provincial sources and has published over 20 articles in refereed journals.

Geraldine Cradduck, BScN (Toronto), MScN (Western Ontario), is currently retired as Director of Public Health Nursing, Director of Healthy Growth and Development Program, Elgin–St. Thomas Health Unit, and Clinical Associate for the Faculty of Nursing, University of Western Ontario. She has served as Chair of the Community Health Nurses Interest Group of the Registered Nurses Association of Ontario and President of the Community Health Nurses Association of Canada. She was also a member of the task force that rewrote the Canadian Public Health Association publication, *Community Health/Public Health Nursing in Canada: Preparation and Practice.* She has been involved in public health nursing practice in both a staff and an administrative capacity for over 16 years at the Elgin–St. Thomas Health Unit.

Dorothy M. Craig, BA, BScN, MScN (Toronto), is Professor Emeritus, Faculty of Nursing, University of Toronto. Her interests lie in health promotion, disease prevention, and program evaluation, particularly with older adults. She has completed research focussed on stressors of older adults and nurses and has evaluated community health nursing programs. Prof. Craig was a Director of Public Health Nursing in Halton Region, Ontario, and is a former president of the Ontario Public Health Association. She is currently a Trustee for the Neuman Systems Model and is a board member of The Dorothy Ley Hospice.

Clémence Dallaire, BScS (Laval), MSc(A) (McGill), PhD (Montréal), is Associate Professor at l'École des Sciences Infirmières, Université Laval. She has extensive experience in various clinical settings (psychiatry, CCU, emergency, and geriatry). She is author of several articles on political action for nurses and also author and co-author of chapters related to the nursing profession. She has an interest in health promotion as a conceptual component of nursing knowledge and nursing practice.

Hélène Denoncourt, RN, is completing a BScN at Université de Montréal. She has been on the Team for the Homeless at the CLSC des Faubourgs in downtown Montréal for five years. She has extensive experience in outpost nursing in the Canadian North, in Switzerland, in emergency clinics, and in community health nursing.

Alba DiCenso, PhD, is a Professor in the School of Nursing at McMaster University in Hamilton, Ontario. She is also an Associate Member of the Department of Clinical Epidemiology and Biostatistics at McMaster, a Clinical Nurse Consultant with the Hamilton–Wentworth Department of Public Health Services Teaching Health Unit, and a Career Scientist with the Ontario Ministry of Health. She is co-editor of *Evidence-Based Nursing*, a journal that was introduced in November 1997. Early in her career as a community health nurse, she was the family planning coordinator for Halton Region in Ontario, providing sex education in schools, running a birth control clinic, and couselling pregnant adolescents. More recently, as a nurse researcher, she has completed a large randomized controlled trial to evaluate an intervention to prevent adolescent pregnancy, a systematic review of studies evaluating adolescent pregnancy prevention strategies, and a series of focus groups of adolescents to learn about their concerns regarding current sexual health services and to identify strategies to improve the delivery of these.

Geraldine Dickson, BScN (Saskatchewan), MPH (Hawaii), PhD (Saskatchewan), is Associate Professor, College of Nursing, University of Saskatchewan. She has extensive experience in international health, community health and development, and Aboriginal health. She is the former Coordinator of the National Native Program to Nursing.

Nancy C. Edwards, BScN (Windsor), MSc (McMaster), PhD (McGill), is an Associate Professor at the University of Ottawa School of Nursing and an Academic Consultant at the Ottawa–Carleton Health Department. She has worked as a community health nurse and researcher in diverse settings, including Newfoundland, Ontario, Pakistan, Sierra Leone, and China. Her current research interests include fall prevention for seniors, tobacco use among multicultural groups, and the prevention of smoking relapse during pregnancy and postpartum. She is Director of the Community Health Research Unit (a systems-linked research unit between the University of Ottawa and the Ottawa–Carleton Health Department), which is funded by the Ontario Ministry of Health. She continues to work in the field of international health and is currently director of two projects in China that are funded by the Canadian International Development Agency.

John C.B. English, CBSc (Dip), MHSc (McMaster), is Associate Professor, School of Health Studies, Brandon University. He has extensive experience in community mental health practice, in educating psychiatric nurses, and in working with registered nurses. He has published in the areas of nursing theory and model development for healthy communities and is also interested in community involvement in establishing hospices for the terminally ill.

Nancy Feeley, BSc(A), MSc(A) (McGill), is a doctoral student at the School of Nursing, McGill University, and a Consultant to the Nursing Department of the Montréal Children's Hospital. Her research has dealt with parents' ways of coping with the death of their infant and with testing of the McGill Model of Nursing. Her work on her chapter for this book was supported in part by doctoral fellowships awarded by the Social Sciences and Humanities Research Council of Canada and the Fonds de la recherche en santé du Québec.

Sheila M. Gallagher, BS (Tufts), MS (Nursing) (Pace), PhD (Alberta), is the Child Health Leader on the North East Community Health Centre (NECHC) Project Planning Team and is cross-appointed to the Faculty of Nursing at the University of Alberta. The NECHC development is guided by the principles of Primary Health Care. She has also worked as a clinician and clinical preceptor in underserved neighbourhoods in New York City. Current research includes the development of models for understanding the delivery of health services to marginal/shadow populations, connections between the ecosystem and human health, the character of technology in contemporary nursing practice, and health policies in Alberta.

Angela J. Gillis, BScN, MAdEd (St. Francis Xavier), PhD (Nursing) (Texas at Austin), is Professor and Chair of the Department of Nursing, St. Francis Xavier University, Antigonish, N.S. She has published extensively on aspects of health promotion and on child and adolescent health. She has served on the boards of the Registered Nurses Association of Nova Scotia, the Canadian Nurses Foundation, and the National Institute of Nutrition. Her current research interests include health promotion in women and in adolescents.

Helen Glass, OC, BScN, MA, EdD (Columbia), LLD (Hon), DSc (Hon), is Professor Emerita and former Director of the Faculty of Nursing, University of Manitoba. She was Coordinator of the first graduate program in nursing at the University of Manitoba, and through her efforts the Manitoba Nursing

Research Institute was initiated. She has served as President of the Manitoba Association of Registered Nurses and of the Canadian Nurses Association (CNA) and as first Vice-President of the International Council of Nurses. Dr. Glass has conducted research in teaching and nursing care and has published widely on research, nursing, and health care issues. Always politically inclined, she was active in bringing about amendments to the *Canada Health Act* and spearheaded a drive to establish Community Nurse Resource Centres in Manitoba. Her numerous awards include Officer of the Order of Canada, the McManus Medal from Columbia University, the Jeanne Mance Award from CNA, and the Mary Tolle Wright Founders Award for Leadership from the Sigma Theta Tau International Honour Society in Nursing. She holds honorary doctorates from Memorial University, University of Western Ontario, St. Francis Xavier University, University of Montréal, and McGill University.

Laurie N. Gottlieb, BN, MSc(A), PhD (McGill), is Professor and Director of the School of Nursing, McGill University, where she holds the Flora Madeline Shaw Chair of Nursing. She is also Editor-in-Chief of the *Canadian Journal of Nursing Research.* Her own research has dealt with understanding how family environments shape young children's psychosocial development and adjustment following the birth of a sibling. She has a special interest in parents and has studied mothers' and fathers' bereavement following the death of an infant, factors that affect quality of parenting. For over 20 years she has been involved in the development and testing of the McGill Model of Nursing.

David M. Gregory, BScN (Ottawa), MN (Manitoba), PhD (Arizona), is Associate Professor, Faculty of Nursing, University of Manitoba, and Clinical Research Associate, Riverview Health Centre, Winnipeg. Dr. Gregory is currently Co-chair, ACTION Research Consortium (ARC), Faculty of Nursing. ARC engages in health services research. Dr. Gregory's other current research interests include suffering in the cancer experience, First Nations health issues, and historical research on men in nursing.

Louise Hagan, BScInf (Montréal), MSc (Laval), PhD (Montréal), is Associate Professor, École des Sciences Infirmières, Université Laval. She teaches baccalaureate and master's students in nursing and community health, including health promotion and, particularly, health education issues. Her publications deal mainly with nursing practice in health education. Her research activities emphasize home health care and nursing practice in Primary Health Care.

Margaret B. Harrison, BN (Dalhousie), MHA (Ottawa), PhD (McMaster), is Nurse Scientist in the Division of Nursing at the Ottawa Hospital and Loeb Health Research Institute, Clinical Epidemiology Unit. As well, she is an

Adjunct Professor in the Faculties of Health Science and Administration at the University of Ottawa. As a former Director, Nursing Professional Development and Research, Children's Hospital of Eastern Ontario, she was actively involved with research development particular to pediatric care. She was co-principal investigator with Dr. Sharon Ogden Burke on the clinical trial to test the effects of a preparation program for parents of repeatedly hospitalized children. Currently holding an Ontario Ministry of Health Career Scientist award, she is engaged in health services research focussed on continuity of care, evidenced-based nursing practice, and supportive care needs.

Margaret J. Harrison, BScN (UBC), MSc (Rhode Island), PhD (Alberta), is Associate Professor, Faculty of Nursing, University of Alberta. She has taught community health nursing in several university settings. Her research focusses on family issues such as parenting premature infants, support for family caregivers, and support for women during different life transitions. Dr. Harrison also is conducting research on the use of nursing diagnosis in community health nursing and is involved in a study of women's health and poverty. She is a member of the Family, Health and Work Research Group, Faculty of Nursing and the Perinatal Research Centre at the University of Alberta.

Sue Hicks, BN, MES, began her career as a public health nurse and since has held positions in research and development, policy development, teaching, and administration. She has been Director of Public Health Nursing, Calgary Health Services; Director of the Women's Health Directorate, Manitoba Health; Assistant Deputy Minister of Healthy Public Policy, Manitoba Health; Assistant Deputy Minister of Community and Mental Health Services, Manitoba Health; and, most recently, Associate Deputy Minister of External Program and Operations, Manitoba Health. She has delivered papers at conferences both nationally and internationally, conducted and published research, and participated in the development of governmental working documents. Throughout her career she has been active academically and has served on national and international committees relating to community health and public policy. She is the recipient of the Outstanding Achievement Award for Nursing from the Manitoba Association of Registered Nurses.

Jean R. Hughes, BN (Dalhousie), MSc (Boston), PhD Candidate (Dalhousie), is Associate Professor in the School of Nursing at Dalhousie University, where she teaches the Mental Health/Psychiatric Nursing course and a course on Advanced Concepts of the Helping Relationship in the Master's Program. Her research activities are interdisciplinary in nature and primarily involve studying the treatment effects of parenting programs in lone-parent families with child-maltreating mothers and young children. Related studies include a program of research on depression in disadvantaged women and a service delivery model comparison on the resilience of at-risk adolescents. Prof. Hughes has participated in professional nursing associations at the provincial and national levels and is also active in other professionally related activities. Currently, she is a member of the Boards of Directors for the Canadian Mental Health Association (National) and the Dartmouth Family Research Centre (local).

Elizabeth Kauffmann, BScN, MEd (Queen's), is Assistant Professor at Queen's University School of Nursing. Her research focusses on families who have a child with a chronic condition and implementation of nursing interventions for such families. She was co-investigator with Dr. Sharon Ogden Burke and Dr. Margaret B. Harrison of a clinical trial to test the effects of a preparation program for parents of repeatedly hospitalized children. Her teaching focusses on nursing assessment and intervention specific to family health. She has published on the topic of families who have a child with a chronic condition and has produced educational modules to assist nurses to implement interventions with a family perspective.

Judith C. Kulig, BScN (Alberta), MSN (Arizona), DNSc (California, San Francisco), is an Associate Professor in the School of Health Sciences at the University of Lethbridge. Dr. Kulig has worked with a variety of cultural groups, including Cambodians, Vietnamese, Central Americans, and Aboriginal peoples in Canada and the United States, as a community health nurse, educator, and researcher. She has published articles and presented papers that illustrate the variety of issues and groups with which she has worked. Dr. Kulig is currently Director for the Regional Centre for Health Promotion and Community Studies at the University of Lethbridge. Recently, she was named an Academic Consultant with her local health region and will assist community health staff in pursuing research applicable to their work.

Shirley Cloutier Laffrey, BSN (Wayne State), MPH (Michigan), PhD (Wayne State), is an Associate Professor, Community Health Nursing, at the University of Texas at Austin. She is a member of the American Nurses Association, American Public Health Association, Association of Community Health Nursing Educators, Sigma Theta Tau International, and Southern Nursing Research Society. Dr. Laffrey has published widely in the area of health conceptions and health promotion; has conducted research to study health promotion and outcomes of public health nursing care among men and women aged 60 and older; and is currently conducting research to study the physiological and psychosocial effects of an exercise intervention with Mexican American women aged 65 and older.

Beverly Leipert, BA, BSN (Saskatchewan), MSN (UBC), PhD Candidate (Nursing, Alberta), is Assistant Professor, Nursing Program, University of Northern British Columbia (UNBC). She teaches community health nursing and women's health courses in the undergraduate BSN program and in the Master of Science in Community Health program at UNBC. Her research focus is on community health nursing and women's health, particularly in geographically isolated settings. Her present doctoral research uses a feminist-grounded approach to explore women's health in Northern B.C. with particular attention to context and the determinants of health. Prof. Leipert is a founding and executive member of the Northern Secretariat for the B.C. Centre of Excellence for Women's Health, located at UNBC. She is a Killam Scholar and has published several articles and two books regarding community health nursing, women's health, and northern health issues.

Marjorie E. Linwood, BSN (Saskatchewan), is Professor, College of Nursing, University of Saskatchewan. She teaches pediatric nursing and nursing of long-term illness to undergraduate nursing students. She has a special interest in child and youth safety and is pursuing studies in this area. She has also been involved in research on workload and on stress in hospitalized children.

Carol L. McWilliam, BN (New Brunswick), MScN (Western Ontario), PhD (Toronto), is an Associate Professor on the Faculty of Health Sciences, School of Nursing, University of Western Ontario. Her major program of research has focussed on promoting the independence of seniors in their pursuit of health care, including investigation of the management of their transition from hospital to care at home; health promotion for chronically ill older persons; and approaches to in-home, medical, and public health care that foster independence. Dr. McWilliam's interests include health promotion, health services delivery, case management, living with chronic illness, and innovation in research methodology, including the application of qualitative methodologies and new approaches to knowledge transfer from research.

Alwyn Moyer, BScN (Ottawa), MSc(A) (McGill), PhD (London), is Nursing Research Consultant and Adjunct Professor, University of Ottawa School of Nursing. Formerly a Community Nurse Specialist with the Teaching Unit of the Ottawa–Carleton Health Department and researcher at the Ottawa Community Health Research Unit, she has considerable experience in the design and evaluation of community-based health promotion programs, using both quantitative and qualitative methods. Her current research interests include the evaluation of community-based diabetes programs and exploration of the concept of community capacity.

Anne Neufeld, BScN (Saskatchewan), MA (Regina), PhD (Saskatchewan), is Professor, Faculty of Nursing, University of Alberta. She has previous experience in community health nursing and has taught in community college and university settings. Her research foci include social support for caregivers in the community and for women during life transitions. She is also conducting research on the use of nursing diagnosis in community health nursing and is involved in a study of women's health and poverty. She is a member of the Family, Health and Work Research Group, Faculty of Nursing, and the University of Alberta Centre for Gerontology. Her previous research has included evaluation of programs for older adults and use of health care services by the elderly.

T.W. (Tom) Noseworthy, MSc, MPH, MD, is Professor and Chair of the Department of Public Health Sciences, Faculty of Medicine and Oral Health Sciences, University of Alberta. He is an internist and critical care physician. He served on the Prime Minister's National Forum on Health, in which he was a member of the Evidence-Based Decision Making and Striking the Balance Working Groups and Chair of the Steering Committee. Dr. Noseworthy's past appointments have included President and Chief Executive Officer and Vice President–Medical Services of the Royal Alexandra Hospital, Edmonton. He currently chairs the Senior Reference Committee on alberta we*ll*net, the province's health information system. Dr. Noseworthy is Co-chair of the Advisory Council on Health Infostructure, reporting to the Minister of Health.

Michel O'Neill, BA, MA (Laval), PhD (Boston), is Professor in Medical Sociology, Community Health and Health Promotion in the Faculty of Nursing of Laval University in Québec City. He is also Co-Director of the GRIPSUL (Groupe de recherche et d'intervention en promotion de la senté de l'Université Laval) and Co-Director of the Québec World Health Organization Collaborating Centre on the Development of Healthy Cities. Dr. O'Neill has been involved in community/public health for 25 years as community health worker, professor, researcher, consultant, and activist. His longstanding teaching and research interests pertain to the political and policy dimensions of health promotion, with a special interest in the Healthy Cities movement in Canada and internationally. He is co-editor of three books, has published extensively in the scientific and professional literature, and has presented numerous papers in scientific and professional meetings in Québec, Canada, and worldwide.

Sandra M. Reilly, BSn (Hunter), MEd, EdD (Columbia), is Associate Professor, Faculty of Nursing, University of Calgary. She teaches public health nursing and conducts research on health promotion, concentrating on the enhancement of parent–infant/child interactions. She has completed a longitudinal study of fussy behaviour in early infancy and undertook, as co-investigator, research into the effects of different soothing interventions on crying by infants, as well as parent–infant interactions. She also wrote the proposal for the Children's Cottage in Calgary, the only nurse-managed crisis nursery and respite centre in Canada.

Linda I. Reutter, BScN, BA (Alberta), MS (Colorado), PhD (Alberta), is Associate Professor, Faculty of Nursing, and Associate Faculty, Centre for Health Promotion Studies, University of Alberta. Dr. Reutter teaches in the area of community health nursing and health promotion. Her research foci relate to social determinants of health and public health nursing. Her research program includes studies on women's health and poverty, programs for low-income women, public perceptions of the relationship between poverty and health, low-income consumers' perspectives of determinants of health service use, and public health nurses' perspectives of their practice. Her previous research has explored public and professional responses to HIV/AIDS.

Ginette Lemire Rodger, BScN (Ottawa), MNAdm (Montréal), PhD (Alberta), is President of Lemire Rodger & Associates and President-Elect of the Canadian Nurses Association. She has had diversified experience in management, education, research, and clinical nursing and has served on commissions and boards of directors of many health, nursing, political, and educational organizations. She has been politically active in promoting the nursing profession at the local, provincial, national, and international levels, lobbying for health care reform with emphasis on health promotion, consumer education, and better use of health professionals in the health care system. Dr. Rodger has received many awards and honorary degrees for her contributions to nursing, education, health, and the *Canada Health Act.*

Laurene E. Sheilds, BSN (University of Victoria), MS, PhD (University of Oregon), is an Associate Professor of Nursing at the University of Victoria, Victoria, B.C. She conducts research and publishes in a variety of areas, including women's health, health promotion, process of change, and participatory/transformative education.

Miriam J. Stewart, BScN (McMaster), MN, PhD (Dalhousie), is Professor in the Faculty of Nursing and in the Department of Public Health Sciences, University of Alberta. She is Director and Chair of the Centre for Health Promotion Studies in Alberta. She was Director of the Atlantic Health Promotion Research Centre funded by NHRD–SSHRC, co-creator of the Maritime Centre of Excellence on Women's Health funded by Health Canada, and an NHRDP–MRC Research Scholar for a program of research on social support and coping. Dr. Stewart has published four books, *Community Health Nursing in Canada* (1985), *Integrating Social Support in Nursing* (1993), *Community Nursing: Promoting Canadians' Health* (1995), and *Chronic Conditions and Caregiving in Canada: Does Support Help?* (1999), as well as some 60 articles. She worked as a public health nurse in Northern Ontario for five years before joining the faculty at Dalhousie, where she held several administrative posts. Dr. Stewart's teaching, publications, research, and professional activities have focussed on issues pertinent to Primary Health Care and community health nursing. In 1999, she was named a Heritage Medical or Health Senior Scholar by the Alberta Heritage Foundation for Medical Research.

Marie-France Castonguay Thibaudeau, BScN (McGill), MScN (Yale), DPH (Montréal), is Professor Emerita, Faculté des sciences infirmières, Université de Montréal. She opened the master's program in psychiatry and mental health nursing in 1968 and served as Dean of the Faculty from 1981 to 1993. She is Past President of the Canadian Association of University Schools of Nursing and current President of the Fondation de recherche en sciences infirmières du Québec. Her research interests include Primary Health Care in CLSCs and the care of poor families and the homeless. She is a member of the Research Consortium on Homelessness at the Université du Québec in Montréal (UQAM). She holds a Doctor Honoris Causa from the Université du Québec, Trois Rivières.

Leslie J. Van Dover, BN (New Brunswick), MScN (Western Ontario), PhD (Michigan), was an Associate Professor at McMaster University School of Nursing for 11 years and is currently Associate Professor and Chair of the Graduate Program at Azusa Pacific University, Azusa, California. Dr. Van Dover has been active in research with the Registered Nurses Association of Ontario and the Canadian Nursing Research Group and chaired the Canadian Nurses Foundation Research Grants Committee for two years. She has clinical experience in parish nursing and has conducted research on adolescent family planning, community-based health promotion, and spiritual aspects of nursing practice.

Lucy D. Willis, BS (British Columbia), MA (Columbia), EdD (Berkeley), is Professor Emerita, College of Nursing, University of Saskatchewan. Dr. Willis taught a research course to senior undergraduate students. Her own research has been on the nursing workforce and on quality assurance. She served on steering committees for research on unit assignment at Royal University Hospital, Saskatoon, and for research on unit–dosage conducted for the Canadian Association of Hospital Pharmacists. In addition, she has given research workshops and served on the initial Special Committee on Research of the Canadian Nurses Association.

Nesta M.W. Wiskin, DipPH (Toronto), is a retired Easter Seal Nurse who worked as a District Nurse in the Eastern region of Ontario from 1967 to 1992. During that time, she also provided a collaborative clinical practice link with Dr. Sharon Ogden Burke's research program and taught undergraduate nursing students at Queen's University School of Nursing. She was a member of the Board of Directors of the Interagency Council for Children and an active participant in the planning and establishment of Almost Home, a low-cost accommodation for families who must travel in order to receive health services. In her retirement, Mrs. Wiskin maintains an active interest in community efforts involving the care of children.

Heather J. Young, BN (Memorial), MScN (Western Ontario), holds the position of Regional Nursing Officer, Medical Services Branch, Alberta Region, Health Canada. She has also held positions of staff nurse at Grenfell Association in Newfoundland; Zone Nursing Officer with Medical Services in Manitoba; Assistant and Acting Director of Public Health Nursing in Nova Scotia; and Acting Director and Director, Public Health, serving Central Health Region in Nova Scotia. Ms. Young obtained her diploma in nursing and midwifery in England. She was a member of the Nova Scotia Task Force on Nursing, is currently a member of the Community Health Nurses Association, and has written on teen health and women's health issues.

Index